A Clinician's Guide to Axial Spondyloarthritis

A Clinician's Guide to Axial Spondyloarthritis

Edited by Donald Keith

AMERICAN
MEDICAL PUBLISHERS
www.americanmedicalpublishers.com

American Medical Publishers,
41 Flatbush Avenue,
1st Floor, New York,
NY 11217, USA

Visit us on the World Wide Web at:
www.americanmedicalpublishers.com

ISBN: 978-1-63927-389-8

Cataloging-in-Publication Data

A clinician's guide to axial spondyloarthritis / edited by Donald Keith.
p. cm.
Includes bibliographical references and index.
ISBN 978-1-63927-389-8
1. Spondyloarthropathies. 2. Arthritis. 3. Spine--Diseases. I. Keith, Donald.
RC935.S67 H36 2022
616.73--dc23

Table of Contents

Preface IX

Chapter 1 **Efficacy, safety, and tolerability of secukinumab in patients with active ankylosing spondylitis: a randomized, double-blind phase 3 study, MEASURE 3** 1
Karel Pavelka, Alan Kivitz, Eva Dokoupilova, Ricardo Blanco, Marco Maradiaga, Hasan Tahir, Luminita Pricop, Mats Andersson, Aimee Readie and Brian Porter

Chapter 2 **Nonradiographic axial spondyloarthritis: clinical and therapeutic relevance** 11
Nilasha Ghosh and Eric M. Ruderman

Chapter 3 **Age and fecal microbial strain-specific differences in patients with spondyloarthritis** 20
Matthew L. Stoll, Pamela F. Weiss, Jennifer E. Weiss, Peter A. Nigrovic, Barbara S. Edelheit, S. Lou Bridges Jr, Maria I. Danila, Charles H. Spencer, Marilynn G. Punaro, Kenneth Schikler, Andreas Reiff, Ranjit Kumar, Randy Q. Cron, Casey D. Morrow and Elliot J. Lefkowitz

Chapter 4 **Feasibility and reliability of the Spondyloarthritis Research Consortium of Canada sacroiliac joint inflammation score in children** 30
Pamela F. Weiss, Walter P. Maksymowych, Robert G. Lambert, Jacob L. Jaremko, David M. Biko, Joel Paschke, Timothy G. Brandon, Rui Xiao and Nancy A. Chauvin

Chapter 5 **Clinical and MRI remission in patients with nonradiographic axial spondyloarthritis who received long-term open-label adalimumab treatment: 3-year results of the ABILITY-1 trial** 37
Désirée van der Heijde, Joachim Sieper, Walter P. Maksymowych, Robert G. Lambert, Su Chen, Maja Hojnik, Jaclyn K. Anderson and Aileen L. Pangan

Chapter 6 **IL-17A induces osteoblast differentiation by activating JAK2/STAT3 in ankylosing spondylitis** 50
Sungsin Jo, Sung Eun Wang, Young Lim Lee, Suman Kang, Bitnara Lee, Jinil Han, Il-Hoon Sung, Ye-Soo Park, Sang-Cheol Bae and Tae-Hwan Kim

Chapter 7 **Are gender-specific approaches needed in diagnosing early axial spondyloarthritis? Data from the SPondyloArthritis Caught Early cohort** 60
Augusta Ortolan, Miranda van Lunteren, Sofia Ramiro, Roberta Ramonda, Robert B. M. Landewé, Hanne Dagfinrud, Lennart T. H. Jacobsson, Désirée van der Heijde and Floris A. van Gaalen

Chapter 8 **Influence of HLA-B27 on the ankylosing spondylitis phenotype: results from the REGISPONSER database** 68
Marta Arévalo, Jordi Gratacós Masmitjà, Mireia Moreno, Joan Calvet, Cristobal Orellana, Desirée Ruiz, Carmen Castro, Pilar Carreto, Marta Larrosa, Eduardo Collantes and Pilar Font

Chapter 9 **Factors related to health-related quality of life in ankylosing spondylitis, overall and stratified by sex** 74
Lucy Law, Jeanette Beckman Rehnman, Anna Deminger, Eva Klingberg, Lennart T. H. Jacobsson and Helena Forsblad-d'Elia

Chapter 10 **Prevalence of peripheral and extra-articular disease in ankylosing spondylitis versus non-radiographic axial spondyloarthritis** 86
Janneke J. de Winter, Leonieke J. van Mens, Désirée van der Heijde, Robert Landewé and Dominique L. Baeten

Chapter 11 **Chondrocyte activity is increased in psoriatic arthritis and axial spondyloarthritis** 97
Natasja Stæhr Gudmann, Heidi Lausten Munk, Anne Friesgaard Christensen, Leif Ejstrup, Grith Lykke Sørensen, Anne Gitte Loft, Morten Asser Karsdal, Anne-Christine Bay-Jensen, Yi He, Anne Sofie Siebuhr and Peter Junker

Chapter 12 **Childhood hospitalisation with infections and later development of ankylosing spondylitis** 106
Ulf Lindström, Sofia Exarchou, Elisabeth Lie, Mats Dehlin, Helena Forsblad-d'Elia, Johan Askling and Lennart Jacobsson

Chapter 13 **Clinical improvement and reduction in serum calprotectin levels after an intensive exercise programme for patients with ankylosing spondylitis and non-radiographic axial spondyloarthritis** 114
Andrea Levitova, Hana Hulejova, Maja Spiritovic, Karel Pavelka, Ladislav Senolt and Marketa Husakova

Chapter 14 **Genome-wide DNA methylation profile analysis identifies differentially methylated loci associated with ankylosis spondylitis** 126
Jiangcan Hao, Yang Liu, Jiawen Xu, Wenyu Wang, Yan Wen, Awen He, Qianrui Fan, Xiong Guo and Feng Zhang

Chapter 15 **Serum levels of leptin and high molecular weight adiponectin are inversely associated with radiographic spinal progression in patients with ankylosing spondylitis: results from the ENRADAS trial** 132
Agnes Hartl, Joachim Sieper, Uta Syrbe, Joachim Listing, Kay-Geert Hermann, Martin Rudwaleit and Denis Poddubnyy

Chapter 16 **Serum biomarkers and changes in clinical/ MRI evidence of golimumab-treated patients with ankylosing spondylitis: results of the randomized, placebo-controlled GO-RAISE study** 143
Robert D. Inman, Xenofon Baraliakos, Kay-Geert A. Hermann, Jürgen Braun, Atul Deodhar, Désirée van der Heijde, Stephen Xu and Benjamin Hsu

Chapter 17 **Comparison of non-radiographic axial spondyloarthritis and ankylosing spondylitis patients–baseline characteristics, treatment adherence, and development of clinical variables during three years of anti-TNF therapy in clinical practice** 150
Johan K. Wallman, Meliha C. Kapetanovic, Ingemar F. Petersson, Pierre Geborek and Lars Erik Kristensen

Chapter 18 **Comparable long-term efficacy, as assessed by patient-reported outcomes, safety and pharmacokinetics, of CT-P13 and reference infliximab in patients with ankylosing spondylitis: 54-week results from the randomized, parallel-group PLANETAS study** 161
Won Park, Dae Hyun Yoo, Janusz Jaworski, Jan Brzezicki, Andriy Gnylorybov, Vladimir Kadinov, Irmgadt Goecke Sariego, Carlos Abud-Mendoza, William Jose Otero Escalante, Seong Wook Kang, Daina Andersone, Francisco Blanco, Seung Suh Hong, Sun Hee Lee and Jürgen Braun

Chapter 19 **Evaluation of the impact of fibromyalgia in disease activity and treatment effect in spondyloarthritis** 172
Natalia Bello, Adrien Etcheto, Caroline Béal, Maxime Dougados and Anna Moltó

Chapter 20 **The prevalence of vertebral fractures in spondyloarthritis: relation to disease characteristics, bone mineral density, syndesmophytes and history of back pain and trauma** 179
Piet Geusens, Liesbeth De Winter, Dana Quaden, Johan Vanhoof, Debby Vosse, Joop van den Bergh and Veerle Somers

Chapter 21 **Is the current ASAS expert definition of a positive family history useful in identifying axial spondyloarthritis? Results from the SPACE and DESIR cohorts** 187
Zineb Ez-Zaitouni, Andrea Hilkens, Laure Gossec, Inger Jorid Berg, Robert Landewé, Roberta Ramonda, Maxime Dougados, Désirée van der Heijde and Floris van Gaalen

Chapter 22 **Work outcome in yet undiagnosed patients with non-radiographic axial spondyloarthritis and ankylosing spondylitis; results of a cross-sectional study among patients with chronic low back pain** 192
Lonneke van Hoeven, Annelies E. R. C. H. Boonen, Johanna M. W. Hazes and Angelique E. A. M. Weel

Chapter 23 **The performance of different classification criteria sets for spondyloarthritis in the worldwide ASAS-COMOSPA study** 200
Pauline Bakker, Anna Moltó, Adrien Etcheto, Filip Van den Bosch, Robert Landewé, Floris van Gaalen, Maxime Dougados and Désirée van der Heijde

Chapter 24 **Mechanistic rationales for targeting interleukin-17A in spondyloarthritis** 208
Siba P. Raychaudhuri and Smriti K. Raychaudhuri

Chapter 25 **Does evaluation of the ligamentous compartment enhance diagnostic utility of sacroiliac joint MRI in axial spondyloarthritis?** 217
Ulrich Weber, Walter P. Maksymowych, Stanley M. Chan, Kaspar Rufibach, Susanne J. Pedersen, Zheng Zhao, Veronika Zubler, Mikkel Østergaard and Robert GW Lambert

Permissions

List of Contributors

Index

Preface

Spondyloarthritis or spondylarthropathy is a group of inflammatory diseases that affect the joints and the entheses where tendons and ligaments attach to bones. It is a major cause of arthritis of the spine and of the peripheral joints, particularly those in the hands, arms, feet and legs. Psoriatic arthritis, ankylosing spondylitis, enteropathic arthritis and reactive arthritis are some of its different forms. It occurs due to genetic factors of inheritance, with close to 30 genes linked with this condition. Spondyloarthritis is characterized with low back pain, which if not controlled, may lead to fusion of the vertebrae and limited spinal mobility. Intermittent joint inflammation accompanied by fatigue, swelling in the arms and legs, osteoporosis, inflammation of the aortic heart valve, psoriasis, redness of the eyes, and intestinal inflammation are some other symptoms of spondyloarthritis. It can be treated with NSAIDs, corticosteroids, disease-modifying antirheumatic drugs, TNF-alpha blockers and antibiotics. This book is a valuable compilation of topics, ranging from the basic to the most complex advancements in the management and treatment of spondyloarthritis. It presents this complex disease in the most comprehensible and easy to understand language. This book will help new researchers by foregrounding their knowledge in this condition.

The information contained in this book is the result of intensive hard work done by researchers in this field. All due efforts have been made to make this book serve as a complete guiding source for students and researchers. The topics in this book have been comprehensively explained to help readers understand the growing trends in the field.

I would like to thank the entire group of writers who made sincere efforts in this book and my family who supported me in my efforts of working on this book. I take this opportunity to thank all those who have been a guiding force throughout my life.

Editor

Preface

1

Efficacy, safety, and tolerability of secukinumab in patients with active ankylosing spondylitis: a randomized, double-blind phase 3 study, MEASURE 3

Karel Pavelka[1*], Alan Kivitz[2], Eva Dokoupilova[3], Ricardo Blanco[4], Marco Maradiaga[5], Hasan Tahir[6], Luminita Pricop[7], Mats Andersson[8], Aimee Readie[7] and Brian Porter[7]

Abstract

Background: Secukinumab, an anti–interleukin-17A monoclonal antibody, improved the signs and symptoms of ankylosing spondylitis (AS) in two phase 3 studies (MEASURE 1 and MEASURE 2). Here, we present 52-week results from the MEASURE 3 study assessing the efficacy and safety of secukinumab 300 and 150 mg subcutaneous maintenance dosing, following an intravenous loading regimen.

Methods: A total of 226 patients were randomized to intravenous secukinumab 10 mg/kg (baseline, weeks 2 and 4) followed by subcutaneous secukinumab 300 mg (IV-300 mg) or 150 mg (IV-150 mg) every 4 weeks, or matched placebo. Patients in the placebo group were re-randomized to subcutaneous secukinumab at a dose of 300 or 150 mg at week 16. The primary endpoint was the Assessment of SpondyloArthritis international Society criteria for 20% improvement (ASAS20) response rate at week 16 in the IV-300 mg or IV-150 mg versus placebo. Other endpoints assessed through week 52 included improvements in ASAS40, ASAS 5/6, Bath Ankylosing Spondylitis Disease Activity Index, and ASAS partial remission responses, as well as the change from baseline in high-sensitivity C-reactive protein levels. Statistical analyses followed a predefined hierarchical hypothesis testing strategy to adjust for multiplicity of testing, with non-responder imputation used for binary variables and mixed-model repeated measures for continuous variables.

Results: The primary efficacy endpoint was met; the ASAS20 response rate was significantly greater at week 16 in the IV-300 mg (60.5%; $P < 0.01$) and IV-150 mg (58.1%; $P < 0.05$) groups versus placebo (36.8%). All secondary endpoints were met at week 16, except ASAS partial remission in the IV-150 mg group. Improvements achieved with secukinumab in all clinical endpoints at week 16 were also sustained at week 52. Infections, including candidiasis, were more common with secukinumab than with placebo during the placebo-controlled period. During the entire treatment period, pooled incidence rates of *Candida* infections and grade 3–4 neutropenia were 1.8% for both of these adverse events in secukinumab-treated patients.

Conclusions: Secukinumab (300 mg and 150 mg dose groups) provided rapid, significant and sustained improvement through 52 weeks in the signs and symptoms of patients with AS. The safety profile was consistent with previous reports, with no new or unexpected findings.

Keywords: Secukinumab, IL-17, Ankylosing spondylitis, Biologic therapy

* Correspondence: pavelka@revma.cz
[1]Institute of Rheumatology and Department of Rheumatology, 1st Faculty of Medicine, Charles University, Prague, Czech Republic
Full list of author information is available at the end of the article

Background

Ankylosing spondylitis (AS) is a chronic inflammatory disease, which is mainly characterized by the involvement of the axial skeleton and the sacroiliac joints [1, 2]. AS is often associated with inflammatory back pain and stiffness, which can lead to functional impairment and reduced quality of life [3, 4].

AS affects up to 1.4% of the population worldwide and is associated with significant morbidity and disability [5, 6]. As per the treatment recommendations of the Assessment of SpondyloArthritis international Society criteria (ASAS)/ European League Against Rheumatism (EULAR)/American College of Rheumatology (ACR), non-steroidal anti-inflammatory drugs (NSAIDs) are the first-line treatment for patients with active, predominantly axial manifestations of spondyloarthritis. Patients with peripheral disease who do not respond to NSAIDs may be treated with conventional disease-modifying anti-rheumatic drugs (DMARDs); nonetheless, DMARDs are not recommended in patients with axial manifestations, due to lack of efficacy [3, 7].

Although, tumor necrosis factor (TNF) inhibitors are the first-line biologic therapy for AS, up to 40% of patients do not respond to them [8, 9], collectively due to primary or secondary treatment failure or intolerance. Therefore, there remains an unmet medical need, particularly in these patients [10, 11].

The interleukin (IL)-23/IL-17 axis is known to be implicated in the pathogenic mechanism of AS [12]. Secukinumab, a fully human anti-IL-17A monoclonal antibody, has shown efficacy in the treatment of patients with AS [12–15], psoriasis [16], and psoriatic arthritis [17–19]. Previous proof-of-concept and phase 3 studies (MEASURE 1 and MEASURE 2) have shown that the inhibition of IL-17A receptor with secukinumab improves signs and symptoms in patients with AS [14, 15]. MEASURE 3 is the first phase 3 study evaluating the 300 mg subcutaneous dose of secukinumab, along with the approved 150 mg dose, in patients with moderate to severe active AS (NCT02008916).

Here, we present the efficacy and safety results of subcutaneous maintenance dosing of secukinumab 300 and 150 mg, following a 10 mg/kg intravenous loading regimen, through 52 weeks from the MEASURE 3 study.

Methods

Patients

Patients aged ≥ 18 years with moderate to severe AS fulfilling the Modified New York criteria for AS were enrolled in the study. Other inclusion criteria included a score of 4 or higher on the Bath Ankylosing Spondylitis Disease Activity Index (BASDAI; scores of 0–10), a spinal pain score ≥4 (out of 10) in the BASDAI item 2, and a total back pain score ≥40 mm on a 100 mm visual analog scale (VAS), despite treatment with the highest recommended dose of NSAIDs with an acceptable side effect profile for the patient.

Patients on scheduled NSAIDs were included if they had received a stable dose for at least 2 weeks before randomization. Previous use of DMARDs and anti-TNF agents was allowed. Washout periods for these agents, other than sulfasalazine and methotrexate, were required before the initiation of study treatment. Patients previously treated with not more than one anti-TNF agent could participate if they had an inadequate response to an approved dose for 3 months or more or had unacceptable side effects following at least one dose (hereafter, collectively referred to as patients with an inadequate response to anti-TNF agents). Patients could continue to receive the following medications at a stable dose: sulfasalazine (≤ 3 g per day), methotrexate (7.5–25 mg per week), prednisone or equivalent (≤ 10 mg per day), and NSAIDs.

Key exclusion criteria were total spinal ankylosis, evidence of infection or cancer on chest radiography, active systemic infection within 2 weeks before the baseline visit, and previous treatment with cell-depleting therapies or biologics other than anti-TNF agents.

Study design

MEASURE 3 is a randomized, double-blind, double-dummy, placebo-controlled, parallel-group, 3-year study, which is being conducted at 54 centers across the USA, Belgium, Czech Republic, Germany, Greece, Mexico, Portugal, Russian Federation, Spain, and the UK. After a 10-week screening period, eligible patients were randomized (1:1:1) using an interactive response technology (IRT) system to one of two secukinumab dose groups (300 mg or 150 mg) or a placebo group. Patients in the secukinumab groups received an intravenous dose of 10 mg/kg body weight (delivered as a 125 mg/5 mL liquid-in-vial formulation) at baseline and weeks 2 and 4, followed by subcutaneous secukinumab in the form of prefilled syringes (PFS) at a dose of either 300 mg (IV-300 mg) or 150 mg (IV-150 mg) every 4 weeks starting at week 8. Patients in the placebo group were treated according to the same intravenous-to-subcutaneous administration schedule (see Additional file 1). At week 16, all patients in the placebo group were re-randomized to receive either secukinumab 300 mg or 150 mg (1:1) subcutaneously every 4 weeks.

The randomization of patients was stratified according to previous anti-TNF therapy (patients who were naïve to anti-TNF therapy (anti-TNF-naïve) or those with a history of inadequate response or intolerance to these agents (anti-TNF-IR)).

The institutional review board at each participating center approved the protocol. The trial was conducted by the study investigators in accordance with the

Declaration of Helsinki and Good Clinical Practice (GCP) guidelines, and was analyzed by the Sponsor. Written informed consent was obtained from all patients. Data from the primary analysis at week 16 and the 1-year follow-up analysis (after all patients had completed the visit at week 52) are presented here.

Outcomes

The primary endpoint was the proportion of patients who met the ASAS20 (improvement of ≥ 20% and absolute improvement of ≥ 1 unit (on a 10-unit scale) in at least three of the four main ASAS domains, with no more than 20% worsening in the remaining domain) response criteria at week 16. Secondary endpoints assessed as part of the predefined hierarchical hypothesis-testing strategy at week 16 included improvement in ASAS40 response criteria (improvement of ≥ 40% and absolute improvement of ≥ 2 units (on a 10-unit scale) in at least three of the four main ASAS domains, with no worsening in the remaining domain), change from baseline in high-sensitivity C-reactive protein (hsCRP) level, ASAS5/6 response (≥ 20% improvement in five of the six ASAS response domains), change from baseline in the total BASDAI score, and proportion of patients achieving ASAS partial remission (a score of ≤ 2 units in each of the four core ASAS domains). Primary and secondary endpoints were assessed at baseline, weeks 1, 2, 4, and every 4 weeks until week 16, thereafter all efficacy endpoints were assessed at weeks 32, 40, and 52.

PFS usability was assessed with the Self-Injection Assessment Checklist and the Possible Hazard Assessment Checklist at weeks 8 and 12. Satisfaction with the PFS was assessed with the Self-Injection Assessment Questionnaire (SIAQ) focusing on three domains: feeling about "self-injections", "self-confidence", and "satisfaction with self-injection". The first part of the SIAQ (the PRE module) was completed before self-injection at baseline and the second part (the POST module) was completed after self-injection at the week 8, 12, and 16 visits.

Pre-specified subgroup analyses on the basis of anti-TNF response status (TNF-naïve vs TNF-IR) were performed for key efficacy endpoints. Safety was evaluated by means of open assessment of adverse events (AEs), serious AEs, electrocardiogram (ECG), vital signs, and routine laboratory values.

For the safety analysis during the entire treatment period (from baseline through the week 52 visit of the last patient), the secukinumab groups included any patients who received the stated dose of secukinumab, including those patients randomized to placebo at baseline who were re-randomized to active treatment at week 16. These secukinumab groups have been denoted as any secukinumab 300 mg, any secukinumab 150 mg, or any secukinumab (which includes all patients who received any dose of secukinumab, whether assigned at baseline or re-randomized to active treatment at week 16).

Statistical analysis

Assuming an ASAS20 response rate of 60% in the secukinumab groups and 20% in the placebo group, including 74 patients in each study group, provided 99% power to reject the primary hypothesis with a 2.5% type I error rate based on Fisher's exact test. This sample-size also provided adequate power for analysis of secondary endpoints ranging from 79% to 99%.

Primary and secondary efficacy endpoint analyses included all patients according to the treatment assigned at baseline randomization. Closed testing procedures were used to maintain a family-wise error rate of 5% across the secukinumab groups and endpoints. The hypotheses for the primary objective in either secukinumab treatment arm vs placebo were tested simultaneously at the $P = 0.025$ level. Based on the rejection of one or both of these hypotheses, secondary endpoint analysis was completed according to a pre-specified hierarchy sequence.

The primary and other binary endpoints were evaluated by means of logistic regression with treatment and anti-TNF response status as factors and weight as a covariate. Missing values, including those due to discontinuation of the study treatment, were imputed as failure to achieve the given response (non-responses).

Between-group differences in continuous variables were evaluated using the mixed-model repeated measures (MMRM) approach, with missing data assumed to be missing at random and with study group, assessment visit, and anti-TNF response status as factors. Weight and baseline values of the endpoints were included in the model as continuous covariates. Interaction terms included study group and baseline value according to the assessment visit. For changes in hsCRP, the log ratio of the post-baseline value to the baseline value was used to normalize the distribution of hsCRP at each assessment.

Safety endpoints were evaluated in the safety set, which included all patients who received at least one dose of the study drug; these endpoints were summarized descriptively. Safety results are presented for the placebo-controlled period (i.e., first 16 weeks of treatment) to reflect the time point at which the primary objective was defined and the entire safety reporting period, which included all safety data up to the date cut-off of the last patient's week 52 clinic visit.

Results

Patients

Of 278 patients screened, 226 (81.3%) underwent randomization to receive an intravenous loading regimen of secukinumab 10 mg/kg body weight at baseline and weeks 2 and 4, followed by subcutaneous secukinumab at a dose of 300 mg (IV-300 mg; N = 76), or 150 mg (IV-150 mg; N = 74) starting from week 8. Placebo-group patients (N = 76) received an intravenous loading regimen of placebo at baseline and weeks 2 and 4, followed by subcutaneous placebo starting from week 8. Of the patients randomized, 222 (98.2%) completed the 16-week evaluation period (Fig. 1). Four patients discontinued the study before week 16 for the reasons outlined in Fig. 1. Demographics and baseline disease characteristics were similar across the study groups (Table 1). Most of the patients (97.8%) were < 65 years of age, with a median age among the groups ranging from 42.0 to 43.0 years. Approximately 24% of patients were anti-TNF-IR, two-thirds (60.2%) of the patients were male, and 72.6% were white.

Pharmacokinetics

Despite the relatively high dose of the intravenous loading regimen (10 mg/kg times three doses, based on previous pharmacokinetic and pharmacodynamics studies [20]) administered to both secukinumab groups, overall drug exposure was higher in the IV-300-mg-dose group (median concentration of 40 mcg/mL) compared to the IV-150-mg-dose group (20 mcg/mL) at week 24.

Efficacy

The primary endpoint was met with both secukinumab groups at week 16; the ASAS20 response rate was 60.5% ($P < 0.01$) with secukinumab IV-300 mg and 58.1% ($P <$ 0.05) with secukinumab IV-150 mg vs 36.8% with placebo (Fig. 2a), with differentiation from placebo seen as early as week 1.

Secondary endpoints were assessed in hierarchical order. ASAS40 response rates at week 16 were significant in both secukinumab groups (42.1% and 40.5% with secukinumab IV-300 and IV-150 mg, respectively) vs placebo (21.1%; $P < 0.05$ for both comparisons vs placebo; Fig. 2b). All other predefined secondary endpoints were also met in both secukinumab groups, except ASAS partial remission in the secukinumab IV-150 mg group. Significantly greater mean decreases from baseline in hsCRP (represented by lower post-baseline to baseline ratios) were observed with both secukinumab groups vs placebo (0.48 for secukinumab IV-300 mg and 0.55 for secukinumab IV-150 mg versus 1.09 for placebo; $P < 0.05$ for both secukinumab groups vs placebo). Both secukinumab groups achieved significantly higher ASAS 5/6 response rates compared with the placebo group at week 16 (39.5% for secukinumab IV-300 mg and 41.9% for secukinumab IV-150 mg vs 14.5% for placebo; $P <$ 0.05 for both secukinumab groups vs placebo). The improvement in total BASDAI score from baseline to week

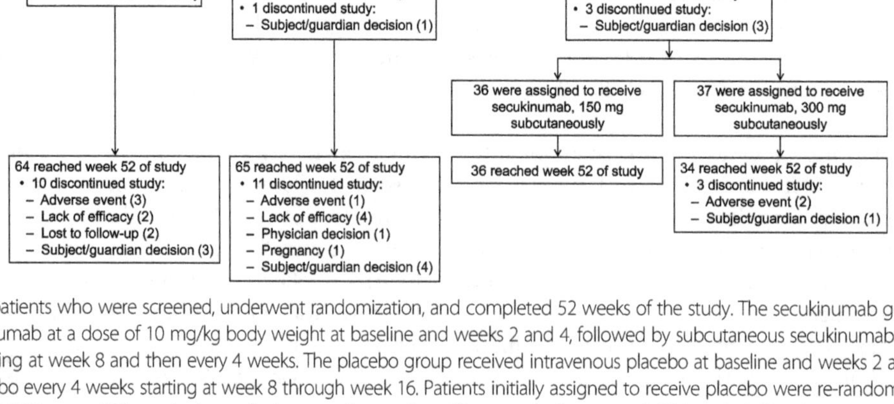

Fig. 1 Number of patients who were screened, underwent randomization, and completed 52 weeks of the study. The secukinumab groups received intravenous secukinumab at a dose of 10 mg/kg body weight at baseline and weeks 2 and 4, followed by subcutaneous secukinumab at a dose of 300 mg or 150 mg, starting at week 8 and then every 4 weeks. The placebo group received intravenous placebo at baseline and weeks 2 and 4, followed by subcutaneous placebo every 4 weeks starting at week 8 through week 16. Patients initially assigned to receive placebo were re-randomized at week 16 to receive secukinumab 300 mg or 150 mg. Analyses of primary and secondary efficacy endpoints at week 16 included all patients according to the assigned study treatment at baseline. The most frequent reasons for screening failure included meeting the exclusion criteria of history of ongoing, chronic or recurrent infectious disease or evidence of tuberculosis infection (n = 11), not meeting the inclusion criteria of: active ankylosing spondylitis assessed by total Bath Ankylosing Spondylitis Disease Activity Index ≥4 (0–10) at baseline (n = 9) and total back pain as measured by visual analog scale ≥40 mm (0–100 mm) at baseline (n = 6)

Table 1 Demographic and baseline characteristics of the patients

Characteristic	Secukinumab IV-300 mg ($N = 76$)	Secukinumab IV-150 mg ($N = 74$)	Placebo ($N = 76$)
Age (years), mean (SD)	42.1 (11.8)	42.9 (11.1)	42.7 (11.4)
Male, *n* (%)	50 (65.8)	46 (62.2)	40 (52.6)
White, *n* (%)	52 (68.4)	54 (73.0)	58 (76.3)
Weight (kg), mean (SD)	82.7 (16.9)	80.3 (19.2)	79.0 (15.5)
Time since AS diagnosis (years), mean (SD)	5.3 (7.3)	6.0 (7.2)	5.2 (6.4)
HLA-B27 positive at baseline, *n* (%)	56 (73.7)	52 (70.3)	53 (69.7)
Anti-TNF-naïve, *n* (%)	57 (75.0)	57 (77.0)	59 (77.6)
Total BASDAI score, mean (SD)	7.0 (1.4)	7.0 (1.4)	6.9 (1.3)
hsCRP (mg/L), median (min–max)	13.3 (0.2–65.1)	21.1 (0.4–111.3)	20.0 (0.2–112.5)
Total back pain score (0–100 mm scale), mean (SD)	74.1 (15.1)	75.2 (14.9)	75 (13.9)
Baseline systemic treatment, *n* (%)			
Methotrexate use at randomization	13 (17.1)	10 (13.5)	6 (7.9)
Sulfasalazine use at randomization	20 (26.3)	14 (18.9)	19 (25.0)
Corticosteroid use at randomization	6 (7.9)	9 (12.2)	14 (18.4)
NSAID use at randomization	63 (82.9)	62 (83.8)	64 (84.2)

n number of patients, *SD* standard deviation, *AS* ankylosing spondylitis, *HLA* human leukocyte antigen, *TNF* tumor necrosis factor, *BASDAI* Bath Ankylosing Spondylitis Disease Activity Index, *hsCRP* high-sensitivity C-reactive protein, *NSAID* non-steroidal anti-inflammatory drugs

16 was also significantly greater for both secukinumab groups compared with the placebo group (−2.69 for secukinumab IV-300 mg and −2.28 for secukinumab IV-150 mg versus −1.45 for placebo; $P < 0.05$ for both secukinumab groups versus placebo). The proportion of patients achieving ASAS partial remission at week 16 was significantly higher in the secukinumab IV-300 mg group (21.1%; $P < 0.05$) compared with the placebo group (1.3%), while the secukinumab IV-150 mg group (9.5%) did not significantly differ from placebo on the basis of hierarchical testing (Table 2).

In pre-specified subgroup analyses at week 16, ASAS20 responses were higher in both secukinumab groups vs placebo, regardless of anti-TNF status. ASAS20 response rates in anti-TNF-naïve patients were 64.9% and 63.2% in the secukinumab IV-300 and IV-150 mg groups, respectively, vs 39.0% with placebo; the corresponding rates in TNF-IR patients were 47.4% and 41.2% vs 29.4%, respectively. In these subgroup analyses, numerical improvements were also observed in both secukinumab groups vs placebo in the secondary efficacy endpoints (ASAS40, hsCRP, ASAS5/6, BASDAI, and ASAS partial remission), regardless of anti-TNF status (Table 3).

Long-term efficacy

A total of 199 (88.1%) patients completed the 52-week evaluation period; 27 patients discontinued the study before week 52 due to the reasons depicted in Fig. 1. ASAS20 and ASAS40 response rates observed at week 16 in both secukinumab groups were sustained through 52 weeks of therapy, on the basis of both observed data and a more conservative estimate of efficacy with missing values imputed as non-response (Fig. 2 and Additional file 2). At week 52, ASAS20 and ASAS40 response rates using non-responder imputations were 68.4% and 53.9%, and 58.1% and 40.5% with secukinumab IV-300 mg and IV-150 mg, respectively. Improvements achieved with secukinumab in all other secondary endpoints at week 16 were also sustained at week 52 (see Additional file 2). Improvements in ASAS20 and ASAS40 response rates, and all other endpoints were observed in placebo-treated patients re-randomized at week 16 to either secukinumab 300 or 150 mg through week 52 (see Additional file 3).

Consistent with the results on usability and satisfaction with the PFS from previous secukinumab studies in patients with psoriatic arthritis and psoriasis [21], all patients reported successful self-administration of study treatment using the PFS at week 12. "Needle stick in a non-critical area" was the only hazard experienced across all treatment groups (total 4.6%). Overall, SIAQ domain scores improved over time across all treatment groups (see Additional file 4).

Safety

The 16-week placebo-controlled period

During the 16-week placebo-controlled period, AEs were reported in 44.7% of patients in the secukinumab IV-300 mg group, 45.9% of patients in the secukinumab IV-150 mg group, and 44.0% of patients in the placebo group. The most frequent treatment-emergent AEs during week

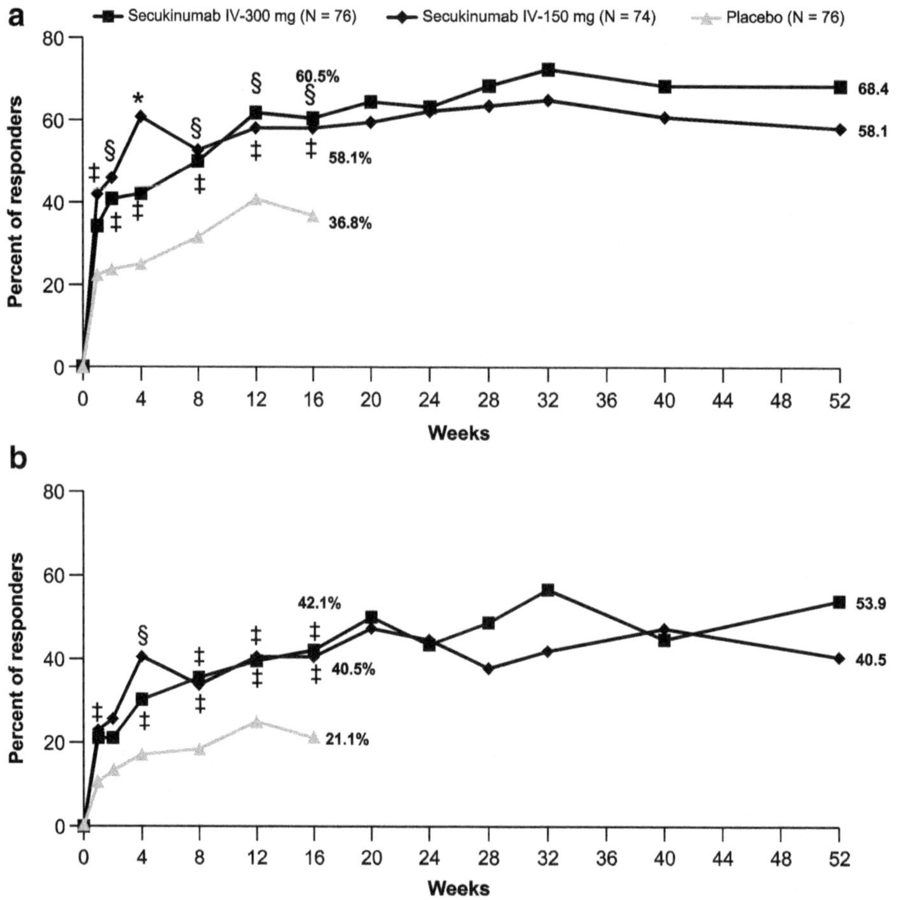

Fig. 2 Response rates through week 16 (placebo-controlled phase) and through week 52. Shown are the proportions of patients with Assessment of SpondyloArthritis international Society 20% improvement (ASAS20) responses (improvement of ≥ 20% and absolute improvement of ≥ 1 unit (on a 10-unit scale) in at least three of the four main ASAS domains, with no worsening of ≥ 20% in the remaining domain (**a**)) and ASAS40 responses (improvement of ≥ 40% and absolute improvement of ≥ 2 units (on a 10-unit scale) in at least three of the four main ASAS domains, with no worsening in the remaining domain (**b**)). Missing data were imputed as non-responses up to week 52. *P* values at week 16 were adjusted for multiplicity of testing: $^{*}P < 0.0001$; $^{§}P < 0.01$; $^{‡}P < 0.05$ versus placebo

16 were nasopharyngitis, diarrhea, headache, and cough. Through week 16, none of the patients discontinued treatment due to an AE. Rates of non-fatal SAEs and discontinuations were low and similar across the study groups (Table 4). Treatment-emergent SAEs were reported in one patient each in the secukinumab IV-300 mg group (ankylosing spondylitis flare) and placebo group (non-serious urinary tract infection), neither of which led to interruption of study treatment.

Entire safety reporting period

During the entire safety reporting period, the maximum duration of exposure to secukinumab in the "any secukinumab" group was 607 days, with a median exposure of 428.0 days. The exposure-adjusted incidence rate of non-fatal SAEs was low and was similar between both secukinumab groups (4.8 events per 100 patient-years in the any secukinumab 300 mg and 150 mg groups).

No cases of adjudicated major adverse cardiovascular events, Crohn's disease, or ulcerative colitis were reported. Two patients (one case each in the any secukinumab 150 mg and any secukinumab 300 mg) group reported grade 3 neutropenia; grade 4 neutropenia was reported in two patients from the any secukinumab 150 mg group. These findings resolved, did not lead to discontinuation of study treatment, and no concomitant infections or infestations were reported. *Candida* infection was reported in two patients each in the any secukinumab 300 mg and 150 mg dose groups. These included one case each of esophageal candidiasis, vulvovaginal candidiasis, genital candidiasis and oral candidiasis. All these cases were mild to moderate in severity and resolved with standard antifungal treatment, without leading to study discontinuation. Uveitis was reported in one patient in the any secukinumab 300 mg group and in two patients in the any secukinumab 150 mg group

Table 2 Efficacy endpoints at week 16 using non-responder imputation

Endpoints	Secukinumab IV-300 mg (*N* = 76)	Secukinumab IV-150 mg (*N* = 74)	Placebo (*N* = 76)
ASAS20, *n* (%)	46 (60.5)§	43 (58.1)‡	28 (36.8)
ASAS40, *n* (%)	32 (42.1)‡	30 (40.5)‡	16 (21.1)
hsCRP (post-baseline/baseline ratio), mean change from baseline ± SE	0.48 ± 1.1‡	0.55 ± 1.1‡	1.09 ± 1.1
ASAS 5/6, *n* (%)	30 (39.5)‡	31 (41.9)‡	11 (14.5)
BASDAI, mean change from baseline ± SE	-2.7 ± 0.3‡	-2.3 ± 0.3‡	-1.5 ± 0.3
ASAS partial remission, *n* (%)	16 (21.1)‡	7 (9.5)	1 (1.3)

Non-responder imputation (binary variables) and mixed-model repeated measures (continuous variables) data are presented
ASAS20 20% response according to criteria of the Assessment of Spondyloarthritis International Society, *ASAS40* 40% response according to ASAS criteria, *hsCRP* high-sensitivity C-reactive protein, *BASDAI* Bath Ankylosing Spondylitis Disease Activity Index
ASAS Assessment of SpondyloArthritis international Society, *BASDAI* Bath Ankylosing Spondylitis Disease Activity Index, *hsCRP* high-sensitivity C-reactive protein, *N* number of patients, *SE* standard error
‡$P < 0.05$, §$P < 0.01$ vs placebo. *P* values were adjusted for multiplicity of testing

Table 3 Efficacy endpoints at week 16 by anti-TNF status

Endpoints	Secukinumab IV-300 mg	Secukinumab IV-150 mg	Placebo
Anti-TNF-naïve	*N* = 57	*N* = 57	*N* = 59
ASAS20, *n* (%)	37 (64.9)§	36 (63.2)‡	23 (39.0)
ASAS40, *n* (%)	25 (43.9)‡	25 (43.9)‡	14 (23.7)
hsCRP (post-baseline/baseline ratio), LS mean change ± SE	0.43 ± 1.1*	0.51 ± 1.1†	0.[illegible]1 ± 1.1
ASAS 5/6, *n* (%)	24 (42.1)‡	26 (45.6)§	11 (18.6)
BASDAI, LS mean change ± SE	-3.2 ± 0.3§	-2.6 ± 0.3	-1.9 ± 0.3
ASAS partial remission, *n* (%)	12 (21.1)§	6 (10.5)	1 (1.7)
Anti-TNF-IR	*N* = 19	*N* = 17	*N* = 17
ASAS20, *n* (%)	9 (47.4)	7 (41.2)	5 (29.4)
ASAS40, *n* (%)	7 (36.8)	5 (29.4)	2 (11.8)
hsCRP (post-baseline/baseline ratio), LS mean change ± SE	0.57 ± 1.2§	0.58 ± 1.3§	1.5 ± 1.2
ASAS 5/6, *n* (%)	6 (31.6)‡	5 (29.4)‡	0
BASDAI, LS mean change ± SE	-1.8 ± 0.6	-2.2 ± 0.6	-0.9 ± 0.6
ASAS partial remission, *n* (%)	4 (21.1)	1 (5.9)	0

Non-responder imputation (binary variables) and mixed-model repeated measures (continuous variables) analyses are presented
TNF tumor necrosis factor, *N* number of patients, *ASAS* Assessment of SpondyloArthritis international Society, *hsCRP* high-sensitivity C-reactive protein, *LS* least squares, *SE* standard error, *BASDAI* Bath Ankylosing Spondylitis Disease Activity Index
‡$P < 0.05$, §$P < 0.01$, †$P < 0.001$, *$P < 0.0001$ vs placebo. *P*-values are unadjusted

(with one new-onset mild event leading to treatment discontinuation, while the other two cases were in patients with a prior history of uveitis). Benign tumor was reported in one patient each in the any secukinumab 300 mg (skin papilloma) and 150 mg (enchondroma) groups.

No other clinically relevant changes were observed in laboratory parameters, vital signs, and ECG findings over the entire safety reporting period. No dose dependence was observed in any safety risk. Treatment-emergent anti-drug antibodies were reported in only one patient in the secukinumab IV-300 mg group, which were not neutralizing to secukinumab and did not lead to loss of efficacy, pharmacokinetic abnormalities, or associated immunogenicity-related AEs. No deaths were reported during the study.

Discussion

Both secukinumab groups (300 mg and 150 mg subcutaneous maintenance dosing, preceded by an intravenous loading regimen) had rapidly reduced signs and symptoms of active AS, further confirming the results from two previous phase 3 studies that used either intravenous or subcutaneous loading [15]. Placebo-treated patients re-randomized to secukinumab at week 16 (no loading regimen) also showed improvements across all efficacy endpoints through 52 weeks of treatment.

As in previous studies, the current trial met the primary endpoint with approximately 60% of patients achieving an ASAS20 response in each secukinumab group, with an early onset of action by week 1 and sustained treatment responses through week 52 [15]. The bulk of the data collection in MEASURE 3 occurred following regulatory approval of secukinumab for the treatment of AS, which could potentially have contributed to increased placebo responses on patient-reported outcome measures (due to patient expectations). If this was the case, changes in objective markers of inflammation, such as hsCRP levels, would not be subject to this same placebo response, which was confirmed by the lack of decrease in hsCRP in the placebo group.

Improvements observed in more stringent ASAS40 and ASAS5/6 response criteria were more than 40% across both secukinumab groups up to 52 weeks of treatment, which provides further evidence of clinically meaningful long-term improvements in AS with secukinumab. Although MEASURE 3 is the first study to assess the efficacy and safety of a 300 mg dose of secukinumab in AS, the intravenous loading regimen used in both the 300 mg and 150 mg dose groups may have obscured dose-dependent differences in efficacy at week 16, although dose-dependent drug exposure was observed by week 24, with the IV-300 mg dose group demonstrating a median secukinumab concentration

Table 4 Safety profile during week 16 (placebo-controlled period) and the entire safety reporting period

Variable	Through week 16 (placebo-controlled period)[a]			Entire safety-data period		
	Secukinumab IV-300 mg (*N* = 76)	Secukinumab IV-150 mg (*N* = 74)	Placebo (*N* = 75)	Any secukinumab 300 mg (*N* = 113)	Any secukinumab 150 mg (*N* = 110)	Any secukinumab (*N* = 223)
Exposure to study treatment, days, mean ± SD	112.9 ± 14.2	117.4 ± 13.1	112.2 ± 19.4	410.7 ± 108.9	425.9 ± 92.4	418.2 ± 101.1
	Number of patients (%)			Number of patients (incidence rate per 100 patient years)		
Any AE	34 (44.7)	34 (45.9)	33 (44.0)	83 (152.7)	90 (179.2)	173 (165.4)
Serious AE	1 (1.3)	0 (0.0)	1 (1.3)	6 (4.8)	6 (4.8)	12 (4.8)
Discontinued due to AEs	0 (0.0)	0 (0.0)	0 (0.0)	4 (3.5)	4 (3.6)	8 (3.6)
Death	0 (0.0)	0 (0.0)	0 (0.0)	0 (0.0)	0 (0.0)	0 (0.0)
Common AEs[a]						
Nasopharyngitis	3 (3.9)	6 (8.1)	2 (2.7)	16 (13.7)	22 (19.6)	38 (16.6)
Diarrhea	3 (3.9)	5 (6.8)	0 (0.0)	8 (6.6)	9 (7.5)	17 (7.0)
Headache	3 (3.9)	5 (6.8)	5 (6.7)	11 (9.1)	12 (10.1)	23 (9.6)
Cough	3 (3.9)	3 (4.1)	1 (1.3)	5 (4.1)	3 (2.4)	8 (3.2)
Pharyngitis	3 (3.9)	1 (1.4)	1 (1.3)	4 (3.2)	3 (2.4)	7 (2.8)
Ear infection	3 (3.9)	0 (0.0)	0 (0.0)	3 (2.4)	0	3 (1.2)
Urinary tract infection	3 (3.9)	0 (0.0)	3 (4.0)	6 (4.9)	3 (2.4)	9 (3..6)
AEs of special interest						
Candida infection	1 (1.4)	1 (1.3)	0 (0.0)	2 (1.8)	2 (1.8)	4 (1.8)
Malignant tumor	0 (0.0)	0 (0.0)	0 (0.0)	1 (0.9)	1 (0.9)	2 (0.9)
Neutropenia						
Grade 3	0 (0.0)	1 (1.4)	0 (0.0)	1 (0.9)	1 (0.9)	2 (0.9)
Grade 4	0 (0.0)	2 (2.7)	0 (0.0)	0 (0.0)	2 (1.8)	2 (0.9)

The entire safety reporting period includes all safety data up to the date cutoff of the last patient's week 52 clinic visit. One patient was excluded from placebo group as no treatment was given after randomization. In the analysis of the entire study period, the secukinumab groups include any patients who received the stated dose of secukinumab, including those who were randomly assigned to the placebo group at baseline and who underwent a second randomization to active treatment at week 16

N number of patients, *AE* adverse event, *SD* standard deviation

[a]AEs with frequency ≥3% in either of the two secukinumab groups during the 16-week placebo-controlled period

that was double that in the IV-150 mg group by this time point. Some differences in efficacy responses were evident by week 52, particularly for higher-hurdle efficacy endpoints such as ASAS40 (IV-300 mg, 53.9%; IV-150 mg, 40.5%) and ASAS partial remission (IV-300 mg, 22.4%; IV-150 mg, 16.2%).

Although TNF inhibitors have shown efficacy in patients with AS, an unmet medical need persists due to primary and secondary treatment failure and intolerance, which has been well-documented in a substantial proportion of patients with AS [10, 22]. Addressing this need, secukinumab has demonstrated efficacy in patients with AS with an inadequate response or intolerance to anti-TNF therapy in this and previous studies in AS [15]. In addition, in patients who were naïve to anti-TNF therapy for whom secukinumab was their first biologic treatment, ASAS20 response rates were approximately 5% higher with secukinumab IV-300 mg and IV-150 mg after 16 weeks of treatment, compared to the overall study population.

The safety profile of secukinumab in this study was consistent with that observed in previous trials of secukinumab in patients with active AS [14, 15] and other indications, including psoriatic arthritis [17, 18] and psoriasis [16]. No new or unexpected safety findings were reported in this study, with lower AE and SAE rates observed than previously reported in the MEASURE 1 or MEASURE 2 studies, despite the use of a higher secukinumab dose (300 mg subcutaneous monthly dosing following three weight-based 10 mg/kg intravenous loading doses), suggesting that secukinumab 300 mg is as well-tolerated as the currently approved 150 mg dose.

The use of immunomodulatory biologics has been associated with an elevated risk of AEs including *Candida* infections [23], uveitis [24], malignancy [25] and neutropenia [24, 26]. TNF inhibitors, in particular, have been associated with an increased risk of serious infections, including reactivation tuberculosis, bacterial sepsis, invasive fungal infections (such as histoplasmosis), and infections due to opportunistic pathogens [27, 28]. In the current study, for the any secukinumab 300-mg and 150-mg dose groups, the exposure-adjusted incidence rates for serious infections were 1.6 and 0.8 per 100 patient-years, respectively, over the entire safety reporting period. Absolute rates of serious infection were also comparable to placebo (secukinumab IV-300 mg, 3.9%; secukinumab IV-150 mg, 5.4%; placebo, 8%) over the first 16 weeks of treatment (placebo-controlled period). Rates of other AEs of clinical interest were similarly reassuring and comparable to placebo, including *Candida* infection, uveitis, malignancy, and grade 3 or 4 neutropenia, with no cases of Crohn's disease or ulcerative colitis reported.

Conclusions

In conclusion, this study reinforces the observation that secukinumab provides rapid, significant, and sustained improvement over 52 weeks in the signs and symptoms of active AS, regardless of prior experience with TNF inhibitors, with response rates that were highest in patients naïve to anti-TNF therapy. Also, the usability of the PFS and acceptability of a liquid-in-vial formulation to deliver intravenous loading doses was confirmed. These 52-week results demonstrate that both the 300 mg and 150 mg doses of secukinumab are efficacious and well-tolerated.

Additional files

Additional file 1: Study design. Randomization was stratified according to whether patients were anti-TNF-naïve or had previous inadequate response or intolerance to anti-TNF therapy. ASAS, Assessment of SpondyloArthritis international Society; ASAS20, 20% improvement in ASAS criteria; BL, baseline; i.v., intravenous; q4wk, every 4 weeks; PBO, placebo; R, randomization; s.c., subcutaneous; TNF, tumor necrosis factor; wk, week. (PDF 817 kb)

Additional file 2: Efficacy endpoints at week 52 using non-responder imputation and observed data. (DOCX 16 kb)

Additional file 3: Efficacy endpoints at week 52 for placebo patients re-randomized to secukinumab using non-responder imputation and observed data. (DOCX 16 kb)

Additional file 4: SIOQ domain scores over week 16. Overall patient experience with secukinumab administration via the pre-filled syringes was assessed over time from baseline (PRE module) to week 16 (POST modules) by SIAQ domains: (a) feeling about self-injection; (b) self-confidence and (c) satisfaction with self-injection. SIAQ, Self-Injection Assessment Questionnaire. (PDF 781 kb)

Additional file 5: List of Independent Ethics Committees (IECs) or Institutional Review Boards (IRBs) that approved study. (DOCX 19 kb)

Additional file 6: List of ethical approval reference numbers for each participating center of this study. (DOCX 23 kb)

Abbreviations

ACR: American College of Rheumatology; AE: Adverse event; AS: Ankylosing spondylitis; ASAS: Assessment of SpondyloArthritis international Society criteria; BASDAI: Bath Ankylosing Spondylitis Disease Activity Index; DMARDs: Disease-modifying anti-rheumatic drugs; ECG: Electrocardiogram; EULAR: European League Against Rheumatism; GCP: Good Clinical Practice; hsCRP: High sensitivity C-reactive protein; IFU: Instructions for use; IL: Interleukin; IRT: Interactive response technology; NSAID: Non-steroidal anti-inflammatory drug; PFS: Pre-filled syringe; SAE: Serious adverse event; SIAQ: Self-Injection Assessment Questionnaire; TNF: Tumor necrosis factor; TNF-IR: Tumor necrosis factor inhibitor inadequate responder; VAS: Visual analog scale

Acknowledgments

The authors thank the patients who participated in this study, the study investigators, and John Gallagher, medical consultant for Novartis Pharma AG, Basel, Switzerland. Manuscript writing support was provided by Vasundhara Pathak, Novartis Healthcare Pvt Ltd, Hyderabad, India.

Funding

Novartis Pharma AG (Basel, Switzerland).

Authors' contributions

KP, AK, ED, RB, MM, and HT contributed to the interpretation of data, and critically reviewed and provided feedback on all versions of the manuscript. LP contributed to the design of the study, data analysis, and interpretation of data, and critically reviewed and provided feedback on all versions of the manuscript. MA conducted the statistical analysis, contributed to interpretation of data, and critically reviewed and provided feedback on all versions of the manuscript. AR contributed to the design of the study, data analysis, and interpretation of data, and critically reviewed and provided feedback on all versions of the manuscript. BP contributed to the design of the study, the data analysis plan, and data interpretation, and critically reviewed and provided feedback on all versions of the manuscript. All authors reviewed and approved the final manuscript.

Ethics approval and consent to participate

The trial was conducted under GCP and ethics approval was confirmed by the Sponsor prior to first patient first visit (FPFV) at each center. The Institutional Review Board (IRB) at each participating center approved the protocol. Further information related to ethics approval can be found at https://www.clinicaltrialsregister.eu/ctr-search/search?query=2013-001090-24. A list of Independent Ethics Committees (IECs) or IRBs that approved study is given in Additional file 5. The list of ethical approval reference numbers for each participating center of this study is given in Additional file 6. The trial was conducted in accordance with the Declaration of Helsinki and GCP guidelines by the study investigators and was analyzed by the Sponsor. Written informed consent was obtained from all patients for participation in trial and for publication.

Competing interests

KP: Speakers bureau - MSD, AbbVie, Roche, UCB, Amgen, Hospira, Egis, Pfizer, Medac, BMS. AK: consulting fees - Celgene, Janssen, Pfizer, Genentech, and Sanofi; Speakers bureau: Celgene, Pfizer, Genentech, and Novartis. ED: no competing interests. RB: research grants - AbbVie, MSD, and Roche; consulting fees - AbbVie, Pfizer, Roche, Bristol-Myers, Janssen, and MSD; Speakers bureau - AbbVie, Pfizer, Roche, Bristol-Myers, Janssen, and MSD. MM: no competing interests. HT: Speakers bureau - Novartis, Eli Lilly, and AbbVie. LP, MA, AR, and BP are employees of Novartis. LP, AR, and BP own Novartis stock.

Author details

[1]Institute of Rheumatology and Department of Rheumatology, 1st Faculty of Medicine, Charles University, Prague, Czech Republic. [2]Altoona Center for Clinical Research, Duncansville, PA, USA. [3]Medical Plus, s.r.o., Uherske Hradiste, Czech Republic. [4]Division of Rheumatology, Hospital Universitario Marqués de Valdecilla, Santander, Spain. [5]Centro de Investigación de Tratamientos Innovadores de Sinaloa, Culiacán, México. [6]Barts Health NHS Trust, London, UK. [7]Novartis Pharmaceuticals Corporation, East Hanover, NJ, USA. [8]Novartis Pharma AG, Basel, Switzerland.

References

1. Dougados M, Baeten D. Spondyloarthritis. Lancet. 2011;377(9783):2127–37.
2. Garg N, van den Bosch F, Deodhar A. The concept of spondyloarthritis: where are we now? Best Pract Res Clin Rheumatol. 2014;28(5):663–72.
3. Braun J, Sieper J. Ankylosing spondylitis. Lancet. 2007;369(9570):1379–90.
4. Kotsis K, Voulgari PV, Drosos AA, Carvalho AF, Hyphantis T. Health-related quality of life in patients with ankylosing spondylitis: a comprehensive review. Expert Rev Pharmacoecon Outcomes Res. 2014;14(6):857–72.
5. Boonen A, van der Linden SM. The burden of ankylosing spondylitis. J Rheumatol Suppl. 2006;78:4–11.
6. Dean LE, Jones GT, MacDonald AG, Downham C, Sturrock RD, Macfarlane GJ. Global prevalence of ankylosing spondylitis. Rheumatology (Oxford). 2014;53(4):650–7.
7. Braun J, van den Berg R, Baraliakos X, Boehm H, Burgos-Vargas R, Collantes-Estevez E, Dagfinrud H, Dijkmans B, Dougados M, Emery P, et al. 2010 update of the ASAS/EULAR recommendations for the management of ankylosing spondylitis. Ann Rheum Dis. 2011;70(6):896–904.
8. van der Heijde D, Schiff MH, Sieper J, Kivitz AJ, Wong RL, Kupper H, Dijkmans BA, Mease PJ, Davis Jr JC. Adalimumab effectiveness for the treatment of ankylosing spondylitis is maintained for up to 2 years: long-term results from the ATLAS trial. Ann Rheum Dis. 2009;68(6):922–9.
9. Braun J, Kiltz U, Heldmann F, Baraliakos X. Emerging drugs for the treatment of axial and peripheral spondyloarthritis. Expert Opin Emerg Drugs. 2015;20(1):1–14.
10. Sieper J. Treatment challenges in axial spondylarthritis and future directions. Curr Rheumatol Rep. 2013;15(9):356.
11. Van Lümig PPM, Lecluse LLA, Driessen RJB, Spuls PI, Boezeman JB, Van De Kerkhof PCM, De Jong EMGJ. Switching from etanercept to adalimumab is effective and safe: results in 30 patients with psoriasis with primary failure, secondary failure or intolerance to etanercept. Br J Dermatol. 2010;163(4):838–46.
12. Lubberts E. The IL-23-IL-17 axis in inflammatory arthritis. Nat Rev Rheumatol. 2015;11(7):415–29.
13. Duarte JH. Spondyloarthropathies: IL-17A blockade ameliorates ankylosing spondylitis. Nat Rev Rheumatol. 2016;12(2):72.
14. Baeten D, Baraliakos X, Braun J, Sieper J, Emery P, van der Heijde D, McInnes I, van Laar JM, Landewe R, Wordsworth P, et al. Anti-interleukin-17A monoclonal antibody secukinumab in treatment of ankylosing spondylitis: a randomised, double-blind, placebo-controlled trial. Lancet. 2013;382(9906):1705–13.
15. Baeten D, Sieper J, Braun J, Baraliakos X, Dougados M, Emery P, Deodhar A, Porter B, Martin R, Andersson M, et al. Secukinumab, an interleukin-17A inhibitor, in ankylosing spondylitis. N Engl J Med. 2015;373(26):2534–48.
16. Langley RG, Elewski BE, Lebwohl M, Reich K, Griffiths CE, Papp K, Puig L, Nakagawa H, Spelman L, Sigurgeirsson B, et al. Secukinumab in plaque psoriasis–results of two phase 3 trials. N Engl J Med. 2014;371(4):326–38.
17. McInnes IB, Mease PJ, Kirkham B, Kavanaugh A, Ritchlin CT, Rahman P, van der Heijde D, Landewe R, Conaghan PG, Gottlieb AB, et al. Secukinumab, a human anti-interleukin-17A monoclonal antibody, in patients with psoriatic arthritis (FUTURE 2): a randomised, double-blind, placebo-controlled, phase 3 trial. Lancet. 2015;386(9999):1137–46.
18. Mease PJ, McInnes IB, Kirkham B, Kavanaugh A, Rahman P, van der Heijde D, Landewe R, Nash P, Pricop L, Yuan J, et al. Secukinumab inhibition of interleukin-17A in patients with psoriatic arthritis. N Engl J Med. 2015; 373(14):1329–39.
19. McInnes IB, Sieper J, Braun J, Emery P, van der Heijde D, Isaacs JD, Dahmen G, Wollenhaupt J, Schulze-Koops H, Kogan J, et al. Efficacy and safety of secukinumab, a fully human anti-interleukin-17A monoclonal antibody, in patients with moderate-to-severe psoriatic arthritis: a 24-week, randomised, double-blind, placebo-controlled, phase II proof-of-concept trial. Ann Rheum Dis. 2014;73(2):349–56.
20. Hueber W, Patel DD, Dryja T, Wright AM, Koroleva I, Bruin G, Antoni C, Draelos Z, Gold MH, Durez P, et al. Effects of AIN457, a fully human antibody to interleukin-17A, on psoriasis, rheumatoid arthritis, and uveitis. Sci Transl Med. 2010;2:52ra72.
21. Gottlieb AB, Blauvelt A, Prinz JC, Papanastasiou P, Pathan R, Nyirady J, Fox T, Papavassilis C. Secukinumab self-administration by prefilled syringe maintains reduction of plaque psoriasis severity over 52 weeks. results of the FEATURE trial. J Drugs Dermatol. 2016;15(10):1226–34.
22. Van den Bosch F, Deodhar A. Treatment of spondyloarthritis beyond TNF-alpha blockade. Best Pract Res Clin Rheumatol. 2014;28(5):819–27.
23. Filler SG, Yeaman MR, Sheppard DC. Tumor necrosis factor inhibition and invasive fungal infections. Clin Infect Dis. 2005;41 Suppl 3:S208–12.
24. Perez-Alvarez R, Perez-de-Lis M, Ramos-Casals M. Biologics-induced autoimmune diseases. Curr Opin Rheumatol. 2013;25(1):56–64.
25. Wolfe F, Michaud K. Biologic treatment of rheumatoid arthritis and the risk of malignancy: analyses from a large US observational study. Arthritis Rheum. 2007;56(9):2886–95.
26. Ottaviani S, Cerf-Payrastre I, Kemiche F, Pertuiset E. Adalimumab-induced neutropenia in a patient with rheumatoid arthritis. Joint Bone Spine. 2009;76(3):312–3.
27. HUMIRA: Highlights of prescribing information. [http://www.rxabbvie.com/pdf/humira.pdf]. Accessed 21 Nov 2016.
28. ENBREL: Highlights of prescribing information. [http://pi.amgen.com/united_states/enbrel/derm/enbrel_pi.pdf]. Accessed 21 Nov 2016.

2

Nonradiographic axial spondyloarthritis: clinical and therapeutic relevance

Nilasha Ghosh and Eric M. Ruderman*

Abstract

Current classification criteria for axial spondyloarthritis (axSpA) provide for the inclusion of patients with a wide range of presentations and manifestations. While not considered a formal subclassification, patients are often divided into radiographic or nonradiographic axSpA based on the presence or absence of radiographic sacroiliitis. This review will focus on nonradiographic axSpA and will discuss clinical manifestations of disease that distinguish, or in many cases do not distinguish, this entity from other individuals with axSpA. This review will also cover treatment paradigms for nonradiographic axSpA, particularly the use of biologic therapies, where current data suggest that nonradiographic disease should be managed largely the same as radiographic disease, or classical ankylosing spondylitis.

Keywords: Axial spondyloarthritis, Nonradiographic axial spondyloarthritis, Disease classification, Therapy, Biologic therapy

Background

Spondyloarthritis (SpA) refers to a family of chronic rheumatic disorders of joint inflammation, including ankylosing spondylitis (AS), psoriatic arthritis, reactive arthritis, and arthritis related to inflammatory bowel disease [1, 2]. Axial spondyloarthritis (axSpA) refers to predominant inflammation in the spine and/or sacroiliac joints and is characterized clinically by inflammatory back pain and stiffness that may be improved with exercise [3]. Sacroiliac changes on conventional radiographs have long been a key element of the classification of AS, now considered a subset of axSpA [4]. With this in mind, some have suggested dividing axSpA into radiographic (r-axSpA) or nonradiographic (nr-axSpA) forms depending on the presence or absence of radiographic changes at the sacroiliac joints; under this schema, patients traditionally classified as AS would be considered r-axSpA. This review will discuss various aspects of axial spondyloarthritis, with a strong focus on nr-axSpA and its current classification in the field of rheumatology. We will review epidemiology, prognosis, current treatments, and potential future therapies.

* Correspondence: e-ruderman@northwestern.edu
Northwestern University Feinberg School of Medicine, 675 North St. Clair, Suite 14-100, Chicago, IL 60611, USA

Search strategy

Information for the review has been drawn from manuscripts in the PubMed database published within the last 10 years. Search terms included "axial spondyloarthritis," "non-radiographic axial spondyloarthritis," "criteria AND axial spondyloarthritis," "inflammatory spinal disease," "[TNF inhibitors OR treatment] of axial spondyloarthritis," "biomarkers AND axial spondyloarthritis," "[predictors OR progression] of axial spondyloarthritis," "fibromyalgia AND axial spondyloarthritis," "therapy + axial spondyloarthritis" and "monitoring tools AND disease activity."

History of axSpA

AxSpA represents a spectrum of inflammatory conditions that primarily affect the axial skeleton and sacroiliac joints. AS is the prototypic disorder, with recognition as a distinct entity in the early 1900s [5]. Among the earliest criteria established for the diagnosis of AS was the modified New York (mNY) criteria, which combined clinical and conventional radiographic findings. The mNY criteria became the most widely used for clinical studies and treatment trials for many years until it was recognized that identifying sacroiliitis on plain film was a late finding in the disease course of many patients [3, 5]. In the 1990s, the Amor and the European Spondyloarthropathy Study Group (ESSG) criteria were established in an effort to capture a wider spectrum of spondyloarthropathies in the hopes of identifying patients in earlier stages of disease [6, 7]. The Amor criteria involved scoring several clinical, radiographic, and treatment response variables to indicate the presence or absence of SpA, whereas the ESSG criteria required the presence of inflammatory spinal pain or synovitis with one additional minor criterion in order to establish the diagnosis of SpA [6]. Because these criteria were designed to capture the entire spectrum of spondyloarthritis, they were too general to specifically identify early axial disease [7]. The next step, therefore, was to build upon the Amor and ESSG criteria to establish the Assessment of SpondyloArthritis International Society (ASAS) criteria [5] with the aim of identifying patients with early axial disease that is not evident on conventional radiographs.

ASAS criteria

In 2009, a study of 71 patients without definite sacroiliitis by the mNY criteria was reviewed by a panel of twenty experts to determine the utility of magnetic resonance imaging (MRI) as an appropriate diagnostic tool in the recognition of early axial disease [8, 9], since bone marrow edema on MRI represents the early stages of inflammation [6]. Based on the patients' histories, data, and imaging, a list of characteristics associated with axSpA was established, thus forming the ASAS criteria for axSpA [5, 8, 9] (Fig. 1). These criteria provide two routes through which the diagnosis can be made: either through a clinical arm (positive testing for human leukocyte antigen (HLA)-B27 plus two additional characteristic features of SpA) or a radiographic/imaging arm (radiographic sacroiliitis or active inflammation of the sacroiliac joints on MRI, plus one other characteristic feature of SpA) [8, 9]. Using MRI as a tool for the diagnosis of axSpA as the basis of the imaging arm criteria yielded high specificity (97.3%); however, sensitivity was compromised at 66.2%, thus missing about a third of the patients with axSpA [5, 8, 9]. The clinical arm alone had a sensitivity and specificity of 83.3% and 84.9%, respectively, in the validation set used for the criteria [5, 8, 9]. When these arms were combined, the overall sensitivity and specificity became 82.9% and 84.4%, respectively, thus ensuring the best combination for the final criteria for axSpA. One of the challenges of these criteria is that the clinical arm is not as specific as the imaging arm. Few would question the accuracy of the classification in patients with sacroiliitis and/or MRI inflammation. However, the clinical arm is potentially much more lenient. In theory, a patient with a positive HLA-B27 and a family history of SpA could be classified as axSpA with a finding of enthesitis or dactylitis, even without a history of inflammatory back pain. As will be discussed below, this has important implications for therapy, where the response to tumor necrosis factor (TNF) inhibitors in the absence of sacroiliitis is clearly associated with the presence of active inflammation, as identified by either MRI findings or an elevated C-reactive protein (CRP) level. While the ASAS criteria

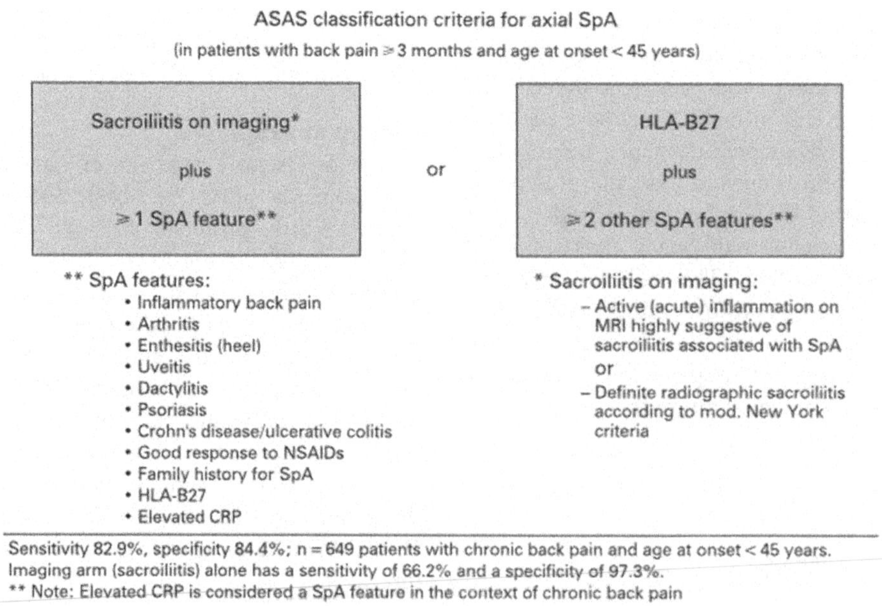

Fig. 1 ASAS classification criteria for axial spondyloarthritis. Published with permission from [9]. *ASAS* Assessment of SpondyloArthritis International Society, *CRP* C-reactive protein, *HLA* human leukocyte antigen, *MRI* magnetic resonance imaging, *NSAIDs* nonsteroidal anti-inflammatory drugs, *SpA* spondyloarthritis

allow for a balance between sensitivity and specificity, some might argue that specificity is the more critical issue when using this classification to consider the use of expensive therapies.

Epidemiology

It has been difficult to determine the exact incidence and prevalence of axSpA in the US. Due to changing criteria and differing recognition of disease not specifically associated with radiographic findings, such as nr-axSpA, diagnostic delay and misdiagnosis can be very common. This is illustrated with differing prevalence data that have been reported in the US. According to the National Health and Nutrition Examination Survey (NHANES), approximately 1.7 million individuals aged 20–69 years in the USA suffer from spondyloarthritis as defined by the Amor and ESSG criteria [10]. However, the SPEED study, one of the first systematic studies to estimate axSpA prevalence using the ASAS criteria, estimated that 0.7% of the population aged 18–44 years is affected, or just under one million individuals [11]. Of these individuals, nr-axSpA and AS each accounted for about half of all axSpA cases in this study.

AS versus nr-axSpA

The inflammation and eventual progression of joint damage in some individuals with axSpA can cause significant impairment in physical function [1]. Both AS and nr-axSpA are frequently associated with both peripheral articular and extra-articular disease; these are equally prevalent in both groups, with the exception of uveitis [12]. Uveitis appears to be more prevalent among patients with AS than nr-axSpA, a difference that is not clearly related to differences in HLA-B27 status [12]. Aside from uveitis, the clinical distinction between the two entities is not very pronounced, although nr-axSpA patients are more likely to be female [13, 14] and less likely to be HLA-B27^{+} [15]. Several studies have shown that patients with AS and nr-axSpA have similar levels of clinical disease as measured by the Bath Ankylosing Spondyloarthritis Disease Activity Index (BASDAI), functional status as measured by the Bath Ankylosing Spondyloarthritis Functional Index (BASFI), and health-related quality of life (HRQOL) measurements [13, 16, 17]. However, it can be argued that AS and nr-axSpA do differ slightly when considering nonclinical factors such as CRP levels and inflammation seen on MRI. In a trial that followed patients with AS and nr-axSpA during the first 2 years from diagnosis, CRP was higher in the AS group than in the nr-axSpA group, potentially indicating a burden of inflammation that was higher in patients with AS [16]. In a cohort of AS and nr-axSpA patients not treated with TNF inhibitors, AS patients with higher CRP levels did not spontaneously achieve low disease activity status as compared with their nr-axSpA counterparts [16]. This higher burden of inflammation is further supported by the finding of higher levels of inflammation seen on MRI in patients with AS [13, 18]. Despite the increased inflammation often seen in AS, response to TNF blockade has been similar between the two groups when inflammation is present [2, 17, 19], further supporting the fact that the two diagnoses are clinically comparable, and some have argued that the distinction may not be relevant when it comes to therapy [20]. Some studies have suggested that higher CRP levels and a higher degree of inflammation seen on MRI may play a role in the degree of treatment response for both AS and nr-axSpA, which could have relevance in AS if signs of inflammation are more prominent [17]. Finally, longer disease duration has also been associated with a divergence between the two entities. In the German Spondyloarthritis Inception Cohort (GESPIC) of patients with AS and nr-axSpA, AS patients (who had longer symptom duration at baseline) had significantly worse functional scores, and this difference was maintained over 2 years of follow-up [16].

Disease monitoring

The BASDAI is a validated instrument for monitoring disease status/activity in patients with AS by assessing fatigue, pain (both axial and peripheral), morning stiffness, and tenderness (Table 1) [21]. While not validated in the broader diagnosis of axSpA, the ASAS group has suggested that BASDAI may be used to assess disease activity in patients across the spectrum of axSpA, including patients with nr-axSpA [3]. Another useful monitoring tool is the BASFI, which measures functional status and the ability to complete activities of daily living (Table 2) [22]. Both tools rely on patient questionnaires and are considered to be purely subjective and patient-oriented [23]. Clinical trials have typically relied on the ASAS response criteria, which measures improvement

Table 1 Items in the Bath Ankylosing Spondylitis Disease Activity Index (BASDAI), scored on a numerical rating scale [17]

How would you describe the overall level of fatigue/tiredness you have experienced?
How would you describe the overall level of ankylosing spondylitis neck, back or hip pain you have had?
How would you describe the overall level of pain/swelling in joints other than neck, back or hips you have had?
How would you describe the overall level of discomfort you have had from any areas tender to touch or pressure?
How would you describe the overall level of morning stiffness you have had from the time you wake up?
How long does your morning stiffness last from the time you wake up?

Table 2 Items in the Bath Ankylosing Spondylitis Functional Index (BASFI), scored on a numerical rating scale [18]

Putting on your socks or tights without help or aids (e.g., sock aid).
Bending forward from the waist to pick up a pen from the floor without an aid.
Reaching up to a high shelf without help or aids (e.g., helping hand).
Getting up out of an armless dining room chair without using your hands or any other help
Getting up off the floor without help from lying on your back.
Standing unsupported for 10 min without discomfort.
Climbing 12 to 15 steps without using a handrail or walking aid. One foot at each step.
Looking over your shoulder without turning your body.
Doing physically demanding activities (e.g., physiotherapy, exercises, gardening or sports).
Doing a full days activities, whether it be at home or at work.

in four domains of patient-reported outcomes: global assessment, spinal pain, function, and inflammation. The BASDAI has been criticized for redundancy in its variables, assessment of only certain aspects of disease activity, and lack of specificity for inflammatory processes [23]. The ASAS response also lacks an objective measure of inflammation. The Ankylosing Spondylitis Disease Activity Score (ASDAS) was created to address these issues, most notably incorporating objective evidence of systemic inflammation in the form of a CRP level and including specific questions on axial and peripheral pain and stiffness drawn from the BASDAI. It has been shown to perform very well as a monitoring tool and is now widely considered superior to the BASDAI [23].

CRP

The biomarker of greatest interest in axial spondyloarthritis has been CRP, although its use and measurement is not without controversy. It general, patients with nr-axSpA have lower levels of CRP than similar patients with AS [13, 16], and this difference remains consistent even after receiving treatment [2, 16]. Despite this finding, some believe that CRP is not sensitive in axSpA [13] and overall has poor correlation with disease activity in both entities [18]. However, CRP has been shown to be a useful in its prognostic value with respect to progression and response to treatment. In studies that followed patients with axSpA over time (including both radiographic and nonradiographic disease), CRP positivity was the strongest risk factor associated with radiographic progression [18, 22, 24, 25]. A number of studies have shown an increased response to therapy, both with nonsteroidal anti-inflammatory drugs (NSAIDs) and TNF inhibitors, when baseline CRP or high-sensitivity CRP (hsCRP) was elevated, for both r-axSpA and nr-axSpA [2, 26, 27]. These findings seem to support the notion that objective findings of increased inflammation at baseline can predict response to TNF inhibitor therapy, which will be discussed in more detail below.

Progression

While nr-axSpA and AS may fall on the same disease spectrum, not all patients with nr-axSpA will develop radiographic sacroiliitis, supporting the notion that nr-axSpA is not simply "early" AS [3, 5]. Additionally, not all patients with radiographic sacroiliitis will develop syndesmophytes [3]. Several observational studies have cited rates of progression from 10–12% of the population within the first 2 years [16, 18], to 20–25% 2–8 years after diagnosis [15], to 26–28% of patients after 10 or more years of observation [28, 29]. More recently, however, a prospective longitudinal study found that rates of progression actually may be lower than previously described. Dougados et al. followed patients from the Devenir des Spondylarthropathies Indifférenciées Récentes (DESIR) cohort for 5 years to evaluate progression of nr-axSpA to AS, and they found that only 5.1% had progressed [30]. Within this cohort, there were actually a few patients who "regressed" from AS to nr-axSpA [30]; as radiographic sacroiliitis should not reverse, this highlights the potential for variability in the interpretation of radiographs.

There are specific characteristics that have been identified as being associated with increased progression from nr-axSpA to AS. In a study comparing the rates of progression in nr-axSpA patients meeting the two diagnostic arms, subjects in the imaging arms were 3.5 times more likely to have progression to AS than those in the clinical arm [29]; elevation of CRP, like MRI that changes an indication of active inflammation, has also been associated with progression [18]. While cohort studies have not found clinical differences between the two arms in terms of disease severity, patients in the imaging arm were more likely to be male, younger, have a higher CRP level, and have a longer disease duration [31]. These risk factors were also demonstrated in the DESIR cohort longitudinal study described above, where bone marrow edema, longer symptom duration, and younger age were predictive of radiographic progression [30].

Besides establishing factors that are associated with the progression of nr-axSpA to AS, it is also important to note the progression of radiographic change within each entity itself. Poddubnyy et al. assessed an early disease patient cohort (GESPIC) that included both AS and nr-axSpA to determine progression and associated risk factors over a period of 2 years. They found that the strongest predictor of progression of radiographic sacroiliitis by at least one grade was an elevated CRP at baseline, which carried an associated increased risk of 3.65

[18]. Males and those with a longer duration of symptoms also had greater progression of sacroiliitis among the AS group, but not among the nr-axSpA group [18].

Gender differences

Among patients with axSpA, gender differences have been identified in the distribution of disease along the spectrum. In general, proportionally more women have nr-axSpA than AS [13] and these women have a lower grade of inflammation seen on MRI [13, 31]. Even among patients with longstanding AS, women have been shown to have less radiographic damage than men [32, 33], as well as slower progression. Women also tend to have a stronger family history for both AS and early axial SpA [31, 33].

A multicenter prospective study (DESIR cohort) that specifically evaluated gender differences in patients with early axSpA found that extra-articular symptoms such as uveitis, enthesitis, psoriasis, and inflammatory bowel disease are more frequent in women [31]. Clinical disease, as measured by the BASDAI and functional scores, was worse in women; however, the ASDAS-CRP, which includes CRP and excludes peripheral symptoms, did not differ [31]. Given the higher degree of extra-articular disease and overall decreased functional status, it is possible that there may be an overdiagnosis of axSpA in women when using the clinical arm of the ASAS criteria [31]. Alternatively, underdiagnosis and undertreatment may also be possible in light of the sometimes atypical presentation in women [34] or the attribution of inflammatory pain to causes other than axSpA [1, 34], such as fibromyalgia. Both scenarios can pose a diagnostic dilemma for women with axSpA, and it may be helpful to be more liberal in the use of imaging to confirm the diagnosis in women with symptoms of inflammatory back pain [31].

There may also be gender differences in the progression of disease. While men with AS have greater rates of radiographic progression than women, men were shown to be have a lower probability of radiographic progression in one small study of sacroiliitis in nr-axSpA [18]. The impact of gender on progression of disease among nr-axSpA patients remains an area of investigation.

Finally, gender may affect response to treatment. In one study, women with nr-axSpA had a lower response rate to TNF inhibition compared to women with AS, a difference that was not seen in men [35]. While this study excluded patients with self-reported fibromyalgia, it is still possible that fibromyalgia or other noninflammatory conditions could be playing a role in clinical outcome measures. Fibromyalgia is considered to be the most common cause of generalized musculoskeletal pain in women aged 20–55 years [36]. In several studies involving patients with axSpA, fibromyalgia has been found to be a highly prevalent and a possible confounder for the diagnosis and assessment of axSpA [32, 33]. Salaffi et al. found that fibromyalgia was present in almost 15% of patients with axSpA, with a higher prevalence among women [37]. Disease monitoring for women with possible concurrent fibromyalgia and axSpA may be a challenge as well. BASDAI scores, which rely strictly on patient-reported outcomes, have been found to be higher in women with primary fibromyalgia than in those with AS [38], which may suggest an important role for ASDAS, rather than BASDAI, for disease monitoring in women with axSpA [37].

Treatments

The mainstays of treatment for axSpA include both nonpharmacologic approaches and pharmacologic options. Nonpharmacologic approaches are largely based on physical therapy and exercise to maintain flexibility and normal posture [39] Additionally, lifestyle changes such as smoking cessation may of be some utility due to its association with disease activity and radiographic progression, possibly mediated through elevated CRP levels [40]. Furthermore, it has been shown that current smoking can impair response to TNF inhibition [41]. These nonpharmacologic interventions can be very useful in patients with axSpA, and they should be used in conjunction with pharmacologic treatments.

NSAIDS and other oral agents

NSAIDs are considered the initial preferred therapy for all patients with symptomatic axSpA, including patients with both nonradiographic disease and AS [3, 39]. Current recommendations are to titrate up to the maximum dose and use these agents on a continuous basis, while taking into account tolerability and risk/benefit profile [3]. Interestingly, an extensive Cochrane review did not find a dose-dependent benefit with NSAIDs [42]. Although some believe that tolerability, and potentially treatment adherence, may be an issue [43], this same Cochrane review found a lack of adverse effects in clinical trials [42], although this must be balanced against recent evidence of cardiovascular risk with even short-term use of NSAIDs [44]. In addition to its symptom-reducing properties, it has also been suggested that NSAIDs may have a disease-modifying effect through bone growth inhibition via prostaglandin inhibition [45]. The clinical trial evidence for this has not been as clear [46, 47], however, and may be limited by the ethical challenge of conducting the long-term placebo-controlled trials necessary to definitively demonstrate a structural effect. One observational study showed that high NSAID use retarding new bone formation was most pronounced in patients with baseline syndesmophytes and elevated CRP levels [25]. Given this finding, it is not surprising that this study also showed that the effect on radiographic change was less prominent in individuals with nr-axSpA [25].

Considering all of this, the latest update to the ASAS recommendations for treatment of axSpA, including nonradiographic disease, recommends a trial of at least 1 month of maximally dosed NSAIDs prior to initiation of a biologic [3], with the caveat that benefits should outweigh the risks for the specific patient. The same recommendations state that purely axial disease should not be treated with conventional disease-modifying antirheumatic drugs (DMARDs), although sulfasalazine may be considered in patients with peripheral arthritis [3]. Steroids are recommended for use only as local injections to sites of musculoskeletal inflammation, such as monoarticular synovitis or enthesitis.

TNF inhibitors

When NSAIDs fail to control disease symptoms, the next step is the use of biologic DMARDs, such as TNF inhibitors. TNF inhibition has been the therapy of choice for patients with established AS. TNF inhibitor use has also been studied in nr-axSpA (Table 3). Prior to the development of the ASAS criteria, which identified patients with axSpA and nonradiographic disease, two trials were completed in this population. One investigated adalimumab for the treatment of patients with axial spondyloarthritis without radiographically defined sacroiliitis and a second studied infliximab for the treatment of MRI-determined early sacroiliitis. Both trials demonstrated a significant improvement in ASAS scores after 12 weeks of treatment [48, 49]. Following publication of the ASAS criteria, the ABILITY-1 study examined the efficacy of adalimumab in patients with axSpA who did not meet criteria for AS (i.e., nr-axSpA). It, too, found improvements in ASDAS, BASDAI, functional scores, and radiographic inflammation in the spine and sacroiliac joints after 12 weeks of treatment compared to placebo [27]. Interestingly, the response to adalimumab in this trial was quite similar to the response to adalimumab in AS (Table 3). Of note, the response to adalimumab was greater in those patients with inflammatory changes on MRI and an elevated CRP; those with neither did not have significant improvement relative to placebo. Similarly, in the early sacroiliitis trial with infliximab, treatment and placebo ASAS40 rates were 61% and 18% at 24 weeks, compared with 47% and 12% in the pivotal ASSERT trial of infliximab in AS [50].

Etanercept has been evaluated for efficacy in the EMBARK study in nr-axSpA. In this study of early (<5 years of symptoms) nr-axSpA patients, Dougados et al. demonstrated benefit with etanercept compared to placebo as early as 2 weeks, with further improvement at 8 and 12 weeks [51]. As with adalimumab, the response to etanercept in the EMBARK study in nr-AxSpA was similar to that seen in the pivotal phase 3 trial in AS (Table 3). In the ESTHER trial, which included patients with both AS and nr-axSpA, etanercept was found to be superior to sulfasalazine in the reduction of inflammation seen on MRI in the spine, sacroiliac joints, and entheseal sites [52]. The clinical response rate for the two groups was similar and for some outcomes even superior for nr-axSpA [17].

Golimumab has also been studied in both AS and nr-axSpA and, again, the response was fairly comparable (Table 3). As with adalimumab, the ASAS40 response rates for golimumab in nrAxSpa were higher for those

Table 3 Phase 3 trials of tumor necrosis factor (TNF) inhibitors in nonradiographic spondyloarthritis and ankylosing spondylitis

Trial	TNF inhibitor	Dose	Primary endpoint	Comparator	Results
nr-axSpA Trials					
ABILITY-1 [27]	Adalimumab	40 mg q 2 weeks	ASAS40 response at week 12	Placebo	ASAS20: 52% vs. 41% ASAS40: 36% vs. 15%
RAPID-axSpA (nr-axSpA subset) [19]	Certolizumab pegol	400 mg q 4 weeks	ASAS20 response at week 12	Placebo	ASAS20: 63% vs. 40% ASAS40: 47% vs. 16%
EMBARK [51]	Etanercept	50 mg q week	ASAS40 response at week 12	Placebo	ASAS20: 52% vs. 36% ASAS40: 33% vs. 15%
GO-AHEAD [26]	Golimumab	50 mg q 4 weeks	ASAS20 response at week 16	Placebo	ASAS20: 72% vs. 40% ASAS40: 57% vs. 23%
AS Trials					
ATLAS [56]	Adalimumab	40 mg q 2 weeks	ASAS20 response at week 12	Placebo	ASAS20: 58% vs. 21% ASAS40: 40% vs. 13%
RAPID-axSpA (AS subset) [19]	Certolizumab pegol	400 mg q 4 weeks	ASAS20 response at week 12	Placebo	ASAS20: 64% vs. 37% ASAS40: 50% vs. 19%
Etanercept phase III [57]	Etanercept	50 mg q week	ASAS20 response at week 12	Placebo	ASAS20: 59% vs. 28% ASAS50: 44% vs. 16%
GO-RAISE [53]	Golimumab	50 mg q 4 weeks	ASAS20 response at week 14	Placebo	ASAS20: 59% vs. 22% ASAS40: 44% vs. 15%

patients with an elevated CRP and inflammatory changes on MRI. At 14 weeks, the ASAS20 response rate for golimumab and placebo was 59%/22%, and the ASAS40 response rate was 44%/15% [53].

Finally, certolizumab has been evaluated in a clinical trial that included both AS and nr-axSpA patients in the same study [19]. In this study, which enrolled 325 patients meeting ASAS criteria for axSpA, 178 also met NY criteria for AS, while 147 were considered nr-axSpA, although all patients were required to have either MRI evidence of inflammation or an elevated CRP at study entry. This trial included two dosing regimens for certolizumab, 200 mg every 2 weeks and 400 mg every 4 weeks. At week 12, the ASAS20 response rates for certolizumab 400 mg every 4 weeks and placebo were 64% and 38%, and the ASAS40 response rates were 49% and 18%. When the results were analyzed by disease criteria, the ASAS20 and ASAS40 response rates for AS were 64% and 50%, and those for nr-axSpA were 63% and 47%.

Data such as these have led to the ASAS recommendation to extend TNF inhibitor treatment to the nr-axSpA subpopulation [19], although this recommendation is not yet accepted by all regulatory agencies worldwide. In Europe, for example, TNF inhibitors are indicated for axSpA, including nonradiographic disease, as long as there is evidence of active inflammation, while in the USA the indication is currently restricted to AS. As noted, several trials have shown that patients with a shorter disease duration (<5 years), elevated CRP, or sacroiliac joint inflammation seen on MRI may have a better response to therapy. Some trials have shown that symptom control remains equivalent between patients with nr-axSpA and AS on TNF inhibitor therapy at the 1-year follow-up [51] and even at a 3-year follow-up [2]. Despite the improvement in symptom and inflammation control, it must be noted that there is no firm evidence that TNF inhibitors are actually disease-modifying for axSpA [3]. This is certainly a relevant concern in AS; it is perhaps somewhat less relevant in nr-axSpA, where many patients may never develop progressive structural changes, and changes may be small in those who do, so that it would be difficult to prove meaningful benefit in this setting even with an agent believed to be truly disease-modifying.

The only other biologic currently approved for the treatment of AS is secukinumab, a monoclonal antibody directed against interleukin (IL)-17A [54]. Trials have shown the drug to be symptomatically effective compared with placebo [55]. Secukinumab has not been studied in nr-axSpA, nor are there any data available on its comparative efficacy relative to TNF inhibitors [54]. At this time, the ASAS recommendations are to treat with a TNF inhibitor after failure of two NSAIDs and to use it for at least 12 weeks [3]. In the event of an inadequate response, switching to another TNF inhibitor or treatment with an IL-17 inhibitor may be considered [3].

Conclusion

The classification of spondyloarthritis remains an evolving topic. While there is general agreement on the current ASAS classification of axSpA, there is remaining uncertainty on whether clinical differences among patients meeting these criteria may have relevance for prognosis, disease progression, and response to therapy. Nonradiographic axSpA has emerged as one subclassification, though it appears to be part of the spectrum of axSpA rather than an entity in itself. As such, it currently seems to have more relevance as a regulatory construct than a disease definition. Other aspects of disease, such as gender, duration, and inflammatory burden, some of which may differ in those patients with nr-axSpA, appear to be more relevant to clinical course and treatment response. As these other demographic elements are better understood, particularly with respect to their impact on therapy, the concept of nr-axSpA will almost certainly become less important.

Abbreviations

AS: Ankylosing spondylitis; ASAS: Assessment of SpondyloArthritis International Society; ASDAS: Ankylosing Spondylitis Disease Activity Score; axSpA: Axial spondyloarthritis; BASDAI: Bath Ankylosing Spondylitis Disease Activity Index; BASFI: Bath Ankylosing Spondylitis Functional Index; CRP: C-reactive protein; DESIR: Devenir des Spondylarthropathies Indifférenciées Récentes; DMARD: Disease-modifying antireheumatic drug; ESSG: European Spondyloarthropathy Study Group; GESPIC: German Spondyloarthritis Inception Cohort; HLA: Human leukocyte antigen; HRQOL: Health-related quality of life; hsCRP: High-sensitivity C-reactive protein; IL: Interleukin; mNY: Modified New York; MRI: Magnetic resonance imaging; NHANES: National Health and Nutrition Examination Survey; nr-axSpA: Nonradiographic axial spondyloarthritis; NSAID: Nonsteroidal anti-inflammatory drug; r-axSpA: Radiographic axial spondyloarthritis; SpA: Spondyloarthritis; TNF: Tumor necrosis factor

Acknowledgments

None.

Funding

No funding was received for this work.

Authors' contributions

NG and EMR both contributed to the research and writing of this work. Both authors read and approved the final manuscript.

Competing interests

EMR has received consulting fees from Amgen, AbbVie, Janssen, Novartis, and Pfizer. NG declares that they have no competing interests.

References

1. Strand V, Singh JA. Evaluation and management of the patient with suspected inflammatory spine disease. Mayo Clinic Proceedings. 2017;92(4): 555–64.
2. Wallman JK, et al. Comparison of non-radiographic axial spondyloarthritis and ankylosing spondylitis patients—baseline characteristics, treatment adherence, and development of clinical variables during three years of anti-TNF therapy in clinical practice. Arthritis Res Ther. 2015;17(1):378.
3. van der Heijde D, et al. 2016 update of the ASAS-EULAR management recommendations for axial spondyloarthritis. Ann Rheum Dis. 2017;76:978–91.
4. Linden SVD, Valkenburg HA, Cats A. Evaluation of diagnostic criteria for ankylosing spondylitis. Arthritis Rheumatol. 1984;27(4):361–8.
5. Sieper J, van der Heijde D. Review: nonradiographic axial spondyloarthritis: new definition of an old disease? Arthritis Rheum. 2013;65(3):543–51.
6. Lipton S, Deodhar A. The new ASAS classification criteria for axial and peripheral spondyloarthritis: promises and pitfalls. Int J Clin Rheumatol. 2012;7(6):675–82.
7. Taylor WJ, Robinson PC. Classification criteria: peripheral spondyloarthropathy and psoriatic arthritis. Curr Rheumatol Rep. 2013;15(4):317.
8. Rudwaleit M, et al. The development of Assessment of SpondyloArthritis international Society classification criteria for axial spondyloarthritis (part I): classification of paper patients by expert opinion including uncertainty appraisal. Ann Rheum Dis. 2009;68(6):770–6.
9. Rudwaleit M, Landewe R, van der Heijde D. SpondyloArthritis international Society (ASAS) classification criteria for axial spondyloarthritis (part II): validation and final selection. Ann Rheum Dis. 2009;68(6):777–83.
10. Reveille JD, Witter JP, Weisman MH. Prevalence of axial spondylarthritis in the United States: estimates from a cross-sectional survey. Arthritis Care Res. 2012;64(6):905–10.
11. Strand V, et al. Prevalence of axial spondyloarthritis in United States rheumatology practices: Assessment of SpondyloArthritis International Society criteria versus rheumatology expert clinical diagnosis. Arthritis Care Res. 2013;65(8):1299–306.
12. de Winter JJ, et al. Prevalence of peripheral and extra-articular disease in ankylosing spondylitis versus non-radiographic axial spondyloarthritis: a meta-analysis. Arthritis Res Ther. 2016;18(1):196.
13. Kiltz U, et al. Do patients with non-radiographic axial spondylarthritis differ from patients with ankylosing spondylitis? Arthritis Care Res. 2012;64(9):1415–22.
14. Rudwaleit M, et al. The early disease stage in axial spondylarthritis: results from the German Spondyloarthritis Inception Cohort. Arthritis Rheum. 2009; 60(3):717–27.
15. Sampaio-Barros PD, et al. Undifferentiated spondyloarthritis: a long-term follow-up. J Rheumatol. 2010;37(6):1195–9.
16. Poddubnyy D, et al. Brief report: clinical course over two years in patients with early nonradiographic axial spondyloarthritis and patients with ankylosing spondylitis not treated with tumor necrosis factor blockers: results from the German Spondyloarthritis Inception Cohort. Arthritis Rheumatol. 2015;67(9): 2369–75.
17. Song I-H, et al. Similar response rates in patients with ankylosing spondylitis and non-radiographic axial spondyloarthritis after 1 year of treatment with etanercept: results from the ESTHER trial. Ann Rheum Dis. 2013;72(6):823–5.
18. Poddubnyy D, et al. Rates and predictors of radiographic sacroiliitis progression over 2 years in patients with axial spondyloarthritis. Ann Rheum Dis. 2011;70(8): 1369–74.
19. Landewe R, et al. Efficacy of certolizumab pegol on signs and symptoms of axial spondyloarthritis including ankylosing spondylitis: 24-week results of a double-blind randomised placebo-controlled phase 3 study. Ann Rheum Dis. 2014;73:39–47.
20. Deodhar A, et al. The term 'non-radiographic axial spondyloarthritis' is much more important to classify than to diagnose patients with axial spondyloarthritis. Ann Rheum Dis. 2016;75:791–4.
21. Garrett S, et al. A new approach to defining disease status in ankylosing spondylitis: the Bath Ankylosing Spondylitis Disease Activity Index. J Rheumatol. 1994;21(12):2286–91.
22. Calin A, et al. A new approach to defining functional ability in ankylosing spondylitis: the development of the Bath Ankylosing Spondylitis Functional Index. J Rheumatol. 1994;21(12):2281–5.
23. Machado P, van der Heijde D. How to measure disease activity in axial spondyloarthritis? Curr Opin Rheumatol. 2011;23(4):339–45.
24. Poddubnyy D, et al. Baseline radiographic damage, elevated acute-phase reactant levels, and cigarette smoking status predict spinal radiographic progression in early axial spondylarthritis. Arthritis Rheum. 2012;64(5):1388–98.
25. Poddubnyy D, et al. Effect of non-steroidal anti-inflammatory drugs on radiographic spinal progression in patients with axial spondyloarthritis: results from the German Spondyloarthritis Inception Cohort. Ann Rheum Dis. 2012;71(10):1616–22.
26. Sieper J, et al. A randomized, double-blind, placebo-controlled, sixteen-week study of subcutaneous golimumab in patients with active nonradiographic axial spondyloarthritis. Arthritis Rheumatol. 2015;67(10):2702–12.
27. Sieper J, et al. Efficacy and safety of adalimumab in patients with non-radiographic axial spondyloarthritis: results of a randomised placebo-controlled trial (ABILITY-1). Ann Rheum Dis. 2013;72(6):815–22.
28. Ruderman E, et al. Spondyloarthritis Epidemiology and Burden Phase 2 [speed 2] Study: Disease progression in axial spondyloarthropathy (SpA). Arthritis Rheum. 2013;65:S1052–3.
29. Wang R, Gabriel SE, Ward MM. Progression of nonradiographic axial spondyloarthritis to ankylosing spondylitis: a population-based cohort study. Arthritis Rheumatol. 2016;68(6):1415–21.
30. Dougados M, Sepriano A, Molto A, Ramiro S, de Hooge M, Van Den Berg R, Navarro Compan V, De Mattei C, Landewé R, Van der Heijde D. Evaluation of the changes in structural damage in axial spondyloarthritis on plain pelvic radiographs: the 5 years data of the DESIR cohort. Ann Rheum Dis. 2017;76(supplement 2):100.
31. Tournadre A, et al. Differences between women and men with recent-onset axial spondyloarthritis: results from a prospective multicenter french cohort. Arthritis Care Res. 2013;65(9):1482–9.
32. Aloush V, et al. Fibromyalgia in women with ankylosing spondylitis. Rheumatol Int. 2007;27(9):865–8.
33. Lee W, et al. Are there gender differences in severity of ankylosing spondylitis? Results from the PSOAS cohort. Ann Rheum Dis. 2007;66(5):633–8.
34. Slobodin G, et al. Recently diagnosed axial spondyloarthritis: gender differences and factors related to delay in diagnosis. Clin Rheumatol. 2011;30(8):1075–80.
35. Ciurea AHM, Weber U, Tamborrini G, Micheroli R, Wildi L, Zufferey P, Nissen MJ, Villiger PM, Bernhard J, van der Heijde D, Landewé RBM, Scherer A, Exer P. In contrast to men, women with nonradiographic axial spondyloarthritis have lower response rates to TNF inhibitors than women with ankylosing spondylitis. ACR. 2016;2016:Abstract 699.
36. Atzeni F, et al. Chronic widespread pain in the spectrum of rheumatological diseases. Best Pract Res Clin Rheumatol. 2011;25(2):165–71.
37. Salaffi F, et al. Fibromyalgia in patients with axial spondyloarthritis: epidemiological profile and effect on measures of disease activity. Rheumatol Int. 2014; 34(8):1103–10.
38. Heikkilä S, et al. Functional impairment in spondyloarthropathy and fibromyalgia. J Rheumatol. 2002;29(7):1415–9.
39. Ward MM, et al. American College of Rheumatology/Spondylitis Association of America/Spondyloarthritis Research and Treatment Network 2015 recommendations for the treatment of ankylosing spondylitis and nonradiographic axial spondyloarthritis. Arthritis Rheumatol. 2016;68(2): 282–98.
40. Poddubnyy D, et al. Cigarette smoking has a dose-dependent impact on progression of structural damage in the spine in patients with axial spondyloarthritis: results from the GErman SPondyloarthritis Inception Cohort (GESPIC). Ann Rheum Dis. 2013;72(8):1430–2.
41. Ciurea A, et al. Impaired response to treatment with tumour necrosis factor α inhibitors in smokers with axial spondyloarthritis. Ann Rheum Dis. 2016;75: 532–9.
42. Kroon FP, et al. Nonsteroidal antiinflammatory drugs for axial spondyloarthritis: a Cochrane review. J Rheumatol. 2016;43(3):607–17.
43. Varkas G, et al. OP0170 treatment of axial spondyloarthritis with an optimal dosage of nsaids: a 6-week follow up study focusing on magnetic resonance imaging of the sacroiliac joints. Ann Rheum Dis. 2015;74 Suppl 2:134.
44. Bally M, et al. Risk of acute myocardial infarction with NSAIDs in real world use: Bayesian meta-analysis of individual patient data. BMJ. 2017;357:j1909.
45. Blackwell KA, Raisz LG, Pilbeam CC. Prostaglandins in bone: bad cop, good cop? Trends Endocrinol Metab. 2010;21(5):294–301.
46. Sieper J, et al. Comparison of two different dosages of celecoxib with diclofenac for the treatment of active ankylosing spondylitis: results of a 12-week randomised, double-blind, controlled study. Ann Rheum Dis. 2008;67(3):323–9.
47. Wanders A, et al. Nonsteroidal antiinflammatory drugs reduce radiographic progression in patients with ankylosing spondylitis: a randomized clinical trial. Arthritis Rheum. 2005;52(6):1756–65.

48. Barkham N, et al. Clinical and imaging efficacy of infliximab in HLA-B27-positive patients with magnetic resonance imaging-determined early sacroiliitis. Arthritis Rheumatol. 2009;60(4):946–54.
49. Haibel H, et al. Efficacy of adalimumab in the treatment of axial spondylarthritis without radiographically defined sacroiliitis: results of a twelve-week randomized, double-blind, placebo-controlled trial followed by an open-label extension up to week fifty-two. Arthritis Rheum. 2008;58(7):1981–91.
50. van der Heijde D, et al. Efficacy and safety of infliximab in patients with ankylosing spondylitis: results of a randomized, placebo-controlled trial (ASSERT). Arthritis Rheumatol. 2005;52(2):582–91.
51. Dougados M, et al. Symptomatic efficacy of etanercept and its effects on objective signs of inflammation in early nonradiographic axial spondyloarthritis: a multicenter, randomized, double-blind, placebo-controlled trial. Arthritis Rheumatol. 2014;66(8):2091–102.
52. Song I, et al. Effects of etanercept versus sulfasalazine in early axial spondyloarthritis on active inflammatory lesions as detected by whole-body MRI (ESTHER): a 48-week randomised controlled trial. Ann Rheum Dis. 2011;70(4):590–6.
53. Inman RD, et al. Efficacy and safety of golimumab in patients with ankylosing spondylitis: results of a randomized, double-blind, placebo-controlled, phase III trial. Arthritis Rheum. 2008;58(11):3402–12.
54. Cheung PP. Anti-IL17A in axial spondyloarthritis—where are we at? Front Med. 2017;4:1.
55. Baeten D, et al. Secukinumab, an interleukin-17A inhibitor, in ankylosing spondylitis. N Engl J Med. 2015;373(26):2534–48.
56. van der Heijde D, et al. Efficacy and safety of adalimumab in patients with ankylosing spondylitis: results of a multicenter, randomized, double-blind, placebo-controlled trial. Arthritis Rheum. 2006;54(7):2136–46.
57. Davis JC, et al. Recombinant human tumor necrosis factor receptor (etanercept) for treating ankylosing spondylitis: a randomized, controlled trial. Arthritis Rheumatol. 2003;48(11):3230–6.

3

Age and fecal microbial strain-specific differences in patients with spondyloarthritis

Matthew L. Stoll[1*], Pamela F. Weiss[2], Jennifer E. Weiss[3], Peter A. Nigrovic[4], Barbara S. Edelheit[5], S. Lou Bridges Jr[1], Maria I. Danila[1], Charles H. Spencer[6], Marilynn G. Punaro[7], Kenneth Schikler[8], Andreas Reiff[9], Ranjit Kumar[1], Randy Q. Cron[1], Casey D. Morrow[1] and Elliot J. Lefkowitz[1]

Abstract

Background: Prior studies have demonstrated abnormalities in the composition of the gastrointestinal microbiota in pediatric and adult patients with spondyloarthritis (SpA). In particular, diminished fecal abundance of *Faecalibacterium prausnitzii* and abnormalities in both directions in the abundance of the *Bacteroides* genus have been identified.

Methods: We obtained fecal specimens from 30 children with treatment-naïve enthesitis-related arthritis (ERA) and 19 healthy controls, as well as specimens from 11 adult patients with longstanding SpA and 10 adult healthy controls. All of the samples underwent sequencing of the 16S ribosomal DNA. A subset of the pediatric fecal samples was subjected to shotgun metagenomics sequencing.

Results: ERA patients had decreased abundance of the anti-inflammatory *F. prausnitzii* A2-165 strain (41 ± 28% versus 54 ± 20% of all sequences matching *F. prausnitzii*, $p = 0.084$) and an increased abundance of the control *F. prausnitzii* L2/6 strain (28 ± 28% versus 15 ± 15%, $p = 0.038$). Similar trends were observed in adults with longstanding SpA (n = 11) and controls ($n = 10$). In contrast, the fecal abundance of *Bacteroides fragilis* was increased in ERA subjects (2.0 ± 4.0% versus 0.45 ± 0.7% of all sequences, $p = 0.045$), yet was diminished in adult subjects (0.2 ± % versus 1.0 ± % of all sequences, $p = 0.106$). Shotgun metagenomics sequencing of the fecal DNA in the pediatric subjects revealed diminished coverage of the butanoate pathway (abundance normalized to controls of 1 ± 0.48 versus 0.72 ± 0.33 in ERA, $p = 0.037$).

Conclusions: The anti-inflammatory *F. prausnitzii* A2-165 strain appears to be depleted in both pediatric and adult SpA. In contrast, *B. fragilis* may be depleted in adult disease yet abundant in pediatric SpA, suggesting developmental effects on the immune system.

Keywords: Microbiota, Spondyloarthritis, Sequencing, Bacteroides, Faecalibacterium

Background

The role of the intestinal microbiota in the pathogenesis of spondyloarthritis (SpA) is gaining widespread interest [1]. Much of this interest was spurred by a large body of literature indicating abnormalities of the microbiota in patients with inflammatory bowel disease (IBD) [2], a condition in which therapeutic alteration of the microbiota in the form of antibiotics, probiotics, and even fecal transplant may be effective [3], along with the clinical and genetic associations between IBD and SpA [4]. Prior studies evaluating fecal or mucosal microbiota of adult patients with SpA demonstrated diminished fecal abundance of *Bacteroides* [5, 6], with one study showing a potential association between the *Dialister* genus and disease severity [6]. There are comparatively few data reported in pediatric SpA. One study showed decreased abundance of *Prevotella* in pediatric SpA [7], and our prior work showed decreased abundance of *Faecalibacterium prausnitzii* [8]. The latter finding is consistent with multiple similar reports in subjects with IBD [9]. Depletion of *F. prausnitzii* may adversely impact intestinal health through diminished production of butyrate and other short chain fatty acids [10], and our previous work has shown diminished abundance of butyrate in the fecal

* Correspondence: mstoll@peds.uab.edu
[1]University of Alabama at Birmingham, Birmingham, AL, USA

water of children with ERA [11]. Both pediatric SpA studies also showed increased abundance of unspecified species within the *Bacteroides* genus, consistent with studies in children with other categories of juvenile idiopathic arthritis (JIA) [12, 13], yet the opposite of findings in adult subjects with rheumatoid arthritis (RA) [14, 15] or SpA [5, 6].

Herein, we studied the intestinal microbiota in children with treatment-naïve SpA in comparison to pediatric healthy controls; to do this, we used a novel bioinformatics tool in combination with the Basic Local Alignment Search Tool (BLAST) that permitted assessment of species and even strain-level identification of certain organisms, as different strains within a species can have dramatically different effects [16, 17]. In order to validate our prior results and to further increase the sample size, we recruited subjects from geographic locations around the country. Prior studies have shown that geography can impact the microbiota in situations in which subjects with highly different environments (e.g., urban versus rural) and ethnicities are compared [18, 19], but there are no data evaluating subjects from different urban areas specifically within the United States. The findings in these subjects were compared with those in adults with longstanding SpA and adult controls, to identify which changes might be common to SpA and which might be unique to pediatric populations. We also performed shotgun metagenomics sequencing on a subset of children with juvenile SpA in order to obtain additional information regarding potential mechanisms whereby the microbiota might predispose to SpA. Herein, we demonstrate that the anti-inflammatory A2-165 strain of *F. prausnitzii* is depleted in both pediatric and adult SpA, and that the microbiota of children with SpA has decreased genetic capacity to synthesize butyrate. We additionally demonstrate that *B. fragilis* is depleted in adult SpA yet abundant in pediatric disease.

Table 1 Demographic and clinical characteristics of pediatric study participants

Characteristic	ERA	Controls
n	30	19
Age (years), mean ± SD	13.5 ± 3.0	13.6 ± 2.7
BMI (kg/m^2), mean ± SD	20.7 ± 4.1	21.5 ± 6.1
Male	19 (63%)	13 (68%)
Race		
Caucasian	23 (77%)	17 (89%)
African-American	3 (10%)	2 (10%)
Asian	2 (6.7%)	0
Other/unknown	2 (6.7%)	0
Site		
UAB (Birmingham, AL, USA)	8 (27%)	9 (47%)
CHOP (Philadelphia, PA, USA)	10 (33%)	4 (21%)
HUMC (Hackensack, NJ, USA)	1 (3.3%)	4 (21%)
CCMC (Hartford, CT, USA)	1 (3.3%)	2 (10%)
BCH (Boston, MA, USA)	4 (13%)	0
NCH (Columbus, OH, USA)	2 (6.7%)	0
TSRH (Dallas, TX, USA)	2 (6.7%)	0
CHLA (Los Angeles, CA, USA)	1 (3.3%)	0
UL (Louisville, KY, USA)	1 (3.3%)	0
HLA-B27$^+$	15/29 (52%)	Not measured
Sacroiliitis	18 (60%)	None
Clinical only	8/18 (44%)	
Imaging	10/18 (56%)	

Data presented as *n* (%) unless stated otherwise
BCH Boston Children's Hospital, *BMI* body mass index, *CHLA* Children's Hospital of Los Angeles, CCMC Connecticut Children's Medical Center, *CHOP* Children's Hospital of Philadelphia, *ERA* enthesitis-related arthritis, *HUMC* Hackensack University Medical Center, *NCH* Nationwide Children's Hospital, *TSRH* Texas Scottish Rite Hospital, *UAB* University of Alabama at Birmingham, *UL* University of Louisville

Methods

Subjects

Pediatric SpA subjects were mostly children with enthesitis-related arthritis (ERA; juvenile SpA) as per the International League of Association for Rheumatology criteria [20]; three with sacroiliitis in the absence of peripheral arthritis met the Assessment of Spondyloarthritis International Society (ASAS) criteria for axial SpA [21]. Pediatric controls were either healthy children recruited through advertisements or children referred to rheumatology for evaluation of arthritis but found to have noninflammatory causes of joint pain or irrelevant laboratory markers, such as a positive antinuclear antibody. None of the controls had any findings suggestive of infectious arthropathies, including Lyme synovitis. Pediatric subjects were recruited from eight sites around the country (Table 1). Exclusion criteria were receipt of antibiotics within 3 months prior to study enrollment and prior treatment with any immunosuppressive agent excluding less than 2 weeks of corticosteroids. None of the pediatric subjects or controls had been included in our prior work [8].

Adult SpA subjects were all recruited at the University of Alabama at Birmingham (UAB). Patients met either the ASAS criteria for peripheral [22] or axial [21] SpA or the Classification Criteria for Psoriatic Arthritis (CASPAR) criteria [23] for psoriatic arthritis (PsA). Sacroiliitis in both children and adults was defined based upon either clinical findings per the judgment of the treating rheumatologist or imaging findings on MRI or radiography; only a single observer was required. Adult controls were healthy volunteers recruited through advertisements or patients with noninflammatory causes of joint pain (Table 2). For the adult subjects, as with the pediatric counterparts, recent antibiotic use was an exclusion criterion; however, for the adult subjects, immunosuppressive therapy was not.

Table 2 Demographic and clinical characteristic of adult study participants

Characteristic	SpA	Controls
n	11	10
Age (years), mean ± SD	52 ± 7.4	47 ± 8.1
BMI (kg/m^2), mean ± SD	32 ± 7.8	28 ± 4.8
Disease duration (years), mean ± SD	11 ± 9.5	Not applicable
Male	4 (36%)	3 (30%)
Race		
Caucasian	9 (82%)	6 (60%)
African-American	2 (18%)	4 (40%)
Diagnosis		Not applicable
Undifferentiated SpA	1 (9.1%)	
Ankylosing spondylitis	6 (54%)	
IBD-associated arthritis	1 (9.1%)	
Psoriatic arthritis	2 (18%)	
Reactive arthritis	1 (9.1%)	
Current medications		
None	2 (18%)	10 (100%)
Traditional DMARDs alone	5 (45%)	
TNFi alone	3 (27%)	
DMARDs plus TNFi	1 (9.1%)	
HLA-B27$^+$	3/3 (100%)	Not measured
Sacroiliitis	8 (73%)	None
Clinical	1 (12%)	
Imaging	7 (88%)	

Data presented as *n* (%) unless stated otherwise
BMI body mass index, *DMARD* disease-modifying anti-rheumatic drug (leflunomide, *n* = 2; methotrexate, *n* = 2; sulfasalazine, *n* = 3), *IBD* inflammatory bowel disease, *SpA* spondyloarthritis, *TNFi* tumor necrosis factor inhibitor

Processing of fecal samples

Subjects collected the samples at home and immediately placed the samples in a 50-ml container filled with Cary-Blair media. Samples were shipped overnight via commercial carrier to the microbiota core at UAB. Microbial genomic DNA was isolated by standard methods using kits from Zymo Research (Irvine, CA, USA) as per the manufacturer's instructions. For 16S sequencing, the Zymo ZR Fecal DNA MiniPrep kit (catalog # D6010) was used; for shotgun metagenomics, the whole genome DNA kit (catalog # D6110) was used.

Sequencing and analysis of 16S ribosomal DNA from the fecal specimens

The purified DNA (~100 ng) underwent PCR amplification using primers designed to the conserved region flanking the V4 region from the 16S ribosomal DNA (rDNA) gene, as described previously [8]. Resulting PCR fragments were run on the Illumina MiSeq (San Diego, CA, USA) at a concentration of 12 pM; read lengths were approximately 250-bp paired-end reads. Initial steps of the analysis were performed with the Divisive Amplicon Denoising Algorithm (DADA2) [24, 25]. Unlike some of the widely used algorithms [26, 27], DADA2 does not cluster similar sequences. Instead, it uses error modeling to distinguish amplification or sequencing errors from true sequences, which are typically referred to as sequence variants (SVs). This assessment is based upon features of the sequence, specifically the distance from its nearest neighbor as measured by the number of nucleotide differences and as influenced by quality scores and specific nucleotide transitions; and its abundance. Thus, a highly abundant sequence may be assessed as a true SV rather than a sequence error, even if it is highly similar to another abundant SV. Consequently, DADA2 can identify unique strains within a species. The output of DADA2 is an abundance table, in which each unique sequence is characterized by its abundance in each sample. Taxonomic information was incorporated into this abundance table with the ribosomal database project naïve Bayesian classifier [28] using the May 2013 version of Greengenes [29]. This abundance table has the same structure as a traditional operational taxonomic unit table that is the analytic unit in the Quantitative Insight Into Microbial Ecology (QIIME) tool suite [26]. Thus, it was incorporated into QIIME with the biom convert script, and assessment of alpha and beta diversity was performed within QIIME. Alpha diversity indexes of richness and evenness were assessed with the Chao1 and Shannon measures respectively; beta diversity was assessed with the Bray Curtis measure, visualized using principal coordinates analysis (PCoA). Variables assessed were presence versus absence of arthritis, and among the ERA patients were geographic location, presence versus absence of sacroiliitis, and HLA-B27 status. Geographic location was assessed both by looking at each site as a separate unit and by pooling into one region the four sites located in the northeast (Boston Children's Hospital, Connecticut Children's Medical Center, Hackensack University Medical Center, and Children's Hospital of Philadelphia), a geographic area that is similar in size to the catchment area of UAB. To identify specific strains within *F. prausnitzii*, the 16S sequences were downloaded from the National Library of Medicine, and the SVs matching *F. prausnitzii* were aligned against the known sequences using BLAST. The code used for the 16S sequence analysis is available in Additional file 1.

Sequencing and analysis of shotgun sequencing from the fecal specimens

The purified DNA was sheared and 500–600-bp fragments were purified by agarose gel electrophoresis. Illumina kits were used for adapter ligation followed by Illumina HiSeq, 125-bp paired-end sequencing. Approximately 25–30 million reads per sample were obtained from each sample. A second set was run on the Illumina MiSeq, yielding 3–7 million reads per sample, approximately 250-bp paired-end sequencing. Quality control of both sets was performed using PRINSEQ [30]. Alignment with the human genome to remove human reads was performed with Bowtie2 [31] using the very-sensitive mode. Conversion of fastq to fasta files was performed with the FASTX tool kit (http://hannonlab.cshl.edu/fastx_toolkit/commandline.html). The remainder of the analysis was performed with the HMP Unified Metabolic Analysis Network (HUMAnN V2) program [32]. A detailed description of the program is available online (http://huttenhower.sph.harvard.edu/humann2). Briefly, the input fasta files were aligned against a functionally annotated pan-genome database of over 4000 species, named ChocoPhlan by the HUMAnN2 investigators, using Bowtie2 [31]. Reads not mapped to ChocoPhlan were subsequently aligned against the UniProt universal proteins database [33] using double index alignment of next-generation sequencing data (DIAMOND) [34], a more efficient alternative to BLASTX. Pathway assignments were performed with MetaCyc [35]; all genes associated with a pathway must be present for the pathway to be considered a match. Gene and pathway abundances were normalized to the sequencing depth prior to any further analyses. Translation from UniProt to Kyoto Encyclopedia of Genes and Genomes (KEGG) [36] was performed with the map_ko_uniref50.txt.gz mapping file made available by the HUMAnN investigators. The output of HUMAnN2 is files containing the abundance of each gene as well as of each pathway, optionally normalized to the sequencing depth of each subject. The code used for the HUMAnN2 analysis is included in Additional file 1.

Statistical analysis

To evaluate whether the samples as a whole clustered according to nominal variables, the permutation multivariate analysis of variance (PERMANOVA) test was run against the distance matrix generated from the Bray Curtis test of beta diversity. The PERMANOVA test partitions a distance matrix among sources of variation (e.g., presence versus absence of arthritis) in order to describe the strength and significance that a categorical variable has in determining the variation of distances [37]. Comparisons in the abundance of specific taxa, as well as assessments of differences in alpha diversity, were performed with Student's t test. Pairwise comparisons performed at each of the phylogenetic levels (e.g., phylum) were corrected for multiple comparisons with the Benjamini–Hochberg false discovery rate (FDR) test [38] with a significance threshold of 0.05.

Results

Subjects

The demographic and clinical features of the pediatric subjects are summarized in Table 1. All were naïve to immunosuppressive therapy, and none had been exposed to systemic antibiotics within 3 months prior to enrollment in the study. The patients and controls were well matched for age and BMI.

16S sequencing

A mean of 129,226 (range 39,741–249,043) paired-end reads were obtained from the 49 subjects. Following quality filtering, merging, and chimera removal, a total of 64,016 (range 23,942–105,497) reads were used. Among the 49 subjects, a total of 1402 unique sequences (sequence variants (SVs)) were obtained; as most of these were rare and unique to specific subjects, the range was 46–236 SVs/subject.

PCoA on the 49 subjects demonstrated clustering by diagnosis (ERA versus control; Fig. 1). This visually evident clustering was confirmed by the PERMANOVA test ($F = 1.45$, $p = 0.046$). Among the ERA patients, no sources of variation were observed on the basis of any single variable, including geographic location (Bray Curtis $F = 1.09$, $p = 0.277$), HLA-B27 status (Bray Curtis $F = 0.902$, $p = 0.652$), or the presence of sacroiliitis (Bray Curtis $F = 0.471$, $p = 1$). Geographic location was assessed both by looking at each site as a separate unit and by pooling into one region the four sites located in the northeast

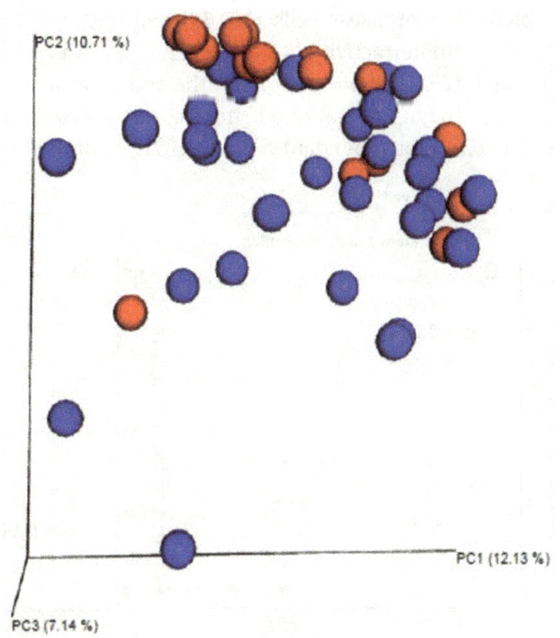

Fig. 1 Principal coordinates analysis of the 16S sequencing results obtained from children with ERA and pediatric healthy controls demonstrating clustering by diagnosis. Blue and red dots reflect ERA patients and controls, respectively

(Boston Children's Hospital, Connecticut Children's Medical Center, Hackensack University Medical Center, and Children's Hospital of Philadelphia), a geographic area that is similar in size to the catchment area of UAB.

Due to the large number of SVs as already indicated, pairwise comparisons at most of the phylogenetic levels failed to identify any groupwise differences following adjustment for multiple comparisons. The only exception was that ERA patients demonstrated decreased abundance of the Actinobacteria phylum as compared to controls (3.4% versus 9.3%, $p = 0.002$ uncorrected, $p = 0.05$ FDR-corrected). This lack of any significant pairwise differences held even after SVs within a species were collapsed into the species, thus reducing the number of unique items to 366. Consequently, based upon previous work in children with ERA [7, 8], the analysis was focused on two organisms: *F. prausnitzii* and the *Bacteroides* genus, particularly *B. fragilis.*

The abundance of *F. prausnitzii* as a whole was nominally higher in the patients (10 versus 7.8%, $p = 0.192$; Fig. 2a), in contrast to our previous results [8]. Twenty-three unique SVs were identified within *F. prausnitzii.* As discussed in Methods, BLAST was used to identify strains within the *F. prausnitzii* SVs identified by DADA2. Of those 23 SVs, one of them was a 100% best match (253/253 bp) with strain A2-165, which has been shown previously to have regulatory effects [39]. Recent studies have demonstrated that even compared to other strains of *F. prausnitzii,* such as L2/6, the A2-165 strain induces increased interleukin-10 production from peripheral blood mononuclear cells [16, 40] and has increased butyrate promoter activity [41]. A separate SV was a 99% best match (252/253 bp) with L2/6, the comparator strain in some of the aforementioned studies. These two strains were the two most abundant SVs matching *F. prausnitzii.* As a proportion of the sequences that matched *F. prausnitzii,* ERA patients had relatively decreased abundance of the regulatory A2-165 strain (41 ± 28% versus 54 ± 20%, $p = 0.084$; Fig. 2b) and a relatively increased abundance of the SV that most closely matched L2/6 (28 ± 28% versus 15 ± 15%, $p = 0.038$; Fic 2c). Thus, the stool samples from pediatric ERA patients contained a decreased ratio of the antiinflammatory, relative to the neutral, strain of *F. prausnitzii.*

ERA patients and controls had similar levels of the *Bacteroides* genus (20 versus 19%). However, among the *Bacteroides* genus, *B. fragilis* is considered to have regulatory properties through its polysaccharide tail [42] and thus was investigated further. Here, consistent with our previous findings [8], ERA patients had a four-fold increased abundance (2.0 ± 4.0% versus 0.45 0.7%, $p = 0.045$; Fig. 3a). There were no significant differences with any of the other species of *Bacteroides.* In summary, children with ERA had diminished abundance of the regulatory A2-165 strain of *F. prausnitzii* as well as increased abundance of *B. fragilis,* compared to healthy control subjects.

To evaluate whether these strain-level and species-level differences between arthritis subjects and controls are unique to pediatric subjects or are potentially a marker of SpA as a whole, 16S sequencing was run on a cohort of 11 adults with longstanding SpA and 10 healthy adult controls. Characteristics of the adult subjects are presented in Table 2; most had longstanding disease, with a mean disease duration of 11 years, and most were on immunosuppressive therapy. As with the pediatric subjects, none of the adult SpA patient or controls had been exposed to systemic antibiotics within 3 months of enrollment.

Among the adults, the opposite trend with respect to *Bacteroides* abundance was seen. Specifically, *Bacteroides* abundance as a proportion of total sequencing depth was

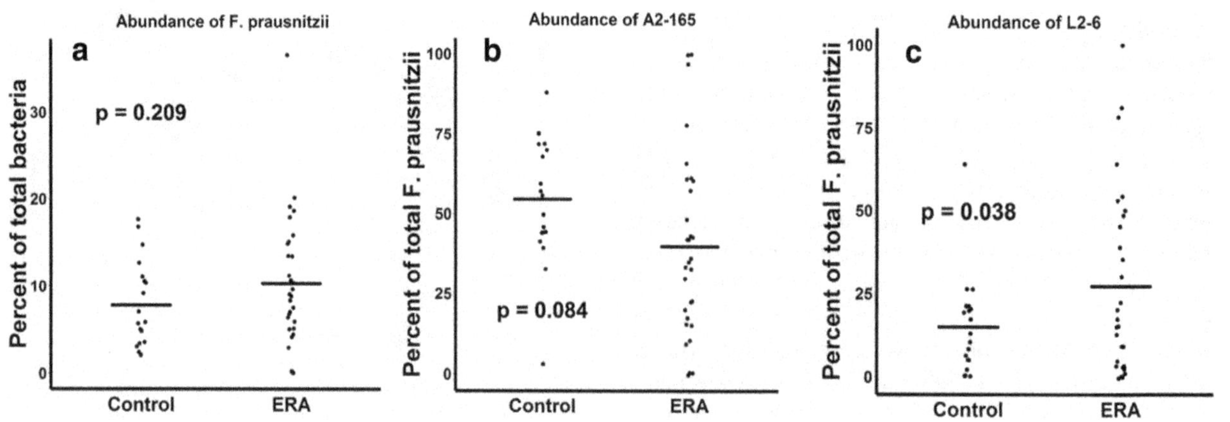

Fig. 2 Strain-level variation in the fecal abundance of *Faecalibacterium prausnitzii* in children with ERA and pediatric controls. Abundance of *F. prausnitzii* as a percentage of total fecal content is similar in patients and controls (**a**). As a percentage of total *F. prausnitzii*, children with ERA have a trend toward decreased fecal abundance of the anti-inflammatory A2-165 strain (**b**) as well as increased abundance of the L2/6 strain (**c**). ERA enthesitis-related arthritis

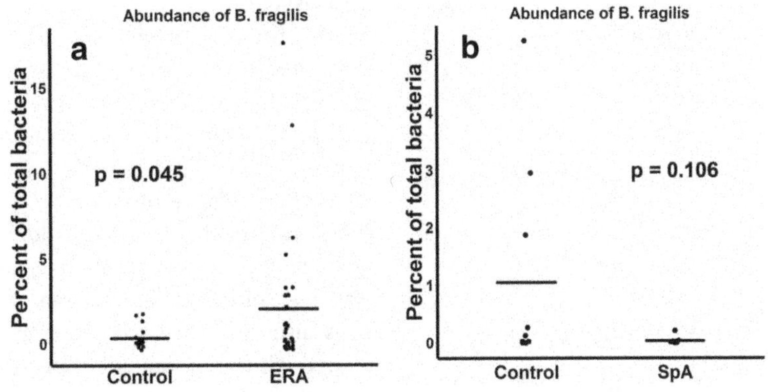

Fig. 3 Fecal abundance of *Bacteroides fragilis* in pediatric and adult subjects with SpA. Increased fecal abundance is observed in ERA patients compared to pediatric controls (**a**), while a trend toward decreased fecal abundance was observed in adult SpA patients compared to adult controls (**b**). ERA enthesitis-related arthritis, SpA spondyloarthritis

11 ± 9% among the patients, compared to 26 ± 18% in the controls ($p = 0.036$), although there were no significant differences in the abundance of *B. fragilis* (0.2 ± 0.6% in patients versus 1 ± 1.8% in controls, $p = 0.106$) (Fig. 3b). In contrast, the trends involving *F. prausnitzii* strains were similar in adults as compared to children (total *F. prausnitzii* 6.9 ± 6.9% in controls versus 10 ± 10% in patients ($p = 0.427$); A2-165 as percentage of *F. prausnitzii* 41 ± 30% in controls versus 25 ± 13% in patients ($p = 0.175$)), although the differences were not statistically significant, possibly due to a smaller sample size. Similar trends for both organisms were observed if the three subjects taking sulfasalazine were excluded (data not shown.)

Finally, the abundance of additional organisms that have emerged as being of interest in SpA was evaluated. Specifically, the Lachnospiraceae family was reduced in children with ERA in our previous work [8], yet was elevated in both biopsy [43] and fecal [44] specimens in prior studies of adults with SpA. There were, however, no differences in the abundance of this family in either the pediatric or the adult subjects (data not shown). A study of ileal biopsies demonstrated that the abundance of the *Dialister* genus correlated with disease activity in treatment-naïve SpA patients [6]; this organism was virtually undetectable (<1%) in the fecal specimens of all subjects in both age groups, likely indicating specificity to mucosal specimens. *Ruminococcus gnavus* was elevated in the feces of adult subjects with SpA in a prior report [44], but the differences of this organism herein were not statistically significant in either age group. Finally, both Stebbings et al. [5] and our group [8] have shown increased abundance of *Bifidobacterium* in the feces of SpA patients; surprisingly, the same genus was depleted among pediatric ERA subjects compared to healthy controls (2.6% versus 7.2%, $p = 0.008$), with no differences among the adult subjects.

Whole genome sequencing

To assess the potential functional consequences of the presented findings, whole genome sequencing of fecal DNA with the HiSeq device was performed on a subset of the aforementioned pediatric patients, consisting of 14 patients each (ERA and healthy controls), supplemented by 12 additional subjects (five controls and seven ERA patients) who were sequenced with the MiSeq device. These subjects were similar with respect to demographic characteristics and BMI (Table 3). A mean of 23 million (range 14.7–38.7 million) high-quality sequences from the Illumina HiSeq sequencer was analyzed, as was a mean of 5.3 million (range 3.5–7.8 million) high-quality sequences from the MiSeq device. There was no obvious clustering based upon diagnosis at either the level of individual genes or whole pathways (data not shown), consistent with a core microbiome not affected by the disease state [45]. In light of our findings in the present study and our previous report [8] showing alterations in the fecal abundance of *F. prausnitzii*, we specifically examined the butanoate pathway (MetaCyc title CENTFERM-PWY pyruvate fermentation to butanoate), which results in synthesis of butyrate from precursors such as pyruvate and acetyl-CoA. With both devices, there was a modest difference in the abundance of this pathway. For both the MiSeq and HiSeq devices, each value was normalized to the mean value for the controls for the respective run, and the two sets were pooled, revealing a statistically significant decreased representation of the butanoate pathway in ERA patients compared to controls (1 ± 0.48 versus 0.72 ± 0.33, $p = 0.037$; Fig. 4.) Thus, our data indicate that the fecal microbiota of ERA patients compared to controls had decreased capacity to synthesize a compound that is generally considered to have anti-inflammatory properties within the intestinal environment [46].

Table 3 Demographic and clinical characteristics of participants undergoing whole genome shotgun sequencing

Characteristic	ERA	Controls
n	21	19
Age (years), mean ± SD	13.6 ± 3.0	12.9 ± 3.0
BMI (kg/m^2), mean ± SD	21.0 ± 5.1	20.4 ± 6.2
Male	12 (57%)	12 (63%)
Race		
Caucasian	14 (67%)	14 (74%)
African-American	5 (24%)	5 (26%)
Asian	2 (9.5%)	0
Site		
UAB (Birmingham, AL, USA)	8 (38%)	11 (58%)
CHOP (Philadelphia, PA, USA)	7 (33%)	2 (10%)
HUMC (Hackensack, NJ, USA)	1 (4.8%)	2 (10%)
CCMC (Hartford, CT, USA)	1 (4.8%)	4 (21%)
BCH (Boston, MA, USA)	4 (19%)	0
HLA-B27$^+$	10/20 (50%)	Not measured
Sacroiliitis	10 (48%)	None
Clinical only	4 (40%)	
Imaging	6 (60%)	

Data presented as *n* (%) unless stated otherwise
BCH Boston Children's Hospital, *BMI* body mass index, *CCMC* Connecticut Children's Medical Center, *CHOP* Children's Hospital of Philadelphia, *ERA* enthesitis-related arthritis, *HUMC* Hackensack University Medical Center, *UAB* University of Alabama at Birmingham

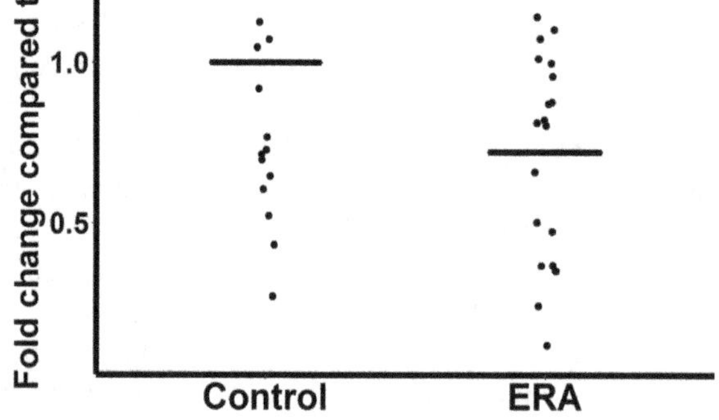

Fig. 4 Fecal abundance of bacterial genes comprising a pathway involved in butyrate synthesis. Results of two separate studies shown. For each, each subject was normalized to the mean of the healthy controls for that study, and the combined results are shown. ERA enthesitis-related arthritis

Discussion

Mechanisms by which an altered microbiota might be associated with inflammatory arthritis are as yet unknown. Animal studies clearly demonstrate a causal relationship, as an animal model of SpA is abrogated in the germ-free environment [47]. Herein, we report strain-level differences in fecal abundance of *F. prausnitzii* between children with ERA and healthy controls. Additionally, at the functional level, decreased genetic abundance of the butanoate pathway was observed in children with ERA. Children with ERA also had increased abundance of *B. fragilis*. Notably, adults with longstanding SpA had similar trends with respect to *F. prausnitzii* abundance, but opposite trends with respect to *Bacteroides*, with decreased abundance of *Bacteroides* genus seen in adult SpA patients compared to adult healthy controls.

This work supports a potential role of *F. prausnitzii* in the pathogenesis of SpA. Although previous studies assessing the microbiota in adults with SpA have not reported alterations in the abundance of this organism [5, 6, 43], this was reported previously in a pediatric study of SpA patients [8]. This particular species is generally considered to have anti-inflammatory effects through production of SCFAs, such as butyrate [10], or by direct effects on cytokine production [39], and our results demonstrated decreased genetic capacity to synthesize butyrate among ERA patients compared to healthy control pediatric subjects. SCFAs serve as major sources of energy for the intestinal enterocytes and also regulate the differentiation of T cells, promoting a regulatory phenotype [46, 48]. A meta-analysis of studies of patients with IBD showed decreased intestinal abundance of *F. prausnitzii* [9]. Our work extends these previous observations, by showing that the specific strain within *F. prausnitzii* may be of particular relevance. Recent studies indicated that the A2-165 strain, as compared to L2/6 and other strains, may have greater capacity to induce IL-10 production [40] and has increased promoter activity at the butyryl-CoA CoA transferase gene, which codes for the enzyme that catalyzes the final step in the butyrate synthesis pathway [41]. Thus, not only did ERA patients demonstrate less representation of the butanoate pathway, but their promoter activity at a key locus determining butyrate production may also be diminished. Not surprisingly in light of these results, a study of fecal metabolomics demonstrated diminished representation of the butanoate pathway in ERA patients compared to controls [11].

Another important finding in this work pertained to the abundance of *Bacteroides*. Consistent with previous observations in children with multiple forms of JIA including ERA [7, 8, 13], this organism was relatively overrepresented among pediatric SpA patients. This finding appears to be uniquely associated with pediatric subjects; several studies in adults with both RA [14, 15, 49] and SpA [5, 6] have shown decreased abundance of *Bacteroides* in patients compared to healthy controls. Similar to these other reports, adult SpA patients in this study showed decreased abundance of *Bacteroides*.

One potential way to reconcile these findings is that *B. fragilis* may contribute to JIA not by directly causing an inflammatory process, but rather through its effects on the ontogeny of the immune system. Vatanen et al. [50] compared the fecal microbiota of children up to age 3 years in areas with high (Estonia and Finland) and low (Russia) incidences of pediatric autoimmunity, finding among the differences decreased fecal abundance of *Bacteroides*, particularly *Bacteroides dorei*, in the Russian children. That the differences in the incidence of autoimmunity may have been related to the abundance of *Bacteroides* was suggested by findings that the lipopolysaccharide (LPS) of *B. dorei* generated a less robust inflammatory reaction than did that of *Escherichia coli* yet failed to induce tolerance to repeated doses of endotoxin; furthermore, the LPS of *B. dorei*, unlike that of *E. coli*, did not prevent development of type 1 diabetes when injected intraperitoneally into young nonobese diabetic mice. Thus, elevated fecal abundance of *Bacteroides* may represent an illustration of the hygiene hypothesis, which posits that abnormal early life microbial exposures result in altered immune priming and consequent increased risk of autoimmune diseases [51].

The findings of our study need to be interpreted in view of its limitations. Despite including subjects from around the country, the sample size was small, and we cannot exclude geographic contributions to the findings. HLA-B27 itself may also have contributed to the variance [52], although among the ERA patients there was no evident clustering based upon the presence versus absence of this marker, and there is to our knowledge no published data indicating that the HLA-B27 allele affects the microbiota in humans. In addition, all adult participants with longstanding SpA had been exposed to a variety of immunosuppressive therapies. Furthermore, three of them had been exposed to sulfasalazine, which is in part an antibiotic; however, excluding them did not alter our findings. We also do not have information on subclinical intestinal inflammation, which is frequently present in patients with SpA [53]. Finally, many of the adult and pediatric controls had been referred to evaluate for arthritis; however, these subjects were evaluated by an attending pediatric or adult rheumatologist, who excluded a diagnosis of arthritis on the basis of the historical and physical examination findings. The strengths of the study are that the pediatric arm was limited to treatment-naïve subjects, we used a novel informatics approach to identify strain-level differences between patients and controls, and we included shotgun sequencing data that corroborated the 16S findings.

Conclusion

Our study supports previous work indicating that decreased fecal abundance of a regulatory strain of *F. prausnitzii* may be at least partly responsible for the pathogenesis of SpA, possibly due to decreased production of butyrate, and that efforts to replenish it in patients with SpA may be a potential therapeutic avenue. In contrast, to the extent that increased abundance of *Bacteroides* or *B. fragilis* in children reflects altered immunologic development rather than direct pathogenicity or the organism, enthusiasm for microbial-based interventions to address this organism may be tempered. Instead, our findings may underscore the necessity for prevention efforts, such as avoiding unnecessary use of antibiotics in healthy children [54, 55].

Abbreviations

ASAS: Assessment of Spondyloarthritis International Society; BLAST: Basic Local Alignment Search Tool; CASPAR: Classification Criteria for Psoriatic Arthritis; DADA: Divisive Amplicon Denoising Algorithm; DIAMOND: double index alignment of next-generation sequencing data; ERA: Enthesitis-related arthritis; FDR: False discovery rate; HUMAnN: HMP Unified Metabolic Analysis; IBD: Inflammatory bowel disease; JIA: Juvenile idiopathic arthritis; KEGG: Kyoto Encyclopedia of Genes and Genomes; LPS: Lipopolysaccharide; PCoA: Principal coordinates analysis; PERMANOVA: Permutation multivariate analysis of variance; PsA: Psoriatic arthritis; QIIME: Quantitative Insight Into Microbial Ecology; RA: Rheumatoid arthritis; rDNA: Ribosomal DNA; SCFA: Short chain fatty acids; UAB: University of Alabama at Birmingham

Acknowledgements

Not applicable.

Funding

MLS was supported by the Childhood Arthritis and Rheumatology Research Alliance, the American College of Rheumatology, and the NIH-NIAMS P60 AR064172. PAN was supported by the Fundación Bechara. MID was supported by NIH-NIAMS K23 AR062100. In addition, the following are acknowledged for their support of the Microbiome Resource at the University of Alabama at Birmingham: School of Medicine, Comprehensive Cancer Center (P30 CA013148), Center for AIDS Research (5P30AI027767), Center for Clinical Translational Science (UL1TR001417), and Heflin Center for Genomic Sciences.

Authors' contributions

MLS designed the study, performed bioinformatics and statistical analyses, and drafted the manuscript. PFW, JEW, PAN, BSE, CHS, MGP, KS, and AR were all PIs at their respective institutions and contributed data on one or more subjects reported herein. MID and SLB recruited adult patients at UAB. RQC supervised all aspects of the study and provided substantial input into the initial draft. CDM runs the Microbiome facility at UAB and oversaw the collection and processing of the samples. RK and EJL met with MLS on a regular basis to provide informatics support. All authors read and approved the final manuscript.

Competing interests

The authors declare that they have no competing interests.

Author details

[1]University of Alabama at Birmingham, Birmingham, AL, USA. [2]Children's Hospital of Philadelphia, Philadelphia, PA, USA. [3]Hackensack University

Medical Center, Hackensack, NJ, USA. [4]Boston Children's Hospital and Brigham and Women's Hospital, Boston, MA, USA. [5]Connecticut Children's Medical Center, Hartford, CT, USA. [6]Nationwide Children's Hospital, Columbus, OH, USA. [7]Texas Scottish Rite Hospital, Dallas, TX, USA. [8]University of Louisville, Louisville, KY, USA. [9]Children's Hospital of Los Angeles, Los Angeles, CA, USA.

References

1. Stoll ML. Gut microbes, immunity, and spondyloarthritis. Clin Immunol. 2015;159(2):134–42.
2. Sheehan D, Shanahan F. The gut microbiota in inflammatory bowel disease. Gastroenterol Clin North Am. 2017;46(1):143–54.
3. Hansen JJ, Sartor RB. Therapeutic manipulation of the microbiome in IBD: current results and future approaches. Curr Treat Options Gastroenterol. 2015;13(1):105–20.
4. van Sommeren S, Janse M, Karjalainen J, Fehrmann R, Franke L, Fu J, et al. Extraintestinal manifestations and complications in inflammatory bowel disease: from shared genetics to shared biological pathways. Inflamm Bowel Dis. 2014;20(6):987–94.
5. Stebbings S, Munro K, Simon MA, Tannock G, Highton J, Harmsen H, et al. Comparison of the faecal microflora of patients with ankylosing spondylitis and controls using molecular methods of analysis. Rheumatology (Oxford). 2002;41(12):1395–401.
6. Tito RY, Cypers H, Joossens M, Varkas G, Van Praet L, Glorieus E, et al. Brief Report: Dialister as a microbial marker of disease activity in spondyloarthritis. Arthritis Rheumatol. 2017;69(1):114–21.
7. Aggarwal A, Sarangi AN, Gaur P, Shukla A, Aggarwal R. Gut microbiome in children with enthesitis-related arthritis in a developing country and the effect of probiotic administration. Clin Exp Immunol. 2017;187(3):480–9.
8. Stoll ML, Kumar R, Morrow CD, Lefkowitz EJ, Cui X, Genin A, et al. Altered microbiota associated with abnormal humoral immune responses to commensal organisms in enthesitis-related arthritis. Arthritis Res Ther. 2014;16(6):486.
9. Cao Y, Shen J, Ran ZH. Association between Faecalibacterium prausnitzii reduction and inflammatory bowel disease: a meta-analysis and systematic review of the literature. Gastroenterol Res Pract. 2014;2014:872725.
10. Hold GL, Schwiertz A, Aminov RI, Blaut M, Flint HJ. Oligonucleotide probes that detect quantitatively significant groups of butyrate-producing bacteria in human feces. Appl Environ Microbiol. 2003;69(7):4320–4.
11. Stoll ML, Kumar R, Lefkowitz EJ, Cron RQ, Morrow CD, Barnes S. Fecal metabolomics in pediatric spondyloarthritis implicate decreased metabolic diversity and altered tryptophan metabolism as pathogenic factors. Genes Immun. 2016;17(7):400–5.
12. Muller PH, De Meij TG, Westedt M, De Groot EF, Allaart CF, Brinkman DM, et al. Disturbance of microbial core species in new-onset juvenile idiopathic arthritis. J Pediatr Infect Dis. 2017;12:131–5.
13. Tejesvi MV, Arvonen M, Kangas SM, Keskitalo PL, Pirttila AM, Karttunen TJ, et al. Faecal microbiome in new-onset juvenile idiopathic arthritis. Eur J Clin Microbiol Infect Dis. 2016;35(3):363–70.
14. Scher JU, Sczesnak A, Longman RS, Segata N, Ubeda C, Bielski C, et al. Expansion of intestinal Prevotella copri correlates with enhanced susceptibility to arthritis. Elife. 2013;2:e01202.
15. Maeda Y, Kurakawa T, Umemoto E, Motooka D, Ito Y, Gotoh K, et al. Dysbiosis contributes to arthritis development via activation of autoreactive T cells in the intestine. Arthritis Rheumatol. 2016;68(11):2646–661.
16. Martin R, Miquel S, Benevides L, Bridonneau C, Robert V, Hudault S, et al. Functional characterization of novel Faecalibacterium prausnitzii strains isolated from healthy volunteers: a step forward in the use of F prausnitzii as a next-generation probiotic. Front Microbiol. 2017;8:1226.
17. Ahern PP, Faith JJ, Gordon JI. Mining the human gut microbiota for effector strains that shape the immune system. Immunity. 2014;40(6):815–23.
18. De Filippo C, Cavalieri D, Di Paola M, Ramazzotti M, Poullet JB, Massart S, et al. Impact of diet in shaping gut microbiota revealed by a comparative study in children from Europe and rural Africa. Proc Natl Acad Sci U S A. 2010;107(33):14691–6.
19. Zhang J, Guo Z, Xue Z, Sun Z, Zhang M, Wang L, et al. A phylo-functional core of gut microbiota in healthy young Chinese cohorts across lifestyles, geography and ethnicities. ISME J. 2015;9(9):1979–90.
20. Petty RE, Southwood TR, Manners P, Baum J, Glass DN, Goldenberg J, et al. International League of Associations for Rheumatology classification of juvenile idiopathic arthritis: second revision, Edmonton, 2001. J Rheumatol. 2004;31(2):390–2.
21. Rudwaleit M, van der Heijde D, Landewe R, Listing J, Akkoc N, Brandt J, et al. The development of Assessment of SpondyloArthritis International Society classification criteria for axial spondyloarthritis (part II): validation and final selection. Ann Rheum Dis. 2009;68(6):777–83.
22. Rudwaleit M, van der Heijde D, Landewe R, Akkoc N, Brandt J, Chou CT, et al. The Assessment of SpondyloArthritis International Society classification criteria for peripheral spondyloarthritis and for spondyloarthritis in general. Ann Rheum Dis. 2011;70(1):25–31.
23. Taylor W, Gladman D, Helliwell P, Marchesoni A, Mease P, Mielants H. Classification criteria for psoriatic arthritis: development of new criteria from a large international study. Arthritis Rheum. 2006;54(8):2665–73.
24. Callahan BJ, McMurdie PJ, Rosen MJ, Han AW, Johnson AJ, Holmes SP. DADA2: high-resolution sample inference from Illumina amplicon data. Nat Methods. 2016;13(7):581–3.
25. Rosen MJ, Callahan BJ, Fisher DS, Holmes SP. Denoising PCR-amplified metagenome data. BMC Bioinformatics. 2012;13:283.
26. Caporaso JG, Kuczynski J, Stombaugh J, Bittinger K, Bushman FD, Costello EK, et al. QIIME allows analysis of high-throughput community sequencing data. Nat Methods. 2010;7(5):335–6.
27. Schloss PD, Westcott SL, Ryabin T, Hall JR, Hartmann M, Hollister EB, et al. Introducing mothur: open-source, platform-independent, community-supported software for describing and comparing microbial communities. Appl Environ Microbiol. 2009;75(23):7537–41.
28. Wang Q, Garrity GM, Tiedje JM, Cole JR. Naive Bayesian classifier for rapid assignment of rRNA sequences into the new bacterial taxonomy. Appl Environ Microbiol. 2007;73(16):5261–7.
29. DeSantis TZ, Hugenholtz P, Larsen N, Rojas M, Brodie EL, Keller K, et al. Greengenes, a chimera-checked 16S rRNA gene database and workbench compatible with ARB. Appl Environ Microbiol. 2006;72(7):5069–72.
30. Schmieder R, Edwards R. Quality control and preprocessing of metagenomic datasets. Bioinformatics. 2011;27(6):863–4.
31. Langmead B, Salzberg SL. Fast gapped-read alignment with Bowtie 2. Nat Methods. 2012;9(4):357–9.
32. Abubucker S, Segata N, Goll J, Schubert AM, Izard J, Cantarel BL, et al. Metabolic reconstruction for metagenomic data and its application to the human microbiome. PLoS Comput Biol. 2012;8(6):e1002358.
33. Pundir S, Martin MJ, O'Donovan C. UniProt Protein Knowledgebase. Methods Mol Biol. 2017;1558:41–55.
34. Buchfink B, Xie C, Huson DH. Fast and sensitive protein alignment using DIAMOND. Nat Methods. 2015;12(1):59–60.
35. Caspi R, Altman T, Billington R, Dreher K, Foerster H, Fulcher CA, et al. The MetaCyc database of metabolic pathways and enzymes and the BioCyc collection of Pathway/Genome Databases. Nucleic Acids Res. 2014; 42(Database issue):D459–71.
36. Kanehisa M, Sato Y, Kawashima M, Furumichi M, Tanabe M. KEGG as a reference resource for gene and protein annotation. Nucleic Acids Res. 2016;44(D1):D457–62.
37. Kelly BJ, Gross R, Bittinger K, Sherrill-Mix S, Lewis JD, Collman RG, et al. Power and sample-size estimation for microbiome studies using pairwise distances and PERMANOVA. Bioinformatics. 2015;31(15):2461–8.
38. Benjamini Y, Hochberg Y. Controlling the false discovery rate: a practical and powerful appraoch to multiple testing. J R Stat Soc B. 1995;57:289–300.
39. Sokol H, Pigneur B, Watterlot L, Lakhdari O, Bermudez-Humaran LG, Gratadoux JJ, et al. Faecalibacterium prausnitzii is an anti-inflammatory commensal bacterium identified by gut microbiota analysis of Crohn disease patients. Proc Natl Acad Sci U S A. 2008;105(43):16731–6.
40. Rossi O, van Berkel LA, Chain F, Tanweer Khan M, Taverne N, Sokol H, et al. Faecalibacterium prausnitzii A2-165 has a high capacity to induce IL-10 in human and murine dendritic cells and modulates T cell responses. Sci Rep. 2016;6:18507.
41. Song H, Yoo Y, Hwang J, Na YC, Kim HS. Faecalibacterium prausnitzii subspecies-level dysbiosis in the human gut microbiome underlying atopic dermatitis. J Allergy Clin Immunol. 2016;137(3):852–60.
42. Round JL, Lee SM, Li J, Tran G, Jabri B, Chatila TA, et al. The Toll-like receptor 2 pathway establishes colonization by a commensal of the human microbiota. Science. 2011;332(6032):974–7.

43. Costello ME, Ciccia F, Willner D, Warrington N, Robinson PC, Gardiner B, et al. Intestinal dysbiosis in ankylosing spondylitis. Arthritis Rheumatol. 2015;67:686–91.
44. Breban M, Tap J, Leboime A, Said-Nahal R, Langella P, Chiocchia G, et al. Faecal microbiota study reveals specific dysbiosis in spondyloarthritis. Ann Rheum Dis. 2017;76(9):1614–622.
45. Turnbaugh PJ, Hamady M, Yatsunenko T, Cantarel BL, Duncan A, Ley RE, et al. A core gut microbiome in obese and lean twins. Nature. 2009;457(7228): 480–4.
46. Hamer HM, Jonkers D, Venema K, Vanhoutvin S, Troost FJ, Brummer RJ. Review article: the role of butyrate on colonic function. Aliment Pharmacol Ther. 2008;27(2):104–19.
47. Taurog JD, Richardson JA, Croft JT, Simmons WA, Zhou M, Fernandez-Sueiro JL, et al. The germfree state prevents development of gut and joint inflammatory disease in HLA-B27 transgenic rats. J Exp Med. 1994;180(6):2359–64.
48. Segain JP, Raingeard De La Bletiere D, Bourreille A, Leray V, Gervois N, Rosales C, et al. Butyrate inhibits inflammatory responses through NFkappaB inhibition: implications for Crohn's disease. Gut. 2000;47(3):397–403.
49. Vaahtovuo J, Munukka E, Korkeamaki M, Luukkainen R, Toivanen P. Fecal microbiota in early rheumatoid arthritis. J Rheumatol. 2008;35(8):1500–5.
50. Vatanen T, Kostic AD, d'Hennezel E, Siljander H, Franzosa EA, Yassour M, et al. Variation in microbiome LPS immunogenicity contributes to autoimmunity in humans. Cell. 2016;165(4):842–53.
51. Rook GA. Hygiene hypothesis and autoimmune diseases. Clin Rev Allergy Immunol. 2012;42(1):5–15.
52. Lin P, Bach M, Asquith M, Lee AY, Akileswaran L, Stauffer P, et al. HLA-B27 and human beta2-microglobulin affect the gut microbiota of transgenic rats. PLoS One. 2014;9(8):e105684.
53. Mielants H, De Keyser F, Baeten D, Van den Bosch F. Gut inflammation in the spondyloarthropathies. Curr Rheumatol Rep. 2005;7(3):188–94.
54. Arvonen M, Virta LJ, Pokka T, Kroger L, Vahasalo P. Repeated exposure to antibiotics in infancy: a predisposing factor for juvenile idiopathic arthritis or a sign of this group's greater susceptibility to infections? J Rheumatol. 2015;42(3):521–6.
55. Horton DB, Scott FI, Haynes K, Putt ME, Rose CD, Lewis JD, et al. Antibiotic exposure and juvenile idiopathic arthritis: a case-control study. Pediatrics. 2015;136(2):e333–43.

4

Feasibility and reliability of the Spondyloarthritis Research Consortium of Canada sacroiliac joint inflammation score in children

Pamela F. Weiss[1,3,4,8*], Walter P. Maksymowych[5,7], Robert G. Lambert[6,7], Jacob L. Jaremko[6], David M. Biko[2], Joel Paschke[7], Timothy G. Brandon[1,3], Rui Xiao[4] and Nancy A. Chauvin[2]

Abstract

Background: Published methods for quantification of magnetic resonance imaging (MRI) evidence of inflammation in the sacroiliac joint lack validation in pediatric populations. We evaluated the reliability and construct validity of the Spondyloarthritis Research Consortium of Canada (SPARCC) sacroiliac joint inflammation score (SIS) in children with suspected or confirmed juvenile spondyloarthritis (JSpA).

Methods: The SPARCC SIS measures the presence, depth, and intensity of bone marrow inflammation on MRI through the cartilaginous part of the joint. Six readers blinded to clinical details except age, participated in two reading exercises, each preceded by a calibration exercise. Inter-observer reliability was assessed using intraclass correlation coefficients (ICCs) and for pre-specified acceptable reliability the inraclass correlation coefficient (ICC) was > 0.8.

Results: The SPARCC SIS had face validity and was feasible to score in pediatric cases in both reading exercises. Cases were mostly male (64%) and the median age at the time of imaging was 14.9 years. After calibration, the median ICC across all readers for the SIS total score was 0.81 (IQR 0.71–0.89). SPARCC SIS had weak correlation with disease activity (DA) as measured by the JSpADA ($r = -0.12$) but discriminated significantly between those with and without elevated C-reactive protein ($p = 0.03$).

Conclusion: The SPARCC SIS was feasible to score and had acceptable reliability in children. The ICC improved with additional calibration and reading exercises, for both experienced and inexperienced readers.

Keywords: Imaging, Spondyloarthritis, Ankylosing spondylitis, Juvenile idiopathic arthritis, Outcomes

Background

Children with spondyloarthritis (SpA) and axial arthritis are at risk of progression to ankylosing spondylitis, an inflammatory disease that causes joint fusion and leads to permanent functional impairment. While there are similarities between juvenile and adult SpA, there are distinct phenotypic differences that warrant specific focus and clinical trials in juvenile disease [1–5]. In order to assess the efficacy and effectiveness of medications for SpA and axial disease in critically needed clinical trials, we need an objective measure to quantify response in the pediatric sacroiliac joint.

There are five Food and Drug Administration (FDA)-approved anti-TNF drugs for ankylosing spondylitis in adults and many more phase III trials underway. There has only been one trial of biologic agents in children with axial arthritis [6]. This trial had several limitations leading to findings that were not statistically significant for the primary outcome. Noteworthy limitations were that imaging was not part of the protocol and the primary outcome was achievement of an Assessment of SpA International Society (ASAS) working group 40 response criteria [7], which has never been validated in

* Correspondence: weisspa@email.chop.edu
[1]Department of Pediatrics, Division of Rheumatology, Children's Hospital of Philadelphia, Philadelphia, PA, USA
[3]Center for Pediatric Clinical Effectiveness (CPCE), Children's Hospital of Philadelphia, Philadelphia, PA, USA

children. Despite the negative results, most pediatric rheumatologists believe TNF inhibitors are effective. This trial experience underscores the importance of identifying clinically meaningful and responsive measures of inflammation in the pediatric sacroiliac joint.

Validated measures to objectively assess inflammation in the adult sacroiliac joint include the modified Berlin magnetic resonance imaging (MRI) method [8] and the SPondylo Arthritis Research Consortium of Canada (SPARCC) Sacroiliac joint Inflammation Score (SIS) [9]. The modified Berlin method grades the proportion of bone marrow edema in each sacroiliac joint according to the percentage of each joint quadrant (grade 1, < 33%; grade 2, ≥ 33–66%; grade 3, > 66%) affected by edema so that the total score for both SIJs ranges from 0 to 24. The SPARCC SIS measures the presence, depth, and intensity of bone marrow inflammation in each sacroiliac joint quadrant in consecutive semi-coronal slices through the joint. The SPARCC SIS has been used successfully in clinical trials of biologic agents in adults with SpA and axial disease [10–14]. Improvements in inflammation on MRI were significantly correlated with change in several clinical measures including composite disease activity measures and C-reactive protein levels [11].

Identification of useful measures of inflammation in the pediatric sacroiliac joint will translate into improved care algorithms and increased opportunities for labeling of emerging targeted medications for these children. We evaluated the reliability and construct validity of the SPARCC SIS in children with suspected or confirmed juvenile SpA.

Methods

This study protocols were reviewed and approved by the Children's Hospital of Philadelphia Committee for the Protection of Human Subjects (16–012641 and 17–013883). Waivers of consent and HIPAA authorization were granted as the procedures represented minimal risk to the subjects and did not adversely affect the rights and welfare of the subjects.

Cases were children with suspected or confirmed SpA who had imaging performed at the Children's Hospital of Philadelphia (Philadelphia, PA, USA) or Stollery Children's Hospital (Edmonton, Alberta, Canada). All images were de-identified prior to scoring and demographics were abstracted from the clinical chart. The imaging protocols at the two institutions varied slightly and minor modifications of the imaging protocols over the time period were noted. The SPARCC SIS scores, however, only require two specific sequences, which were uniformly performed on all included studies with the T1-weighted and short-tau inversion recovery (STIR) coronal oblique sequences. One of the advantages of the SPARCC tool is that as long as these two sequences are present, subtle differences in MRI procedure amongst institutions do not impact its applicability.

The SPARCC SIS assesses the presence, depth and intensity of bone marrow edema on consecutive fluid sensitive coronal oblique slices through the cartilaginous part of the joint (Table 1). Six consecutive semi-coronal slices through the cartilaginous portion of the joint are scored for bone marrow edema (BME; Fig. 1). The presence or absence of edema is scored for each joint quadrant (total score per slice 0–8). The presence or absence of bone marrow signal intensity (present if intensity is the same or greater than the presacral veins) and depth ≥1 cm are scored dichotomously for each sacroiliac joint. T1-weighted and STIR sequences are viewed simultaneously to help the reader define the anatomy but only STIR sequences are scored. The total score ranges from 0 to 72 with higher scores indicating more inflammation. We completed two calibration modules and two reading exercises over the course of approximately 18 months.

All training and scoring exercises were performed within a web-based environment (CaREArthritis.com) by six readers (three pediatric radiologists, one pediatric rheumatologist, one adult radiologist and one adult rheumatologist). Two of the readers were SPARCC SIS developers (WM and RL). Before completing reading exercise 1, all readers reviewed a pediatric PowerPoint training module that included scoring instructions and examples of bone marrow edema and bright subchondral signal on STIR scans that may be easily confused with inflammation. The reference for normal bone marrow signal intensity in children was the iliac crests, edges of the vertebral bodies, tri-radiate cartilage and ischial pubic synchondrosis. Each reader, blinded to clinical details except age, subsequently used the online viewing and scoring system to score 30 digital imaging and communication in medicine (DICOM)-based studies that included semi-coronal T1-weighted and STIR sequences.

Table 1 Scoring system used to evaluate six consecutive semi-coronal magnetic resonance imaging slices (total score range 0–72)

Feature	Definition	Score range per slice	Maximum score
Bone marrow edema	Hyperintense signal on short-tau inversion recovery	Score 4 quadrants in each sacroiliac joint 0/1, range per slice is 0–8	48
Bone marrow intensity	Hyperintensity of marrow edema using the presacral veins as reference	Score each sacroiliac joint 0/1, range per slice is 0–2	12
Bone marrow depth	Homogeneous increase of marrow signal ≥1 cm from the articular surface within either sacroiliac joint	Score each sacroiliac joint 0/1, range per slice is 0–2	12

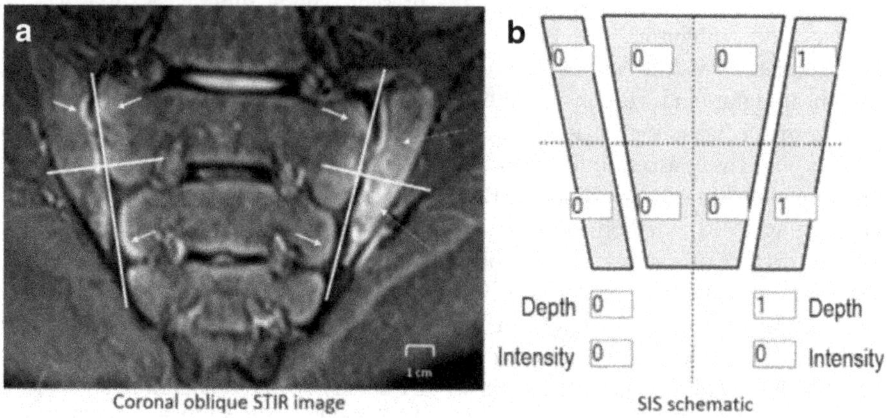

Fig. 1 Sample slice and scoring methods for sacroiliac joint inflammation score (SIS). **a** Coronal oblique short-tau inversion recovery (STIR) image of the sacroiliac joints shows each joint divided into four quadrants. There is normal bright subchondral signal along both sides of the right sacroiliac joint and along the periarticular region of the left sacrum (solid arrows) in this skeletally immature patient. On the left, there is abnormal signal consistent with bone marrow edema within the periarticular region of the left ilium in both the upper and lower quadrants (dashed arrows). **b** Scoring schematic demonstrates a "1" within the left iliac bone in both the upper and lower quadrants representing bone marrow edema. An additional score of "1" is given as the depth of the bone marrow edema extends > 1 cm from the articular surface. The patient received a total score of "3" for this image slice

The data for reading exercises 1 and 2 were based on data from a single time point.

After reading exercise 1, all readers, except WM and RL (SPARCC SIS developers), completed an interactive calibration module comprising 40 adult cases, each with studies of T1-weighted and STIR scans from baseline and 2 years after initiation of TNF inhibitor therapy (https://www.carearthritis.com/mriportal/sparccsij/index/). Each study was scored in pairs, blinded to time point. Readers received instantaneous feedback on concordance/discordance of scoring with the expert readers (WM and RL) after scoring each individual semi-coronal slice in the first 20 cases. Feedback on the next 20 cases was provided after scoring the entire case. The intraclass correlation coefficient (ICC) for concordance with the expert readers was calculated after the first 20 cases were completed, again after the next 10 cases, and finally after all 40 cases had been scored. The *a priori* score deemed acceptable for this calibration was an ICC >0.8 for the total SPARCC SIS score. After the interactive training module, we conducted a second reading exercise based on DICOM images comprising T1-weighted and STIR scans from 30 pediatric studies, which were a mix of 15 studies from the first exercise and 15 new studies.

Face and content validity were established through discussion during the creation of the pediatric PowerPoint training module and initial calibration exercise. Face and content validity is demonstrated if the criteria are sensible on face value to physicians who utilize them in their field. Feasibility was assessed by asking the raters to estimate the time it took to score each case and to rate the ease with which it was performed.

Inter-observer reliability was assessed using ICC. The ICCs are presented as agreement for all readers together, SPARCC developers (n = 2), pediatric radiologists (n = 3) and rheumatologists (n = 2). We applied the pre-specified ICC target from the interactive adult calibration module to the interpretation of the results from the two reading exercises (> 0.8 for the total score).

Construct validity was tested using Spearman's rho, measuring correlation between the mean SPARCC SIS developers' status scores from reading exercise 2 and disease activity as measured by the juvenile SpA disease activity (JSpADA) index (range 0–8) [15] and physician global disease activity assessment (visual analogue scale, range 0–10). The JSpADA index is a disease activity measure that is scored 0 to 8, with higher scores indicating more active disease. The components of the score are weighted equally and consist of the following measures: arthritis, enthesitis, patient pain assessment, inflammatory markers, morning stiffness, clinical sacroiliitis, uveitis and back mobility. Discrimination was tested by comparing the mean SPARCC SIS developers' scores with laboratory values (C-reactive protein ≥1 or <1 mg/dl and erythrocyte sedimentation rate ≥21 or <21 mm/h) and patients with and without inflammatory back pain. Laboratory values were included if available +/− 60 days from the date of the MRI.

Results

Subjects

Demographic and clinical characteristics of the cases included in the two reading exercises are shown in Table 2. In total there were 45 unique cases from two tertiary care centers that were utilized for the two reading exercises.

Table 2 Case characteristics

	Number	Frequency (%)/median (IQR)
Age (years)	45	14.9 (12.7–16.5)
Sex-male	45	29 (64.4%)
HLA-B27+	39	25 (64.1%)
Race	39	
Caucasian		32 (82.1%)
African American		5 (12.8%)
Other		2 (5.1%)
Active joint count	36	0 (0–1)
Tender enthesis count	36	0 (0–5)
Patient-reported pain[a] (VAS; range 0–10)	32	3.8 (1–6)
Patient-reported disease activity (VAS; range 0–10)	31	3 (0.5–5.1)
Physician global disease activity (VAS; range 0–10)	31	3 (2–4)
CRP (≥1.0 mg/dL)	28	17 (60.7%)
ESR (≥21 mm/h)	29	12 (41.4%)

There were 45 unique cases assessed in the two reading exercises
VAS visual analogue scale, *CRP* C-reactive protein, *ESR* erythrocyte sedimentation rate
[a]General pain recorded on a visual analogue scale

There were 29 (64%) male patients and median age at the time of imaging was 14.9 years (IQR 12.7–16.5, range 6.8–18.7 years). At the time of imaging, most children and adolescents had minimal peripheral disease activity (median active joint and tender entheses counts of 0) but moderate self-reported pain (median 4) and self-reported and physician-reported disease activity (3 and 3, respectively).

Feasibility and interobserver reliability

The SPARCC SIS had acceptable face validity and was feasible to score. The time required to assess a case for the presence, depth and intensity of lesions for a single case less than 15 min. All readers felt the online scoring platform was easy to use.

In exercise 1, 140 (78%) studies read by all six readers had a SPARCC SIS ≥2 and the median SPARCC SIS was 14 (IQR 3–29). The ICCs for the SPARCC SIS total score from both reading exercises are shown in Fig. 2. In the first exercise, both the SPARCC developers and pediatric radiologists achieved the pre-specified target of > 0.8 for the total score. The ICC amongst all readers was 0.63 (IQR 0.45–0.78).

In between the first and second reading exercises, the four readers who were not SPARCC SIS developers (PW, JJ, DB and NC) completed an interactive calibration module comprising 40 adult cases. Three of the four readers rated the scoring platform for the calibration module as easy to use and the time to score each case ranged from 4 to 15 min. All four readers achieved an ICC status score >0.82 (range 0.82–0.99).

In exercise 2, 133 (74%) of the studies had a SPARCC SIS ≥2. Median SPARCC SIS was 7.5 (IQR 1–24.5). The ICC amongst all six readers surpassed the pre-specified target of 0.8. When assessed by different rater backgrounds, only the SPARCC developers achieved the pre-specified target of > 0.8 for the total score. The ICCs amongst pediatric radiologists and rheumatologists were 0.77 and 0.79, respectively (Fig. 2).

Construct validity

Correlation between disease activity, as measured by the JSpADA index and physician global disease activity, and the SPARCC SIS developers' mean scores for all unique patients was weak ($r = -0.12$, $p = 0.64$ and $r = 0.09$, $p = 0.65$, respectively). The SPARCC SIS discriminated well between those children with and without elevated C-reactive protein ($p = 0.03$) but not between children with and without inflammatory back pain ($p = 0.92$).

Discussion

Identification of reliable, objective, and quantifiable measures of response in children with axial disease is critical. Without measures to objectively quantify the severity of disease in the pediatric sacroiliac joint, assessment of interval change and response to medication in efficacy or effectiveness studies is not possible. This is the first evaluation of the feasibility and reliability of the SPARCC SIS in children. The SPARCC SIS was feasible to score and achieved the pre-specified target for acceptable reliability (ICC ≥0.8) in children. The ICC improved and surpassed the pre-specified acceptable reliability threshold with additional calibration and reading exercises, even for readers with limited experience. The SPARCC SIS did not have convergent validity with clinical measures of disease activity, highlighting that imaging and clinical evaluations provide complimentary but non-overlapping information. The SPARCC SIS did discriminate between those children with and without elevated C-reactive protein but did not discriminate between children with and without back pain.

Our findings indicate that readers with various levels of imaging experience can have their reading calibrated to acceptable levels of reliability using a relatively simple calibration module that provides iterative real-time feedback on the concordance/discordance of their scoring with the expert readers at the level of individual sacroiliac joint quadrants. This is promising as this means that radiologists (both adult and pediatric) from geographically isolated institutions can have their reading calibrated for the purposes of both efficacy and effectiveness studies. In the first reading exercise both the pediatric radiologists ($n = 3$) and SPARCC developers (n

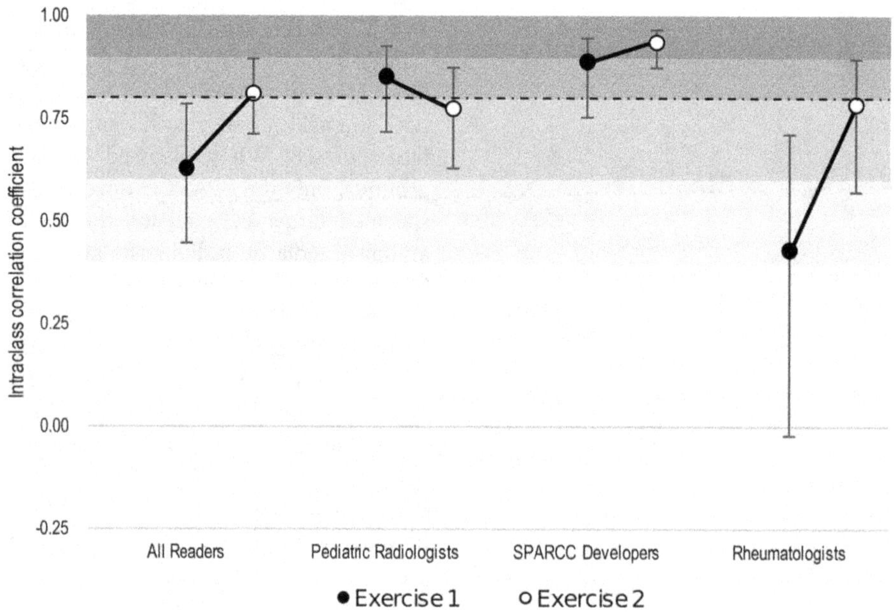

Fig. 2 Intraclass correlation coefficients of the Spondyloarthritis Research Consortium of Canada (SPARCC) sacroiliac joint inflammation score across two exercises

= 2) attained an ICC >0.8 yet the overall ICC was lower (0.63). The lower total group ICC was likely secondary to inclusion of an inexperienced reader (PW) and to systematic differences in the way in which the pediatric radiologists and the SPARCC developers approach evaluation of these studies. The subsequent calibration exercises were meant to reduce these betwee-group differences and heighten overall agreement or reliability, which they did. Interestingly, the ICC in the pediatric radiology group dropped slightly in the second reading exercise, which might signal that each of the pediatric radiologists adjusted his/her interpretations slightly differently and that perhaps with additional training the total ICC can improve even more. It would be ideal in the future to develop an interactive calibration module based solely on pediatric imaging studies.

In adults, the SPARCC SIS has been shown to significantly correlate with the magnitude of C-reactive protein and other measures of clinical disease activity [11] that have not been validated in children. We did not see correlation with disease activity measures, perhaps secondary to the relatively small sample size or the lack of validated specific measures of axial disease activity to use as reference standards. One measure specifically designed to assess clinical disease activity in juvenile SpA is the JSpADA index [15], but this is an assessment of overall SpA disease activity and axial disease activity accounts for only two of eight variables contributing to the score. No other validated juvenile arthritis disease activity tools assess axial disease activity. The SPARCC SIS did discriminate between those with and without elevated C-reactive protein. This is not entirely surprising given the results from the aforementioned adult studies [11] and the pediatric studies demonstrating increased predictive probability of sacroiliitis with elevated C-reactive protein [4]. Discrimination was not uniform across multiple clinical attributes as it did not discriminate those with and without back pain. This latter finding may be a problem unique to pediatric SpA in which back pain has been shown to be poorly correlated with the presence of axial arthritis in multiple studies [4, 16].

There are several limitations to our study that should be considered. First, the number of pediatric studies was limited, largely due to missing semi-coronal sequences which are essential for SPARCC scoring. The limited number of studies necessitated re-evaluation during the second exercise of some cases used in the first reading exercise. We do not believe using the same studies more than once impacted our results because the cases were not discussed amongst the readers after the first reading exercise and the two reading exercises were separated by approximately 15 months. The limited number of studies also means we could not assess the minimal detectable difference or change in scores; this will be a focus of future work. Second, the studies utilized in the reading and calibration exercises were primarily from only two North American hospitals. Data collection from only two hospitals frequently leads to overrepresentation of regional demographics and a cohort that may not be typical of the entire disease population; however, this limitation is mitigated by the fact that both of these institutions are large referral centers, so the studies included are likely to be representative of cases evaluated in a wide variety of geographic areas. Third, some physician and patient-reported assessments were missing, which is expected in a retrospective study. Fourth, specific clinical measures of axial disease activity were not available as they are neither validated nor routinely collected in pediatric clinical care. Although these latter two issues limited the assessment of construct and discriminative validity, they do not affect the feasibility or reliability assessment. These relatively minor limitations are to be expected in the first systematic assessment of the feasibility and reliability of a new tool. Fifth, there was no gold standard by which to assess construct validity of the tool. The closest constructs to measure clinical (not radiographic) disease activity were the juvenile SpA disease activity index and the physician global assessment of disease activity. At most, we hypothesized there would be modest correlation. The absence a current gold standard should not preclude assessment of the feasibility and reliability utility of the tool.

Conclusions

We have demonstrated the feasibility and reliability of the SPARCC sacroiliac joint inflammation scoring methodology in children with established or suspected spondyloarthritis. This scoring system is based upon dichotomous scoring of lesions on consecutive slices through the cartilaginous part of the sacroiliac joint. We have not only established feasibility but also demonstrated that inexperienced readers can have their reading calibrated using standardized definitions, DICOM reference cases and an interactive calibration module. Further work is needed to assess the responsiveness and prognostic significance of the SPARCC SIS in evaluating MRI lesions in children.

Abbreviations

ASAS: Assessment of SpA International Society; CRP: C-reactive protein; *DICOM*: Digital Imaging and Communication in Medicine; *ICC*: Intraclass correlation coefficients; *JSpA*: Juvenile spondyloarthritis; *JSpADA*: Jjuvenile SpA disease activity index; *MRI*: magnetic resonance imaging; *SIS*: sacroiliac joint inflammation score; *SpA*: spondyloarthritis; *SPARCC*: Spondyloarthritis Research Consortium of Canada; *STIR*: Short-tau inversion recovery; *TNF*: Tumor necrosis factor

Acknowledgements

Dr Jaremko and Dr Lambert are supported by Medical Imaging Consultants, Edmonton.

Funding

Dr Weiss' work was supported by the Rheumatology Research Foundation. Dr Jaremko is supported by the Capital Health Chair in Diagnostic Imaging.

Disclosures

Dr. Weiss has served as a consultant for Lilly.

Authors' contributions

PW designed the study, participated in the reading exercise, analyzed the results and drafted the manuscript. WPM contributed to the design of the study, participated in the reading exercise and interpretation of the results and helped revise the manuscript. RGL participated in the reading exercise, interpretation of the results and manuscript revision. JLJ participated in the reading exercise, interpretation of the results and manuscript revision. DMB participated in the reading exercise, interpretation of the results and manuscript revision. JP was responsible for feasibility and coordination of data acquisition and participated in data analysis. TGB participated in study design, coordination, data analysis, interpretation and drafting of the manuscript. RX participated in data analysis and drafting of the manuscript. NAC participated in the reading exercise, interpretation of the results and manuscript revision. All authors read and approved the final manuscript.

Competing interests

The authors declare that they have no competing interests.

Author details

[1]Department of Pediatrics, Division of Rheumatology, Children's Hospital of Philadelphia, Philadelphia, PA, USA. [2]Department of Radiology, Children's Hospital of Philadelphia, Philadelphia, PA, USA. [3]Center for Pediatric Clinical Effectiveness (CPCE), Children's Hospital of Philadelphia, Philadelphia, PA, USA. [4]Center for Clinical Epidemiology and Biostatistics, Perelman School of Medicine at the University of Pennsylvania, Philadelphia, PA, USA. [5]Department of Medicine, University of Alberta, Edmonton, AB, Canada. [6]Department of Radiology and Diagnostic Imaging, University of Alberta, Edmonton, AB, Canada. [7]Canadian Research and Education (CaRE) Arthritis Organization, Edmonton, AB, Canada. [8]The Children's Hospital of Philadelphia, Roberts Center for Pediatric Research, 2716 South Street, Room 11121, Philadelphia, PA 19146, USA.

References

1. Jadon DR, Shaddick G, Jobling A, Ramanan AV, Sengupta R. Clinical outcomes and progression to orthopedic surgery in juvenile- versus adult-onset ankylosing spondylitis. Arthritis Care Res. 2015;67(5):651–7.
2. Lin YC, Liang TH, Chen WS, Lin HY. Differences between juvenile-onset ankylosing spondylitis and adult-onset ankylosing spondylitis. J Chin Med Assoc. 2009;72(11):573–80.
3. Gensler LS, Ward MM, Reveille JD, Learch TJ, Weisman MH, Davis JC Jr. Clinical, radiographic and functional differences between juvenile-onset and adult-onset ankylosing spondylitis: results from the PSOAS cohort. Ann Rheum Dis. 2008;67(2):233–7.
4. Weiss PF, Xiao R, Biko DM, Chauvin NA. Assessment of sacroiliitis at diagnosis of juvenile spondyloarthritis by radiography, magnetic resonance imaging, and clinical examination. Arthritis Care Res. 2016;68(2):187–94.
5. O'Shea FD, Boyle E, Riarh R, Tse SM, Laxer RM, Inman RD. Comparison of clinical and radiographic severity of juvenile-onset versus adult-onset ankylosing spondylitis. Ann Rheum Dis. 2009;68(9):1407–12.
6. Horneff G, Fitter S, Foeldvari I, Minden K, Kuemmerle-Deschner J, Tzaribacev N, Thon A, Borte M, Ganser G, Trauzeddel R, et al. Double-blind, placebo-controlled randomized trial with adalimumab for treatment of juvenile onset ankylosing spondylitis (JoAS): significant short term improvement. Arthritis Res Ther. 2012;14(5):R230.
7. Lukas C, Landewe R, Sieper J, Dougados M, Davis J, Braun J, van der Linden S, van der Heijde D. Assessment of SpondyloArthritis international S. Development of an ASAS-endorsed disease activity score (ASDAS) in patients with ankylosing spondylitis. Ann Rheum Dis. 2009;68(1):18–24.
8. Althoff CE, Sieper J, Song IH, Haibel H, Weiss A, Diekhoff T, Rudwaleit M, Freundlich B, Hamm B, Hermann KG. Active inflammation and structural change in early active axial spondyloarthritis as detected by whole-body MRI. Ann Rheum Dis. 2013;72(6):967–73.
9. Maksymowych WP, Lambert RG, Brown LS, Pangan AL. Defining the minimally important change for the SpondyloArthritis Research Consortium of Canada Spine and sacroiliac joint magnetic resonance imaging indices for ankylosing spondylitis. J Rheumatol. 2012;39(8):1666–74.

10. Pedersen SJ, Poddubnyy D, Sorensen IJ, Loft AG, Hindrup JS, Thamsborg G, Asmussen K, Hendricks O, Norregaard J, Piil AD, et al. Course of magnetic resonance imaging-detected inflammation and structural lesions in the sacroiliac joints of patients in the randomized, double-blind, placebo-controlled Danish multicenter study of adalimumab in spondyloarthritis, as assessed by the Berlin and Spondyloarthritis Research Consortium of Canada Methods. Arthritis Rheum. 2016;68(2):418–29.
11. Maksymowych WP, Dougados M, van der Heijde D, Sieper J, Braun J, Citera G, Van den Bosch F, Logeart I, Wajdula J, Jones H, et al. Clinical and MRI responses to etanercept in early non-radiographic axial spondyloarthritis: 48-week results from the EMBARK study. Ann Rheum Dis. 2016;75(7):1328–35.
12. Lambert RG, Salonen D, Rahman P, Inman RD, Wong RL, Einstein SG, Thomson GT, Beaulieu A, Choquette D, Maksymowych WP. Adalimumab significantly reduces both spinal and sacroiliac joint inflammation in patients with ankylosing spondylitis: a multicenter, randomized, double-blind, placebo-controlled study. Arthritis Rheum. 2007;56(12):4005–14.
13. Sieper J, van der Heijde D, Dougados M, Mease PJ, Maksymowych WP, Brown MA, Arora V, Pangan AL. Efficacy and safety of adalimumab in patients with non-radiographic axial spondyloarthritis: results of a randomised placebo-controlled trial (ABILITY-1). Ann Rheum Dis. 2013;72(6):815–22.
14. Sieper J, van der Heijde D, Dougados M, Maksymowych WP, Scott BB, Boice JA, Berd Y, Bergman G, Curtis S, Tzontcheva A, et al. A randomized, double-blind, placebo-controlled, sixteen-week study of subcutaneous golimumab in patients with active nonradiographic axial spondyloarthritis. Arthritis Rheum. 2015;67(10):2702–12.
15. Weiss PF, Colbert RA, Xiao R, Feudtner C, Beukelman T, DeWitt EM, Pagnini I, Wright TB, Wallace CA. Development and retrospective validation of the juvenile spondyloarthritis disease activity index. Arthritis Care Res. 2014; 66(12):1775–82.
16. Stoll ML, Bhore R, Dempsey-Robertson M, Punaro M. Spondyloarthritis in a pediatric population: risk factors for sacroiliitis. J Rheumatol. 2010;37(11):2402–8.

5

Clinical and MRI remission in patients with nonradiographic axial spondyloarthritis who received long-term open-label adalimumab treatment: 3-year results of the ABILITY-1 trial

Désirée van der Heijde[1*], Joachim Sieper[2], Walter P. Maksymowych[3], Robert G. Lambert[3], Su Chen[4], Maja Hojnik[5], Jaclyn K. Anderson[4] and Aileen L. Pangan[4]

Abstract

Background: Adalimumab was effective in treating patients with nonradiographic axial spondyloarthritis (nr-axSpA) in the 12-week ABILITY-1 trial. We present long-term efficacy and safety results of adalimumab from the open-label ABILITY-1 extension, including the relationship between clinical and magnetic resonance imaging (MRI) remission and impact of sustained clinical remission on physical function.

Methods: Patients received adalimumab 40 mg every other week or placebo for 12 weeks, then open-label adalimumab for up to 144 weeks. Clinical and safety data were collected through 3 years, and MRI data were collected until 2 years. Analyses were performed in the total population and subpopulation with positive MRI and/or elevated C-reactive protein (MRI/CRP-positive) at baseline. Clinical and MRI remission definitions included Ankylosing Spondylitis Disease Activity Score inactive disease (ASDAS ID; score < 1.3) and Spondyloarthritis Research Consortium of Canada (SPARCC) MRI score < 2 for sacroiliac joints (SIJs), spine, or both. Physical function was assessed using the Bath Ankylosing Spondylitis Functional Index.

Results: Overall, 185 patients were included in the total population and 142 in the MRI/CRP-positive subpopulation; 65% and 68%, respectively, completed 3 years. Clinical, functional, and MRI improvements were similar and equally sustainable in both populations. At year 3, the percentages of patients in ASDAS ID in the MRI/CRP-positive subpopulation were 30%/33% (nonresponder imputation) and 46%/49% (observed) for those initially receiving adalimumab/placebo. At years 1 and 2, patients in ASDAS ID vs not had significantly greater improvements in SPARCC SIJ scores from baseline ($P < 0.001$). Among patients with baseline MRI scores ≥ 2 who achieved ASDAS ID at year 2, 44–68% also had MRI remission. Significantly more patients with sustained ASDAS ID through year 2 or 3 vs without achieved normal physical function (100% vs 48%; 100% vs 44%; both $P < 0.001$). No new safety concerns were observed.

Conclusions: In the ABILITY-1 study of nr-axSpA, adalimumab therapy provided sustained clinical and functional improvements through 3 years, as well as suppression of MRI axial inflammation, which was greater in patients who achieved clinical remission. Sustained clinical remission was associated with increased attainment of normal physical function. The safety profile of adalimumab was consistent with prior studies.

Keywords: Anti-TNF, Axial spondyloarthritis, Adalimumab

* Correspondence: mail@dvanderheijde.nl
[1]Leiden University Medical Center, PO Box 9600, Leiden 2300 RC, The Netherlands
Full list of author information is available at the end of the article

Background

Patients with axial spondyloarthritis (axSpA) include those with radiographic axSpA (also termed *ankylosing spondylitis* [AS]), which requires radiographic evidence of sacroiliitis according to the modified New York criteria [1], and those with nonradiographic axial spondyloarthritis (nr-axSpA) [2], who have similar signs and symptoms but without such radiographic changes. Magnetic resonance imaging (MRI) is increasingly used as an imaging tool in patients with axSpA [3, 4] for diagnosis, classification, and monitoring of disease activity [5–7]. Thus, there is a need to better understand the relationship between inflammation assessed by MRI and disease activity assessed clinically, as well as their impact on long-term physical function in patients with axSpA.

Therapeutic targets are emerging for axSpA. Clinical remission or inactive disease has been recommended as a major treatment target in the most recent updates of the Assessment of SpondyloArthritis international Society (ASAS)/European League Against Rheumatism management recommendations for axSpA and treat-to-target recommendations for spondyloarthritis [8, 9]. Once this goal is achieved, clinical remission should ideally be maintained over time. Ankylosing Spondylitis Disease Activity Score inactive disease (ASDAS ID) is the preferred definition of clinical remission [9]; however, more data on the long-term impact of remission status on physical function and quality of life are needed [8].

Treatment options for axSpA include nonsteroidal anti-inflammatory drugs (NSAIDs) and biologic disease-modifying antirheumatic drugs that target tumor necrosis factor (TNF)-α (i.e., anti-TNF agents) [10] or interleukin (IL)-17 (i.e., anti-IL-17) [11, 12]. Only anti-TNFs have proven efficacy in patients with nr-axSpA to date [8]. Adalimumab was effective for the treatment of patients with nr-axSpA in the ABILITY-1 trial [13]. Greater improvements in disease activity, physical function, and health-related quality of life, as well as reduction of sacroiliac joint (SIJ) and spine inflammation, based on MRI findings were demonstrated after 12 weeks of adalimumab therapy compared with placebo. Positive week 12 results were further supported by sustained clinical response and remission data through year 2 of the study [14].

This paper reports the final efficacy and safety data from the open-label extension (OLE) of the ABILITY-1 study in patients with nr-axSpA who received adalimumab for up to 3 years. Specifically, we evaluated the relationship between clinical and MRI remission, as well as the impact of sustained clinical remission on long-term physical function.

Methods

Patients

Patients were ≥ 18 years old with nr-axSpA and fulfilled the ASAS classification criteria for axSpA [2] but did not meet the modified New York criteria for AS [1]. Patients had active disease based on a Bath Ankylosing Spondylitis Disease Activity Index (BASDAI) score ≥ 4 (0–10 score) and total back pain score ≥ 4 on a 0- to 10-cm visual analogue scale (VAS; ≥ 40 on a 0- to 100-mm VAS). Patients must have also had an inadequate response or intolerance to at least one NSAID or a contraindication for NSAIDs. More detailed inclusion and exclusion criteria are published elsewhere [13].

Study design

ABILITY-1 (ClinicalTrials.gov, NCT00939003) was a phase 3, multicenter, randomized, double-blind, placebo-controlled trial conducted at 37 sites in Australia, Europe, and North America. It was designed to evaluate the efficacy and safety of adalimumab in patients with nr-axSpA [13]. Data were collected from August 2009 through August 2013. Patients were randomized to subcutaneous adalimumab 40 mg every other week or placebo during a 12-week double-blind period, followed by a 144-week OLE in which patients received adalimumab 40 mg every other week for a total of 3 years of study participation. Study visits occurred at weeks 2 and 4, then every 4 weeks until week 28, every 8 weeks until week 68, every 12 weeks until week 140, and at week 156. The study was conducted with the approval of the appropriate institutional ethics review boards and with voluntary written informed patient consent, as well as in accordance with the International Conference on Harmonization good clinical practice guideline and the Declaration of Helsinki.

Clinical and safety assessments

The efficacy and safety outcomes through week 12 of treatment were previously published [13]. Clinical disease activity was measured using the BASDAI and the Ankylosing Spondylitis Disease Activity Score (ASDAS) based on C-reactive protein (CRP). Criteria for clinical remission included ASDAS ID, defined as ASDAS < 1.3 [15], and ASAS partial remission (ASAS PR), defined as a score < 2 (0–10 scale) for each of the four components of the ASAS response criteria [16]. Sustained clinical remission was defined as meeting the remission criteria of interest (ASDAS ID) at all available study visits during the respective study period: year 2 (between weeks 52 and 104), year 3 (between weeks 104 and 156), and during both years 2 and 3 (between weeks 52 and 156). Clinical response is presented using ASAS20 and ASAS40, defined as ≥ 20% and ≥ 40% improvement, respectively, and an absolute improvement from baseline of ≥ 1 and ≥ 2 units, respectively, in at least three of the following four domains without worsening (defined as ≥ 20% worsening and net worsening from baseline ≥ 1 unit for ASAS20 and no worsening at all for ASAS40) in the remaining domain: patient global assessment of disease activity (0- to 10-cm VAS), total back pain (0- to 10-cm VAS), Bath Ankylosing Spondylitis Functional Index (BASFI; 0- to 10-cm VAS), and inflammation/morning stiffness (mean score of items 5 and 6 of the BASDAI [0- to 10-cm VAS]) [17]. Physical function was measured using BASFI [18]; normal/patient acceptable physical function was defined as BASFI ≤ 3 [19].

MRI of the SIJ and spine was performed at baseline and weeks 12, 52, and 104. Two central readers blinded to radiographs, treatment, and time point independently scored all MRIs of an individual patient, first scoring the SIJ using the Spondyloarthritis Research Consortium of Canada (SPARCC) method for SIJ (0–72) [20], followed by the SPARCC six-discovertebral unit method for spine (0–108) [21]. MRI remission was defined as a SPARCC score < 2 for the SIJ, spine, or both. Treatment-emergent adverse events (AEs) were defined as AEs that began or worsened after the first dose of study medication through 70 days after the last dose.

Statistical methods

Clinical outcomes during the OLE were summarized in two ways: (1) by an observed case analysis of completers and (2) nonresponder imputation (NRI) for categorical variables or last observation carried forward (LOCF) analyses for continuous variables in the total efficacy population, which consisted of all randomized patients who received at least one dose of study drug (adalimumab or placebo). Subgroup analyses using the same methods were performed in patients with objective evidence of inflammation at baseline, defined as a SPARCC MRI score ≥ 2 for either the SIJ or spine or both, or elevated CRP (referred to as the *MRI/CRP-positive subpopulation*). In addition, key long-term clinical outcomes were also analyzed in the subgroup of patients without objective evidence of inflammation at baseline (referred to as the *MRI- and CRP-negative subpopulation*).

Mean changes from baseline in SPARCC MRI scores were calculated at weeks 52 and 104 for patients who achieved clinical remission at the same time points and compared with those who did not, using observed case analysis and analysis of variance. To assess the impact of sustained clinical remission on physical function, patients in the MRI/CRP-positive subpopulation with normal/abnormal physical function at baseline were grouped by achieving or not achieving sustained clinical remission during year 2, year 3, or throughout years 2 and 3 combined, and the proportions of patients with normal or abnormal physical function at years 2 and 3 (weeks 104 and 156) were compared by chi-square test (or Fisher's exact test if ≥ 20% of the cells had expected counts ≤ 5).

The safety population consisted of all randomized patients who received at least one dose of adalimumab during the study. AEs were summarized as the number and percentage of patients experiencing AEs and number of events per 100 patient-years of adalimumab exposure using the Medical Dictionary for Regulatory Activities (MedDRA®) version 15.1 system organ classes and preferred terms.

Results

Patient disposition and characteristics

Overall, 185 patients were included in the total efficacy population (adalimumab, n = 91; placebo, n = 94), and 142 patients were included in the MRI/CRP positive subpopulation (adalimumab, n = 69; placebo, n = 73) [13]; 42 patients had confirmed absence of MRI inflammation and normal CRP at baseline (MRI- and CRP-negative subpopulation); 1 patient who had normal CRP at baseline but missing baseline MRI assessment was excluded from the MRI- and CRP-negative subpopulation analyses but was included in the baseline data (Table 1). A total of 179 patients (adalimumab, n = 87 [96%]; placebo, n = 92 [98%]) from the total efficacy population and 139 patients (adalimumab, n = 68 [99%]; placebo, n = 71 [97%]) from the MRI/CRP-positive subpopulation completed the double-blind period and entered the OLE (Fig. 1). Similar proportions of patients in the total efficacy population (81%, 71% and 65%) and MRI/CRP-positive subpopulation (81%, 72%, and 68%) completed years 1, 2, and 3 of the OLE, respectively (Fig. 1). In the MRI- and CRP-negative subgroup, 57% of patients completed year 3.

The demographic and clinical characteristics were similar between the total efficacy population and the MRI/CRP-positive subpopulation (Table 1). Slightly more than half were female (55% and 54%, respectively), mean age was 38 years, and mean symptom duration was approximately 10 years. Patients had similar disease activity and impairment in physical function (Table 1). Among the 43 patients in the MRI- and CRP-negative population, including the 1 patient with normal CRP but missing MRI at baseline, mean ASDAS was slightly lower (most likely due to lower CRP), symptom duration was shorter, and a smaller proportion of patients were human leukocyte antigen (HLA)-B27-positive at baseline compared with the MRI/CRP-positive subpopulation (Table 1).

Maintenance of clinical and functional improvements through 3 years

The improvements in ASDAS and BASDAI with adalimumab treatment were similar and sustained in the MRI/CRP-positive subpopulation and the total efficacy population (Fig. 2). At week 156, mean (SD) ASDAS was 1.9 (1.2) and BASDAI was 3.3 (2.7) in the initial adalimumab group of the MRI/CRP-positive subpopulation (LOCF)

Table 1 Baseline demographics and disease characteristics

Characteristic, mean (SD)	Total efficacy population *(N* = 185)	MRI/CRP-positive subpopulation *(n* = 142)	MRI- and CRP-negative subpopulation *(n* = 43)[a]
Female, n (%)	101 (54.6)	77 (54.2)	24 (55.8)
Age, years	38.0 (10.8)	38.3 (11.1)	37.2 (10.1)
Symptom duration, years	10.0 (8.9)[b]	10.5 (9.4)[c]	8.3 (6.6)[d]
HLA-B27 positive, n (%)	145 (78.4)	114 (80.3)	31 (72.1)
BASDAI (0–10)	6.5 (1.5)	6.4 (1.5)	6.7 (1.5)
ASDAS (0–10)	3.3 (0.8)[e]	3.4 (0.8)[f]	2.9 (0.6)[d]
Patient Global Assessment of Disease Activity (0–10 cm VAS)	6.8 (1.8)	6.8 (1.9)	6.8 (1.8)
Physician Global Assessment of Disease Activity (0–10 cm VAS)	5.7 (1.6)[g]	5.6 (1.6)	6.1 (1.7)[h]
Total back pain (0–10 cm VAS)	6.9 (1.8)	6.8 (1.8)	7.3 (1.5)
BASFI (0–10)	4.7 (2.1)[g]	4.7 (2.2)[i]	4.8 (2.0)
Inflammation/morning stiffness[j] (0–10 cm VAS)	6.6 (2.0)	6.6 (2.1)	6.7 (1.7)
Elevated baseline CRP,[k] n (%)	48 (33.6)[l]	48 (46.2)[m]	0
CRP, [k] mg/L	7.2 (11.0)	9.0 (12.0)	1.4 (1.1)
SPARCC MRI score, SIJ	4.9 (9.7)[n]	6.3 (10.7)[c]	0.4 (0.5)[h]
SPARCC MRI score, spine	4.3 (5.8)[o]	5.5 (6.1)[p]	0.5 (0.6)[h]
HAQ-S (0–3)	1.0 (0.6)	1.0 (0.5)	1.1 (0.6)
BASMI linear (0–10)	2.7 (1.2)[g]	2.7 (1.3)[i]	2.7 (1.1)

Abbreviations: ASDAS Ankylosing Spondylitis Disease Activity Score, *BASDAI* Bath Ankylosing Spondylitis Disease Activity Index, *BASFI* Bath Ankylosing Spondylitis Functional Index, *BASMI* Bath Ankylosing Spondylitis Metrology Index, *CRP* C-reactive protein, *HAQ-S* Health Assessment Questionnaire for the Spondyloarthropathies, *HLA-B27* human leukocyte antigen B27, *MRI* Magnetic resonance imaging, *SPARCC* Spondyloarthritis Research Consortium of Canada, *VAS* Visual analogue scale
[a]The baseline data for the MRI- and CRP-negative subpopulation includes 42 patients with confirmed absence of MRI inflammation and normal CRP at baseline and 1 patient with normal CRP but missing baseline MRI,[b]*n* = 180,[c]*n* = 140,[d]*n* = 40,[e]*n* = 178,[f]*n* = 138,[g]*n* = 184,[h]*n* = 42,[i]*n* = 141,[j]Mean of BASDAI questions 5 and 6,[k]Based on either standard or high-sensitivity CRP values,[l]*n* = 143,[m]*n* = 104,[n]*n* = 182,[o]*n* = 181,[p]*n* = 139

(Figs. 2a and c); the mean (SD) changes from baseline to week 156 were – 1.4 [1.3] for ASDAS and – 3.1 [2.6] for BASDAI. Similar improvements in ASDAS and BASDAI were noted for the MRI- and CRP-negative subpopulation; at week 156, the mean (SD) ASDAS was 1.8 (1.0) and BASDAI was 3.7 (2.6), and the mean (SD) changes from baseline to week 156 were – 1.1 (1.0) for ASDAS and – 2.9 (2.7) for BASDAI (LOCF).

In the MRI/CRP-positive subpopulation, ASAS40 response was achieved by approximately half (NRI) or two-thirds (observed) of the patients through years 1, 2, and 3 (Additional file 1: Figure S1). Similar ASAS40 responses were observed in the total efficacy population, whereas ASAS40 response was lower in the MRI- and CRP-negative subpopulation (Additional file 1: Figure S1).

The improvements in physical function were also sustained with adalimumab treatment through 3 years. In the MRI/CRP-positive subpopulation, the mean (SD) BASFI score at week 156 was 2.8 (2.6) and mean (SD) change from baseline to week 156 was – 1.7 (2.2) in the initial adalimumab group (LOCF) (Fig. 3a). Improvements in physical function were comparable in the total efficacy population (Fig. 3b) and in the MRI- and CRP-negative subpopulation (mean [SD] BASFI at week 156, 3.0 [2.5]; mean [SD] change from baseline to week 156, – 1.9 [2.5]; LOCF).

Maintenance of MRI improvements through 2 years

There was a significant reduction in both SPARCC MRI SIJ and spinal inflammation scores from baseline to 1 and 2 years in the MRI/CRP-positive subpopulation and total efficacy population (all $P < 0.001$). Among patients in both populations who had both year 1 and year 2 MRI scans available, sustained improvements in MRI inflammation were evident through year 2 (Table 2).

Clinical and MRI remission achievement and agreement

Clinical remission rates were maintained through 3 years in both the MRI/CRP-positive subpopulation and the total efficacy population (Fig. 4). In the MRI/CRP-positive subpopulation among patients receiving adalimumab throughout 3 years, 32% and 30% of patients achieved ASAS PR and 35% and 30% achieved ASDAS ID at years 2 and 3, respectively, using NRI analysis. The rates were 45% and 46% for ASAS PR and 49% and 46% for ASDAS ID at years 2 and 3, respectively, by observed data (Fig. 4a and c). In the MRI- and CRP-negative subpopulation, 14% and 17% of patients achieved ASAS PR (NRI) at years 2 and 3, respectively, and 29% and 24%, respectively, achieved ASDAS ID (NRI).

The mean SIJ SPARCC MRI scores decreased significantly more ($P < 0.001$) from baseline to years 1 and 2 in patients in clinical remission (ASDAS ID) than in

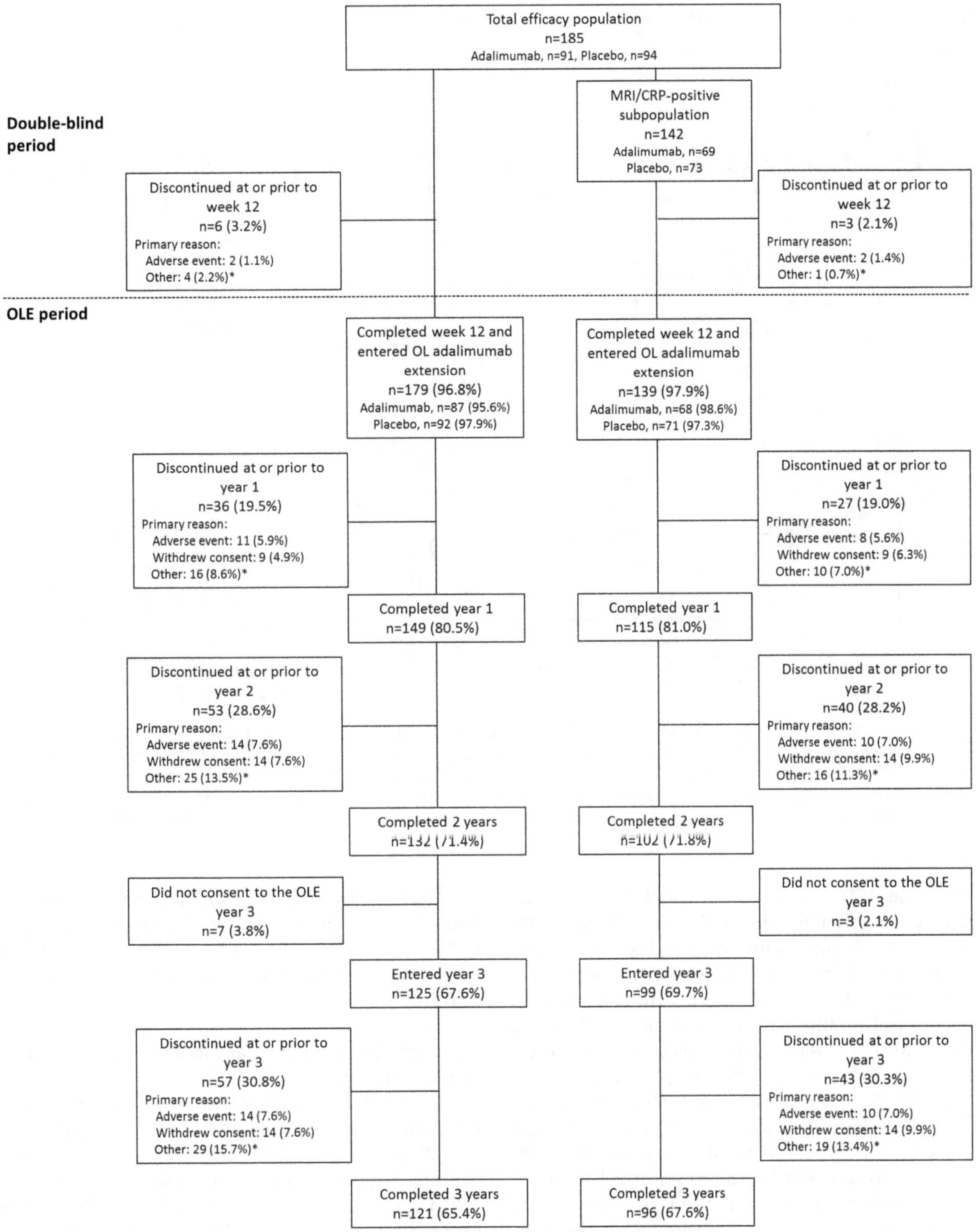

Fig. 1 Patient disposition in the total efficacy and MRI/CRP-positive populations over 3 years. *Other reasons included lack of efficacy, pregnancy, investigator decision, patient moved, and protocol violation. OL Open label, OLE Open-label extension

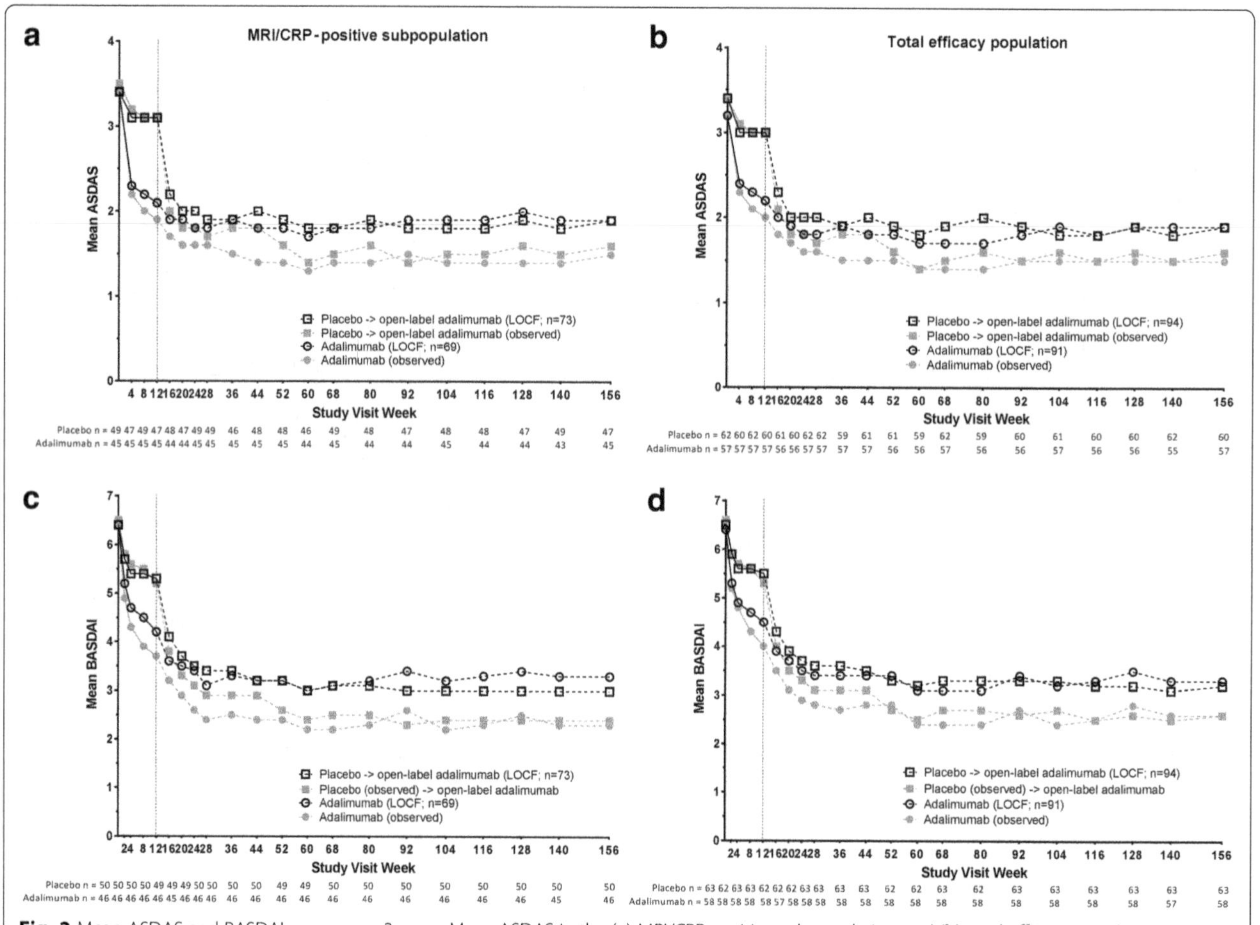

Fig. 2 Mean ASDAS and BASDAI scores over 3 years. Mean ASDAS in the (**a**) MRI/CRP-positive subpopulation and (**b**) total efficacy population and mean BASDAI in the (**c**) MRI/CRP-positive subpopulation and (**d**) total efficacy population. Observed data (closed gray symbols) and LOCF data (open black symbols) through 3 years of OLE. Dashed line represents the start of the open-label adalimumab period; n values below the x-axis are for observed data at each visit, and n values in the figure legend are for the LOCF data. ASDAS Ankylosing Spondylitis Disease Activity Score, BASDAI Bath Ankylosing Spondylitis Disease Activity Index, CRP C-reactive protein, LOCF last observation carried forward, MRI magnetic resonance imaging

those not in ASDAS ID at years 1 and 2 (Fig. 5a and b). The reductions from baseline in the spine SPARCC MRI scores were not significantly different between patients who achieved clinical remission and those who did not.

Among patients in the MRI/CRP-positive subpopulation who had positive baseline MRI for the SIJ, spine, or both, MRI remission in the respective location was achieved by 65%, 48%, and 41% of patients at year 1, and by 71%, 52%, and 50% at year 2 (observed). Among patients in clinical remission (ASDAS ID) who had positive baseline MRI for the SIJ, spine, or both, MRI remission was achieved by 73%, 53%, and 40% of patients, respectively, at year 1, and by 68%, 68%, and 44% at year 2 (Additional file 1: Figure S2a). Similarly, among patients in MRI remission who had positive baseline MRI for the SIJ, spine, or both, clinical remission (ASDAS ID) was achieved by 67%, 50%, and 67%, respectively, at year 1, and by 58%, 63%, and 62% at year 2 (Additional file 1: Figure S2b). Of the patients who had positive baseline MRI for the SIJ, spine, or both, and who did not achieve clinical remission, 56%, 43%, and 44% had MRI remission of the SIJ, spine, or both, respectively, at year 1, as did 74%, 35%, and 56% at year 2.

Sustained clinical remission and its impact on long-term physical function

Sustained clinical remission (defined as ASDAS ID at all time points) was achieved by 34 of 142 (24%) patients in year 2 (between weeks 52 and 104), 32 of 142 (23%) patients in year 3 (between weeks 104 and 152), and 25 of 142 (18%) patients through both years 2 and 3 (between weeks 52 and 156) in the MRI/CRP-positive subpopulation (NRI analysis). At baseline, 102 patients in the MRI/CRP-positive subpopulation had abnormal physical function (BASFI score > 3); among these patients, normal function was achieved by 48 of 78 (62%) patients at year 2 and 42 of 71 (59%) patients at year 3. Among patients with

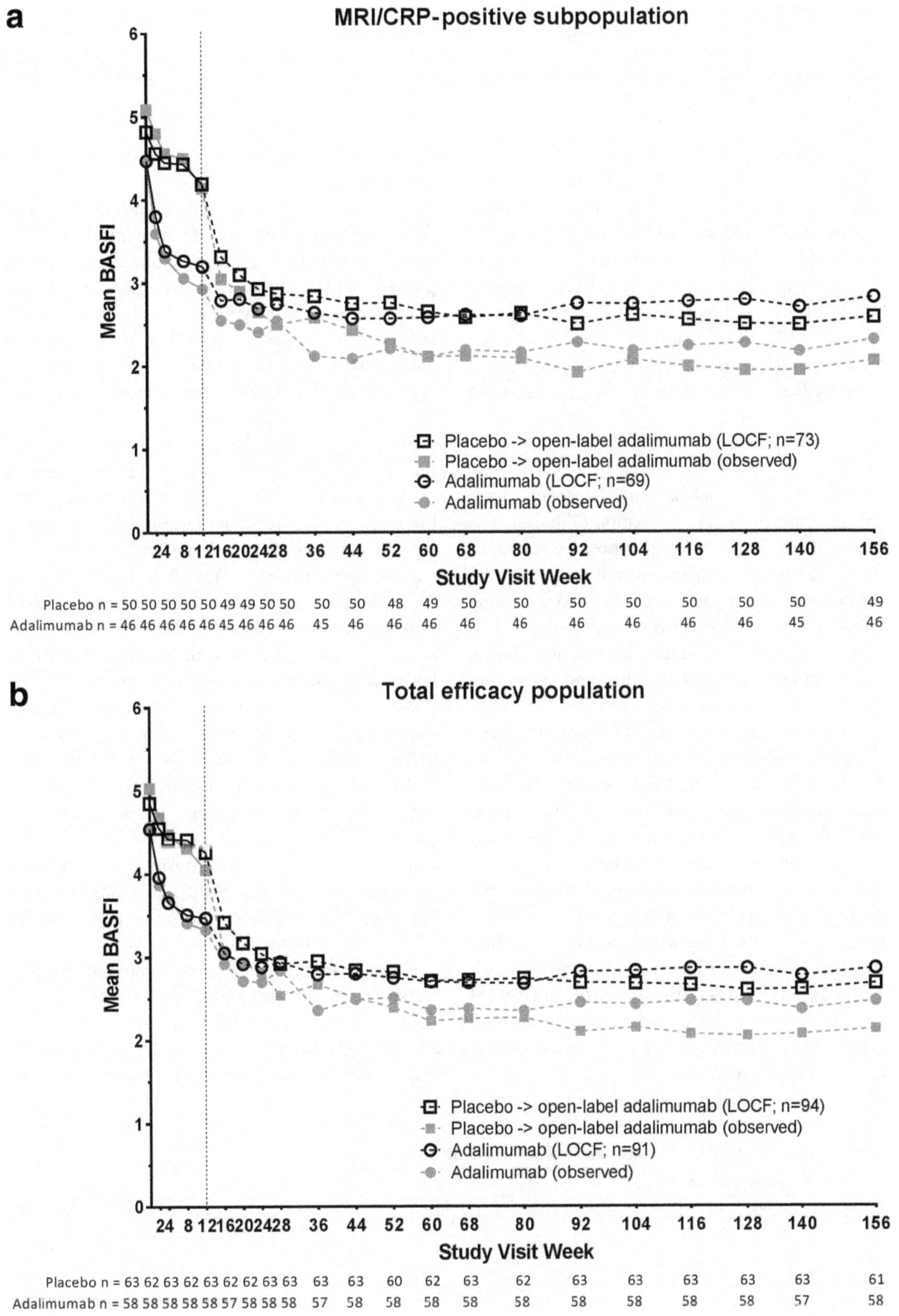

Fig. 3 (See legend on next page.)

(See figure on previous page.)

Fig. 3 Mean BASFI scores over 3 years. Mean BASFI in the (**a**) MRI/CRP-positive subpopulation and (**b**) total efficacy population. Observed data (closed gray symbols) and LOCF data (open black symbols) through 3 years of OLE. Dashed lines represent the start of the open-label adalimumab period; n values below the x-axis are for observed data at each visit, and n values in the figure legend are for the LOCF data. BASFI Bath Ankylosing Spondylitis Functional Index, CRP C-reactive protein, LOCF last observation carried forward, MRI magnetic resonance imaging

abnormal physical function at baseline, all patients in sustained clinical remission during year 2, year 3, or through both years 2 and 3 achieved normal function (20 of 20, 19 of 19, and 14 of 14, respectively) compared with less than half of the patients not in sustained clinical remission (28 of 58 [48%], 23 of 52 [44%], and 28 of 57 [49%], respectively; all $P < 0.001$) (Fig. 6). All patients with normal physical function at baseline (n = 39) maintained normal function at years 2 and 3, regardless of being in remission or not.

Safety

Over 400 patient-years of adalimumab exposure were included in the long-term safety evaluation (Table 3). The types and rates of AEs in the MRI/CRP-positive subpopulation were similar to those in the overall study population. No incidents of malignancy, vasculitis, demyelinating disease, or reactivation of hepatitis B were reported.

One patient experienced a lupus-like reaction during the OLE, presenting with facial flushing and joint pain associated with a positive antinuclear antibody and anti-double-stranded DNA. Adalimumab was discontinued because of the event, and symptoms improved. One patient with a family history of deep vein thrombosis (DVT), who was receiving hormonal birth control and had a prior event of DVT during the study, developed a pulmonary embolism. The patient discontinued the hormonal contraceptive device and was able to restart open-label adalimumab treatment after a temporary interruption.

There were two deaths. One was a suicide of a man with a history of heavy alcohol use and anxiety; his death occurred 40 days after discontinuation of open-label adalimumab. Another patient died of cardiorespiratory failure related to recreational opiate toxicity during open-label adalimumab treatment.

Discussion

The results of the long-term extension of the ABILITY-1 study demonstrated sustained clinical and functional improvements through 3 years of adalimumab therapy in patients with nr-axSpA. Furthermore, there was a sustained reduction in MRI axial inflammation, which was significantly greater in the SIJ of patients who achieved clinical remission than in those not in remission. Sustained clinical remission was associated with attainment of normal physical function.

In contrast to AS, there is still limited understanding of the disease course and appropriate long-term management of patients with nr-axSpA. The present work adds to the body of evidence that clinical and MRI improvements can be maintained with long-term anti-TNF therapy in patients with nr-axSpA classified by ASAS criteria [22, 23]. Further, it provides important insights into the relationship between clinical and MRI remission in nr-axSpA, as well as the significance of sustained clinical remission for achieving normal physical function.

We evaluated the efficacy outcomes separately in the total efficacy population (n = 185) and subpopulation of patients with objective signs of inflammation at baseline (MRI/CRP-positive subpopulation; n = 142) for whom anti-TNF therapy, including adalimumab, is currently approved. No major differences were observed in the results, with the MRI/CRP-positive subpopulation representing 77% of the total efficacy population. For completeness, we also provided information for the MRI- and CRP-negative subpopulation.

Throughout the OLE, approximately two-thirds (as observed) or nearly half (NRI) of the patients in the MRI/CRP-positive subpopulation achieved ASAS40 response. Almost half (observed) or around one-third (NRI) of patients were in clinical remission measured as either ASAS

Table 2 Mean baseline and changes from baseline in SPARCC MRI SIJ and spine scores

Mean (95% CI)	MRI/CRP-positive subpopulation		Total efficacy population	
	SPARCC MRI SIJ (n = 102)	SPARCC MRI spine (n = 101)	SPARCC MRI SIJ (n = 131)	SPARCC MRI spine (n = 130)
Baseline	6.2 (4.1–8.2)	4.3 (3.3–5.4)	5.0 (3.3–6.6)	3.5 (2.6–4.3)
Change from baseline to:				
Year 1	− 5.0 (− 6.9 to − 3.1)	− 1.9 (− 2.8 to − 1.0)	− 3.9 (− 5.5 to − 2.4)	− 1.3 (− 2.1 to − 0.5)
Year 2	− 4.8 (− 6.9 to − 2.8)	− 2.0 (− 2.9 to − 1.1)	− 3.8 (− 5.4 to − 2.2)	− 1.4 (− 2.2 to − 0.7)

Abbreviations: CRP C-reactive protein, *MRI* Magnetic resonance imaging, *SIJ* Sacroiliac joint, *SPARCC* Spondyloarthritis Research Consortium of Canada
Data for patients in the MRI/CRP-positive subpopulation and total efficacy population with MRI scans available at all time points

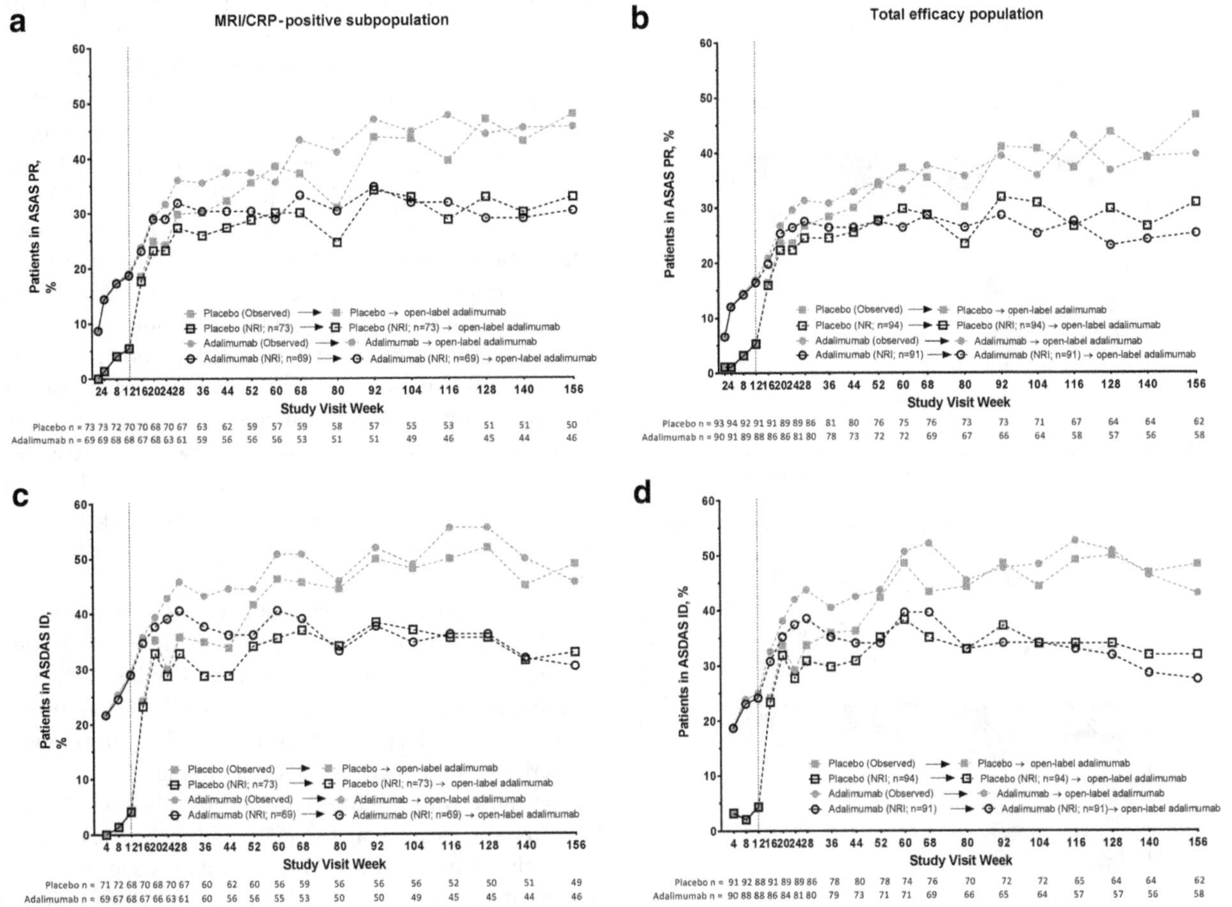

Fig. 4 Proportion of patients achieving clinical remission over 3 years. ASAS partial remission in the (**a**) MRI/CRP-positive subpopulation and (**b**) total efficacy population and ASDAS ID (ASDAS < 1.3) in the (**c**) MRI/CRP-positive subpopulation and (**d**) total efficacy population. Observed data are shown with closed gray symbols and NRI data with open black symbols; the dashed line represents the start of the open-label adalimumab period. n Values below the x-axis are for observed data at each visit. n Values in the figure legend are for NRI data; patients who permanently discontinued at or prior to week 12 (double-blind phase) were excluded from open-label phase analyses (MRI/CRP-positive subpopulation, $n = 3$; total efficacy population, $n = 6$). ASAS Assessment of SpondyloArthritis international Society, ASDAS Ankylosing Spondylitis Disease Activity Score, CRP C-reactive protein, ID Inactive disease, MRI Magnetic resonance imaging, NRI Nonresponder imputation

PR or ASDAS ID at the end of the study. Furthermore, sustained clinical remission, defined as achieving ASDAS ID at all available visits, was seen in nearly one-fourth of patients through each of year 2 and year 3, with 18% of patients in sustained ASDAS ID throughout both years 2 and 3.

Although the clinical improvements observed in the small MRI- and CRP-negative subpopulation ($n = 42$) were generally smaller than in the MRI/CRP-positive subpopulation, it appears that some patients without objective evidence of inflammation at baseline responded to adalimumab treatment and maintained clinical improvements through 3 years. However, interpretation should be done with caution because of the small number of patients in this group.

MRI scans taken at 1 and 2 years showed a significant and sustained suppression of inflammation in both the SIJ and spine. An interesting observation was an apparent better responsiveness of the MRI inflammation in the SIJ than in the spine to adalimumab treatment. The reductions in the mean SPARCC MRI scores were relatively larger, and a higher proportion of patients achieved MRI remission (SPARCC MRI score < 2) in the SIJ than in the spine among patients with positive MRI at baseline; SIJ vs spine MRI remission rates were 65% vs 48% and 71% vs 52% at years 1 and 2, respectively. There also seemed to be a better numerical agreement between clinical and MRI remission in the SIJ than in the spine. Among patients with positive baseline MRI, a larger proportion of patients in clinical remission (ASDAS ID) reached MRI remission in the SIJ than in the spine at year 1 (73% vs 53%). Furthermore, significantly greater mean improvements from baseline were observed at years 1 and 2 for the SIJ SPARCC MRI scores

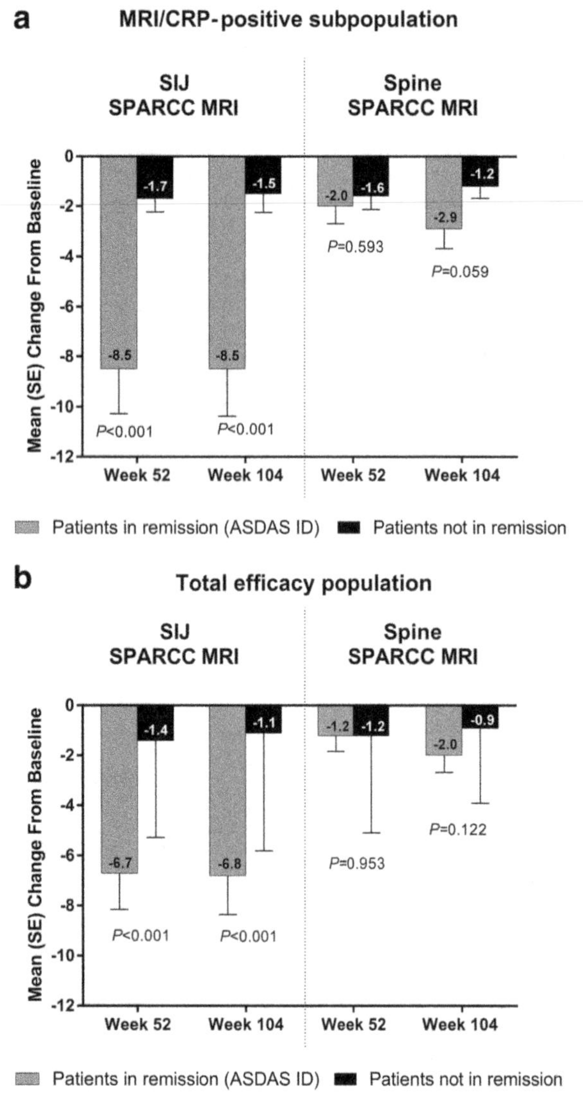

Fig. 5 Change from baseline in SPARCC MRI scores among patients who achieved clinical remission. Mean (SE) change from baseline in the SIJ and spine SPARCC MRI scores in patients who achieved ASDAS ID vs those who did not in the (**a**) MRI/CRP-positive subpopulation and (**b**) total efficacy population at years 1 and 2. Observed data. *P* values for comparison of patients in remission vs patients not in remission from analysis of variance. ASDAS ID Ankylosing Spondylitis Disease Activity Score inactive disease, CRP C-reactive protein, MRI Magnetic resonance imaging, SIJ Sacroiliac joint, SPARCC Spondyloarthritis Research Consortium of Canada

in patients achieving ASDAS ID than in those not in ASDAS ID. The differences between patients in ASDAS ID vs those not in ASDAS ID were not significant for the spine SPARCC MRI scores.

Of note, the baseline MRI scores were numerically greater in the SIJ than in the spine, especially in the MRI/CRP-positive subpopulation, in spite of the mean symptom duration of around 10 years in this nr-axSpA population. It is generally believed that axial inflammation starts in the SIJ and then involves the spine in axSpA [24], but there was still considerable inflammation in the SIJ in this nr-axSpA study population. Another possible explanation for the somewhat lower effect on the spine MRI scores is that not all the lesions detected in the spine were specific for axSpA [25] or were responsive to anti-TNF treatment. It is also interesting that in the EMBARK study with etanercept in nr-axSpA, more patients achieved MRI remission in the spine than in SIJ after 2 years in a cohort with much shorter symptom duration (mean 2.4 years) [23]. However, the differences between the proportions of patients achieving either remission in the SIJ or spine were not significant between those with or without sustained ASDAS ID or low disease activity in that study. The definitions of MRI remission were less stringent, especially for the spine, in the EMBARK study than in the ABILITY-1 study [23].

A discordance between clinical and MRI disease activity in axSpA has been noted before [26–28]. In our study, only 40% and 44% of patients with positive baseline MRI who achieved ASDAS ID also attained overall MRI remission (both in SIJ and spine) at years 1 and 2, respectively. Numerically more patients achieving overall MRI remission among those with positive baseline MRI also met ASDAS ID criteria at years 1 and 2 (67% and 62%, respectively). Currently, clinical and not MRI remission is suggested as a treatment target [8, 9] because the impact of persistent MRI inflammation in the SIJ or spine on long-term physical function or structural progression in patients with axSpA who are in clinical remission is unknown. Further studies are needed in this area.

Evidence that has accumulated over the past few years in AS suggests a direct relationship of clinical disease activity with physical function and syndesmophyte formation [29–31]. The long-term impact of achieving and maintaining clinical remission in nr-axSpA has not previously been evaluated. Our results demonstrate the importance of sustained clinical remission (defined as ASDAS ID) for achieving normal physical function over time. All patients in sustained clinical remission achieved normal physical function at years 2 and 3, as compared with only 44–49% of patients not in sustained clinical remission. All patients with normal physical function at baseline maintained it until the end of the OLE with adalimumab, regardless of achieving sustained clinical remission or not. The total number of patients with normal physical function at baseline was small, however, and no definite conclusions can be drawn on the importance of sustained clinical remission for the maintenance of normal physical function. It also needs to be noted that our definition of sustained clinical remission was very strict, requiring ASDAS ID at all study visits. Our findings lend further

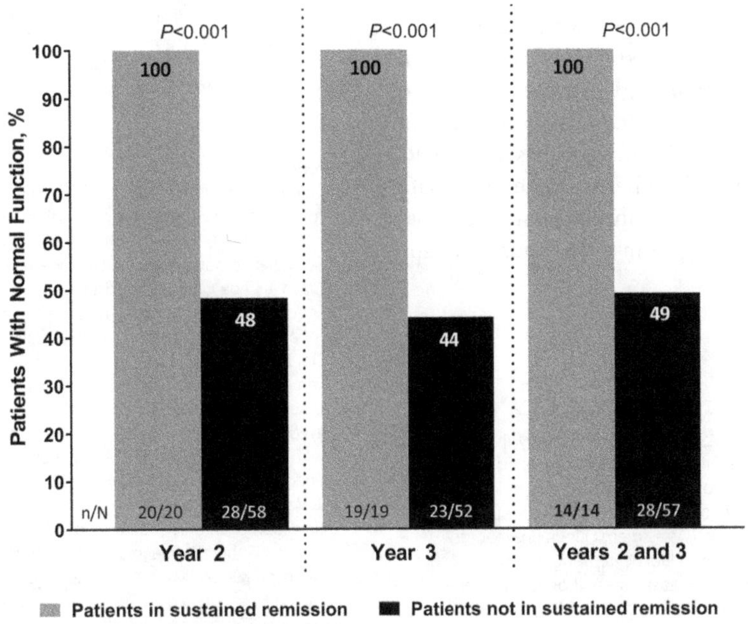

Fig. 6 Patients in sustained remission achieving normal physical function at years 2 and 3. Analysis of patients in the MRI/CRP-positive subpopulation with abnormal physical function at baseline (normal function defined as BASFI ≤ 3). Sustained clinical remission was defined as achieving ASDAS < 1.3 at all available visits during year 2 (from week 52 to week 104), during year 3 (from week 104 to week 156), and during both years 2 and 3 (from week 52 to week 156). ASDAS Ankylosing Spondylitis Disease Activity Score, BASFI Bath Ankylosing Spondylitis Functional Index, CRP C-reactive protein, MRI Magnetic resonance imaging

support to ASDAS ID as a clinically meaningful definition of clinical remission [32]. They also substantiate the treat-to-target recommendation that once the target of clinical remission is achieved, remission should ideally be maintained throughout the patient's disease course [9].

It is known that the extent of structural damage along with the degree of inflammation measured by disease activity determine physical function in AS [28, 29]. Limitations of our analyses include the lack of assessment of structural damage, which made it impossible to correlate sustained clinical remission or MRI remission with structural progression. MRI was also not performed at year 3, limiting the analyses of MRI findings to the years 1 and 2 time points. Safety data collected over 3 years did not reveal new safety concerns in nr-axSpA compared with the known safety profile of adalimumab in other immune-mediated inflammatory diseases, particularly in AS [33].

Table 3 Rates of adverse events of interest through 3 years of treatment

AE	Overall safety population (*n* = 190; 412.2 patient-years)		MRI/CRP-positive safety subpopulation (*n* = 145; 320.9 patient-years)	
	No. (%)	Events/100 patient-years	No. (%)	Events/100 patient-years
Serious AEs	33 (17.4)	10.9	25 (17.2)	9.7
Serious infection	8 (4.2)	2.4	6 (4.1)	2.2
Tuberculosis	1 (0.5)	0.2	1 (0.7)	0.3
Lupus-like reaction and systemic lupus erythematosus	1 (0.5)	0.2	1 (0.7)	0.3
Pulmonary embolism	1 (0.5)	0.2	1 (0.7)	0.3
New-onset psoriasis	2 (1.1)	0.5	1 (0.7)	0.3
Hepatic-related AEs	2 (1.1)	0.5	1 (0.7)	0.3
Diverticulitis	1 (0.5)	0.2	1 (0.7)	0.3
Death	2 (1.1)	0.5	2 (1.4)	0.6

Abbreviations: AE Adverse event, *CRP* C-reactive protein, *MRI* Magnetic resonance imaging

Includes all patients who received at least one dose of adalimumab, including patients who were excluded from the efficacy analyses because of noncompliance at the investigative site

Conclusions

Treatment of patients with nr-axSpA with adalimumab over 3 years demonstrated sustained clinical remission in a substantial proportion of patients, which was associated with the achievement or maintenance of normal physical function. Clinical remission and remission based on MRI were only partly concordant. Together with the safety data from the ABILITY-1 study, our findings support the favorable benefit-risk profile of long-term adalimumab therapy in patients with nr-axSpA.

Abbreviations

AE: Adverse event; AS: Ankylosing spondylitis; ASAS: Assessment of SpondyloArthritis international Society; ASDAS: Ankylosing Spondylitis Disease Activity Score; axSpA: Axial spondyloarthritis; BASDAI: Bath Ankylosing Spondylitis Disease Activity Index; BASFI: Bath Ankylosing Spondylitis Functional Index; BASMI: Bath Ankylosing Spondylitis Metrology Index; CRP: C-reactive protein; DVT: Deep vein thrombosis; HAQ-S: Health Assessment Questionnaire for the Spondyloarthropathies; HLA-B27: Human leukocyte antigen B27; ID: Inactive disease; IL: Interleukin; LOCF: Last observation carried forward; MedDRA: Medical Dictionary for Regulatory Activities; MRI: Magnetic resonance imaging; nr-axSpA: Nonradiographic axial spondyloarthritis; NRI: Nonresponder imputation; NSAID: Nonsteroidal anti-inflammatory drug; OLE: Open-label extension; PR: Partial remission; SIJ: Sacroiliac joint; SPARCC: Spondyloarthritis Research Consortium of Canada; TNF: Tumor necrosis factor; VAS: Visual analogue scale

Acknowledgements

Medical writing support was provided by Kathleen V. Kastenholz, PharmD, MS, of AbbVie, and by Maria Hovenden, PhD, and Tiffany Brake, PhD, of Complete Publication Solutions, LLC. This support was funded by AbbVie.

Funding

AbbVie funded the study (ClinicalTrials.gov, NCT00939003); contributed to its design; and was involved in the collection, analysis, and interpretation of the data, as well as in the writing, review, and approval of the publication.

Authors' contributions

ALP, JS, DvdH, WPM, and RGL conceived of and designed the study. ALP, JKA, and RGL acquired data. SC performed statistical analysis. All authors analyzed and interpreted data, drafted the manuscript, and critically revised the manuscript for important intellectual content. All authors read and approved the final manuscript.

Competing interests

DvdH has received consulting fees from AbbVie, Amgen, Astellas, AstraZeneca, BMS, Boehringer Ingelheim, Celgene, Daiichi, Eli Lilly, Galapagos, Gilead, GlaxoSmithKline, Janssen, Merck, Novartis, Pfizer, Regeneron, Roche, Sanofi, Takeda, and UCB and is director of Imaging Rheumatology B.V. JS has received research grants, consulting fees, and speaker's fees from AbbVie, Merck, Pfizer, and UCB. WPM has received research grants and consulting fees from AbbVie, Amgen, Eli Lilly, Janssen, Merck, Novartis, Pfizer, SYNARC, and UCB and is chief medical officer of CaRE Arthritis. RGL has received consulting or advisory board fees from AbbVie, BioClinica, Janssen, Parexel, and UCB. SC, MH, JKA, and ALP are full-time employees of AbbVie and may hold stock and/or options.

Author details

[1]Leiden University Medical Center, PO Box 9600, Leiden 2300 RC, The Netherlands. [2]Charité Universitätsmedizin Berlin, Berlin, Germany. [3]University of Alberta, Edmonton, AB, Canada. [4]AbbVie Inc., North Chicago, IL, USA. [5]AbbVie Inc., Ljubljana, Slovenia.

References

1. van der Linden S, Valkenburg HA, Cats A. Evaluation of diagnostic criteria for ankylosing spondylitis: a proposal for modification of the New York criteria. Arthritis Rheum. 1984;27(4):361–8.
2. Rudwaleit M, van der Heijde D, Landewé R, Listing J, Akkoc N, Brandt J, Braun J, Chou CT, Collantes-Estevez E, Dougados M, et al. The development of Assessment of SpondyloArthritis international Society classification criteria for axial spondyloarthritis (part II): validation and final selection. Ann Rheum Dis. 2009;68(6):777–83.
3. van der Heijde D, Machado P, Braun J, Hermann KG, Baraliakos X, Hsu B, Baker D, Landewé R. MRI inflammation at the vertebral unit only marginally predicts new syndesmophyte formation: a multilevel analysis in patients with ankylosing spondylitis. Ann Rheum Dis. 2012;71(3):369–73.
4. Poddubnyy D, Gaydukova I, Hermann KG, Song IH, Haibel H, Braun J, Sieper J. Magnetic resonance imaging compared to conventional radiographs for detection of chronic structural changes in sacroiliac joints in axial spondyloarthritis. J Rheumatol. 2013;40(9):1557–65.
5. Hermann KG, Baraliakos X, van der Heijde DM, Jurik AG, Landewé R, Marzo-Ortega H, Ostergaard M, Rudwaleit M, Sieper J, Braun J, et al. Descriptions of spinal MRI lesions and definition of a positive MRI of the spine in axial spondyloarthritis: a consensual approach by the ASAS/OMERACT MRI study group. Ann Rheum Dis. 2012;71(8):1278–88.
6. Rudwaleit M, Jurik AG, Hermann KG, Landewé R, van der Heijde D, Baraliakos X, Marzo-Ortega H, Ostergaard M, Braun J, Sieper J. Defining active sacroiliitis on magnetic resonance imaging (MRI) for classification of axial spondyloarthritis: a consensual approach by the ASAS/OMERACT MRI group. Ann Rheum Dis. 2009;68(10):1520–7.
7. Weber U, Lambert RG, Ostergaard M, Hodler J, Pedersen SJ, Maksymowych WP. The diagnostic utility of magnetic resonance imaging in spondylarthritis: an international multicenter evaluation of one hundred eighty-seven subjects. Arthritis Rheum. 2010;62(10):3048–58.
8. van der Heijde D, Ramiro S, Landewé R, Baraliakos X, Van den Bosch F, Sepriano A, Regel A, Ciurea A, Dagfinrud H, Dougados M, et al. 2016 Update of the ASAS-EULAR management recommendations for axial spondyloarthritis. Ann Rheum Dis. 2017;76(6):978–91.
9. Smolen JS, Schols M, Braun J, Dougados M, FitzGerald O, Gladman DD, Kavanaugh A, Landewé R, Mease P, Sieper J, et al. Treating axial spondyloarthritis and peripheral spondyloarthritis, especially psoriatic arthritis, to target: 2017 update of recommendations by an international task force. Ann Rheum Dis. 2018;77(1):3–17.
10. van der Heijde D, Sieper J, Maksymowych WP, Dougados M, Burgos-Vargas R, Landewé R, Rudwaleit M, Braun J. Assessment of SpondyloArthritis international Society. 2010 Update of the international ASAS recommendations for the use of anti-TNF agents in patients with axial spondyloarthritis. Ann Rheum Dis. 2011;70(6):905–8.
11. Baeten D, Sieper J, Braun J, Baraliakos X, Dougados M, Emery P, Deodhar A, Porter B, Martin R, Andersson M, et al. Secukinumab, an interleukin-17A inhibitor, in ankylosing spondylitis. N Engl J Med. 2015;373(26):2534–48.
12. Lubrano E, Perrotta FM. Secukinumab for ankylosing spondylitis and psoriatic arthritis. Ther Clin Risk Manag. 2016;12:1587–92.
13. Sieper J, van der Heijde D, Dougados M, Mease PJ, Maksymowych WP, Brown MA, Arora V, Pangan AL. Efficacy and safety of adalimumab in patients with non-radiographic axial spondyloarthritis: results of a randomised placebo-controlled trial (ABILITY-1). Ann Rheum Dis. 2013;72(6):815–22.
14. Sieper J, Baeten DL, Van den Bosch F, Rathmann SS, Anderson J, Pangan AL. Sustained clinical remission in patients with non-radiographic axial spondyloarthritis after two years of adalimumab treatment [abstract]. Rheumatology. 2014;53(Suppl 1):i140.
15. Machado P, Landewé R, Lie E, Kvien TK, Braun J, Baker D, van der Heijde D. Assessment of SpondyloArthritis international Society. Ankylosing Spondylitis Disease Activity Score (ASDAS): defining cut-off values for disease activity states and improvement scores. Ann Rheum Dis. 2011;70(1):47–53.

16. Anderson JJ, Baron G, van der Heijde D, Felson DT, Dougados M. Ankylosing spondylitis assessment group preliminary definition of short-term improvement in ankylosing spondylitis. Arthritis Rheum. 2001;44(8):1876–86.
17. Sieper J, Rudwaleit M, Baraliakos X, Brandt J, Braun J, Burgos-Vargas R, Dougados M, Hermann KG, Landewé R, Maksymowych W, et al. The Assessment of SpondyloArthritis international Society (ASAS) handbook: a guide to assess spondyloarthritis. Ann Rheum Dis. 2009;68(Suppl 2):ii1–44.
18. Calin A, Garrett S, Whitelock H, Kennedy LG, O'Hea J, Mallorie P, Jenkinson T. A new approach to defining functional ability in ankylosing spondylitis: the development of the Bath Ankylosing Spondylitis Functional Index. J Rheumatol. 1994;21(12):2281–5.
19. Maksymowych WP, Gooch K, Dougados M, Wong RL, Chen N, Kupper H, van der Heijde D. Thresholds of patient-reported outcomes that define the patient acceptable symptom state in ankylosing spondylitis vary over time and by treatment and patient characteristics. Arthritis Care Res (Hoboken). 2010;62(6):826–34.
20. Maksymowych WP, Inman RD, Salonen D, Dhillon SS, Williams M, Stone M, Conner-Spady B, Palsat J, Lambert RG. Spondyloarthritis Research Consortium of Canada magnetic resonance imaging index for assessment of sacroiliac joint inflammation in ankylosing spondylitis. Arthritis Rheum. 2005;53(5):703–9.
21. Maksymowych WP, Inman RD, Salonen D, Dhillon SS, Krishnananthan R, Stone M, Conner-Spady B, Palsat J, Lambert RG. Spondyloarthritis Research Consortium of Canada magnetic resonance imaging index for assessment of spinal inflammation in ankylosing spondylitis. Arthritis Rheum. 2005;53(4):502–9.
22. van der Heijde D, Dougados M, Landewé R, Sieper J, Maksymowych WP, Rudwaleit M, Van den Bosch F, Braun J, Mease PJ, Kivitz AJ, et al. Sustained efficacy, safety and patient-reported outcomes of certolizumab pegol in axial spondyloarthritis: 4-year outcomes from RAPID-axSpA. Rheumatology (Oxford). 2017;56(9):1498–509.
23. Dougados M, van der Heijde D, Sieper J, Braun J, Citera G, Lenaerts J, van den Bosch F, Wei JC, Pedersen R, Bonin R, et al. Effects of long-term etanercept treatment on clinical outcomes and objective signs of inflammation in early non-radiographic axial spondyloarthritis: 104-week results from the EMBARK study. Arthritis Care Res (Hoboken). 2017;69(10):1590–8.
24. Sieper J, van der Heijde D. Nonradiographic axial spondyloarthritis: new definition of an old disease? Arthritis Rheum. 2013;65(3):543–51.
25. de Hooge M, de Bruin F, de Beer L, Bakker P, van den Berg R, Ramiro S, van Gaalen F, Fagerli K, Landewé R, van Oosterhout M, et al. Is the site of back pain related to the location of magnetic resonance imaging lesions in patients with chronic back pain? Results from the Spondyloarthritis Caught Early Cohort. Arthritis Care Res (Hoboken). 2017;69(5):717–23.
26. Lambert RG, Salonen D, Rahman P, Inman RD, Wong RL, Einstein SG, Thomson GT, Beaulieu A, Choquette D, Maksymowych WP. Adalimumab significantly reduces both spinal and sacroiliac joint inflammation in patients with ankylosing spondylitis: a multicenter, randomized, double-blind, placebo-controlled study. Arthritis Rheum. 2007;56(12):4005–14.
27. Kiltz U, Baraliakos X, Karakostas P, Igelmann M, Kalthoff L, Klink C, Krause D, Schmitz-Bortz E, Florecke M, Bollow M, et al. The degree of spinal inflammation is similar in patients with axial spondyloarthritis who report high or low levels of disease activity: a cohort study. Ann Rheum Dis. 2012;71(7):1207–11.
28. Machado P, Landewé RB, Braun J, Baraliakos X, Hermann KG, Hsu B, Baker D, van der Heijde D. MRI inflammation and its relation with measures of clinical disease activity and different treatment responses in patients with ankylosing spondylitis treated with a tumour necrosis factor inhibitor. Ann Rheum Dis. 2012;71(12):2002–5.
29. Landewé R, Dougados M, Mielants H, van der Tempel H, van der Heijde D. Physical function in ankylosing spondylitis is independently determined by both disease activity and radiographic damage of the spine. Ann Rheum Dis. 2009;68(6):863–7.
30. Ramiro S, van der Heijde D, van Tubergen A, Stolwijk C, Dougados M, van den Bosch F, Landewé R. Higher disease activity leads to more structural damage in the spine in ankylosing spondylitis: 12-year longitudinal data from the OASIS cohort. Ann Rheum Dis. 2014;73(8):1455–61.
31. Poddubnyy D, Protopopov M, Haibel H, Braun J, Rudwaleit M, Sieper J. High disease activity according to the Ankylosing Spondylitis Disease Activity Score is associated with accelerated radiographic spinal progression in patients with early axial spondyloarthritis: results from the GErman SPondyloarthritis Inception Cohort. Ann Rheum Dis. 2016;75(12):2114–8.
32. van der Heijde D, Joshi A, Pangan AL, Chen N, Betts K, Mittal M, Bao Y. ASAS40 and ASDAS clinical responses in the ABILITY-1 clinical trial translate to meaningful improvements in physical function, health-related quality of life and work productivity in patients with non-radiographic axial spondyloarthritis. Rheumatology (Oxford). 2016;55(1):80–8.
33. Burmester GR, Panaccione R, Gordon KB, McIlraith MJ, Lacerda AP. Adalimumab: long-term safety in 23 458 patients from global clinical trials in rheumatoid arthritis, juvenile idiopathic arthritis, ankylosing spondylitis, psoriatic arthritis, psoriasis and Crohn's disease. Ann Rheum Dis. 2013;72(4):517–24.

6

IL-17A induces osteoblast differentiation by activating JAK2/STAT3 in ankylosing spondylitis

Sungsin Jo[1], Sung Eun Wang[2], Young Lim Lee[1], Suman Kang[1], Bitnara Lee[1], Jinil Han[3], Il-Hoon Sung[4], Ye-Soo Park[5], Sang-Cheol Bae[1,6] and Tae-Hwan Kim[1*]

Abstract

Background: IL-17A has recently emerged as a potential target that regulates the extensive inflammation and abnormal bone formation observed in ankylosing spondylitis (AS). Blocking IL-17A is expected to inhibit bony ankylosis. Here, we investigated the effects of anti IL-17A agents in AS.

Methods: TNFα, IL-17A, and IL-12/23 p40 levels in serum and synovial fluid from patients with ankylosing spondylitis (AS), rheumatoid arthritis (RA), osteoarthritis (OA), or healthy controls (HC) were measured by ELISA. Bone tissue samples were obtained at surgery from the facet joints of ten patients with AS and ten control (Ct) patients with noninflammatory spinal disease. The functional relevance of IL-17A, biological blockades, Janus kinase 2 (JAK2), and non-receptor tyrosine kinase was assessed in vitro with primary bone-derived cells (BdCs) and serum from patients with AS.

Results: Basal levels of IL-17A and IL-12/23 p40 in body fluids were elevated in patients with AS. JAK2 was also highly expressed in bone tissue and primary BdCs from patients with AS. Furthermore, addition of exogenous IL-17A to primary Ct-BdCs promoted the osteogenic stimulus-induced increase in ALP activity and mineralization. Intriguingly, blocking IL-17A with serum from patients with AS attenuated ALP activity and mineralization in both Ct and AS-BdCs by inhibiting JAK2 phosphorylation and downregulating osteoblast-involved genes. Moreover, JAK2 inhibitors effectively reduced JAK2-driven ALP activity and JAK2-mediated events.

Conclusions: Our findings indicate that IL-17A regulates osteoblast activity and differentiation via JAK2/STAT3 signaling. They shed light on AS pathogenesis and suggest new rational therapies for clinical AS ankylosis.

Keywords: Ankylosing spondylitis, Osteoblastic activity and differentiation, IL-17A, JAK2/STAT3 signaling

Background

A key feature of ankylosing spondylitis (AS) is chronic inflammation of the spine, leading to bony ankylosis. The development of tumor necrosis factor (TNF) blockade strategies for inflammatory diseases such as rheumatoid arthritis (RA) and AS was a significant treatment breakthrough [1]. However, effective and safe therapeutic approaches to AS remain a substantial clinical challenge, as the suitability of TNF blockade for preventing new bone formation is yet controversial [2–8]. Thus, it may be fruitful to investigate inflammatory cytokines involved in new bone formation as therapeutic targets.

The interleukin (IL)-23/17 axis has emerged as a key player in AS pathogenesis and has been suggested to induce osteoblastogenesis directly, resulting in bony ankyloses [9–11]. IL-17 and 23, which exhibit properties of proinflammatory cytokines, are predominantly produced by T helper (Th)-17 cells, dendritic cells, and other immune cells [12, 13]. These cytokines are highly expressed in AS and have been associated with rapid differentiation toward mature osteoblasts. Notably, anti-IL-17A-targeting therapies have been shown to be effective for the treatment of AS [14, 15]. However, the mechanisms by which blocking IL-17 in inflammation contributes to the regulation of new bone formation are not understood.

* Correspondence: thkim@hanyang.ac.kr
[1]Department of Rheumatology, Hanyang University Hospital for Rheumatic Diseases, 222-1, Wangsimni-ro, Seongdong-gu, Seoul 04763, Republic of Korea

Janus kinase (JAK)-mediated signaling transduction is connected to surface receptors for multiple cytokines and plays an important role in bone development and metabolism, as demonstrated by knockout mice for individual JAKs [16]. Since AS is characterized by extensive inflammation and altered osteoblastic differentiation, small molecules targeting JAK, such as tofacitinib, have been used. In this context, the concept of targeting JAK in AS is now being tested in clinical trials [17]. Therefore, cytokine-mediated JAK stimulation is integral to osteoblast activation, differentiation and function; suppression of JAK signaling may ameliorate the microenvironment of ankylosis.

Understanding the mechanisms that regulate differentiation and hyperactivation of osteoblasts in AS is critical for developing new therapeutic medications. Although the ability of IL-17A blocking to achieve a cure has been emphasized in previous studies, the regulatory mechanism by which IL-17A modulates bony ankylosis remains unknown. Thus, clarification of the intercellular mechanisms underlying the negative regulation of cytokine-induced osteoblastic activity could provide important clues toward understanding bony ankylosis.

Methods

Human patient serum, synovial fluid, and bone tissue

All patients and healthy serum donors were male. Serum was collected from 27 patients with AS who met the modified New York criteria [18]. Eighteen serum samples from patients with RA who met 2010 RA classification criteria [19] were provided through the Korean Observational Study Network for Arthritis (KORONA) [20]. Thirty healthy donors were obtained as controls. Synovial fluid samples were collected from 27 patients with RA, seven patients with osteoarthritis (OA) who met the classification of OA of the knee [21], and 24 patients with AS. Bone tissue was obtained from ten patients with AS and ten patients with non-inflammatory spinal disease as disease controls. Serum samples that were used to treat bone tissue were obtained from nine patients with active AS.

ELISA analysis of human body fluid

Serum was collected in separator tubes and allowed to clot for 2-4 h at 4 °C before centrifugation for 15 min at approximately 3000 rpm. For synovial fluid, 10 ml of fluid was aspirated and incubated with 1.5 mg hyaluronidase (Sigma-Aldrich, St Louis, MO, USA; H3506) for 15 min at 37 °C. After this incubation, the mixture was spun by centrifugation at 3000 rpm at 4 °C. All body fluids were immediately divided into aliquots and stored at − 80 °C. The levels of human TNF-α (Biolegend, San Diego, CA, USA; 430,204), human IL-17A (Biolegend; 433,914), and human IL-12/23 p40 (Biolegend; 430,704) in the body fluid samples were determined using commercial ELISA kits according to the manufacturers' protocols.

Human primary BdCs

Primary bone-derived cells (BdCs) were isolated and cultured as previously described [22, 23]. All primary BdCs were used for experiments in the second or fourth passage. All isolated BdCs were checked for mycoplasma using a PCR-based method (Takara, Tokyo, Japan 6601) before experiments were performed and before long-term storage in liquid nitrogen.

In vitro osteogenic differentiation

Osteogenic differentiation of primary BdCs was performed as previously described [24]. Briefly, the cells were seeded in growth medium (GM) and then stimulated with osteogenic conditional medium including ascorbic acid, beta-glycerol phosphate, and dexamethasone. Osteogenic medium (OM) was changed every 3 days. Alkaline phosphatase (ALP) activity and staining were assessed at early time points after stimulation with OM. Alizarin red (ARS) staining was performed at late time points after stimulation with OM.

Reagents and biologics

Recombinant human IL-17A (200-17), TNF-α (300-01A), and interleukin-12/23 p40 subunit (IL-12/23 p40) (200-12p40) were purchased from Pepprotech (Rocky Hill, NJ, USA). Golimumab (Janssen, New Brunswick, NJ, USA), secukinumab (Novartis, Basel, Switzerland), and ustekinumab (Janssen) were obtained.

ALP promoter assay

A plasmid with the ALP promoter was a generous gift from Dr. KwangYoul Lee (College of Pharmacy, Chonnam National University, Gwangju, Korea) [25]. 293T cells were co-transfected with the ALP promoter plasmid and the firefly luciferase gene using Lipofectamine 3000, after which luciferase activity was assessed according to the manufacturer's protocol (Promega, Madison, WI, USA; E1500). Luciferase activity was measured with a luminometer (Berthold, Oak Ridge, TN, USA).

Other methods

Quantitative reverse transcriptase-PCR (qRT-PCR), immunoblotting, immunofluorescence, immunohistochemistry, and measurement of cell vitality and toxicity procedures are described in detail in the Additional file 1 [22, 24, 26]. The primers and antibodies information used in the experiments are listed in Additional file 1: Table S1 and Table S2, respectively.

Statistical analysis

GraphPad Prism version 6 (GraphPad Software, San Diego, CA, USA) was used to analyze and present the reported data. All values are expressed as means ± standard deviations (SDs). The statistical significance of differences between two groups was assessed using the nonparametric Mann-Whitney *U* test; one-way ANOVA analysis of variance with Bonferroni's post hoc test was used for multiple comparisons.

Results

Demographic findings

All serum donors were male. Serum was collected from 27 patients with AS (mean age 37.3 ± 2.6 years), 18 patients with RA (34.4 ± 7.0 years), and 30 healthy donors (32.1 ± 5.2 years). Synovial fluid samples were collected from 24 patients with AS (20 males and 4 females; 38.4 ± 10.2 years), 27 patients with RA (3 males and 24 females; 53.4 ± 16.5 years), and 7 patients with OA (2 males and 5 females; 61.4 ± 6.7 years).

The serum samples that were incubated with BdCs were obtained from nine patients with active AS. All patients were male, and the mean age was 30 years. The mean erythrocyte sedimentation rate (ESR) and C-reactive protein (CRP) level were 40.33 mm/h and 3.15 mg/dl, respectively. The mean Bath Ankylosing Spondylitis Disease Activity Index BASDAI was 7.23.

Elevated IL-17A and IL-12/23 p40 levels in body fluid from patients with AS

IL-17A and IL-12/23 p40 (but not TNF-α) concentrations were significantly higher in sera from patients with AS (hereafter referred to as "AS sera") compared to sera from healthy controls (HC) or patients with RA as a disease control (Fig. 1a). In addition, the IL-17A concentration in synovial fluid was even higher in patients with AS only. IL-12/23 p40 and TNF-α concentrations were also higher in AS sera and RA sera than in OA sera (Fig. 1b). Cumulatively, these data indicate that IL-17A concentrations were higher in body fluids from patients with AS compared to the corresponding controls.

JAK2 is highly expressed in patients with AS

JAK2 was highly expressed in bone tissue from patients with AS, as assessed by immunohistochemistry (Fig. 2a, upper panel) and quantitative RT-PCR (Fig. 2b, left panel), whereas, signal transducer and activator of transcription 3 (*STAT3*) mRNA expression did not change statistically in both bone tissue (Fig. 2b. right panel). IL-17A-positive cells were observed in the bone marrow but not in bone-lining cells (Fig. 2a, lower panel). Moreover, high JAK2 expression but not STAT3 was confirmed in primary bone-derived cells BdCs from patients with AS by immunoblotting (Fig. 2c), quantitative RT-PCR (Fig. 2d), and immunostaining (Fig. 2e). Thus, JAK2 is expressed more

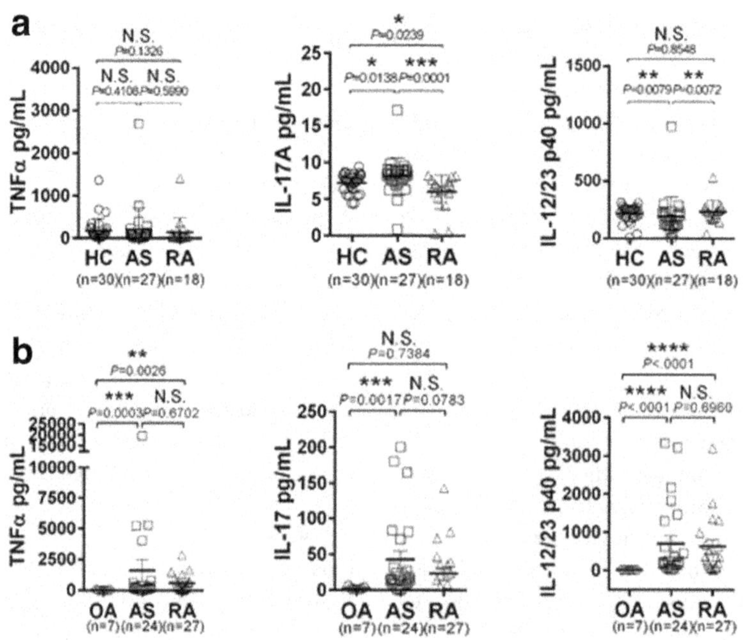

Fig. 1 IL-17A and IL-12/23 p40 concentrations are elevated in body fluid from patients with AS. **a** Serum and (**b**) synovial fluid levels of TNFα, IL-17A, and IL-12/23 p40 in patients with ankylosing spondylitis (AS), patients with rheumatoid arthritis (RA), patients with osteoarthritis (OA), and healthy donors (HC). The Mann-Whitney *U* test was performed to determine statistical significance. Data are presented as means ± SDs. *P* values indicate significant differences between the two groups. N.S., not significant; * $P < 0.05$; ** $P < 0.01$, *** $P < 0.001$; **** $P < 0.0001$

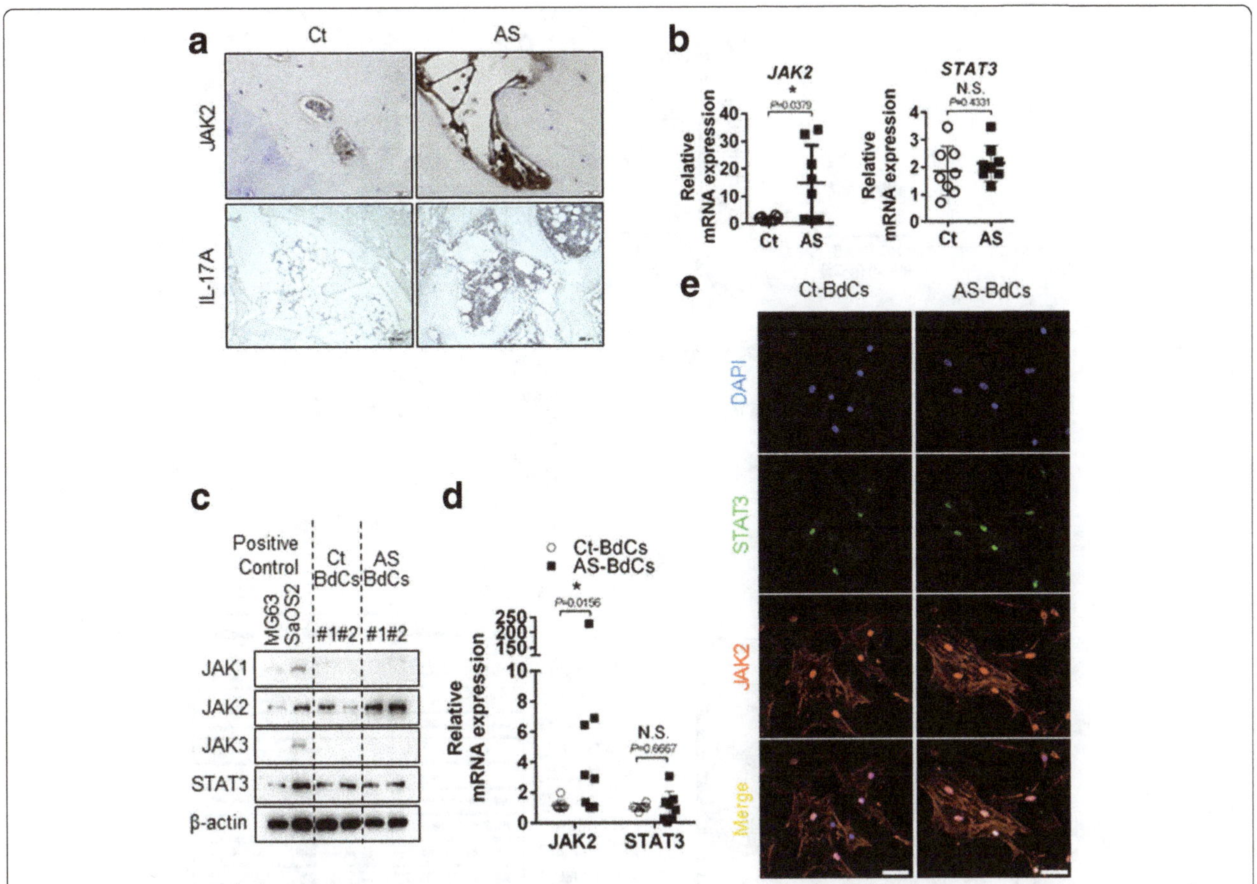

Fig. 2 JAK2 expression levels are highly upregulated in patients with AS. **a** JAK2 and IL-17A expression levels were detected by immunohistochemistry (Ct = 3 and AS = 7). Representative image are shown. Scale bar, JAK2 and IL-17A images; 50 μm and 200 μm, respectively. **b** JAK2 and STAT3 expression in bone tissue were determined by quantitative RT-PCR (Ct = 8 and AS = 8). JAK2 and STAT3 expression levels in BdCs were detected by (**c**) immunoblotting (Ct-BdCs = 2 and AS-BdCs = 2), (**d**) quantitative RT-PCR (Ct-BdCs = 8 and AS-BdCs = 8), and (**e**) immunostaining. Scale bars of confocal image is 50 μm. The Mann-Whitney *U* test was performed to determine statistical significance. Data are presented as means ± SDs. *P* values indicate significant differences between the two groups. N.S., not significant; * $P < 0.05$

highly in bone tissue and BdCs from patients with AS compared to controls.

IL-17A enhances osteogenic activity and differentiation in AS

Elevated ALP levels were observed in patients with AS (Fig. 3a). Moreover, ALP secretion and levels of anchored ALP were high in AS-BdCs (Fig. 3b and c). We additionally assessed three cytokines (TNF-α, IL-17A, and IL-12/23 p40) to determine the origin of the increased ALP promoter activity. The ALP promoter was not responsive to TNF-α, but it did respond to IL-17A. It also responded to IL-12/23, albeit to a lesser extent (Fig. 3d). Thus, we stimulated control (Ct)-BdCs with IL-17A in a dose-dependent manner during osteogenic differentiation. We observed that IL-17A induced a significant increase in ALP activity (Fig. 3e) and mineralization as assessed by ARS staining (Fig. 3f). As seen in Fig. 3g, treatment of Ct-BdCs with IL-17A also led to increases in phos-JAK2, total JAK2, phos-STAT3(Y705), phos-CCAAT/enhance-binding protein beta (C/EBPβ), total C/EBPβ, and RUNX2 expression, despite the fact that these levels decreased upon non-IL-17A stimulation. These findings indicate that IL-17A induces expression driven by the ALP promoter and also promotes osteoblastic differentiation by upregulating JAK2/STAT3, C/EBPβ, and RUNX2 expression.

Blocking IL-17A postpones osteogenic differentiation of AS-BdCs

We found that the levels of IL-17A and IL-12/23 p40 were higher in AS sera; the level of TNF-α also tended to be higher, although not significantly so. Thus, we stimulated primary Ct-BdCs and AS-BdCs with AS sera, with the rationale that AS serum is a strong inducer that mimics the inflammatory condition in AS. We then applied three additional blocking agents. Interestingly, we found that secukinumab and ustekinumab treatment both attenuated ALP staining (Fig. 4a, upper panel), ARS staining (which reflects mineralization) (Fig. 4a, lower panel), and intracellular

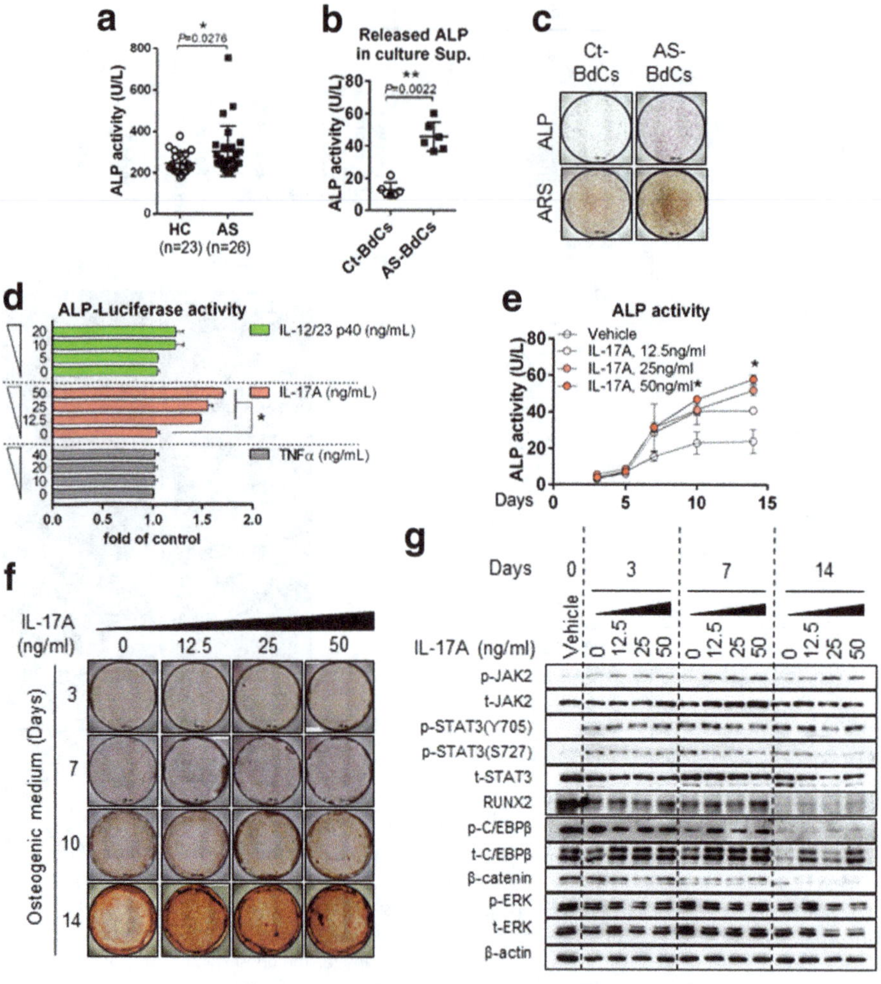

Fig. 3 IL-17A enhances osteogenic activity and differentiation in AS. **a** ALP activity in serum samples (HC = 23 and AS = 26). **b** ALP activity in cultured supernatants of Ct-BdCs and AS-BdCs (Ct-BdCs = 6 and AS-BdCs = 6). **c** ALP and ARS staining of Ct-BdCs and AS-BdCs. **d** 293 T cells were transfected with ALP-luciferase plasmids and treated with the indicated cytokine for 24 h, after which luciferase activity was analyzed. Representative data are shown ($n = 4$). Ct-BdCs were seeded and stimulated with various concentrations of IL-17A in the presence of osteogenic medium. Osteogenic changes were then observed by (**e**) intracellular ALP activity, (**f**) ARS staining, and (**g**) immunoblotting for the indicated proteins. The Mann-Whitney *U* test and one-way ANOVA were performed to determine statistical significance. Data are presented as means ± SDs. *P* values indicate significant differences between the two groups. N.S., not significant; * $P < 0.05$; ** $P < 0.01$

ALP activity (Fig. 4b) in both types of BdCs. In contrast, golimumab did not have these effects. We also assessed changes on the molecular level in both Ct- and AS-BdCs using the same experimental setup. AS-BdCs were more sensitive to Ct-BdCs, as assessed by JAK2, STAT3, and smad2/3 levels. In particular, secukinumab treatment (but not ustekinumab treatment) decreased the levels of phos-JAK2 and phos-C/EBPβ in AS-BdCs (Fig. 4c). This finding indicates that the serum samples regulated osteoblast differentiation-related genes (*ALP*, bone morphogenic protein 2 [*BMP2*], collagen type 1 alpha 1 chain [*COL1A1*], collagen type 1 alpha 2 chain [*COL1A2*], osteocalcin [*OCN*], and osteopontin [*OPN*]). Collectively, the data suggest that secukinumab effectively suppressed osteoblastic activity and osteoblast-related genes, whereas ustekinumab inhibited osteoblastic activity.

Inhibition of JAK2 suppresses the increase in ALP activity mediated by AS serum

To conclusively demonstrate that JAK2 is the main cytokine responsible for ALP activity, we evaluated the effects of tyrophostin tyrosine kinase inhibitor (AG490), a selective JAK2 inhibitor, in concert with six serum samples from patients with active AS in an ALP promoter assay. AS sera induced an increase in ALP promoter activity in a dose-dependent manner (Fig. 5a), whereas AG490 induced a decrease (Fig. 5b). AG490 treatment resulted in no significant change in viability and toxicity of both Ct- and AS-BdCs (Additional file 1:

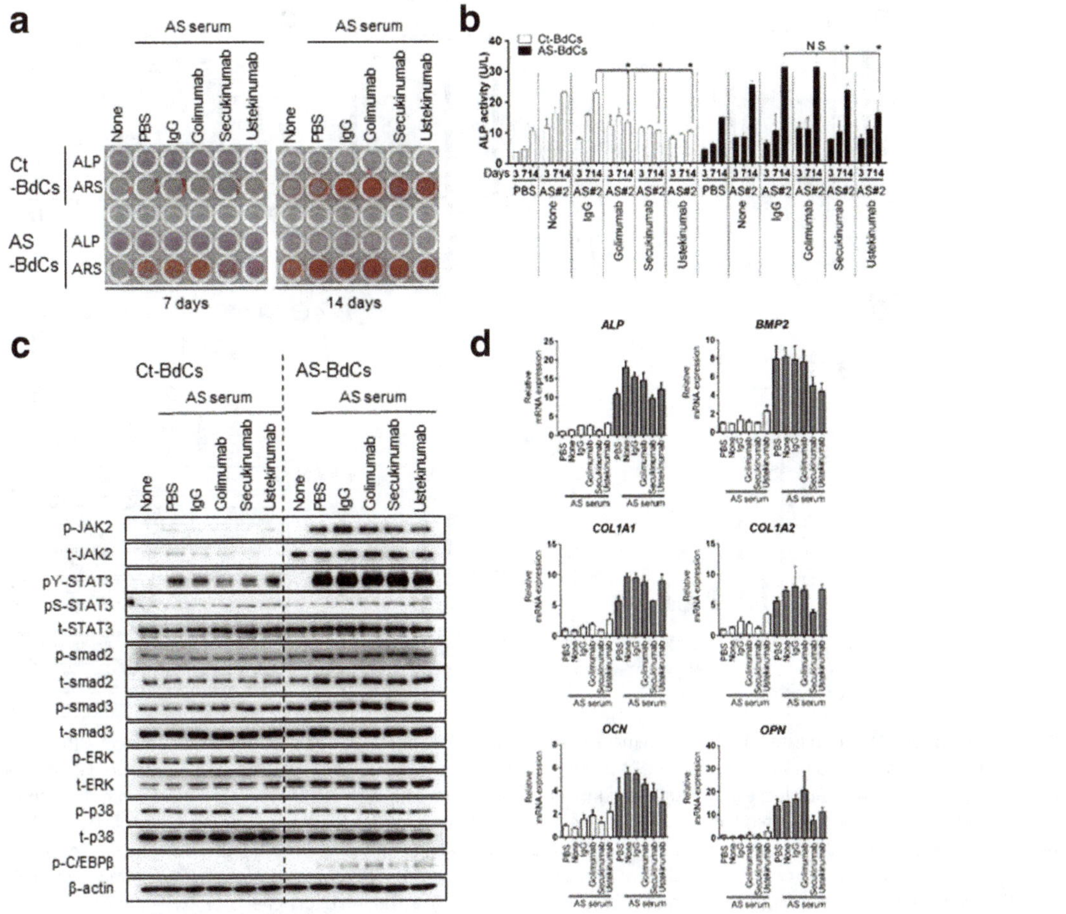

Fig. 4 Targeting IL-17A delays osteogenic differentiation of AS BdCs. Ct and AS-BdCs were stimulated with or without IL-17A blockade (10 μg/mL) in the presence of AS serum (1/10 dilution) in osteogenic medium. On the indicated day, osteogenic differentiation was assessed by (**a**) ALP (*upper*) and ARS (*lower*) staining, (**b**) ALP activity assays. The stimulated cells for 7 days were subjected to (**c**) immunoblotting of the indicated proteins and (**d**) quantitative RT-PCR of the indicated genes. Representative data are shown ($n = 6$). One-way ANOVA analysis was performed to determine statistical significance. Data are presented as means ± SDs. N.S., not significant; $^*P < 0.05$ indicates significant differences between the two groups

Figure S6). Moreover, treatment with AG490 reduced intracellular ALP activity in both Ct- and AS-BdCs and was also a more effective inhibitor in both cell types at early time points compared to late time points (Fig. 5c, d left and right panels). We also observed that AG490 decreased the expression of phos-JAK2 and phosY-STAT3 in both Ct- and AS-BdCs (Fig. 5e). These results demonstrate that JAK2 inhibition ameliorates patient serum-inducible ALP activity and JAK2/STAT3 signaling.

Discussion

In this study, we found that IL-17A and IL-12/23 p40 levels were elevated in AS sera and synovial fluid. Furthermore, the addition of IL-17A under osteoblast stimuli promoted alkaline phosphatase (ALP) activity; mineralization; and JAK2, RUNX2, and C/EBPβ phosphorylation, thereby promoting osteoblastic activity and differentiation. JAK2 was also highly expressed in bone tissue and primary bone-derived cells (BdCs) from patients with AS. IL-17A induced osteoblast activity and differentiation in BdCs through JAK2/STAT3 signaling (Fig. 6). We found that the blocking of IL-17A or JAK2 by AG490 dramatically suppressed AS sera-induced hyperactivation of osteoblasts. Taken together, these data indicate that active inflammation in AS leads to elevated proinflammatory cytokine levels, cytokine-mediated JAK2/STAT3 activation, and increased osteoblastic activity.

We previously characterized the physiology of bone tissue-derived BdCs from patients with AS and assessed IL-23 p19 secretion due to endoplasmic reticulum (ER) stress in these cells [24]. In this study, we demonstrated the mechanism by which IL-17-mediated JAK2 activation leads to osteoblast differentiation and bone formation; this mechanism may be similar to that of ankylosis progression. Moreover, specific blockade of IL-17A and chemical inhibition of JAK2 both inhibited primary Ct- and AS-BdCs. These findings are of particular interest in the context of developing novel strategies for inhibiting

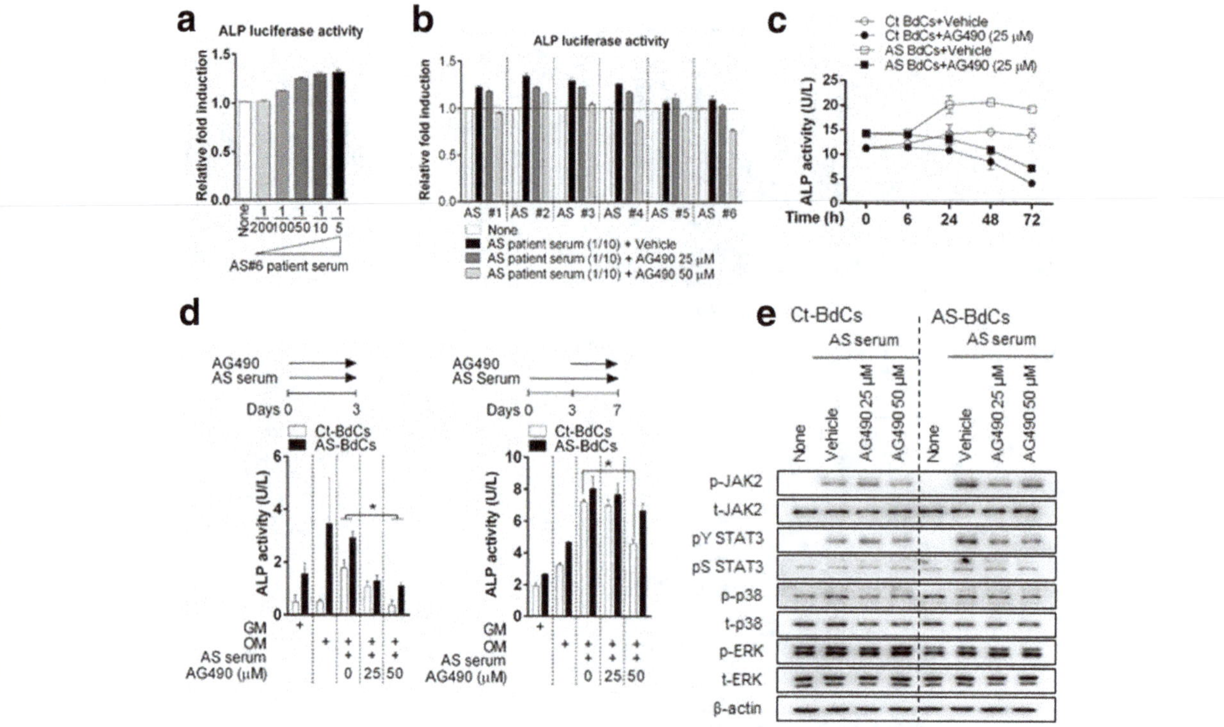

Fig. 5 Inhibition of JAK2 suppresses the AS serum-mediated increase in ALP activity. **a** 293 T cells were transfected with ALP-luciferase plasmids and treated with various volumes of AS serum for 24 h, after which luciferase activity was analyzed. Representative data are shown ($n = 3$). **b** Ct-BdCs were transfected with ALP-luciferase plasmids and then stimulated for 24 h with serum from six patients with AS, with or without AG490. Ct-BdCs and AS-BdCs were stimulated with or without AG490 in the presence of OM for the indicated number of days. **c** The inhibitory effects of AG490 on Ct-BdCs and AS-BdCs were analyzed by assessing intracellular ALP activity over time. Representative data are shown ($n = 4$). **d** The inhibitory effects of AG490 on AS serum (1/10 dilution)-stimulated Ct-BdCs and AS-BdCs were analyzed by measuring intracellular ALP activity at early (*left*) and late (*right*) time points. Representative data are shown ($n = 3$). **e** The inhibitory effects of AG490 on Ct-BdCs and AS-BdCs were assessed by stimulating cells for 3 days and then analyzing the levels of the indicated proteins by immunoblotting. Representative data are shown ($n = 5$). One-way ANOVA analysis was performed to determine statistical significance. Data are presented as means ± SDs. *$P < 0.05$ indicates significant differences between the two groups

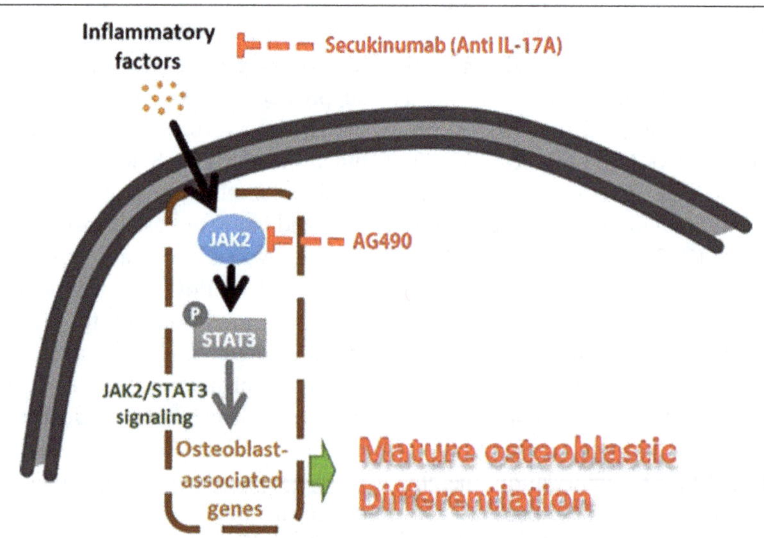

Fig. 6 Schematic model of inflammation-mediated osteoblast activation underlying JAK2/STAT3 expression

bony ankylosis. Thus, our findings suggest that targeting proinflammatory cytokines in AS sera and modulating the response to surface molecules are both essential for stabilizing osteoblast activation induced by the inflammatory environment, which is important for inhibiting bony ankylosis.

In this study, we isolated and cultured primary bone-derived cells (BdCs) from surgically obtained bone from patients with AS and disease controls. Using differentiation-inducing drugs, we then differentiated these cells into osteoblasts. Consistent with another report [27], AS-BdCs exhibited dramatically increased ALP activity and mineralization, which are both features of terminally differentiated osteoblasts (Additional file 1: Figure S1) [28–31].

The correlations between IL-17 and disease markers including ESR, CRP, and BASDAI were varied as shown in Additional file 1: Figures S2 and S3 (ESR: $r = -0.10$, CRP: $r = -0.38$, and BASDAI: $r = -0.06$ in AS sera and ESR: $r = 0.46$, CRP: $r = -0.08$, and BASDAI: $r = 0.43$ in AS synovial fluid). Our data support the notion that IL-17 contributes to osteogenesis and bone formation [32, 33]. ALP is known to be early marker of osteogenesis and sustains during osteogenic differentiation. Introduction of IL-17A and AS patients serum with higher IL-17 concentration accompanied increase in ALP promoter, activity, and staining with phosphorylation of JAK2 and STAT3. It has been shown that modulation of JAK2/STAT3 by IL-17A could play a critical role in osteoblast differentiation proceed with qPCR result [34]. On the basis of these results and reported articles, we suggest that IL-17 drives osteoblast involved genes via phosphorylation of JAK2/STAT3 pathway.

IL-17A concentrations were significantly higher in body fluid from patients with AS. Exogenous treatment of Ct-BdCs with IL-17A promoted osteoblastic activity and differentiation through the JAK2/STAT3 pathway. Moreover, phosphorylation of JAK and tyrosine phosphorylation of STAT3 but not serine by AS sera treatment could be inhibited by IL-17 blockade dose-dependent manner (Additional file 1: Figure S4). The determined IL-17 blockade dose obviously suppressed IL-17A cytokine-induced ALP activity in Ct-BdCs with osteogenic condition (Additional file 1: Figure S5). In particular, blocking IL-17A dramatically decreased AS sera induced-osteoblastic activity in Ct-BdCs, but only mildly suppressed this effect in AS-BdCs. A potential explanation for this finding is that the osteoblasts in AS-BdCs were already influenced by chronic inflammation and were more susceptible to ankylosis. For this reason, IL-17A had a milder effect on AS-BdCs than on Ct-BdCs. While it is well established that TNF inhibitors stabilize inflammation and reduce AS pathogenesis, their effect on bony ankylosis has been controversial. A few studies reported that TNF inhibitors have the potential to reduce bony ankylosis in early AS, i.e. before the development of spinal ankylosis [5, 8, 35]. Taken together, our results and those of previous studies suggest that effective patient treatment could consist of stabilizing and inhibiting proinflammatory cytokines in inflammation at the early stage of AS, but that this approach may not be effective in more advanced stages of disease.

The finding that JAK2 expression is high in AS bone tissue is particularly interesting in the context of developing alternative strategies for protecting patients with AS. We designed the experiments such that the specific JAK2 inhibitor AG490 was added at the time of stimulation. Upon treatment with AG490, the patient serum response to ALP activity was significantly decreased in Ct-BdCs (Fig. 5c). However, this difference was not significant in AS-BdCs at later time points (Fig. 5d, right panel). This finding indicates that the drug did not affect the tissue after osteoblast calcification occurred. In conclusion, AG490 was a more effective inhibitor in the early stage for AS sera responsive to ALP activity than it was in the late. Our results with AG490 may serve as a foundation for future research exploring the efficacy of AG490 for treatment of patients with AS.

Our study has certain limitations. First, we utilized AS sera and primary BdCs to mimic ankylosis in an in vitro system. As shown in Fig. 1, proinflammatory cytokine levels were higher in synovial fluid than in sera. Although we treated BdCs with synovial fluid samples, the fluid viscosity disrupted the cellular response and osteoblastic gene expression and ALP activity could not be analyzed in BdCs. Also, we collected sera from healthy participants and treated BdCs, but no cellular response was observed. Thus, we used AS serum as a strong stimulus for activating BdCs and conducted this experiment using serum from patients with active AS. Another limitation was that all the patients with AS were HLA-B27-positive in this study, but the patients in the other disease group and the healthy group were all HLA-B27-negative. It is considerably difficult to obtain sera from HLA-B27-negative patients with AS and HLA-B27-positive healthy participants. Furthermore, since HLA-B27 is strongly correlated with AS, the role of HLA-B27 must be studied further.

Conclusions

In summary, here we provide evidence for crosstalk between osteoblasts and proinflammatory cytokines during inflammation. We showed that the concentration of IL-17A, the most abundant cytokine in AS sera and synovial fluid, correlates with osteoblast differentiation. Furthermore, blocking IL-17A delayed the patient serum response to ALP activity and mineralization with osteogenic differentiation through JAK2/STAT3 signaling. We also showed that a specific JAK2 inhibitor suppressed stimulus-driven ALP activity, possibly by inhibiting terminal differentiation of BdCs.

Additional file

Additional file 1: Figure S1. Effect of osteogenic differentiation on both Ct-BdCs and AS-BdCs. **Figure S2.** Correlation of IL-17 levels in AS patients with ESR, CRP, and BASDAI levels. **Figure S3.** Correlation of IL-17 levels in RA patients with ESR and CRP levels. **Figure S4.** Secukinumab inhibits AS serum-induced phosphorylation status of JAK2/STAT3 in Ct-BdCs. **Figure S5.** Secukinumab suppresses IL-17A dose-dependent ALP activation in Ct-BdCs. **Figure S6.** Effect of JAK2 inhibitor (AG490) treatment on viability and toxicity of both Ct- and AS-BdCs. **Table S1.** Primer Sequences for qPCR. **Table S2.** Primary antibodies used in Immunoblotting (IB), Immunostaining (IF), and Immunohistochemistry (IHC). (DOCX 826 kb)

Abbreviations

AG490: Tyrphostin JAK2 inhibitor; ALP: Alkaline phosphatase; ARS: Alizarin Red S; AS: Ankylosing spondylitis; BASDAI: Bath Ankylosing Spondylitis Disease Activity Index; BdCs: Bone-derived Cells; BMP2: Bone morphogenic protein 2; C/EBPβ: CCAAT/enhance-binding protein beta; COL1A1: Collagen type 1 alpha 1 chain; COL1A2: Collagen type 1 alpha 2 chain; CRP: C-reactive protein; Ct: Controls; ESR: Erythrocyte sedimentation rate (ESR); GM: Growth medium; HC: Healthy controls; HLA-B27: Human leukocyte antigen B27; IL-12/23 p40: Interleukin-12/23 p40 subunit; IL-17A: Interleukin-17A; JAK2: Janus kinase 2; OA: Osteoarthritis; OCN: Osteocalcin; OM: Osteogenic medium; OPN: Osteopontin; RA: Rheumatoid arthritis; STAT3: Signal transducer and activator of transcription 3; TNF-α: Tumor necrosis factor alpha

Acknowledgements

We would like to thank all participants in this study and members of the Hanyang University Rheumatic Disease staff for helping to collect synovial fluid from patients. We also thank Prof. Young Wha Koh (Department of Pathology, Ajou University School of Medicine, Suwon, Republic of Korea) for evaluating the histologic specimens and Dr. Sang-Hoon Yi for help with confocal imaging. Immunoflurosence images were analyzed by confocal (Leica Microsystems, Wetzlar, Germany) installed at Hanyang LINC Analytical Equipment Center (Seoul, Korea).

Funding

This work was supported by the Basic Science Research Program through the National Research Foundation of Korea (NRF) funded by the Ministry of Science, ICT and Future (NRF-2016R1A2B4008606) and the Ministry of Education (2017R1A6A3A11034394). It was also supported by a Korea Health Technology R&D grant through the Korea Health Industry Development Institute (KHIDI), which is funded by the Ministry of Health and Welfare, Republic of Korea (HI17C0888).

Authors' contributions

SJ designed and performed the experiments and wrote the manuscript. SW, YL, SK, and BL assisted with the laboratory work. JH assisted with statistical analysis and consulting in clinical samples. I-LS and Y-SP provided and evaluated the human bone samples. S-CB provided the patients serum with RA. T-HK conceived the project and was responsible for the overall design and oversight of the project. All authors read and approved the final manuscript.

Competing interests

The authors declare that they have no competing interests.

Author details

[1]Department of Rheumatology, Hanyang University Hospital for Rheumatic Diseases, 222-1, Wangsimni-ro, Seongdong-gu, Seoul 04763, Republic of Korea. [2]Hanyang Biomedical Research Institute, Hanyang University, Seoul, Republic of Korea. [3]Gencurix, Inc, Hanhwan Bizmetro 1, Guro 3-dong, Guro-gu, Seoul, Republic of Korea. [4]Department of Orthopedic Surgery, Hanyang University Hospital, Seoul, Republic of Korea. [5]Department of Orthopedic Surgery, Hanyang University Hospital, Guri, Republic of Korea. [6]Clinical Research Center for Rheumatoid Arthritis (CRCRA), Seoul, Republic of Korea.

References

1. Sieper J, Poddubnyy D. New evidence on the management of spondyloarthritis. Nat Rev Rheumatol. 2016;12:282–95.
2. van der Heijde D, Landewe R, Einstein S, Ory P, Vosse D, Ni L, et al. Radiographic progression of ankylosing spondylitis after up to two years of treatment with etanercept. Arthritis Rheum. 2008;58:1324–31.
3. van der Heijde D, Landewe R, Baraliakos X, Houben H, van Tubergen A, Williamson P, et al. Radiographic findings following two years of infliximab therapy in patients with ankylosing spondylitis. Arthritis Rheum. 2008;58:3063–70.
4. van der Heijde DM, Revicki DA, Gooch KL, Wong RL, Kupper H, Harnam N, et al. Physical function, disease activity, and health-related quality-of-life outcomes after 3 years of adalimumab treatment in patients with ankylosing spondylitis. Arthritis Res Ther. 2009;11:R124.
5. Haroon N, Inman RD, Learch TJ, Weisman MH, Lee M, Rahbar MH, et al. The impact of tumor necrosis factor alpha inhibitors on radiographic progression in ankylosing spondylitis. Arthritis Rheum. 2013;65:2645–54.
6. Baraliakos X, Haibel H, Listing J, Sieper J, Braun J. Continuous long-term anti-TNF therapy does not lead to an increase in the rate of new bone formation over 8 years in patients with ankylosing spondylitis. Ann Rheum Dis. 2014;73:710–5.
7. Maas F, Arends S, Brouwer E, Essers I, van der Veer E, Efde M, et al. Reduction in spinal radiographic progression in ankylosing spondylitis patients receiving prolonged treatment with tumor necrosis factor inhibitors. Arthritis Care Res (Hoboken). 2017;69:1011–9.
8. Molnar C, Scherer A, Baraliakos X, de Hooge M, Micheroli R, Exer P, et al. TNF blockers inhibit spinal radiographic progression in ankylosing spondylitis by reducing disease activity: results from the Swiss Clinical Quality Management cohort. Ann Rheum Dis. 2018;77:63–9.
9. Kenna TJ, Davidson SI, Duan R, Bradbury LA, McFarlane J, Smith M, et al. Enrichment of circulating interleukin-17-secreting interleukin-23 receptor-positive gamma/delta T cells in patients with active ankylosing spondylitis. Arthritis Rheum. 2012;64:1420–9.
10. Raychaudhuri SP, Raychaudhuri SK. Mechanistic rationales for targeting interleukin-17A in spondyloarthritis. Arthritis Res Ther. 2017;19:51.
11. Lubberts E. The IL-23-IL-17 axis in inflammatory arthritis. Nat Rev Rheumatol. 2015;11:415–29.
12. Mei Y, Pan F, Gao J, Ge R, Duan Z, Zeng Z, et al. Increased serum IL-17 and IL-23 in the patient with ankylosing spondylitis. Clin Rheumatol. 2011;30:269–73.
13. Wendling D, Cedoz JP, Racadot E. Serum and synovial fluid levels of p40 IL12/23 in spondyloarthropathy patients. Clin Rheumatol. 2009;28:187–90.
14. Baeten D, Baraliakos X, Braun J, Sieper J, Emery P, van der Heijde D, et al. Anti-interleukin-17A monoclonal antibody secukinumab in treatment of ankylosing spondylitis: a randomised, double-blind, placebo-controlled trial. Lancet. 2013;382:1705–13.
15. Braun J, Baraliakos X, Deodhar A, Baeten D, Sieper J, Emery P, et al. Effect of secukinumab on clinical and radiographic outcomes in ankylosing spondylitis: 2-year results from the randomised phase III MEASURE 1 study. Ann Rheum Dis. 2017;76:1070–7.
16. Li J. JAK-STAT and bone metabolism. JAKSTAT. 2013;2:e23930.
17. van der Heijde D, Deodhar A, Wei JC, Drescher E, Fleishaker D, Hendrikx T, et al. Tofacitinib in patients with ankylosing spondylitis: a phase II, 16-week, randomised, placebo-controlled, dose-ranging study. Ann Rheum Dis. 2017;76:1340–7.
18. van der Linden S, Valkenburg HA, Cats A. Evaluation of diagnostic criteria for ankylosing spondylitis. A proposal for modification of the New York criteria. Arthritis Rheum. 1984;27:361–8.
19. Aletaha D, Neogi T, Silman AJ, Funovits J, Felson DT, Bingham CO 3rd, et al. 2010 Rheumatoid arthritis classification criteria: an American College of

Rheumatology/European League Against Rheumatism collaborative initiative. Arthritis Rheum. 2010;62:2569–81.
20. Sung YK, Cho SK, Choi CB, Park SY, Shim J, Ahn JK, et al. Korean Observational Study Network for Arthritis (KORONA): establishment of a prospective multicenter cohort for rheumatoid arthritis in South Korea. Semin Arthritis Rheum. 2012;41:745–51.
21. Altman R, Asch E, Bloch D, Bole G, Borenstein D, Brandt K, et al. Development of criteria for the classification and reporting of osteoarthritis. Classification of osteoarthritis of the knee. Diagnostic and Therapeutic Criteria Committee of the American Rheumatism Association. Arthritis Rheum. 1986;29:1039–49.
22. Jo S, Koo BS, Lee B, Kwon E, Lee YL, Chung H, et al. A novel role for bone-derived cells in ankylosing spondylitis: focus on IL-23. Biochem Biophys Res Commun. 2017;491:787–93.
23. Jo S, Lee JK, Han J, Lee B, Kang S, Hwang KT, et al. Identification and characterization of human bone-derived cells. Biochem Biophys Res Commun. 2017; https://doi.org/10.1016/j.bbrc.2017.11.155.
24. Jo S, Kang S, Han J, Choi SH, Park YS, Sung IH, et al. Accelerated osteogenic differentiation of human bone-derived cells in ankylosing spondylitis. J Bone Miner Metab. 2017; https://doi.org/10.1007/s00774-017-0846-3.
25. Choi YH, Kim YJ, Jeong HM, Jin YH, Yeo CY, Lee KY. Akt enhances Runx2 protein stability by regulating Smurf2 function during osteoblast differentiation. FEBS J. 2014;281:3656–66.
26. Lee EJ, Lee EJ, Chung YH, Song DH, Hong S, Lee CK, et al. High level of interleukin-32 gamma in the joint of ankylosing spondylitis is associated with osteoblast differentiation. Arthritis Res Ther. 2015;17:350.
27. Xie Z, Wang P, Li Y, Deng W, Zhang X, Su H, et al. Imbalance between bone morphogenetic protein 2 and noggin induces abnormal osteogenic differentiation of mesenchymal stem cells in ankylosing spondylitis. Arthritis Rheumatol. 2016;68:430–40.
28. Beck GR Jr, Zerler B, Moran E. Phosphate is a specific signal for induction of osteopontin gene expression. Proc Natl Acad Sci U S A. 2000;97:8352–7.
29. Boonrungsiman S, Gentleman E, Carzaniga R, Evans ND, McComb DW, Porter AE, et al. The role of intracellular calcium phosphate in osteoblast-mediated bone apatite formation. Proc Natl Acad Sci U S A. 2012;109:14170–5.
30. Dimai HP, Linkhart TA, Linkhart SG, Donahue LR, Beamer WG, Rosen CJ, et al. Alkaline phosphatase levels and osteoprogenitor cell numbers suggest bone formation may contribute to peak bone density differences between two inbred strains of mice. Bone. 1998;22:211–6.
31. Franceschi RT, Iyer BS. Relationship between collagen synthesis and expression of the osteoblast phenotype in MC3T3-E1 cells. J Bone Miner Res. 1992;7:235–46.
32. Osta B, Lavocat F, Eljaafari A, Miossec P. Effects of interleukin-17A on osteogenic differentiation of isolated human mesenchymal stem cells. Front Immunol. 2014;5:425.
33. Huang H, Kim HJ, Chang EJ, Lee ZH, Hwang SJ, Kim HM, et al. IL-17 stimulates the proliferation and differentiation of human mesenchymal stem cells: implications for bone remodeling. Cell Death Differ. 2009;16:1332–43.
34. Noh M. Interleukin-17A increases leptin production in human bone marrow mesenchymal stem cells. Biochem Pharmacol. 2012;83:661–70.
35. Barkham N, Keen HI, Coates LC, O'Connor P, Hensor E, Fraser AD, et al. Clinical and imaging efficacy of infliximab in HLA-B27-Positive patients with magnetic resonance imaging-determined early sacroiliitis. Arthritis Rheum. 2009;60:946–54.

Are gender-specific approaches needed in diagnosing early axial spondyloarthritis? Data from the SPondyloArthritis Caught Early cohort

Augusta Ortolan[1,2], Miranda van Lunteren[1], Sofia Ramiro[1], Roberta Ramonda[2], Robert B. M. Landewé[3,4], Hanne Dagfinrud[5], Lennart T. H. Jacobsson[6], Désirée van der Heijde[1] and Floris A. van Gaalen[1*]

Abstract

Background: Although gender differences have been observed in the severity of axial spondyloarthritis (axSpA), gender differences in disease presentation of early axSpA have not been thoroughly investigated. In particular, their impact on the diagnostic process is unknown.

Methods: Baseline data from the SPondyloArthritis Caught Early cohort, which includes patients with chronic back pain (CBP; duration ≥ 3 months and ≤ 2 years, age of onset < 45 years), were analysed. Patients underwent a full diagnostic work-up, including MRI and radiograph of the sacroiliac joints (MRI-SIJ and X-SIJ), to establish a diagnosis of axSpA. Characteristics of male and female patients with a certain diagnosis of axSpA (confidence level by the physician ≥ 7 on a 0–10 rating scale) were compared. Regression models were built for: the whole CBP cohort stratified by gender, to study which SpA features were associated most with diagnosis in each gender; and for axSpA patients, to test whether gender was associated with imaging positivity (MRI-SIJ$^+$ and/or X-SIJ$^+$).

Results: Of the 719 CBP patients, 275 were male. With 146/275 males and 155/444 females diagnosed as axSpA, males were more likely to be diagnosed with axSpA (OR 2.1, 95% CI 1.5–2.9). Despite similar symptom duration, male axSpA patients were younger at diagnosis (27.4 ± 7.5 vs 29.5 ± 7.8 years; $p = 0.02$). Presence of SpA features was similar in male and female axSpA patients, except for HLA-B27 and imaging positivity that were more common in male axSpA patients (80% vs 60%; $p < 0.01$ and 78% vs 64%; $p = 0.01$). Nevertheless, these SpA features were still more prevalent in female axSpA patients than in no-axSpA patients, both females (HLA-B27$^+$ 23%, positive imaging 7%) and males (HLAB27$^+$ 34%, positive imaging 11%) (all $p < 0.01$). Moreover, in multivariable models with diagnosis of axSpA as outcome, HLA-B27 and imaging positivity were associated with the diagnosis in both sexes. In models with imaging positivity as outcome, male gender and HLA-B27 were both independently associated with MRI$^+$ and/or X-SI$^+$.

Conclusions: While our data show clear gender differences in early axSpA, they highlight that HLA-B27 and imaging are still key elements for diagnosis in both genders. Our study does not suggest that separate diagnostic strategies for men and women are required.

Keywords: Spondyloarthritis, Gender, Diagnosis, Imaging

* Correspondence: f.a.van_gaalen@lumc.nl
[1]Department of Rheumatology, Leiden University Medical Center, Leiden, the Netherlands
Full list of author information is available at the end of the article

Background

Spondyloarthritis (SpA) refers to a group of chronic inflammatory diseases that, according to the Assessment of SpondyloArthritis international Society (ASAS) classification criteria, may be divided by the predominant site of involvement into axial SpA (axSpA) and peripheral SpA [1, 2]. In addition, axSpA can be further split into radiographic axSpA (r-axSpA, also known as ankylosing spondylitis), characterised by typical radiographic changes in sacroiliac joints (SIJ) [3], and non-radiographic axSpA, a form of the disease in which structural damage in the SIJ is not (yet) present.

Although axSpA affects both men and women, r-axSpA is more common in males, with a reported male to female ratio of 2–3:1 [4–6]. The higher incidence of r-axSpA in males compared to females has stimulated research on gender differences in this disease. In patients with longstanding r-axSpA, males have more severe radiographic damage and often more inflammation [7–11]. On the other hand, some authors have reported that female r-axSpA patients more often have cervical spine involvement, peripheral pain, and worse patient-reported outcomes (PROs) [7, 10, 12, 13]. Moreover, a longer time frame between symptom onset (based on patient history) and diagnosis has been repeatedly noticed in female r-axSpA patients [9, 14]. This finding poses the question of whether there is an earlier presentation of the disease in males or an earlier detection of the disease after its onset. If there were phenotypical gender differences at the start or diagnosis of the disease, with less typical findings in women, this could result in a delayed diagnosis. The importance of gender differences in the entire axSpA spectrum has only recently been appreciated, especially since an earlier diagnosis of axSpA has become more feasible. Few studies have been performed in cohorts with early disease such as the German Spondyloarthritis Inception Cohort (GESPIC) and the DEvenir des Spondylarthropathies Indifférenciées Récentes (DESIR) cohort [15, 16], with only one report specifically focusing on possible gender differences [16]. In the GESPIC cohort, composed of patients with a certain diagnosis of axSpA and a mean disease duration approaching 4 years, male gender was independently associated with more radiographic damage [15]. In the DESIR cohort, which includes patients with a high likelihood of SpA (inflammatory back pain highly suspected of axSpA), in the subgroup of patients who fulfilled the ASAS criteria, males were younger at diagnosis, had higher C-reactive protein (CRP) levels, and more often had radiographic sacroiliitis and/or signs of inflammation of SIJ and the spine on magnetic resonance imaging (MRI) [16]. Both studies include only patients with an established (or at least very likely) diagnosis and do not have subjects without axSpA for comparison.

Given the clear gender difference in established r-axSpA, it would be important to know whether differences between male and female axSpA patients are already present early in the disease. If so, different diagnostic strategies may be needed for males and females, considering that diagnostic delay is reported to be higher in females [17, 18]. Therefore, we set out to analyse gender differences at the moment of diagnosis of axSpA in a large inception cohort of chronic back pain (CBP) patients of unknown origin. Our aim was to assess differences in disease presentation between males and females in early axSpA, and to determine whether different SpA features are important for the diagnosis of axSpA in the two genders, possibly demanding separate diagnostic strategies.

Methods

Study design and population

The SPondyloArthritis Caught Early (SPACE) cohort is an ongoing prospective multicentre study which was initiated in January 2009 and has been described in detail elsewhere [19]. In brief, patients with CBP (≥ 3 months and ≤ 2 years of duration) of unknown origin and age of onset < 45 years are included. Patients have been recruited from six different rheumatology outpatient clinics in the Netherlands (Amsterdam, Gouda, Leiden), Norway (Oslo), Sweden (multiple sites), and Italy (Padua). For the present analysis, baseline data were available for 740 patients (SPACE database lock, March 2017). Patients with missing information on clinical diagnosis or imaging were excluded (n = 21), resulting in 719 patients who could be included in the current analyses.

Patients enrolled in the cohort underwent a full diagnostic work-up, including the assessment of SpA features according to the definitions of the ASAS criteria [2]. Consequently, the actual presence or history of the following SpA features was ascertained: inflammatory back pain (IBP), good response to non-steroidal anti-inflammatory drugs (NSAIDs), positive family history of SpA (family history in first or second-degree relatives of r-axSpA, uveitis, reactive arthritis, inflammatory bowel disease, or psoriasis), peripheral arthritis, dactylitis, enthesitis, acute anterior uveitis, inflammatory bowel disease, and psoriasis. Additional details from the patient history were recorded, including their smoking history which was treated as a categorical variable (yes/no/past smoker). The clinical examination included tender/swollen joint and the Maastricht Ankylosing Spondylitis Enthesitis Score (MASES) [20].

In addition to the clinical SpA features, CRP, the erythrocyte sedimentation rate (ESR), and human leukocyte antigen (HLA)-B27 were measured, and plain radiographs of the pelvis (X-SIJ) in the anteroposterior view and MRI-SIJ were performed. Each centre interpreted X-SIJ and MRI-SIJ with respect to the presence or absence of sacroiliitis using global assessment as part of routine clinical practice (local reading), with radiologists and rheumatologists whom had specifically been asked whether there was evidence of sacroiliitis.

Moreover, radiographs of the spine (X-spine) in the sagittal view were taken and centrally scored by three well-trained readers. A syndesmophyte was considered present if detected at the same vertebral corner by at least two readers.

Based on the collected local information, rheumatologists provided a diagnosis of 'axSpA' or 'no axSpA'. In addition, they were requested to provide a level of confidence for their diagnosis on an 11-point numerical rating scale ranging from 0 (not confident at all) to 10 (very confident).

In this study, we considered as 'axSpA patients' those who received a diagnosis of axSpA by the rheumatologist with a level of confidence ≥ 7. This subgroup is hereafter simply referred to as axSpA. 'No-axSpA patients' included patients with a diagnosis of 'no axSpA' and patients with an uncertain diagnosis of axSpA (level of confidence < 7).

Statistical analysis

Patient and disease characteristics were compared between male and female patients, in both groups of axSpA and no-axSpA patients, using the Mann–Whitney *U* test or *t* test for continuous variables and the chi-square or Fisher exact test, as appropriate. Results are presented as frequency (%) or mean (standard deviation (SD)). In order to evaluate which SpA features contributed most to the clinical diagnosis of axSpA, multivariable logistic regression models were built using the whole SPACE cohort stratified by gender. SpA features were used as the independent variables of interest, and a certain diagnosis of axSpA as the outcome. The SpA features were forced into the multivariable regression models, regardless of their significance in univariable analyses.

Furthermore, in axSpA patients, the relationship between gender and imaging abnormalities was investigated through logistic models with X-SIJ$^+$, MRI-SIJ$^+$ or any positive imaging (X-SIJ$^+$ and/or MRI-SIJ$^+$) as the outcomes. Independent variables, apart from gender, consisted of possible determinants of the outcome or potential confounders based on previous studies [21, 22], namely positive family history of SpA, elevated CRP or ESR, and variables that had shown a statistically significant difference between male and female axSpA patients in our baseline data. The independent variables showing an association with the outcome in univariable analyses with $p < 0.10$ were subsequently included in the multivariable model.

Results of regression analyses were expressed in terms of odds ratio (OR) and 95% confidence interval (95% CI).

Data analysis was performed using STATA SE version 14 (StataCorp, College Station, TX, USA) and $p \leq 0.05$ was considered significant.

Results

A total of 719 patients with CBP were analysed. Their mean age was 29.0 (SD 8.2) years, and the mean CBP duration was 13.2 (6.9) months. The majority of patients (n = 444, 62%) were females, with a male to female ratio of 1:1.6. The clinical, laboratory, and imaging characteristics of the CBP population are presented in Table 1.

Out of the 719 CBP patients, 301 patients (42%) were diagnosed with axSpA by the rheumatologist with a level of confidence (LoC) ≥ 7 (axSpA patients). An additional 82 patients (35% males) out of 719 received a diagnosis of axSpA with a level of confidence in diagnosis < 7 (here included in the no-axSpA group).

Of the 275 male CBP patients, 146 (53%) received a certain diagnosis of axSpA, and of the 444 female CBP patients, 155 (35%) received a certain diagnosis of axSpA, showing that male patients with CBP were significantly more likely to be diagnosed with axSpA (OR

Table 1 Baseline characteristics and SpA features of chronic back pain patients included in the SPACE cohort (n = 719)

Characteristic	Value
Male gender, *n* (%)	275 (38)
Age at CBP onset (years), mean (SD)	29.0 (8.0)
Duration of CBP (months), mean (SD)	13.2 (6.9)
Alternating buttock pain, *n* (%) (N = 454[a])	225 (55)
IBP, *n* (%)	499 (70)
Response to NSAIDs, *n* (%)	316 (45)
Family history of SpA, *n* (%)	305 (43)
Peripheral arthritis, *n* (%)	111 (15)
Heel enthesitis, *n* (%)	142 (20)
Dactylitis, *n* (%)	39 (5)
Uveitis, *n* (%)	58 (8)
Psoriasis, *n* (%)	88 (12)
IBD, *n* (%)	48 (6)
HLA-B27$^+$, *n* (%)	315 (44)
Elevated CRP/ESR, *n* (%)	217 (30)
MRI-SIJ$^+$, *n* (%)	234 (32)
X-SIJ$^+$, *n* (%)	91 (12)
Any positive imaging,[b] *n* (%)	250 (34)

SpA spondyloarthritis, *SPACE* SPondyloArthritis Caught Early, *CBP* chronic back pain, *IBP* inflammatory back pain, *NSAID* non-steroidal anti-inflammatory drug, *IBD* inflammatory bowel disease, *HLA* human leukocyte antigen, *CRP* C-reactive protein, *ESR* erythrocyte sedimentation rate, *MRI-SIJ* magnetic resonance imaging of sacroiliac joints, *X-SIJ* plain radiograph of sacroiliac joints
[a]Missing data < 5% unless otherwise indicated
[b]MRI-SIJ$^+$ and/or X-SIJ$^+$

2.1, 95% CI 1.5–2.9). When the patients with a low certainty diagnosis of axSpA (LoC < 7) were removed from the no-SpA group and added to the axSpA group, the gender difference remained the same (OR 2.0, 95% CI 1.5–2.7).

In the axSpA group, the mean age was 28.5 (7.8) years and the mean CBP duration was 13.3 (7.0) months. The male to female ratio was 1:1.1, with 146 (48%) males and 155 (52%) females. Male axSpA patients were younger than female axSpA patients at the time of diagnosis (27.4 (7.5) years vs 29.5 (7.8) years, $p = 0.02$; Table 2).

Among axSpA patients, most SpA features were similarly distributed between the two genders. However, males were significantly more often HLA-B27⁺ (80% vs 60%; $p < 0.001$) and more often had imaging abnormalities (any positive imaging 78% vs 64%; $p = 0.007$) than axSpA female patients. The latter was mainly due to the fact that more males than females had both a positive MRI-SI and a positive X-SI (30% vs 17%; $p = 0.006$). Moreover, although syndesmophytes were uncommon in these patients with early disease, more males than females had syndesmophytes present (8% vs 1%; $p = 0.02$). In contrast, psoriasis appeared to be more common in females (24% vs 15%), although this difference was not statistically significant ($p = 0.051$). Interestingly, the total number of SpA features without HLA-B27 and imaging was not different between males and females (3.5 (1.7) vs 3.5(1.6); $p = 0.99$). Females were less frequently smokers than males (10% vs 22%; $p = 0.02$).

In both genders, all SpA features were significantly more common in axSpA patients as compared to no-axSpA patients except for IBD and family history. The latter was actually more common in male axSpA patients compared to male no-axSpA patients, but such a difference was not observed in female patients. Interestingly, HLA-B27 and positive imaging were still more prevalent in female axSpA patients than in no-axSpA patients, both females (HLA-B27⁺ 23% and positive

Table 2 Characteristics of patients without ($n = 418$) and with ($n = 301$) certain diagnosis of axSpA stratified by gender

	No axSpA		*p* value	axSpA		*p* value
	Male (*N* = 129)	Female (*N* = 289)		Male (*N* = 146)	Female (*N* = 155)	
Age at CBP onset (years), mean (SD)	29.3 (8.6)	29.4 (8.2)	0.9	**27.4 (7.5)**	**29.5 (7.8)**	**0.02**
Duration of CBP (months), mean (SD)	12.8 (6.9)	13.4 (7.0)	0.5	13.3 (7.1)	13.4 (7.0)	0.5
Alternating buttock pain, *n* (%) (*N* = 454[a])	**23 (43)**	**100 (59)**	**0.03**	65 (60)	64 (51)	0.2
IBP, *n* (%)	83 (57)	164 (64)	0.2	123 (84)	129 (84)	1.0
Response to NSAIDs, *n* (%)	45 (37)	81 (29)	0.1	92 (64)	98 (66)	0.8
Family history of SpA, *n* (%)	44 (34)	124 (44)	0.1	68 (46)	69 (45)	0.8
Peripheral arthritis, *n* (%)	15 (12)	25 (9)	0.3	37 (25)	34 (22)	0.5
Heel enthesitis, *n* (%)	17 (13)	28 (10)	0.3	46 (31)	51 (33)	0.7
Dactylitis, *n* (%)	3 (2)	4 (1)	0.5	16 (11)	16 (10)	0.9
Uveitis, *n* (%)	7 (5)	12 (4)	0.6	19 (13)	20 (13)	1.0
Psoriasis, *n* (%)	6 (5)	23 (8)	0.2	22 (15)	37 (24)	0.051
IBD, *n* (%)	11 (8)	15 (5)	0.2	10 (7)	12 (8)	0.8
HLA-B27⁺, *n* (%)	**43 (34)**	**66 (23)**	**0.02**	**114 (80)**	**92 (60)**	**< 0.001**
Elevated CRP/ESR, *n* (%)	21 (16)	61 (21)	0.2	71 (49)	64 (42)	0.2
SpA features without imaging or HLA-B27, mean (SD)	2.4 (0.1)	2.1 (0.1)	0.3	3.5 (1.7)	3.5 (1.6)	1.0
MRI-SIJ⁺/X-SIJ⁻, *n* (%)	7 (5)	19 (6)	0.6	65 (44)	68 (44)	0.9
MRI-SIJ⁻/X-SIJ⁺, *n* (%)	2 (1)	4 (1)	0.9	5 (3)	5 (3)	0.9
MRI-SIJ⁺/X-SIJ⁺, *n* (%)	**5 (4)**	**0 (0)**	**0.01**	**44 (30)**	**26 (17)**	**0.006**
Any positive imaging,[b] *n* (%)	14 (10)	23 (7)	0.3	**114 (78)**	**99 (64)**	**0.007**
Number of syndesmophytes, mean (SD) (*N* = 182[a])	n/a	n/a	–	0.1 (0.4)	0.0 (0.1)	0.5
Patients with syndesmophytes, *n* (%) (*N* = 182[a])	n/a	n/a	–	**7/83 (8)**	**1/99 (1)**	**0.02**
Current smokers, *n* (%)	33 (28)	54 (19)	**0.1**	**31 (22)**	**15 (10)**	**0.02**

Modified Stoke ankylosing spondylitis Spine Score available for 182/301 axSpA patients. Bold data indicate significant results

axSpA axial spondyloarthritis, *CBP* chronic back pain, *IBP* inflammatory back pain, *NSAID* non-steroidal anti-inflammatory drug, *SpA* spondyloarthritis, *IBD* inflammatory bowel disease, *HLA* human leukocyte antigen, *CRP* C-reactive protein, *ESR* erythrocyte sedimentation rate, *MRI-SIJ* magnetic resonance imaging of sacroiliac joints, *X-SIJ* plain radiograph of of sacroiliac joints

[a]Missing data < 5% unless otherwise indicated

[b]MRI-SIJ⁺ and/or X-SIJ⁺

imaging 7%) and males (HLAB27$^+$ 34% and positive imaging 11%) (all $p < 0.01$).

The multivariable regression model in male CBP patients, with a certain diagnosis of axSpA as an outcome, showed that HLA-B27 positivity, elevated CRP and/or ESR, and MRI-SIJ$^+$ were independently associated with the diagnosis of axSpA (Table 3).

In the female CBP population, HLA-B27 positivity, MRI-SIJ$^+$, and X-SIJ$^+$ were independently associated with the diagnosis of axSpA in the multivariable model, but also other SpA features emerged as independent predictors of diagnosis; specifically a positive history or current presence of inflammatory back pain, uveitis, psoriasis, heel enthesitis, dactylitis, IBD, and response to NSAIDs (Table 4).

In axSpA patients, the relationship between gender and imaging abnormalities was investigated. In the univariable regression analysis with positive imaging (MRI-SIJ$^+$ and/or X-SIJ$^+$) as the outcome (Table 5), an independent positive association ($p < 0.05$) was found for male gender, lower age at CBP onset, and HLA-B27 positivity. In the multivariable model, male gender and HLA-B27 positivity were independently and positively associated with imaging positivity. A positive family history of SpA showed a negative association in both the univariable analysis and the multivariable model.

Table 3 Multivariable model with certain diagnosis of axSpA (level of confidence ≥ 7/10) as an outcome and SpA features as independent variables in male CBP population

Independent variable	OR (95% CI) (*N* = 262[a])	*p* value
HLA-B27$^+$	**3.8 (1.7–8.8)**	**< 0.001**
IBP	2.1 (0.8–5.6)	0.1
Uveitis	1.7 (0.5–6.0)	0.3
Psoriasis	2.7 (0.6–11.2)	0.2
Heel enthesitis	2.3 (0.8–6.5)	0.09
Dactylitis	0.3 (0.0–2.4)	0.3
IBD	1.8 (0.4–7.6)	0.4
Peripheral arthritis	1.9 (0.6–6.0)	0.3
Response to NSAIDs	1.5 (0.6–3.3)	0.4
Family history of SpA	1.5 (0.7–3.6)	0.3
Elevated CRP/ESR	**2.5 (1.0–6.1)**	**0.05**
MRI-SIJ$^+$	**24.3 (9.7–60.6)**	**< 0.001**
X-SIJ$^+$	2.7 (0.7–9.4)	0.1

Bold data indicate significant results
axSpA axial spondyloarthritis, *SpA* spondyloarthritis, *CBP* chronic back pain, *OR* odds ratio, *CI* confidence interval, *HLA* human leukocyte antigen, *IBP* inflammatory back pain, *IBD* inflammatory bowel disease, *NSAID* non-steroidal anti-inflammatory drug, *CRP* C-reactive protein, *ESR* erythrocyte sedimentation rate, *MRI-SIJ* magnetic resonance imaging of sacroiliac joints, *X-SIJ* plain radiograph of of sacroiliac joints
[a]Number of patients with complete data on all variables

Table 4 Multivariable model with certain diagnosis of axSpA (level of confidence ≥ 7/10) as an outcome and SpA features as independent variables in female CBP population

Independent variable	OR (95% CI) (*N* = 424[a])	*p* value
HLA-B27$^+$	**6.7 (3.2–14.0)**	**< 0.001**
IBP	**4.0 (1.7—8.9)**	**0.001**
Uveitis	**3.1 (1.0–9.2)**	**0.04**
Psoriasis	**4.6 (1.8–12.0)**	**0.002**
Heel enthesitis	**4.3 (1.9–9.7)**	**< 0.001**
Dactylitis	**5.2 (1.0–26.9)**	**0.05**
IBD	**4.7 (1.5–14.8)**	**0.009**
Peripheral arthritis	1.4 (0.5–3.7)	0.5
Response to NSAIDs	**3.1 (1.6–6.0)**	**0.001**
Family history of SpA	0.9 (0.4–1.8)	0.8
Elevated CRP/ESR	1.7 (0.8–3.5)	0.2
MRI-SIJ$^+$	**32.6 (14.2–75.0)**	**< 0.001**
X-SIJ$^+$	**6.9 (1.4–32.7)**	**0.02**

Bold data indicate significant results
axSpA axial spondyloarthritis, *SpA* spondyloarthritis, *CBP* chronic back pain, *OR* odds ratio, *CI* confidence interval, *HLA* human leukocyte antigen, *IBP* inflammatory back pain, *IBD* inflammatory bowel disease, *NSAID* non-steroidal anti-inflammatory drug, *CRP* C-reactive protein, *ESR* erythrocyte sedimentation rate, *MRI-SIJ* magnetic resonance imaging of sacroiliac joints, *X-SIJ* plain radiograph of of sacroiliac joints
[a]Number of patients with complete data on all variables

Male gender was also positively associated with MRI-SIJ$^+$ alone (OR 1.6, 95% CI 1.0–2.8) and with X-SIJ$^+$ alone (OR 1.9, 95% CI 1.1–3.3) in the multivariable models having MRI-SIJ$^+$ and X-SIJ$^+$ separately as outcomes (data not shown).

Patient-reported outcomes, metrological indices, and disease activity indices of axSpA patients were recorded in the cohort and are presented in Additional file 1: Table S1. Bath Ankylosing Spondylitis Disease Activity Index (BASDAI) scores as well as the percentage of patients presenting with BASDAI > 4 were higher in females (4.5 (2.2) vs 3.4 (1.9) and 57% vs 34%; both $p <$ 0.001). The Bath Ankylosing Spondylitis Functional Index (BASFI) and Short Form (SF)-36 outcomes were not significantly different between genders. Disease activity based on the Ankylosing Spondylitis Disease Activity Score (ASDAS) was similar in terms of absolute value, but females more frequently had a high or very high disease activity (ASDAS ≥ 2.1, 65% vs 46%; $p = 0.004$). Similarly, total MASES was similar between males and females, but the percentage of patients with current entheseal involvement (MASES > 0) was higher in females (70% vs 41%; $p < 0.001$). Finally, more female than male axSpA patients (43% vs 20%; $p = 0.002$) had an extreme BASDAI score (score ≥ 7 on a 0–10 scale in at least three questions of the BASDAI).

Table 5 Factors associated with positive imaging (MRI-SIJ+ and/or X-SIJ+) in patients with certain diagnosis of axial spondyloarthritis (level of confidence ≥ 7/10)

Independent variables	Univariable analysis $N = 289^a$		Multivariable model $N = 289^a$	
	OR (95% CI)	p	OR (95% CI)	p
Male gender	**2.0 (1.2, 3.3)**	**0.007**	**1.8 (1.0, 3.1)**	**0.05**
Age at CBP onset	**1.0 (0.9, 1.0)**	**0.04**	1.0 (0.9, 1.0)	0.052
HLA-B27+	**2.0 (1.2, 3.4)**	**0.01**	**1.8 (1.0, 3.3)**	**0.04**
Positive family history of SpA[b]	**0.4 (0.3, 0.7)**	**0.002**	**0.4 (0.2, 0.7)**	**0.001**
Elevated CRP/ESR	1.6 (1.0, 2.7)	0.06	1.5 (0.9, 2.7)	0.1
Smoking (N=284[c])	1.1 (0.8, 1.6)	0.4	NI	-

Data presented as odds ratio (95% confidence interval). Bold data indicate significant results

MRI-SIJ magnetic resonance imaging of sacroiliac joints, *X-SIJ* plain radiograph of of sacroiliac joints, *CBP* chronic back pain, *HLA* human leukocyte antigen, *SpA* spondyloarthritis, *CRP* C-reactive protein, *ESR* erythrocyte sedimentation rate, *NI* not included in multivariable model because $p > 0.1$ at univariate analysis and no confounder

[a]Number of patients with complete data on all variables

[b]Family history of spondyloarthritis according to the Assessment of SpondyloArthritis international Society includes family history in first or second-degree relatives of ankylosing spondylitis, uveitis, reactive arthritis, inflammatory bowel disease, or psoriasis

[c]Smoking data unavailable in five additional patients

Discussion

The analysis of gender differences in this large CBP cohort with short duration of complaints allowed us to conclude that, while females are the majority of patients in the original CBP population, males were twice as likely to be diagnosed with axSpA. At the moment of diagnosis of axSpA, males were younger and more often presented with HLA-B27 positivity and imaging abnormalities, including a higher prevalence of syndesmophytes, even though symptom duration was similar to female patients. However, the prevalence of most other SpA features was equally distributed between genders.

Although we noticed differences in disease presentation, the results of our study suggest that similar elements are relevant for the diagnosis of male and female axSpA patients. In fact, despite HLA-B27 positivity and imaging abnormalities being more common in male axSpA patients, they were significantly associated with diagnosing axSpA in both genders. We believe this is this first study to examine the possible relevance of different SpA features in making a diagnosis stratified for gender. This is the first report showing in a CBP cohort that males have a higher probability to be diagnosed with axSpA. Since all patients, suspected of axSpA or not, in our cohort underwent the same protocol (including extensive imaging), the gender difference cannot be attributed to differences in the diagnostic process.

Nevertheless, it is obvious that early axSpA does not have such a clear male gender skewing as r-axSpA, since female patients still represent nearly half of the axSpA population, as previously noted [15, 16]. This suggests that specific gender disparities (e.g. radiographic evidence of sacroiliitis) may become more apparent later in the disease course.

Our finding of male patients being younger at disease onset is in line with findings in the DESIR cohort [16]; considering the strict age span allowed by the inclusion criteria and given that males and females in our cohort had similarly short symptom duration, this likely reflects a true difference in the disease onset, rather than a better recognition of the disease in males. Previous reports on age of onset in male and female axSpA patients mainly concern longstanding disease, and some of them reported that males seemed to have an earlier onset [12, 23, 24]. The mechanism behind this is unclear and deserves further investigation.

The results of this study also confirm that imaging abnormalities are more frequently found in male axSpA patients, already at the beginning of the disease [15, 16, 24]. Moreover, we show that male sex is independently associated with positive imaging, both in terms of MRI inflammation and radiographic sacroiliitis. Remarkably, syndesmophytes were more common in males at baseline, showing that differences in radiographic damage between genders, which have been repeatedly observed in r-axSpA [7, 10, 11], can already be found in very early disease. Also, radiographic or MRI sacroiliitis was the most important item for diagnosis in women, and was significantly more common in both male and female axSpA patients compared to no-axSpA patients.

HLA-B27 was also more common in male axSpA patients, and the overall prevalence of HLA-B27 in axSpA patients in our study was similar to other early axSpA cohorts [25]. However, it has to be noted that in other axSpA populations, such as those of the clinical trials, where axSpA patients are included only if they fulfil ASAS criteria and not based solely on the rheumatologist diagnosis, often display higher percentages of HLA-B27$^+$ patients [26, 27].

In studying the factors associated with sacroiliitis in patients with axSpA, a positive family history was protective of positive imaging even in univariate analysis. At present we have no clear explanation for this observation. Little is known about differences in axial spondyloarthritis between patients with and without a familial history. One study reported that familial ankylosing spondylitis was significantly milder than sporadic disease [28], while another found no difference in disease phenotype [29].

Although PROs were not the main outcome of our study, it is interesting to observe how, in line with data from the literature, female patients in our cohorts presented with a higher subjective disease burden [7, 10, 12, 13]. Unfortunately, our cohort lacks assessment of fibromyalgia, but the observation of female axSpA patients presenting with more extreme PROs than males suggests that fibromyalgia could have been a frequent co-morbidity for our axSpA patients, possibly influencing the degree of symptom complaint in females. Indeed, it has been described that about a third of axSpA patients could have a neuropathic pain component [30].

A clear limitation in our analysis is that our diagnostic models for axSpA do not truly reflect a normal diagnostic work-up in clinical practice, in which looking for—and excluding—other causes of CBP is pivotal. However, the validity of our observations derives from the fact that all of the information included in the model was available to the rheumatologist and was used at the moment of making the diagnosis (axSpA/no axSpA). On the other hand, rheumatologists certainly performed a diagnosis according to their background knowledge and beliefs, and therefore there could have been a tendency towards a specific interpretation of the results (e.g. women could have been under-diagnosed if the rheumatologists interpreted axSpA as a predominantly male disease). Finally, we cannot exclude that possible referral bias may have interfered with the proportion of males and females in the study population or with other results such as the nearly significant prevalence of psoriasis in females. Indeed, the reasons why GPs or medical specialists referred CBP patients to the rheumatologists is unknown, but they could have been more prone to refer a female CBP patient if SpA features (besides HLA-B27 and imaging) were already present or because they had worse symptoms, thus a channelling mechanism cannot be excluded. However, other cohorts have reported a higher frequency of CBP in females [31]; moreover, the male to female ratio in our axSpA population is in line with previous findings [15, 16].

Conclusions

In summary, in patients with CBP of unknown origin, males are more likely to be diagnosed with axSpA. In addition, significant differences between genders, including age at onset and imaging abnormalities, already exist at a very early disease stage. Nevertheless, HLA-B27 and imaging are still key elements for a diagnosis of axSpA in both genders, and therefore our data do not support the need for gender-specific diagnostic strategies for early axSpA patients.

Abbreviations

AS: Ankylosing spondylitis; ASAS: Assessment of SpondyloArthritis international Society; ASDAS: Ankylosing Spondylitis Disease Activity Score; axSpA: Axial spondyloarthritis; BASDAI: Bath Ankylosing Spondylitis Disease Activity Index; BASFI: Bath Ankylosing Spondylitis Functional Index; CBP: Chronic back pain; CRP: C-reactive protein; DESIR: DEvenir des Spondylarthropathies Indifférenciées Récentes; ESR: Erythrocyte sedimentation rate; GESPIC: German Spondyloarthritis Inception Cohort; HLA: Human leukocyte antigen; IBP: Inflammatory back pain; MASES: Maastricht Ankylosing Spondylitis Enthesitis Score; MRI: Magnetic resonance imaging; NSAID: Non-steroidal anti-inflammatory drug; PRO: Patient-reported outcome; SF-36: Short Form-36; SIJ: Sacroiliac joints; SpA: Spondyloarthritis; SPACE: SPondyloArthritis Caught Early; X-SIJ: X-rays of sacroiliac joints; X-spine: X-rays of the spine

Funding

The study has partly been funded by the Dutch Rheumatism Association (Reumafonds).

Authors' contributions

AO contributed to the study design, participated in the acquisition and interpretation of data, performed the statistical analysis, and drafted and revised the manuscript. MvL participated in the acquisition and interpretation of data and revised the manuscript. SR participated in the interpretation of data and revised the manuscript. RBML contributed to the acquisition and interpretation of data and revised the manuscript. RR, LTHJ, and HD contributed to the acquisition of data and revised the manuscript. DvdH made substantial contributions to conception and design, interpretation of data, and revision of the manuscript. FAvG made substantial contributions to conception and design, participated in the acquisition and interpretation of data, and drafted and revised the manuscript. All of the authors gave final approval of this version.

Competing interests

The authors declare that they have no competing interests.

Author details

[1]Department of Rheumatology, Leiden University Medical Center, Leiden, the Netherlands. [2]Rheumatology Unit, Department of Medicine (DIMED), University of Padua, Padua, Italy. [3]Department of Rheumatology, Amsterdam Rheumatology and Immunology Center, Amsterdam, the Netherlands. [4]Department of Rheumatology, Zuyderland Medical Center, Heerlen, the Netherlands. [5]Department of Rheumatology, Diakonhjemmet Hospital, Oslo, Norway. [6]Department of Rheumatology, University of Gothenburg, Gothenburg, Sweden.

References

1. Rudwaleit M, van der Heijde D, Landewe R, Akkoc N, Brandt J, Chou CT, et al. The Assessment of SpondyloArthritis International Society classification criteria for peripheral spondyloarthritis and for spondyloarthritis in general. Ann Rheum Dis. 2011;70:25–31.
2. Rudwaleit M, van der Heijde D, Landewe R, Listing J, Akkoc N, Brandt J, et al. The development of Assessment of SpondyloArthritis International Society classification criteria for axial spondyloarthritis (part II): validation and final selection. Ann Rheum Dis. 2009;68:777–83.

3. van der Linden S, Valkenburg HA, Cats A. Evaluation of diagnostic criteria for ankylosing spondylitis. A proposal for modification of the New York criteria. Arthritis Rheum. 1984;27:361–8.
4. Carbone LD, Cooper C, Michet CJ, Atkinson EJ, O'Fallon WM, Melton LJ 3rd. Ankylosing spondylitis in Rochester, Minnesota, 1935-1989. Is the epidemiology changing? Arthritis Rheum. 1992;35:1476–82.
5. Kennedy LG, Will R, Calin A. Sex ratio in the spondyloarthropathies and its relationship to phenotypic expression, mode of inheritance and age at onset. J Rheumatol. 1993;20(11):1900–4.
6. Will R, Edmunds L, Elswood J, Calin A. Is there sexual inequality in ankylosing spondylitis? A study of 498 women and 1202 men. J Rheumatol. 1990;17:1649–52.
7. Ibn Yacoub Y, Amine B, Laatiris A, Hajjaj-Hassouni N. Gender and disease features in Moroccan patients with ankylosing spondylitis. Clin Rheumatol. 2012;31:293–7.
8. van der Horst-Bruinsma IE, Zack DJ, Szumski A, Koenig AS. Female patients with ankylosing spondylitis: analysis of the impact of gender across treatment studies. Ann Rheum Dis. 2013;72:1221–4.
9. Lee W, Reveille JD, Weisman MH. Women with ankylosing spondylitis: a review. Arthritis Rheum. 2008;59:449–54.
10. Webers C, Essers I, Ramiro S, Stolwijk C, Landewe R, van der Heijde D, et al. Gender-attributable differences in outcome of ankylosing spondylitis: long-term results from the outcome in ankylosing spondylitis international study. Rheumatology. 2016;55:419–28.
11. Ramiro S, Stolwijk C, van Tubergen A, van der Heijde D, Dougados M, van den Bosch F, et al. Evolution of radiographic damage in ankylosing spondylitis: a 12 year prospective follow-up of the OASIS study. Ann Rheum Dis. 2015;74:52–9.
12. Roussou E, Sultana S. Spondyloarthritis in women: differences in disease onset, clinical presentation, and Bath Ankylosing Spondylitis Disease Activity and Functional indices (BASDAI and BASFI) between men and women with spondyloarthritides. Clin Rheumatol. 2011;30:121–7.
13. Lee W, Reveille JD, Davis JC Jr, Learch TJ, Ward MM, Weisman MH. Are there gender differences in severity of ankylosing spondylitis? Results from the PSOAS cohort. Ann Rheum Dis. 2007;66:633–8.
14. Jung YO, Kim I, Kim S, Suh CH, Park HJ, Park W, et al. Clinical and radiographic features of adult-onset ankylosing spondylitis in Korean patients: comparisons between males and females. J Korean Med Sci. 2010; 25:532–5.
15. Rudwaleit M, Haibel H, Baraliakos X, Listing J, Marker-Hermann E, Zeidler H, et al. The early disease stage in axial spondylarthritis: results from the German Spondyloarthritis Inception Cohort. Arthritis Rheum. 2009;60:717–27.
16. Tournadre A, Pereira B, Lhoste A, Dubost JJ, Ristori JM, Claudepierre P, et al. Differences between women and men with recent-onset axial spondyloarthritis: results from a prospective multicenter French cohort. Arthritis Care Res. 2013;65:1482–9.
17. Feldtkeller E, Khan MA, van der Heijde D, van der Linden S, Braun J. Age at disease onset and diagnosis delay in HLA-B27 negative vs. positive patients with ankylosing spondylitis. Rheumatol Int. 2003;23:61–6.
18. Feldtkeller E, Bruckel J, Khan MA. Scientific contributions of ankylosing spondylitis patient advocacy groups. Curr Opin Rheumatol. 2000;12:239–47.
19. van den Berg R, de Hooge M, van Gaalen F, Reijnierse M, Huizinga T, van der Heijde D. Percentage of patients with spondyloarthritis in patients referred because of chronic back pain and performance of classification criteria: experience from the Spondyloarthritis Caught Early (SPACE) cohort. Rheumatology. 2013;52:1492–9.
20. Heuft-Dorenbosch L, Spoorenberg A, van Tubergen A, Landewe R, van ver Tempel H, Mielants H, et al. Assessment of enthesitis in ankylosing spondylitis. Ann Rheum Dis. 2003;62:127–32.
21. Blachier M, Canoui-Poitrine F, Dougados M, Lethuaut A, Fautrel B, Ferkal S, et al. Factors associated with radiographic lesions in early axial spondyloarthritis. Results from the DESIR cohort. Rheumatology. 2013;52: 1686–93.
22. Chung HY, Machado P, van der Heijde D, D'Agostino MA, Dougados M. Smokers in early axial spondyloarthritis have earlier disease onset, more disease activity, inflammation and damage, and poorer function and health-related quality of life: results from the DESIR cohort. Ann Rheum Dis. 2012; 71:809–16.
23. Landi M, Maldonado-Ficco H, Perez-Alamino R, Maldonado-Cocco JA, Citera G, Arturi P, et al. Gender differences among patients with primary ankylosing spondylitis and spondylitis associated with psoriasis and inflammatory bowel disease in an iberoamerican spondyloarthritis cohort. Medicine. 2016;95:e5652.
24. de Carvalho HM, Bortoluzzo AB, Goncalves CR, da Silva JA, Ximenes AC, Bertolo MB, et al. Gender characterization in a large series of Brazilian patients with spondyloarthritis. Clin Rheumatol. 2012;31:687–95.
25. Chung HY, Machado P, van der Heijde D, D'Agostino MA, Dougados M. HLA-B27 positive patients differ from HLA-B27 negative patients in clinical presentation and imaging: results from the DESIR cohort of patients with recent onset axial spondyloarthritis. Ann Rheum Dis. 2011;70:1930–6.
26. Maksymowych WP, Dougados M, van der Heijde D, Sieper J, Braun J, Citera G, et al. Clinical and MRI responses to etanercept in early non-radiographic axial spondyloarthritis: 48-week results from the EMBARK study. Ann Rheum Dis. 2016;75:1328–35.
27. Sieper J, van der Heijde D, Dougados M, Maksymowych WP, Scott BB, Boice JA, et al. A randomized, double-blind, placebo-controlled, sixteen-week study of subcutaneous golimumab in patients with active nonradiographic axial spondyloarthritis. Arthritis Rheumatol. 2015;67:2702–12.
28. Calin A, Kennedy LG, Edmunds L, Will R. Familial versus sporadic ankylosing spondylitis. Two different diseases? Arthritis Rheum. 1993;36:676–81.
29. Paardt MV, Dijkmans B, Giltay E, van der Horst-Bruinsma I. Dutch patients with familial and sporadic ankylosing spondylitis do not differ in disease phenotype. J Rheumatol. 2002;29:2583–4.
30. Gok K, Cengiz G, Erol K, Ozgocmen S. Neuropathic pain component in axial spondyloarthritis and the influence on disease burden. J Clin Rheumatol. 2018;24:324–327.https://doi.org/10.1097/RHU.0000000000000711.
31. Gouveia N, Rodrigues A, Eusebio M, Ramiro S, Machado P, Canhao H, et al. Prevalence and social burden of active chronic low back pain in the adult Portuguese population: results from a national survey. Rheumatol Int. 2016; 36:183–97.

8

Influence of HLA-B27 on the ankylosing spondylitis phenotype: results from the REGISPONSER database

Marta Arévalo[1], Jordi Gratacós Masmitjà[1*], Mireia Moreno[1], Joan Calvet[1], Cristobal Orellana[1], Desirée Ruiz[2], Carmen Castro[2], Pilar Carreto[2], Marta Larrosa[1], Eduardo Collantes[2], Pilar Font[2] and REGISPONSER group

Abstract

Objective: To assess HLA-B27 influence on the clinical phenotype of Ankylosing Spondylitis (AS) patients.

Method: An observational, cross-sectional and descriptive study of AS patients from the Spanish REGISPONSER database was performed. Demographic, clinical, disease activity (Bath Ankylosing Spondylitis Disease Activity Index (BASDAI), Bath Ankylosing Spondylitis Functional Index (BASFI), erythrocyte sedimentation rate (ESR), and C-reactive protein (CRP)), and radiographic data (Bath Ankylosing Spondylitis Radiology Index (BASRI) score) were compared regarding HLA-B27 status. A univariate and multivariate analysis was performed to identify variables independently related to the presence of HLA-B27.

Results: Data from 1235 patients (74.8% male) were analyzed; 1029 were HLA-B27 positive (83%). HLA-B27-positive patients showed higher family aggregation and an earlier onset of disease compared with those who were HLA-B27 negative. HLA-B27-negative patients presented statistically higher BASDAI and BASFI scores and higher prevalence of arthritis, dactylitis, and extra-articular manifestations (psoriasis and inflammatory bowel disease (IBD)) but not anytime uveitis compared with those who were HLA-B27 positive.
In the multivariate analysis, family history (odds ratio (OR) 2.10, 95% confidence interval (CI) 1.27–3.49), younger age at diagnosis (OR 0.97, 95% CI 0.96–0.98), presence of peripheral arthritis (OR 0.53, 95% CI 0.32–0.89), dactylitis (OR 0.16, 95% CI 0.05–0.56), psoriasis (OR 0.45, 95% CI 0.26–0.78), and IBD (OR 0.22, 95% CI 0.12–0.40) were the main variables independently related to the presence or not of HLA-B27.

Conclusion: In Caucasian AS patients, the presence of HLA-B27 is related to an earlier disease onset and higher family aggregation. Absence of HLA-B27 is related to a higher frequency of peripheral arthritis, dactylitis, and extra-articular manifestations. Being HLAB27 positive is not related to a higher burden of disease or anytime uveitis.

Keywords: Ankylosing Spondylitis, HLA-B27, Structural damage, Phenotype, Uveitis

Background

Axial Spondyloarthritis (AxSpA) includes an heterogeneous group of rheumatisms characterized by their strong association with HLA-B27 and axial skeleton involvement. Ankylosing Spondylitis (AS) is the main disease of this group and is clinically defined by inflammatory back pain, but it can also involve other sites such as peripheral arthritis, enthesitis, dactylitis, and extra-articular manifestations as uveitis, psoriasis, and inflammatory bowel disease (IBD). Frequently, disease onset occurs in patients 20–30 years of age and, if no effective treatment is given, it can lead to severe disability in nearly a third of individuals [1]. Its prevalence is around 0.2–0.3% depending on the geographical distribution of HLA-B27 [2, 3]. HLA-B27, since its discovery in 1973 [4], constitutes the main genetic factor related to disease etiopathogenesis. However, nearly 10–20% of patients with defined AS do not carry HLA-B27, which increases to 40% when analyzing nonradiographic

* Correspondence: jgratacosmas@gmail.com
[1]Rheumatology Department, Consorci Corporació Sanitària Parc Taulí, Institut d'Investigació i Innovació Parc Taulí I3PT, Universitat Autònoma de Barcelona, Parc Taulí s/n, 08208 Sabadell, Barcelona, Spain

axial spondyloarthritis (nrAxSpA) [5]. Previous studies suggest a relationship between HLA-B27 and axial manifestations including structural progression in early AxSpA [5]. Moreover, a younger age of onset, more family history [5, 6], and less prevalence of psoriasis and IBD [5] have also been reported. Nevertheless, there are few studies evaluating the role of HLA-B27 in defined AS patients [7–9], with some of them focused on radiographic progression [10–12] and reporting controversial results [13]. The main objective of the present study was to evaluate the HLA-B27 influence on the clinical expression of defined AS patients. For this purpose, we reviewed data from the REGISPONSER database [14] which includes more than 1000 AS patients, of whom about 20% are HLA-B27 negative.

Material and methods

This is a comparative, cross-sectional study including all patients fulfilling AS New York modified criteria from the REGISPONSER. REGISPONSER is a Spanish registry that includes 2367 patients who fulfilled European Spondyloarthropathy Study Group (ESSG) criteria for spondyloarthritis. Of these, 1422 had radiographic sacroiliitis as per New York modified criteria, with 1270 of these having HLA-B27 typing available, and finally 1235 of these having no data of interest missing (Fig. 1). Recruitment of patients started in March 2004 and finished in March 2007. All patients included signed an informed consent form, and the project was approved by the ethical committee of all participant hospitals. More information about the methodology and data inclusion are detailed in a previous publication by Collantes et al. [14].

The study included the following clinical and biological variables: age (in years), gender, the presence of HLA-B27, age at disease onset (in years), disease duration (in years), diagnosis delay (in years), axial symptoms, peripheral involvement (peripheral arthritis, coxitis, enthesitis, and dactylitis), extra-articular manifestations confirmed by a specialist (uveitis, IBD, psoriasis, palmoplantar pustulosis, balanitis, prostatitis), clinical disease activity (Bath Ankylosing Spondylitis Disease Activity Index (BASDAI), 0–10 cm), clinical disability (Bath Ankylosing Spondylitis Functional Index (BASFI), 0–10 cm), biological disease activity (erythrocyte sedimentation rate (ESR) and C-reactive protein (CRP)), and structural damage (Bath Ankylosing Spondylitis Radiology Index (BASRI)) assessed by a local radiologist and confirmed by an experienced rheumatologist.

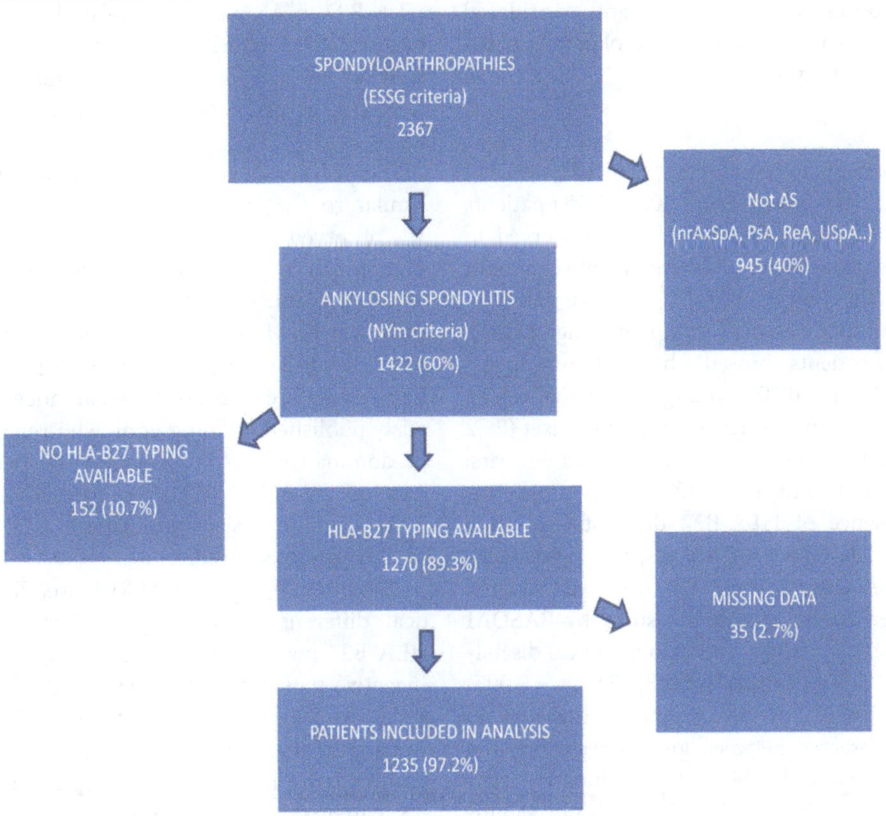

Fig. 1 Flow chart of patients included in the study from the REGISPONSER database. AS Ankylosing Spondylitis, ESSG European Spondyloarthropathy Study Group, nrAxSpA nonradiographic axial spondyloarthritis, NYm New York modified, PsA psoriatic arthritis, ReA reactive arthritis, USpA undifferentiated spondyloarthritis

Statistical analysis

A descriptive analysis of the variables was performed using absolute and relative frequencies for qualitative variables and mean with standard deviation for the quantitative variables. A 95% confidence interval (CI) was calculated. For bivariate analysis the Chi-squared test was used, and the Student *t* test was used for independent data. Finally, a multiple logistic regression model was performed including the following variables: gender, age, age at onset, disease duration, signs and symptoms at onset and during follow-up, peripheral and extra-articular manifestations, BASDAI, BASFI, BASRI, ESR, and CRP. The degree of association was expressed as the odds ratio (OR) and Cornfield confidence interval was established at 95% using Wald statistics. Variables with $p \geq 0.15$ were suppressed from the model one by one (backward stepwise procedure). Comparison between the reduced model and the one including suppressed variables was made using the likelihood ratio test (G statistic). A scale of continuous variables was evaluated with the Bow Tidwell test. Possible interactions between variables were studied as possible confounding factors, considering them if the percentage change of coefficients was higher than 20%. The Hosmer Lemeshow statistic was performed to assess the goodness of fit. All contrasts were bilateral and considered significant when $p < 0.05$. Data were collected, processed, and analyzed using SPSS v.17.

Results

Data from 1235 patients were collected, with 1029 (83.3%) patients being HLA-B27 positive and 206 (17.7%) patients being HLA-B27 negative. Male gender was observed in 924 (74.8%) patients with no differences between both groups (74.7% of males in the HLA-B27-positive group vs. 75.2% in the HLA-B27-negative group; not significant). HLA-B27-positive patients showed a higher family aggregation (22.1% vs 12%; $p = 0.002$), younger age (47.9 vs 50.4 years; $p = 0.012$), and younger age at symptom onset (26.2 vs 30.6 years; $p < 0.001$) and at diagnosis (33.9 vs 39 years; $p < 0.001$) compared with HLA-B27-negative patients. However, the absence of HLA-B27 did not lead to a greater diagnosis delay (7.8 vs. 8.5 years; not significant). Analyzing disease activity, HLA-B27-negative patients expressed a higher disease activity measured by BASDAI (4.1 ± 2.3 vs 4.4 ± 2.4; $p = 0.047$) and higher clinical disability measured by BASFI (3.8 ± 2.7 vs 4.3 ± 2.9; $p = 0.005$) compared with HLA-B27-positive patients. However, no differences were observed between groups regarding the biological markers analyzed (ESR and CRP), nor in structural damage expressed by BASRI (7.2 vs 7.4; not significant). Moreover, HLA-B27-negative patients showed a higher prevalence of peripheral arthritis (15.4% vs 21.8%; $p = 0.023$), dactylitis (0.8% vs 3.9%; $p = 0.001$), and extra-articular manifestations, especially psoriasis (5.9% vs 14.6%; $p < 0.001$) and IBD (3.6% vs 11.7%; $p < 0.001$) compared with HLA-B27-positive patients. On the other hand, this study did not find any statistical differences regarding axial clinical disease expression (neck pain, low back pain, and sacroiliac joint symptoms), the presence of enthesitis (present in 6.1% of subjects) or uveitis (22.4% in HLA-B27-positive and 19.4% in HLA-B27-negative patients; not significant).

In the multivariate analysis, family history (OR 2.10, 95% CI 1.27–3.49; $p = 0.004$), younger age at diagnosis (OR 0.97, 95% CI 0.96–0.98; $p < 0.001$), and the presence of peripheral arthritis (OR 0.53, 95% CI 0.32–0.89; $p = 0.016$), dactylitis (OR 0.16, 95% CI 0.05–0.56; $p = 0.004$), psoriasis (OR 0.45, 95% CI 0.26–0.78; $p = 0.005$), and IBD (OR 0.22, 95% CI 0.12–0.40; $p < 0.001$) were the main variables independently related to the presence or not of HLA-B27. All results are shown in Table 1.

Discussion

This is the most extensive study performed comparing clinical characteristics of Caucasian AS patients regarding HLA-B27. The study confirms the association of HLA-B27 with earlier disease onset and family aggregation. Moreover, the study proves that the absence of HLA-B27 in AS patients is related to a higher frequency of peripheral arthritis, psoriasis, and IBD. Finally, our data do not support the relationship between HLA-B27 and the severity of axial structural damage in AS patients.

The prevalence of HLA-B27 in our study reaches 83%, similar to that previously reported in AS patients [2]. We observed a male:female ratio of 3:1, comparable with that shown in previous studies in AS patients regardless of the presence of HLA-B27 [15], but clearly different from the previously reported gender ratio in nrAxSpA patients where there is not a male predominance [5, 6]. Our results are also not in accordance with those previously published by Yang et al. who reported a clear male predominance in AS patients associated with the presence of HLA-B27 [9]. However, that study was performed in an Asian population, and race differences need to be considered.

Our study, using the BASRI score, did not show statistical differences regarding axial structural damage in HLA-B27-positive AS patients compared with HLA-B27 -negative patients. In this sense, our data are in accordance with those reported in the GESPIC cohort [6]. Previous data regarding the influence of HLA-B27 on the progression and extent of radiographic axial damage in AS patients are controversial due to heterogeneity in published series and the methods used when measuring structural damage [9–13]. In the DESIR cohort, the authors observed higher radiographic damage in early

Table 1 Univariate and multivariate analysis between the HLA-B27-positive and HLA-B27-negative groups

	B27 negative		B27 postive		Univariate analysis	Multivariate analysis		
	n (= 206)	Mean ± SD or %[a]	*n* (= 1029)	Mean ± SD or %[a]	*p*	OR	95% CI	*p*
Men	155	75.2	769	74.7	NS			
Family history	22	12	216	22.1	0.002	2.1	1.27–3.49	0.004
Age (years), mean ± SD	206	50,4 ± 12,9	1025	47,9 ± 13	0,012			
Age at onset (years), mean ± SD	204	30.6 ± 12.3	1010	26.2 ± 9.9	< 0.001			
Age at diagnosis (years), mean ± SD	199	39 ± 12.3	1002	33.9 ± 11.5	< 0.001	0.97	0.96–0.98	< 0.001
Disease duration since first symptom (years), mean ± SD	204	19.8 ± 12.8	1013	21.9 ± 13.1	0.038			
Diagnosis delay (years), mean ± SD	198	8.5 ± 9.6	993	7.8 ± 9.2	NS			
Disease duration since diagnosis (years), mean ± SD	199	11.3 ± 9.3	1004	14 ± 10.6	0.001			
Axial manifestations								
Cervicalgia	28	13.6	103	10	NS			
Lumbalgia	148	71.8	741	72	NS			
Sacroiliac syndrome	85	41.3	435	42.3	NS			
Peripheral manifestations								
Peripheral arthritis	45	21.8	158	15.4	0.023	0.53	0.32–0.89	0.016
Coxitis	6	2.9	32	3.1	NS			
Enthesitis	10	4.9	65	6.3	NS			
Dactylitis	8	3.9	8	0.8	0.001	0.16	0.05–0.56	0.004
Extra-articular manifestations								
Psoriasis	30	14.6	61	5.9	< 0.001	0.45	0.26–0.78	0.005
Inflammatory bowel disease	24	11.7	37	3.6	< 0.001	0.22	0.12–0.4	< 0.001
Urethritis, cervicitis, diarrhea	4	1.9	7	0.7	NS			
Anterior uveitis	40	19.4	230	22.4	NS			
Palmoplantar pustulosis	6	2.9	4	0.4	0.002	0.12	0.02–0.64	0.013
Balanitis	4	1.9	4	0.4	0.022			
Prostatitis	1	0.5	7	0.7	NS			
BASRI score, mean ± SD	194	7.4 ± 4.1	974	7.2 ± 3.9	NS			
BASDAI score, mean ± SD	206	4.4 ± 2.4	1029	4.1 ± 2.3	0.047			
BASFI score, mean ± SD	206	4.3 ± 2.9	1028	3.8 ± 2.7	0.005	0.94	0.88–1	0.037
ESR (mm/1 h), mean ± SD	174	19 ± 15.98	977	18.3 ± 16.3	NS			
CRP (mg/L), mean ± SD	174	10.2 ± 17.7	975	9.2 ± 13.7	NS			

BASDAI Bath Ankylosing Spondylitis Disease Activity Index, *BASFI* Bath Ankylosing Spondylitis Functional Index, *BASRI* Bath Ankylosing Spondylitis Radiology Index, *CRP* C-reactive protein, *ESR* erythrocyte sedimentation rate, *NS* not significant

[a] For qualitative variables as percentage (%) and for quantitative variables as mean ± standard deviation (SD)

AxSpA patients related to the presence of HLA-B27, but only in the sacroiliac joints [5]. No differences in radiographic spine damage measured by the modified Stoke Ankylosing Spondylitis Spine Score (mSASSS) were found. When looking at studies including definite AS patients, our results differ from those reported by Yang et al. [9], who found a higher radiographic extent of structural damage in Asian AS patients and also in the HLA-B27-positive compared to the HLA-B27-negative patients. We do not have any precise explanation for these observed differences, but we cannot exclude some unknown variables related to the genetic and/or environmental factors when comparing different genetic populations. Moreover, since male gender seems to be a strong predictive factor for radiographic damage [6, 16] and the male ratio in HLA-B27-positive AS patients was clearly higher in the study by Yang et al. compared with our study [9], we need to consider this variable as a potential explanation for the differences observed between both studies. Finally, it is also interesting to remark that disease duration was significantly higher in HLA-B27-positive AS patients than the other group. Given that disease duration is one of the main factors related to structural damage, the data reported here do not support a major role of HLA-B27 in the extension of the structural damage in defined AS patients.

Our data appear to confirm previous studies suggesting that HLA-B27 is associated with a younger disease onset and greater family aggregation in AS patients [9, 13]. Similar results were also described in early forms of HLA-B27-positive patients from the DESIR [5] and GESPIC [6] cohorts, in such a way that HLA-B27 seems to anticipate the clinical manifestations and disease onset. Although HLA-B27 is the strongest genetic factor related to familiar aggregation of the disease, we observed that 12% of our HLA-B27-negative patients also had a familial background. As this is much higher than that observed in the general population, these data support the existence of unknown genetic factors other than HLA-B27 that have a role in the familial aggregation of the disease.

We did not observe differences in axial symptoms regardless of the presence or not of HLA-B27. However, we observed a significantly higher frequency of peripheral arthritis, dactylitis, psoriasis, and IBD in HLA-B27-negative AS patients. This association has also been previously described in early forms of AxSpA [5] in which the proportion of HLA-B27-negative patients is much higher than in definite AS patients. Moreover, our data do not support a higher clinical burden of disease in AS patients regarding the presence of HLA-B27. In this sense, HLA-B27-negative AS patients showed significantly higher BASDAI and BASFI scores, even though there were no differences in biologic parameters (ESR and CRP).

Around a fifth of patients included in the analysis had at least one episode of uveitis, this being the most frequent extra-articular manifestation as has been shown in previous studies [17]. Classically, HLA-B27 has been related to the presence of uveitis regardless of the presence or not of a definite AS [18, 19]; thus, in this sense our data are unexpected. However, the results previously reported analyzing the potential association between HLA-B27 in AS patients and the presence of uveitis are quite controversial [7, 9, 13]. It is important to note that 19.4% of HLA-B27-negative AS patients had at least one episode of uveitis. These results, together with the absence of an association between episodes of uveitis and axial inflammation in AS patients, suggest the need for further studies to evaluate the etiopathogenesis of uveitis in AS patients.

Finally, we did not observe any differences in the frequency of coxitis between both groups, in contrast to the data reported by Yang et al. [9]. However, the prevalence of coxitis in our study was low (3.1 and 2.9%, respectively) which makes it difficult to draw any conclusions on this matter.

This study has some limitations. This is a cross-sectional study, and the implications between the observed data and outcomes must be interpreted with caution. Our study did not support a higher percentage of uveitis in the presence or not of HLA-B27. However, we only evaluated the presence or not as a dichotomic measure, and thus we cannot exclude a higher frequency of uveitis flares in AS HLA-B27-positive patients compared with negative patients. The BASRI score was used instead of the mSASSS, which is a more sensitive score to evaluate axial structural changes [20]. Moreover, we do not have data on axial magnetic resonance imaging (MRI), and thus we could not evaluate the influence of bone marrow edema on the potential progression of structural damage. We evaluated only definite AS patients with a long disease evolution (around 8 years) and thus we cannot exclude a potential influence on radiographic progression of HLA-B27 in the early stages of the disease. In this sense, it is not possible to extrapolate these results to nrAxSpA. However, the data observed suggest that, despite HLA-B27 typing, other genetic or environmental factors might play a major role in bone structural damage in AS patients. Finally, given that BASDAI scores were not recorded separately, the Ankylosing Spondylitis Disease Activity score could not be calculated.

Conclusion

In summary, this is the most extensive study analyzing differences in Caucasian AS patients regarding their HLA-B27 status. This study confirms the previously reported association in AS patients between HLA-B27 and an earlier disease onset and greater family aggregation. However, and interestingly, we do not support an association between HLA-B27 and the extent of axial structural damage, or a higher clinical burden of the disease. Moreover, we cannot prove an association between the presence of anytime uveitis and HLA-B27 in definite AS patients. On the other hand, the absence of HLA-B27 is related, in AS patients, to a higher frequency of peripheral arthritis, dactylitis, and extra-articular manifestations.

Abbreviations

AS: Ankylosing Spondylitis; AxSpA: Axial spondyloarthritis; BASDAI: Bath Ankylosing Spondylitis Disease Activity Index; BASFI: Bath Ankylosing Spondylitis Functional Index; BASRI: Bath Ankylosing Spondylitis Radiology Index; CI: Confidence interval; CRP: C-reactive protein; ESR: Erythrocyte sedimentation rate; ESSG: European Spondyloarthropathy Study Group; IBD: Inflammatory bowel disease; mSASSS: Modified Stoke Ankylosing Spondylitis Spine Score; nrAxSpA: Nonradiographic axial spondyloarthritis; OR: Odds ratio

Acknowledgements

REGISPONSER group - listed below are the principal investigator.
HU REINA SOFÍA- Eduardo Collantes Estévez à Main center and ethical committee
H BELLVITGE-Xavier Juanola Roura
HU JUAN CANALEJO-Jose Luis Fernández Sueiro
HU GREGORIO MARAÑÓN- Carlos González Fernández
H. PARC TAULÍ-Jordi Gratacós Masmitjá
CLÍNICA PUERTA HIERRO-Juan Mulero Mendoza
H. MONTE NARANCO-Juan Carlos Torre Alonso
H DOCE DE OCTUBRE- Pilar Fernández Dapica
H RAMÓN Y CAJAL- Mª Elia Brito Brito

HU ALICANTE-Enrique Batlle Gualda
H VIRGEN DE LA ARRIXACA- Luis F. Linares Ferrando
H. VIRGEN DEL PERPETUO SOCORRO- Enrique Judez Navarro
H.G. SAN JORGE- Carlos Vázquez Galeano
H. DE PALAMÓS- Teresa Clavaguera Poch
H. MOSTOLES- Mª Cruz Fernández Espartero
HU CARLOS HAYA- Enrique Calero Secall
H. MUTUA DE TERRASSA- Manuel Pujol Busquets
H. DOCTOR NEGRÍN- Carlos Rodríguez Lozano
H. SANTA MARÍA DEL ROSELL- Manuel J. Moreno Ramos
HU PRÍNCIPE DE ASTURIAS- Eduardo Cuende Quintana
HU DE GUADALAJARA- Manuel Fernández Prada
HU CENTRAL DE ASTURIAS- Rubén Queiro Silva
H. SAN RAFAEL- Estefanía Moreno Ruzafa
HU VIRGEN DE LA VEGA- Carlos Montilla Morales
H. VIRGEN DEL ROCÍO- Alicia García López
HU MIGUEL SERVET- Eugenio Giménez Úbeda
H. FUNDACIÓN SON LLATZER- Antonio Juan Más
H. INTERNACIONAL MERIMAR- Cristina Medrano Le Quement
HU NAVARRA- Enrique Ornilla

Declarations

We confirm that the article has not been published before and is not under consideration for publication elsewhere, and that it is approved by all the authors listed.

Authors' contributions

MA analyzed the data and wrote the paper; JGM, ML, and MM supervised and directed paper writing, and JC and EC reviewed the paper. CO corrected the paper translation. DR, CC, and PC reviewed the database and contributed to the statistical analysis; PF performed the main statistical analysis. All authors read and approved the final manuscript.

Competing interests

The authors declare that they have no competing interests.

Author details

[1]Rheumatology Department, Consorci Corporació Sanitària Parc Taulí, Institut d'Investigació i Innovació Parc Taulí I3PT, Universitat Autònoma de Barcelona, Parc Taulí s/n, 08208 Sabadell, Barcelona, Spain. [2]Rheumatology Department, Hospital General Universitario Reina Sofía/IMIBIC/Universidad de Córdoba Córdoba, Spain.

References

1. Castillo-Ortiz R, Landewé v d H, Dougados v d B, et al. Work outcome in patients with Ankylosing Spondylitis: results from a 12-year follow-up of an international study. Arthritis Care Res. 2016;68:544–52.
2. Khan M. HLA-B27 and its subtypes in world populations. Curr Opin Rheumatol. 1995;7:263–9.
3. Stolwijk C, van Onna M, Boonen A, van Tubergen A. Global prevalence of spondyloarthritis: a systematic review and meta-regression analysis. Arthritis Care Res. 2016;68:1320–31.
4. Caffrey MF, James DC. Human lymphocyte antigen association in Ankylosing Spondylitis. Nature. 1973;242(5393):121.
5. Chung H, Machado P, van der Heijde D, D'Agostino M-A, Dougados M. HLA-B27 positive patients differ from HLA-B27 negative patients in clinical presentation and imaging: results from the DESIR cohort of patients with recent onset axial spondyloarthritis. Ann RheumDis. 2011;70:1930–6.
6. Rudwaleit M, Haibel H, Baraliakos X, Listing J, Märker-Hermann E, Zeidler H, et al. The early disease stage in axial spondyloarthritis: results from the German spondyloarthritis inception cohort. Arthritis Rheumatism. 2009;60: 717–27.
7. Khan M, Kushner I, Braun W. Comparison of clinical features in HLA-B27 positive and negative patients with Ankylosing Spondylitis. Arthritis Rheumatism. 1977;20:909–12.
8. Feldtkeller E, Khan M, van der Heijde D, van der Linden S, Braun J. Age at disease onset and diagnosis delay in HLA-B27 negative vs. positive patients with Ankylosing Spondylitis. Rheumatol Int. 2002;23:61–6.
9. Yang M, Xu M, Pan X, Hu Z, Li Q, Wei Y, et al. Epidemiological comparison of clinical manifestations according to HLA-B*27 carrier status of Chinese Ankylosing Spondylitis patients. Tissue Antigen. 2013;82(5):338–43.
10. Ward MM, Hendrey MR, Malley JD, Learch TJ, Davis JC Jr, Reveille JD, et al. Clinical and immunogenetic prognostic factors for radiographic severity in Ankylosing Spondylitis. Arthritis Rheum. 2009;61(7):859–66.
11. Xiong J, Chen J, Tu J, Ye W, Zhang Z, Liu Q, et al. Association of HLA-B27 status and gender with sacroiliitis in patients with Ankylosing Spondylitis. Pak J Med Sci. 2014;30:22–7.
12. Cortes A, Maksymowych WP, Wordsworth BP, Inman RD, Danoy P, Rahman P, et al. Association study of genes related to bone formation and resorption and the extent of radiographic change in Ankylosing Spondylitis. Ann Rheum Dis. 2015;74(7):1387–93.
13. Akkoç N, Yarkan H, Kenar G, Khan M. Ankylosing Spondylitis: HLA-B*27-positive versus HLA-B*27-negative disease. Curr Rheumatol Rep. 2017;19:26.
14. Collantes E, Zarco P, Muñoz E, Juanola X, Mulero J, Fernández-Sueiro JL, et al. Disease pattern of spondyloarthropathies in Spain: description of the first registry (REGISPONSER). Rheumatology. 2007;46:1309–15.
15. Stolwijk C, van Tubergen A, Castillo-Ortiz JD, Boonen A. Prevalence of extra-articular manifestations in patients with Ankylosing Spondylitis: a systematic review and meta-analysis. Ann Rheum Dis. 2015;74(1):65–73.
16. Ramiro S, Stolwijk C, van Tubergen A, van der Heijde D, Dougados M, van den Bosch F, et al. Evolution of radiographic damage in Ankylosing Spondylitis: a 12 year prospective follow-up of the OASIS study. Ann Rheum Dis. 2015;74(1):52-9.
17. Winter J, Mens L, Heijde D, Landewé R, Baeten D. Prevalence of peripheral and extra-articular disease in Ankylosing Spondylitis versus non-radiographic axial spondyloarthritis: a meta-analysis. Arthritis Res Ther. 2016;18:196.
18. D'Ambrosio EM, La Cava M, Tortorella P, Gharbiya M, Campanella M, Iannetti L. Clinical features and complications of the HLA-B27-associated acute anterior uveitis: a meta-analysis. Semin Ophthalmol. 2016;12:1–13.
19. Valls Pascual E, Fontanilla Ortega P, Vicens Bernabeu E, Martínez-Costa L, Blanco Alonso R. Características clínicas, tratamiento y complicaciones oculares de uveítis anterior asociada y no asociada a HLA-B27. Reumatol Clin. 2016;12:244–7.
20. Creemers MC, Franssen MJ, van't Hof MA, Gribnau FW, van de Putte LB, van Riel PL. Assessment of outcome in Ankylosing Spondylitis: an extended radiographic scoring system. Ann Rheum Dis. 2005;64:127–9.

Factors related to health-related quality of life in ankylosing spondylitis, overall and stratified by sex

Lucy Law[1], Jeanette Beckman Rehnman[1], Anna Deminger[2], Eva Klingberg[2], Lennart T. H. Jacobsson[2] and Helena Forsblad-d'Elia[1,2*]

Abstract

Background: Ankylosing spondylitis (AS) begins early in life and often leads to reduced physical function, but less is known about the impacts it has on health-related quality of life (HRQoL). The aims of this study were to assess HRQoL using the Short Form-36 (SF-36) in a cohort of patients with AS compared with controls and to examine associations between SF-36 scores and spinal radiographic changes, physical function, disease activity and demographic data overall and stratified by sex.

Methods: A cohort of patients with AS from Western Sweden were assessed using the Modified Stoke Ankylosing Spondylitis Spine Score (mSASSS) with spinal radiographs, clinical examination and questionnaires, including the Bath Ankylosing Spondylitis Metrology Index, Bath Ankylosing Spondylitis Functional Index (BASFI), Ankylosing Spondylitis Disease Activity Score-C-reactive protein (ASDAS-CRP), Bath Ankylosing Spondylitis Disease Activity Index, Bath Ankylosing Spondylitis Patient Global (BASG) and SF-36. Each patient's SF-36 results were compared with those of five age-matched and sex-matched persons ($n = 1055$) from the SF-36 Swedish normative population database. Associations between SF-36 physical component summary (PCS) and mental component summary (MCS) scores and disease-related and demographic factors were investigated using univariate and multivariable ogistic regression analyses with PCS and MCS below/above their respective median values as dependent variables.

Results: A total of 210 patients, age (median, IQR) 49.0 (21.2) years, symptom duration 24.0 (21.0) years, men 57.6% and HLAB27 87.1% were included. Patients with AS scored significantly lower ($p < 0.001$) compared to controls in all SF-36 domains and component summaries; PCS 42.4 (14.5) in AS versus 52.4 (11.8) in controls and MCS 47.9 (20.0) in AS versus 54.1 (10.1) in controls. Both men and women scored significantly lower in PCS compared with MCS. Multivariable logistic regression analyses revealed that living without a partner (OR 2.38, 95% CI 1.00–5.67), long symptom duration (year in decade OR 1.66, 95% CI 1.16–2.37), higher BASFI (OR 1.98, 95% CI 1.46–2.70) and ASDAS ≥ 2.1 (OR 3.32, 95% CI 1.45–7.62) were associated with worse PCS, while living without a partner (OR 3.04, 95% CI 1.34–6.91), fatigue (visual analogue scale for global fatigue greater than the median (OR 6.36, 95% CI 3.06–13.19) and ASDAS ≥ 2.1 (OR 2.97, 95% CI 1.41–6.25) with worse MCS. Some differences between sexes were observed in the results.

(Continued on next page)

* Correspondence: helena.forsblad.delia@umu.se
[1]Department of Public Health and Clinical Medicine, Rheumatology, Umeå University, 901 87 Umeå, Sweden
[2]Department of Rheumatology and Inflammation Research, Sahlgrenska Academy at University of Gothenburg, Box 480, 405 30 Gothenburg, Sweden

(Continued from previous page)

Conclusions: The patients with AS had significantly lower HRQoL compared with controls. PCS was more affected compared to MCS in both sexes. Both disease-related and demographic factors were associated with HRQoL, partly overlapping for PCS and MCS. Factors associated with HRQoL showed some differences between sexes. By modifying factors, such as ASDAS-CRP and fatigue, HRQoL may potentially be improved.

Keywords: Ankylosing spondylitis, Health-related quality of life, Medical outcome survey short form-36, Disease activity, Fatigue, Cross-sectional study, Observational study

Background

Ankylosing spondylitis (AS) is a chronic inflammatory rheumatic disease primarily affecting the sacroiliac joints and spine [1]. Inflammation of the spinal structures and progressive spinal changes in the vertebrae and surrounding tissue, is largely responsible for the decreased physical function and mobility experienced by patients with AS [2]. Studies of AS often describe functional disabilities and measures of disease activity, however, they less often report the quality of life experienced by patients with AS and how this is related to AS disease characteristics. Health-related quality of life (HRQoL) is a multi-dimensional concept including not only a person's physical wellbeing, but also a person's mental health and physical ability, both as an individual and as a participating member of the community. The Medical Outcome Survey Short Form-36 (SF-36) was designed for use in clinical practice and research, health policy evaluations, and general population surveys and is utilised in many different countries [3–6]. Yang et al. recently performed a meta-analysis based on of 38 studies assessing HRQoL using the SF-36 in patients with AS and found that they had significantly worse HRQoL compared to persons from general populations and that to measure HRQoL should be regarded as an essential part of the overall assessment of patients with AS [7]. The SF-36 is grouped into eight domains reflecting physical and mental health and two summary scores, a physical component summary (PCS) and a mental component summary (MCS) score. Yang et al. reported that pooled mean scores ranged from 45.9 to 58.2 in the physical health domains and from 47.5 to 62.5 in the mental health domains in their meta-analysis of patients with AS [7] as compared to 72.5 to 85.2 and 60.0 to 84.6, respectively, in the normative general population database from Norway, one of the databases used for comparison with AS [8]. The Bath Ankylosing Spondylitis Disease Activity Index (BASDAI) and Bath Ankylosing Spondylitis Functional Index (BASFI) have been found to be negatively associated with some domains of the SF-36 [7, 9–13]. The relationship between HRQoL, laboratory markers of inflammation, the Ankylosing Spondylitis Disease Activity Score (ASDAS), Bath Ankylosing Spondylitis Metrology Index (BASMI) and spinal radiographic changes, as assessed by the modified Stoke Ankylosing Spondylitis Spinal Score (mSASSS), is less studied. Since the AS phenotype differs between sexes, with men generally displaying more AS spinal radiographic changes compared to women, it is of importance to investigate factors related to HRQoL overall and also stratified by sex to be able to better personalize the care of patients with AS [14, 15].

The objectives of this study were to investigate the following in patients with AS: (1) HRQoL assessed by the SF-36 compared with HRQoL in controls from the general population, (2) HRQoL in relation to age and (3) to examine associations between the SF-36 scores and spinal radiographic changes, physical function, mobility, disease activity and demographic data overall and stratified by sex.

Methods

Patients and controls

Patients were recruited from three sites in Western Sweden [14, 16]. This cross-sectional study focuses on HRQoL assessed by the SF-36 questionnaire. The inclusion criteria for the study were a diagnosis of AS according to the modified New York criteria [17] and age ≥ 18 years. The exclusion criteria were difficulties in understanding the Swedish language, dementia and pregnancy. Patients with psoriasis or inflammatory bowel disease (IBD) were also excluded in order to create a more homogenous cohort of patients with typical AS. All patients with AS meeting the study criteria were invited to participate and of these, 211 patients were initially included.

Results of the SF-36 questionnaires completed by the patients with AS ($n = 211$) were compared to those of five age-matched and sex-matched persons, per AS patient ($n = 1055$), randomly drawn from the SF-36 Swedish normative population database [5]. One of the included patients was later found to have psoriasis and was excluded from further analysis, leaving 210 patients to take part in this study. Figure 1 summarises the process of patient inclusion.

This study was approved by the Regional ethical committee at the University of Gothenburg, Sweden and

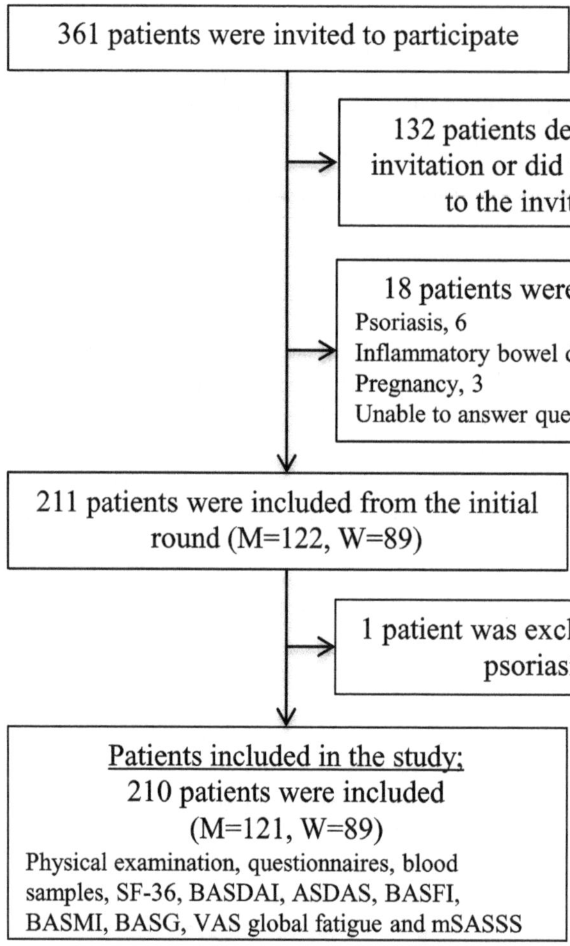

Fig. 1 Process of inclusion of the patients with ankylosing spondylitis. M, men; W, women; BASDAI, Bath Ankylosing Spondylitis Disease Activity Index; ASDAS, Ankylosing Spondylitis Disease Activity Score; BASFI, Bath Ankylosing Spondylitis Functional Index; BASMI, Bath Ankylosing Spondylitis Metrology Index; BAS-G, Bath Ankylosing Spondylitis Patient Global; VAS, visual analogue scale; mSASSS, modified Stoke Ankylosing Spondylitis Spinal Score

was performed in accordance with the Declaration of Helsinki.

The SF-36 questionnaire

HRQoL was assessed using the self-reported SF-36 questionnaire, an instrument consisting of 36 questions grouped into eight domains [3–6]. The eight domains include physical functioning (PF; 10 items), role physical (RP; 4 items), bodily pain (BP; 2 items), general health (GH; 5 items), vitality (VT; 4 items), social functioning (SF; 2 items), role emotional (RE; 3 items) and mental health (MH; 5 items). In addition, a further single item concerns reported health transition over the past year. The response alternatives for the role limitation domains (physical and emotional) are dichotomous (yes/no), and the other items have three to six response choices. The items within each domain contribute to an overall domain score between 0 and 100, with 0 representing worst and 100 excellent health. The questions reflect the individuals' health status during the last 4 weeks. The eight domains are also combined to produce two summary scores. The first four aforementioned domains, PF, RP, BP and GH, give an overall physical component summary (PCS) score and the second four domains, VT, SF, RE and MH, give an overall mental component summary (MCS) score. The component summary scores are standardised combined scores, with a mean of 50 and standard deviation of 10.

Other questionnaires

Participants also answered additional questionnaires including the BASDAI and the BASFI. The BASDAI estimates the patient's disease activity and the BASFI estimates the functional limitations during the last week. Higher values indicate higher disease activity and respectively worse physical function [18].

The Ankylosing Spondylitis Disease Activity Score, including C-reactive protein (ASDAS-CRP), was calculated for each patient. The disease activity is divided into inactive disease (ASDAS < 1.3), low disease activity (1.3 ≤ ASDAS < 2.1), high disease activity (2.1 ≤ ASDAS ≤ 3.5) and very high disease activity (ASDAS > 3.5) [18, 19]. The patients also answered the Bath Ankylosing Spondylitis Patient Global (BAS-G) [18]. A visual analogue scale (VAS) for global fatigue was used to evaluate fatigue experienced over the last few days graded from not at all (0) to extreme fatigue (100). In addition, the patients answered a questionnaire about lifestyle habits, medical history and medication.

Physical examination

The patients' mobility was measured using the BASMI. A higher BASMI score indicates less spinal mobility [18]. Physical examinations were performed by one physician (EK).

Radiography

Spinal radiographic changes were assessed from the lateral projection of the spinal radiographs and were graded using the mSASSS. Anterior corners of vertebra C2–T1 and T12–S1 were graded with a score between 0 and 3 (0 = normal, 1 = erosion, sclerosis or squaring, 2 = syndesmophyte, 3 = bridging syndesmophyte). The overall scoring scale ranges from 0 to 72, with 72 representing complete ankylosis [20]. To have a mSASSS ≥ 2 at a vertebral corner was classified as having a syndesmophyte. Severe spinal radiographic change was defined as ≥ 3 consecutive intervertebral bridges in the cervical spine and/or the lumbar spine, similar to the definition of grade 4 = severe in the Bath Ankylosing Spondylitis Radiology Index (BASRI) [21]. The majority of x-rays were performed within a couple of months after the study inclusion and < 5% of the patients were examined up to 6 months after the inclusion. One experienced radiologist scored all radiographs.

Laboratory tests

Erythrocyte sedimentation rate (ESR) and C-reactive protein (CRP) were analysed consecutively by standard laboratory techniques at the different hospitals.

Statistics

Non-parametrical statistical tests were applied because not all data were normally distributed. The median, 25th percentile (Q1) and 75th percentile (Q3) or interquartile range (IQR) or mean with standard deviation (SD) were presented for continuous data and frequency with percentage for categorical data. Data were compared using the Mann–Whitney U test or chi square test, as appropriate. The Kruskal–Wallis test was used to compare multiple groups and the Mann–Whitney U test was applied for post hoc analyses with a Bonferroni-corrected p value (<0.008). Univariate logistic regression analyses were conducted with dichotomised PCS and MCS below (coded 1) and above (coded 0) their respective median values as dependent variables and demographic and disease-related variables of interest as covariates. Age and symptom duration were stratified into decades and BASMI and BASFI into whole units. BASDAI was dichotomised into ≥ 4 (coded 1) and < 4 (coded 0) and ASDAS-CRP into ≥ 2.1 (coded 1) and < 2.1 (coded 0). mSASSS+ 1 was log-transformed in order to improve the distribution. Variables with p values ≤0.2 in the univariate analyses (Additional file 1: Tables S4 and S5) were chosen first to potentially be entered into the multivariable logistic regression models, the enter method. Thereafter, variables were excluded if the variable of interest by definition was a part of another variable, for instance, ASDAS-CRP was chosen as a variable reflecting disease activity instead of the BASDAI and CRP. The BASG was excluded as the ASDAS-CRP was chosen. The VAS for global fatigue was chosen instead of the BASDAI. The remaining variables were thereafter checked for multicollinearity and variables with the lowest p value in the univariate analysis were kept and entered into the multivariable models. In the multivariable logistic regression analyses, PCS and MCS were dichotomised as described above and were the dependent variables, while the other variables formed the independent variables (Tables 2 and 3). A p value <0.05 was considered statistically significant. All statistical analyses were performed using SPSS version 24 (SPSS Inc., IBM, Chicago, USA).

Results

For the enrolment process see Fig. 1. A total of 210 patients with AS, 121 (57.6%) men and 89 (42.4%) women, with a median age of 49.0 years (40.0, 61.2) and a median symptom duration of 24.0 years (13.0, 34.0), were included in this report. HLA-B27 was present in 183 (87.1%) of the patients with AS. The mSASSS median and mean values were 5.0 (0.0, 20.0) and 13.9 ± 19.0, respectively. Concerning biological drugs, 43 (20.5%) patients were treated with a TNF-inhibitor (TNFi) out of which 32 (15.2%) were used in combination with a conventional synthetic disease modifying anti-rheumatic drug (csDMARD). In total, 73 (34.8%) patients were on a TNFi and/or a csDMARD. Characteristics of all the patients and stratified by sex are displayed in Table 1. Comparisons between men and women showed that the age and symptom duration did not differ significantly between sexes. Women with AS had a significantly higher ESR and VAS for global fatigue compared to the men. Men with AS had significantly higher mSASSS and body mass index (BMI) than the women. More men carried HLA-B27 and had ≥ 1 prevalent syndesmophyte compared to the women. Only men had severe radiographic changes in the spine, defined as ≥ 3 consecutive intervertebral bridges in the cervical spine

Table 1 Characteristics of the patients with ankylosing spondylitis, overall and stratified and compared by sex

Variables	All, $n = 210$	Men, $n = 121$ (57.6)	Women, $n = 89$ (42.4)	P value
Age, years	49.0 (40.0, 61.2)	49.0 (39.5, 61.0)	49.0 (41.5, 62.0)	0.48
BMI, kg/m^2	25.2 (22.8, 28.4)	25.8 (23.6, 28.9)	24.0 (21.8, 27.5)	**0.003**
Civil state: single	58 (27.6)	34 (28.1)	24 (27.0)	0.86
in a relationship	152 (72.4)	87 (71.9)	65 (73.0)	0.87
Years in school: < 13	98 (46.9)[a]	62 (51.7)[a]	36 (40.4)	0.11
≥ 13 years	111 (53.1)	58 (48.3)	53 (59.6)	0.11
Ever smoker	105 (50.0)	65 (53.7)	40 (44.9)	0.21
VAS global fatigue, score	59.0 (27.0, 74.0)	50.0 (20.5, 68.0)	64.0 (42.5, 76.0)	**0.002**
Duration of symptoms, years	24.0 (13.0, 34.0)[c]	23.0 (13.0, 33.0)[b]	24.0 (12.5, 34.0)[a]	0.80
Duration of disease, years	12.0 (5.0, 23.0)[a]	12.5 (6.0, 24.0)[a]	11.0 (4.0, 18.5)	0.11
ESR, mm/h	11.0 (7.0, 19.0)	10.0 (5.0, 17.0)	14.0 (10.0, 22.5)	**0.001**
CRP, mg/L	3.0 (1.0, 7.0)[a]	3.0 (1.0, 7.0)[a]	2.0 (1.0, 7.5)	0.38
HLA-B27 positive	183 (87.1)	112 (92.6)	71 (79.8)	**0.006**
History of anterior uveitis	108 (51.5)	69 (57.0)	39 (43.8)	0.058
TNFi and/or csDMARD	73 (34.8)	45 (37.2)	28 (31.5)	0.39
BASMI, score	3.0 (2.0, 4.0)	3.0 (1.8, 4.3)	2.8 (2.2, 3.8)	0.34
BASFI, score	2.3 (1.0, 3.8)[c]	2.3 (1.0, 3.7)[a]	2.3 (1.0, 4.2)[b]	0.73
BASDAI, score	3.5 (1.7, 5.3)[d]	2.9 (1.5, 5.2)[c]	3.7 (1.9, 5.6)[a]	0.079
ASDAS-CRP, score	2.1 (1.4, 2.9)[a]	2.0 (1.3, 2.9)[a]	2.2 (1.5, 2.8)	0.70
BAS-G, score	2.90 (1.15, 5.45)	2.6 (1.0, 5.0)	3.5 (1.3, 5.7)	0.28
mSASSS, score	5.0 (0.0, 20.0)	8.0 (2.0, 34.0)	2.0 (0.0, 9.5)	**< 0.001**
Syndesmophyte and/or	98 (46.7)	71 (58.7)	27 (30.3)	**< 0.001**
≥ 3 intervertebral bridges consecutively, cervical and/or lumbar spine	29 (13.8)	29 (24)	0	**< 0.001**
PF, score	80.0 (65.0, 90.0)	80.0 (69.4, 90.0)	75.0 (60.6, 90.0)	**0.023**
	74.4 ± 21.4	76.7 ± 21.5	71.2 ± 21.0	
RP, score	75.0 (25.0, 100.0)	75.0 (25.0, 100.0)	75.0 (0.0, 100.0)	0.12
	59.3 ± 41.1	63.1 ± 40.3	54.2 ± 41.8	
BP, score	51.0 (41.0, 64.0)	51.0 (41.0, 72.0)	51.0 (41.0, 62.0)	0.19
	54.1 ± 21.9	55.8 ± 22.8	51.7 ± 20.4	
GH, score	62.0 (40.0, 77.0)	62.0 (40.0, 77.0)	60.0 (40.0, 76.0)	0.78
	57.1 ± 22.8	56.6 ± 23.7	57.7 ± 21.8	
VT, score	50.0 (30.0, 70.0)	55.0 (30.0, 75.0)	50.0 (30.0, 65.0)	**0.010**
	50.6 ± 23.6	54.3 ± 24.1	45.5 ± 22.0	
SF, score	75.0 (65.2, 100.0)	87.5 (62.5, 100.0)	75.0 (62.5, 100.0)	0.10
	75.8 ± 25.0	77.7 ± 25.6	73.3 ± 24.1	
RE, score	100.0 (33.3, 100.0)[b]	100.0 (33.3, 100.0)[a]	100.0 (33.3, 100.0)[a]	0.16
	68.8 ± 40.8[b]	71.9 ± 39.8[a]	64.4 ± 41.9[a]	
MH, score	76.0 (63.0, 88.0)	76.0 (64.0, 88.0)	72.0 (60.0, 84.0)	**0.039**
	71.9 ± 19.8	73.7 ± 20.7	69.5 ± 18.3	
PCS, score	42.4 (34.3, 48.7)[b]	43.6 (35.4, 49,4)[a]	41.8 (32.6, 47.5)[a]	0.16
	41.4 ± 10.0[b]	42.1 ± 10.0[a]	40.4 ± 10.2[a]	
MCS, score	48.0 (35.6, 55.2)[b]	49.2 (39.9, 56.1)[a]	46.0 (33.4, 53.8)[a]	0.13
	44.8 ± 12.5[b]	45.9 ± 12.3[a]	43.3 ± 12.8[a]	

Values are median and 25th percentile (Q1) and 75th percentile (Q3), numbers of patients and percent (%) or mean ± SD. Comparisons between men and women are assessed by Mann-Whitney U-test or Chi-square test. Significant differences are in bold text

BMI body mass index, *VAS* visual analogue scale, *ESR* erythrocyte sedimentation rate, *CRP* C-reactive protein, *TNFi* TNF inhibitor, *csDMARD* conventional synthetic disease modifying anti-rheumatic drug, *BASMI* Bath Ankylosing Spondylitis Metrology Index, *BASFI* Bath Ankylosing Spondylitis Functional Index, *BASDAI* Bath Ankylosing Spondylitis Disease Activity Index, *ASDAS-CRP* Ankylosing Spondylitis Disease Activity Score-CRP, *BAS-G* Bath Ankylosing Spondylitis Patient Global, *mSASSS* Modified Stoke Ankylosing Spondylitis Spine Score, *PF* physical function, *RP* role physical, *BP* bodily pain, *GH* general health, *VT* vitality, *SF* social function, *RE* role emotional, *MH* mental health, *PCS* physical component summary, *MCS* mental component summary

Number of missing data values: [a]$n = 1$; [b]$n = 2$;[c]$n = 3$; [d]$n = 4$

and/or the lumbar spine. Otherwise, baseline characteristics were similar between sexes.

Health related quality of life in patients with ankylosing spondylitis and in the general population

The patients with AS had significantly lower SF-36 scores in all domains and the component summary scores, PCS and MCS, when compared to five age-matched and sex-matched controls from the general population per AS patient ($p < 0.001$) (Fig. 2a, Additional file 1: Table S1). The mean PCS score ± SD was 41.3 ± 10.1 in AS versus 49.1 ± 9.8 in controls and the mean MCS score was 44.6 ± 12.7 in AS versus 50.5 ± 10.4 in controls. The mean age ± SD was 50.1 ± 12.9 years in the patients with AS versus 50.1 ± 12.8 years in the controls, and the sex-distribution was exactly the same, due to the matched selection of controls.

Comparison of SF-36 physical domain scores between sexes in AS showed that women had a significantly lower PF score compared to men ($p = 0.023$). Regarding the mental domains, women had significantly lower VT and MH scores compared to men ($p = 0.010$ and $p = 0.039$, respectively) (Fig. 2b, Table 1). No significant differences were found in PCS or MCS between men and women with AS. PCS was significantly lower compared with MCS in the total AS group ($p < 0.001$), a difference also seen in both women and men in the sex-stratified analyses ($p = 0.027$ and $p = 0.002$ respectively) (Fig. 2b).

Health-related quality of life in relation to age

The patients were divided into four different age groups: ≤ 40 years ($n = 53$), 41–50 years ($n = 57$), 51–60 years ($n = 44$) and ≥ 61 years ($n = 56$), in order to study the

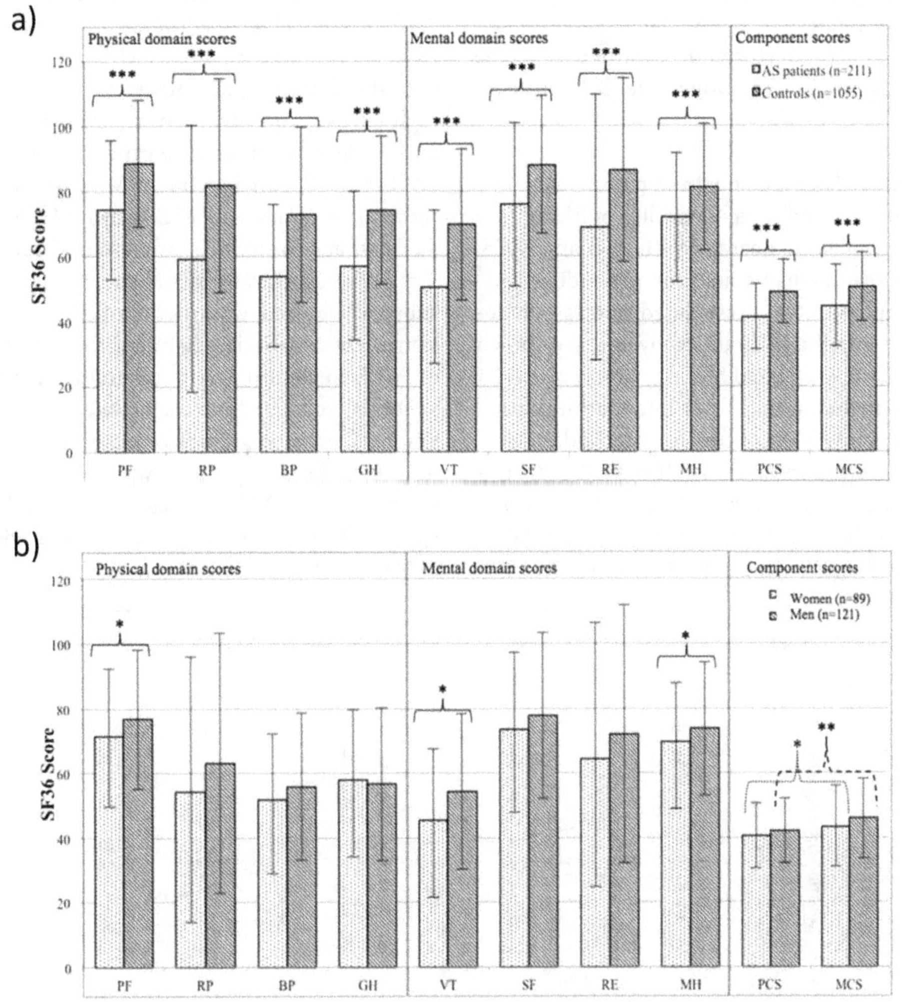

Fig. 2 Short form-36 (SF-36) in 211 patients with ankylosing spondylitis (AS) compared to 1055 age-matched and sex-matched controls from the general population (**a**) and 210 patients with AS, stratified by sex (**b**). Mean ± SD are shown. physical component summary (PCS) and mental component summary (MCS) are standardized scores with a mean of 50 and SD of 10. The other domains score between 0 and 100 with 0 = worst and 100 = best health. PF, physical function; RP, role physical; BP, bodily pain; GH, general health; VT, vitality; SF, social function; RE, role emotional; MH, mental health. Mann-Whitney U test and Wilcoxon rank sum tests were used for comparisons; *$p < 0.05$, **$p < 0.01$, ***$p < 0.001$

impact of age on the SF-36 summary scores. There was a difference in the PCS score between the four age groups ($p < 0.001$), and post hoc analysis showed that the PCS score was significantly lower in the age group ≥ 61 years compared to the age group ≤ 40 years ($p < 0.001$). No difference in the MCS score between the 4 age groups was found, Fig. 3. Correlation analyses revealed an inverse association between PCS score and age ($r_s = -0.29$, $p < 0.001$), and when stratified by sex, there was significant association in men ($r_s = -0.34$, $p < 0.001$) and a trend in women ($r_s = -0.20$, $p = 0.066$). There was no significant correlation between MCS and age.

Comparison between patients with ankylosing spondylitis with higher and lower health-related quality of life scores

The patients were divided into groups according to the median values of PCS and MCS scores and different characteristics were compared between patients with lower versus higher PCS and MCS scores. The comparisons were also performed stratified by sex. The results are shown in Additional file 1: Tables S2 and S3.

Logistic regression analyses demonstrating factors associated with worse health-related quality of life

Univariate logistic regression analyses with PCS and MCS, below their respective median values, as dependent variables and demographic and disease-related factors as independent variables, overall and stratified by sex, are shown in Additional file 1: Tables S4 and S5.

The process for including variables into the multivariable regression analyses is described in "Methods". Multivariable logistic regression analyses showed that to live alone without a partner was a significant factor associated with a worse PCS score (OR 2.38, 95% CI 1.00–5.67). To have a longer symptom duration (decades) (OR 1.66, 95% CI 1.16–2.37), higher BASFI (OR 1.98 per unit, 95% CI 1.46–2.70) and ASDAS-CRP ≥ 2.1 (OR 3.32, 95% CI 1.45–7.62) was also associated with a worse PCS score. The sex-stratified analyses revealed that, in men, the most important determinants for a worse PCS score were a high BASFI and an ASDAS-CRP ≥ 2.1, compared to a high BASFI in women (Table 2). In men, to have severe spinal radiographic changes was associated with a worse PCS score in the univariate but not in the multivariable logistic regression analysis. In a sensitivity analysis, age in decades was inserted into the models instead of symptom duration in decades. Age in decades was not a significant factor in these models, thus symptom duration in decades was kept in the models according to the criteria described in "Methods".

To live alone (OR 3.04, 95% CI 1.34–6.91), to have VAS global fatigue greater than the median value (OR 6.36, 95% CI 3.06–13.19) and ASDAS-CRP ≥ 2.1 (OR 2.97, 95% CI 1.41–6.25), were significant determinants associated with a worse MCS score (Table 3). The sex-stratified analyses revealed that longer education, high fatigue, and no severe radiographic changes in men, and to live without a partner, have high fatigue and ASDAS-CRP ≥ 2.1 in women were the most important determinants of a worse MCS score (Table 3). In sensitivity analysis, age in decades was inserted into the models but was not a significant factor and did not alter the models substantially and was therefore not used. There was no significant association between the mSASSS and the PCS or MCS in the univariate or multivariable logistic regression analyses. Further sensitivity analyses based on demographics, excluding disease-related variables, revealed that to live without a partner was still associated with both worse PCS and MCS scores, and age in decades was associated with a worse PCS score but not with a worse MCS score (Additional file 1: Table S6).

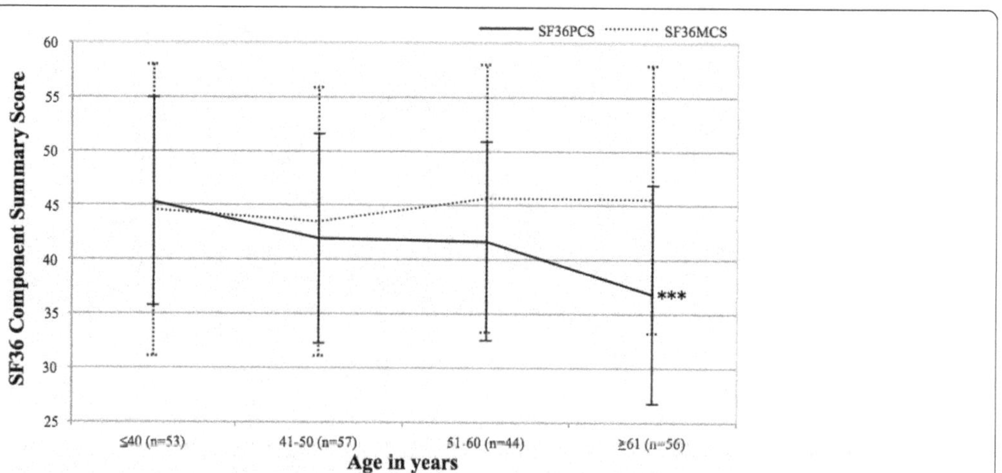

Fig. 3 Patients with ankylosing spondylitis (n = 210) divided in four age groups displaying Short Form-36 (SF-36) physical component summary (PCS) and mental component summary (MCS) scores. Mean ± SD are shown; ***$p < 0.001$, n, number of patients

Table 2 Multivariable logistic regression analyses with PCS score below the median value as dependent variable

	All, $n = 210$ PCS < median PCS 42.4			Men, $n = 121$ PCS < median PCS 43.6			Women, $n = 89$ PCS < median PCS 41.8		
Variables	OR	95% CI	*P* value	OR	95% CI	*P* value	OR	95% CI	*P* value
BMI, kg/m²	1.03	0.93 to 1.14	0.55	0.98	0.84 to 1.14	0.78			
Civil state, single	2.38	1.00 to 5.67	**0.049**	3.28	0.94 to 11.52	0.063	3.07	0.83 to 11.40	0.094
Years in school, < 13 years	1.12	0.50 to 2.48	0.79	1.40	0.43 to 4.55	0.57			
Ever smoker	0.77	0.35 to 1.73	0.53	0.55	0.16 to 1.89	0.34			
VAS global fatigue, > median	1.04	0.46 to 2.38	0.92	2.23	0.66 to 7.56	0.20			
Duration of symptoms, decades	1.66	1.16 to 2.37	**0.005**	1.36	0.81 to 2.30	0.24	1.69	0.99 to 2.90	0.055
ESR, > median	0.98	0.45 to 2.10	0.95						
BASMI, units							0.72	0.38 to 1.34	0.30
Lateral spinal flexion, cm	0.99	0.90 to 1.09	0.86	0.92	0.80 to 1.06	0.27			
BASFI, unit	1.98	1.46 to 2.70	**< 0.001**	2.09	1.29 to 3.41	**0.003**	2.25	1.42 to 3.57	**0.001**
ASDAS-CRP, ≥ 2.1	3.32	1.45 to 7.62	**0.005**	4.87	1.46 to 16.27	**0.010**	1.83	0.51 to 6.53	0.36
Log10mSASSS + 1, score	0.74	0.36 to 1.54	0.43						
≥ 3 intervertebral bridges consecutively (only men)[a]				0.57	0.12 to 2.70	0.48			

Significant differences are in bold text. The independent variables were defined by having a univariate association with PCS (p-value ≤0.2) and not demonstrating collinearity. Due to some missing data, the models are based on an overall 203 patients and in stratified analyses 115 men and 86 women
PCS physical component summary, *OR* odds ratio, *CI* confidence interval, *BMI* body mass index, *VAS* visual analogue scale, *ESR* erythrocyte sedimentation rate, *BASMI* Bath Ankylosing Spondylitis Metrology Index, *BASFI* Bath Ankylosing Spondylitis Functional Index, *ASDAS-CRP* Ankylosing Spondylitis Disease Activity Score C-reactive protein, *mSASSS* Modified Stoke Ankylosing Spondylitis Spine Score [a]Cervical and/or lumbar spine

Discussion

In this study, we have used the generic instrument SF-36 to evaluate HRQoL in a well-characterised cohort of patients with AS. The patients with AS had significantly lower HRQoL compared with controls. PCS was more affected compared to MCS in both sexes. Both disease-related and demographic factors were associated with HRQoL. Also, for the first time, to the best of our knowledge, we identified determinants of worse HRQoL separately in men and in women with AS and we found that the factors associated with HRQoL differed in part between the sexes.

We showed that the patients with AS had significantly lower SF-36 scores compared to 1055 age-matched and sex-matched controls from the general population. The patients with AS scored lower in all SF-36 domains and component summary scores. Our findings are in line with results from other countries in which SF-36 in AS

Table 3 Multivariable logistic regression analyses with MCS score below the median value as dependent variable

	All, $n = 210$ MCS < median MCS 48.0			Men, $n = 121$ MCS < median MCS 49.2			Women, $n = 89$ MCS < median MCS 46.0		
Variables	OR	95% CI	*P* value	OR	95% CI	-value	OR	95% CI	*P* value
BMI, kg/m²	1.01	0.93 to 1.09	0.86						
Civil state, single	3.04	1.34 to 6.91	**0.008**	2.24	0.76 to 6–61	0.14	13.21	2.13 to 81.96	**0.006**
Years in school, < 13 years				0.36	0.13 to 0.96	**0.042**			
Ever smoker	1.26	0.61 to 2.58	0.53				1.35	0.38 to 4.76	0.64
VAS global fatigue, > median	6.36	3.06 to 13.19	**< 0.001**	7.73	2.63 to 22.76	**< 0.001**	17.29	3.82 to 78.23	**< 0.001**
Lateral spinal flexion, cm	1.02	0.95 to 1.09	0.64				0.94	0.81 to 1.10	0.44
BASFI, unit	1.18	0.93 to 1.50	0.16	1.41	0.99 to 2.00	0.057	1.07	0.73 to 1.57	0.72
ASDAS-CRP, ≥ 2.1	2.97	1.41 to 6.25	**0.004**	2.62	0.89 to 7.70	0.080	6.74	1.76 to 25.85	**0.005**
Log10mSASSS + 1, score							1.17	0.29 to 4.66	0.82
≥ 3 intervertebral bridges consecutively (only men)[a]				0.17	0.044 to 0.65	**0.01**			

Significant differences are in bold text. The independent variables were defined by having a univariate association with MCS (p-value ≤0.2) and not demonstrating collinearity. Due to some missing data, the models are based on overall 204 patients and in stratified analyses 117 men and 86 women
MCS mental component summary, *OR* odds ratio, *CI* confidence interval, *BMI* body mass index, *VAS* visual analogue scale, *BASFI* Bath Ankylosing Spondylitis Functional Index, *ASDAS-CRP* Ankylosing Spondylitis Disease Activity Score C-reactive protein, *mSASSS* Modified Stoke Ankylosing Spondylitis Spine Score, [a]Cervical and/or lumbar spine

has been compared indirectly with results from the general population [9, 22–24] and with the meta-analysis by Yang et al. who compared SF-36 scores in AS using two normative general-population databases of the SF-36. They stated also that HRQoL in AS was lower than in type II diabetes mellitus, and comparable with rheumatoid arthritis [7]. Thus, these results underline the importance of taking HRQoL into consideration in the management of patients with AS.

Furthermore, we observed that the PCS score was more affected compared to the MCS score. This was noted in the whole cohort and also in men and in women analysed individually. Yang et al. reported a pooled mean PCS score of 37.5 and MCS score of 44.7 [7]. Our results were similar, with a mean PCS score ± SD of 41.4 ± 10.0 and MCS score of 44.8 ± 12.5 ($n = 210$). This suggests that AS has a larger impact on physical components of HRQoL compared to mental components, although both dimensions are reduced compared to the general population.

It is known that the phenotype of AS differs between the sexes. For instance, at a group level, men with AS have more AS-related spinal radiographic changes [25]. This finding is one reason why it could be hypothesized that there should be more effect on HRQoL in men than in women with AS. However, we found that the women with AS scored worse in two mental domains and one physical domain compared to the men with AS. Similar sex differences in SF-36 scores have been reported previously [22, 26, 27]. Interestingly, results from the SF-36 Swedish normative population database, consisting of 8930 persons from the general population in different parts of Sweden, showed a clear difference in mean scores between men and women, with women generally reporting lower HRQoL. This indicates a general phenomenon that women report worse HRQoL compared to men [4].

We also explored the impact of age on the PCS and MCS scores. Concerning the MCS, the median MCS score was stable among the four different age groups in our study and was not correlated with age. However, the median PCS score was significantly worse in the age group with the oldest patients (≥ 61 years) compared to the group with the youngest patients (≤ 40 years). The pattern was similar in the SF-36 Swedish and Norwegian normative population databases displaying associations with age and the physical health domains but small differences for the mental domains across age groups [4, 28].

The multivariable logistic regression analysis in our study revealed that a patient was twice as likely to have a worse PCS score if they lived without a partner, and three times more likely to have a worse PCS score if they had ASDAS-CRP ≥ 2.1 vs ASDAS-CRP < 2.1. A longer symptom duration and higher BASFI were also associated with a worse PCS score. Analyses by sex revealed that a high BASFI and ASDAS-CRP were the most important determinants of a worse PCS score in the men, while in the women high BASFI/reduced physical function was associated with a worse PCS score. Salaffi et al. also found that high disease activity and chronic comorbidity were significantly associated with a lower PCS [9], and Özdemir reported inverse correlation between BASDAI, BASFI and most of the SF-36 domains [12]. We found that the pattern was somewhat different for the MCS score. A global fatigue score above the median value was associated with a six-fold increase in the risk of a worse MCS score. Patients living without a partner and patients who had an ASDAS-CRP ≥ 2.1 were three times more likely to have a worse MCS score. In analyses stratified by sex the same variables were significant in women, while in men, high levels of fatigue, longer education and absence of severe spinal radiographic changes, defined as ≥ 3 consecutive intervertebral bridges in the cervical spine and/or the lumbar spine were factors associated with worse MCS score. Opposite results on the level of education have previously been reported by some, with a low level of education or ≤ 12 years of education associated with worse HRQoL [9, 22, 26]. The discrepancy may have to do with our sex-stratified analyses and differences in selection and demographics between studies. We did not find the mSASSS for radiographic changes or the presence of syndesmophytes in the spine to be significant determinants of SF-36 scores, but severe spinal radiographic changes in men, defined as ≥ 3 consecutive intervertebral bridges in the cervical spine and/or the lumbar spine, were associated with better mental health, with MCS in multivariable analyses and with worse physical health, worse physical health, PCS in univariate but not in multivariable analyses. Importantly, it was only men in our study that had ≥ 3 consecutive intervertebral bridges in the cervical spine and/or the lumbar spine. Only a few previous studies have addressed if there is a relation between radiographic changes in the spine and HRQoL in AS. A Chinese study conducted in 245 patients with AS found that patients with severe kyphosis had a significantly worse PF domain score compared to patients with milder kyphosis [10]. In a study of 962 patients with AS, Bodur et al. identified weak but significant inverse correlation between the Bath Ankylosing Spondylitis Radiology Index (BASRI) and some of the SF-36 domains (PF, GH and MH) [29] similar to findings in a study of 100 patients with AS from Morocco [30]. Weak significant correlation was identified between the BASRI and worse Ankylosing Spondylitis Quality of Life questionnaire (ASQoL) scores in univariate but not in multivariate regression analyses in early axial SpA [31]. Conversely, a small study conducted in 36 patients with AS found no significant correlation between the mSASSS and SF-36 scores [32] and Machado et al. did not find significant association between the PCS or MCS scores and the mSASSS [13], while a higher mSASSS was significantly associated with better ASQoL in another study [33]. In a longitudinal study, the mSASSS at baseline was not associated with worse ASQoL over time [34]. In summary, previous results are not consistent, which can be explained by the use of different methods for grading spinal radiographic changes; the mSASSS, BASRI, kyphosis and ≥ 3 consecutive intervertebral bridges, different questionnaires assessing HRQoL; SF-36 and ASQoL, different statistical approaches; univariate and multivariable analyses and differences in methods of recruiting the patients etc. However, there seems to be some direct association between HRQoL and AS-related spinal radiographic changes. Interestingly, for the first time, to the best of our knowledge, we found that men who had severe spinal radiographic changes had better mental health compared to men without such changes and we hypothesize that it can be explained by adaptive coping strategies in patients with a longstanding chronic disease [35].

The impact on HRQoL of living alone and/or to be unmarried has previously been investigated in other diseases and in the general population, and to the best of our knowledge, for the first time in this study of patients with AS. The literature displays inconsistent results. In patients with chronic diseases such as cancer and multiple sclerosis, living alone is mostly associated with worse HRQoL, which is in line with the findings in our study [36–38]. However, in a longitudinal study, decline in the MCS score in patients with diabetes mellitus was associated with not living alone [39]. In a study from China, participants living alone had worse HRQoL [40], while the opposite was reported from another part of China, Shanghai [41]. Women in the Nurses' Health Study who lived alone had lower risk of decline in the MH and VT domains compared with those living with a spouse. Furthermore, contact with friends and relatives and level of social engagement significantly protected against a decline in MH in women living alone but not among women living with a partner [42]. Thus, the influence of living alone on HRQoL is complex and seems to be related to the persons' state of health, culture and gender, among other factors.

The sex-stratified analyses in our study revealed some differences; the disease activity seemed to be a more important factor in the physical component of HRQoL in men while the civil state was more important for the mental component of HRQoL in women, which are aspects that can be taken into account in the management of the patients with AS.

There are some limitations to be acknowledged; first this study is cross-sectional and thus we cannot draw any conclusions about the variables identified as associated with worse HRQoL and causality. To investigate this a longitudinal study is required. Second, the SF-36 Swedish normative population database was created in the 1990s and HRQoL in the general population might have changed over the years. However, HRQoL in the general population assessed by the SF-36 was stable from 1996 to 2004 in Norway [43], our neighbouring country, indicating that the difference in time may not be a significant problem. Third, we chose to divide the patients with AS according to their median values of PCS and MCS. Since there is no established cutoff for better or worse HRQoL we used this pragmatic approach. Furthermore, the modest number of subjects in the sex-stratified analyses result in broad confidence intervals and thus results need to be interpreted with some caution. Strengths of this study comprise first, a well-characterised patient cohort with an adequate number of patients allowing subgroup analyses of the sexes to be carried out for the first time. Second, SF-36 scores in patients with AS were compared to those in a large sample of controls from the general population who were precisely matched on sex and age.

Possible implications of our findings include that we have identified variables associated with worse HRQoL, which are modifiable. Even though our study is cross-sectional, and thus not able to show causality, by using these variables as a guide, patients may be treated more efficiently, leading to reduction in disease activity, pain and fatigue, thus potentially improving both the PCS and MCS scores as has been shown in some clinical trials [44–46]. To live alone without a partner was also associated with worse HRQoL in particular in women in the MCS score. A focus on social activities and community support for women with AS might help to improve MCS scores in this subset of patients with AS.

Conclusions

In this study we show that the patients with AS had significantly lower HRQoL when assessed by the SF-36, compared with the general population. The PCS score was more affected than the MCS score in both sexes. Both demographic and disease-related factors were associated with worse HRQoL, with partial overlap for the PCS and MCS. There were some differences between sexes in the factors associated with HRQoL. By modifying factors such as ASDAS-CRP and fatigue, HRQoL may potentially be improved. There is a need for longitudinal studies investigating predictors related to the development of HRQoL in AS over time. We intend to investigate factors related to the change in HRQoL over a 5-year period in this same cohort of patients with AS in a future study.

Additional files

Additional file 1: Table S1. Results of the SF-36 in patients with ankylosing spondylitis and in controls from the general population. **Table S2.** Comparisons of variables in patients with ankylosing spondylitis with scores below or above the median PCS score. **Table S3.** Comparisons of variables in patients with ankylosing and spondylitis scores below or above the median MCS score. **Table S4.** Univariate logistic regression analyses with PCS score below the median values as dependent variable and all assessed variables as covariates. **Table S5.** Univariate logistic regression analyses with MCS score below the median values as dependent variable and all assessed variables as covariates. **Table S6.** Multivariable logistic regression analyses with PCS and MCS scores below their median values as dependent variables and demographics as covariates. (DOCX 92 kb)

Abbreviations

AS: Ankylosing spondylitis; ASAS: Assessment of SpondyloArthritis International Society; ASDAS: Ankylosing Spondylitis Disease Activity Score; BASDAI: Bath Ankylosing Spondylitis Disease Activity Index; BASFI: Bath Ankylosing Spondylitis Functional Index; BASG: Bath Ankylosing Spondylitis Patient Global; BASMI: Bath Ankylosing Spondylitis Metrology Index; BASRI: Bath Ankylosing Spondylitis Radiology Index; BMI: Body mass index; BP: Bodily pain; CI: Confidence interval; CRP: C-reactive protein; DMARD: Disease-modifying anti-rheumatic drug; ESR: Erythrocyte sedimentation rate; GH: General health; HLA-B27: Human leukocyte antigen B27; HRQoL: Health-related quality of life; IBD: Inflammatory bowel disease; MCS: Mental component summary; MH: Mental health; mSASSS: Modified Stoke Ankylosing Spondylitis Spine Score; NSAID: Non-steroid anti-inflammatory drug; OR: Odds ratio; PCS: Physical component summary; PF: Physical functioning; RE: Role emotional; RP: Role physical; SD: Standard deviation; SF: Social functioning; SF-36: Short form-36; TNFi: Tumor necrosis factor inhibitor; VAS: Visual analogue scale; VT: Vitality

Acknowledgements
We wish to thank all the patients who participated in the study.

Funding
This study was supported by grants from the Health and Medical Care Executive Board of the Västra Götaland, Göteborg's Association Against Rheumatism, Västerbotten's Association Against Rheumatism, The Swedish Research Council, The Swedish Association Against Rheumatism, The Swedish Society of Medicine, The Göteborg Medical Society, the Region Västra Götaland and the County of Västerbotten (agreement concerning research and education of doctors).

Authors' contributions

LL and JBR participated in analysis and interpretation of data and drafting the manuscript, AD and EK participated in the design of the study and acquisition, analysis and interpretation of data. LTHJ participated in drafting the manuscript and interpretation of data. HFd'E participated in the conception and design of the work, acquisition, analysis and interpretation of data and drafting the manuscript. All authors critically reviewed the manuscript and approved the final version to be published.

Competing interests

LTHJ has received Advisory Board Fees from Novartis, Celgene and MSD, outside the submitted work. HFd'E has received Advisory Board Fees from Sandoz, Novartis and Abbvie outside the submitted work and an unrestricted grant from Novartis. LL, JRB, AD and EK report no competing interests.

References

1. Braun J, Sieper J. Ankylosing spondylitis. Lancet. 2007;369(9570):1379–90.
2. Baraliakos X, Listing J, Rudwaleit M, Haibel H, Brandt J, Sieper J, Braun J. Progression of radiographic damage in patients with ankylosing spondylitis: defining the central role of syndesmophytes. Ann Rheum Dis. 2007;66(7): 910–5.
3. Ware JE Jr, Sherbourne CD. The MOS 36-item short-form health survey (SF-36). I. Conceptual framework and item selection. Med Care. 1992; 30(6):473–83.
4. Sullivan M, Karlsson J. The Swedish SF-36 Health Survey III. Evaluation of criterion-based validity: results from normative population. J Clin Epidemiol. 1998;51(11):1105–13.
5. Sullivan M, Karlsson J, Ware JE Jr. The Swedish SF-36 Health Survey–I. Evaluation of data quality, scaling assumptions, reliability and construct validity across general populations in Sweden. Soc Sci Med. 1995;41(10): 1349–58.
6. Persson LO, Karlsson J, Bengtsson C, Steen B, Sullivan M. The Swedish SF-36 Health Survey II. Evaluation of clinical validity: results from population studies of elderly and women in Gothenborg. J Clin Epidemiol. 1998;51(11): 1095–103.
7. Yang X, Fan D, Xia Q, Wang M, Zhang X, Li X, Cai G, Wang L, Xin L, Xu S, et al. The health-related quality of life of ankylosing spondylitis patients assessed by SF-36: a systematic review and meta-analysis. Qual Life Res. 2016;25(11):2711–23.
8. Ribu L, Hanestad BR, Moum T, Birkeland K, Rustoen T. A comparison of the health-related quality of life in patients with diabetic foot ulcers, with a diabetes group and a nondiabetes group from the general population. Qual Life Res. 2007;16(2):179–89.
9. Salaffi F, Carotti M, Gasparini S, Intorcia M, Grassi W. The health-related quality of life in rheumatoid arthritis, ankylosing spondylitis, and psoriatic arthritis: a comparison with a selected sample of healthy people. Health Qual Life Outcomes. 2009;7:25.
10. Huang JC, Qian BP, Qiu Y, Wang B, Yu Y, Zhu ZZ, Hu J, Qu Z. Quality of life and correlation with clinical and radiographic variables in patients with ankylosing spondylitis: a retrospective case series study. BMC Musculoskelet Disord. 2017;18(1):352.
11. Vesovic-Potic V, Mustur D, Stanisavljevic D, Ille T, Ille M. Relationship between spinal mobility measures and quality of life in patients with ankylosing spondylitis. Rheumatol Int. 2009;29(8):879–84.
12. Ozdemir O. Quality of life in patients with ankylosing spondylitis: relationships with spinal mobility, disease activity and functional status. Rheumatol Int. 2011;31(5):605–10.
13. Machado P, Landewe R, Braun J, Hermann KG, Baraliakos X, Baker D, Hsu B, van der Heijde D. A stratified model for health outcomes in ankylosing spondylitis. Ann Rheum Dis. 2011;70(10):1758–64.
14. Klingberg E, Carlsten H, Hilme E, Hedberg M, Forsblad-d'Elia H. Calprotectin in ankylosing spondylitis–frequently elevated in feces, but normal in serum. Scand J Gastroenterol. 2012;47(4):435–44. https://doi.org/10.3109/00365521.2011.648953
15. Lee W, Reveille JD, Davis JC Jr, Learch TJ, Ward MM, Weisman MH. Are there gender differences in severity of ankylosing spondylitis? Results from the PSOAS cohort. Ann Rheum Dis. 2007;66(5):633–8.
16. Klingberg E, Geijer M, Gothlin J, Mellstrom D, Lorentzon M, Hilme E, Hedberg M, Carlsten H, Forsblad-D'Elia H. Vertebral fractures in ankylosing spondylitis are associated with lower bone mineral density in both central and peripheral skeleton. J Rheumatol. 2012;39(10):1987–95.
17. van der Linden S, Valkenburg HA, Cats A. Evaluation of diagnostic criteria for ankylosing spondylitis. A proposal for modification of the New York criteria. Arthritis Rheum. 1984;27(4):361–8.
18. Sieper J, Rudwaleit M, Baraliakos X, Brandt J, Braun J, Burgos-Vargas R, Dougados M, Hermann KG, Landewe R, Maksymowych W, et al. The Assessment of SpondyloArthritis international Society (ASAS) handbook: a guide to assess spondyloarthritis. Ann Rheum Dis. 2009;68(Suppl 2):ii1–44.

19. Machado PM, Landewe R, Heijde DV, Assessment of SpondyloArthritis international S. Ankylosing Spondylitis Disease Activity Score (ASDAS): 2018 update of the nomenclature for disease activity states. Ann Rheum Dis. 2018;77(10):1539–40.
20. Creemers MC, Franssen MJ, van't Hof MA, Gribnau FW, van de Putte LB, van Riel PL. Assessment of outcome in ankylosing spondylitis: an extended radiographic scoring system. Ann Rheum Dis. 2005;64(1):127–9.
21. MacKay K, Mack C, Brophy S, Calin A. The Bath Ankylosing Spondylitis Radiology Index (BASRI): a new, validated approach to disease assessment. Arthritis Rheum. 1998;41(12):2263–70.
22. Dagfinrud H, Mengshoel AM, Hagen KB, Loge JH, Kvien TK. Health status of patients with ankylosing spondylitis: a comparison with the general population. Ann Rheum Dis. 2004;63(12):1605–10.
23. Singh JA, Strand V. Spondyloarthritis is associated with poor function and physical health-related quality of life. J Rheumatol. 2009;36(5):1012–20.
24. Davis JC, van der Heijde D, Dougados M, Woolley JM. Reductions in health-related quality of life in patients with ankylosing spondylitis and improvements with etanercept therapy. Arthritis Rheum. 2005;53(4):494–501.
25. Klingberg E, Lorentzon M, Mellstrom D, Geijer M, Gothlin J, Hilme E, Hedberg M, Carlsten H, Forsblad-d'Elia H. Osteoporosis in ankylosing spondylitis - prevalence, risk factors and methods of assessment. Arthritis Res Ther. 2012;14(3):R108.
26. Ward MM. Health-related quality of life in ankylosing spondylitis: a survey of 175 patients. Arthritis Care Res. 1999;12(4):247–55.
27. Webers C, Essers I, Ramiro S, Stolwijk C, Landewe R, van der Heijde D, van den Bosch F, Dougados M, van Tubergen A. Gender-attributable differences in outcome of ankylosing spondylitis: long-term results from the Outcome in Ankylosing Spondylitis International Study. Rheumatology (Oxford). 2016; 55(3):419–28.
28. Loge JH, Kaasa S. Short form 36 (SF-36) health survey: normative data from the general Norwegian population. Scand J Soc Med. 1998;26(4):250–8.
29. Bodur H, Ataman S, Rezvani A, Bugdayci DS, Cevik R, Birtane M, Akinci A, Altay Z, Gunaydin R, Yener M, et al. Quality of life and related variables in patients with ankylosing spondylitis. Qual Life Res. 2011;20(4):543–9.
30. Ibn Yacoub Y, Amine B, Laatiris A, Abouqal R, Hajjaj-Hassouni N. Health-related quality of life in Moroccan patients with ankylosing spondylitis. Clin Rheumatol. 2011;30(5):673–7.
31. Fernandez-Carballido C, Navarro-Compan V, Castillo-Gallego C, Castro-Villegas MC, Collantes-Estevez E, de Miguel E, Esperanza Study G. Disease activity as a major determinant of quality of life and physical function in patients with early axial spondyloarthritis. Arthritis Care Res (Hoboken). 2017; 69(1):150–5.
32. Cho H, Kim T, Kim TH, Lee S, Lee KH. Spinal mobility, vertebral squaring, pulmonary function, pain, fatigue, and quality of life in patients with ankylosing spondylitis. Ann Rehabil Med. 2013;37(5):675–82.
33. Lopez-Medina C, Garrido-Castro JL, Castro-Jimenez J, Gonzalez-Navas C, Calvo-Gutierrez J, Castro-Villegas MC, Ortega-Castro R, Escudero-Contreras A, Font-Ugalde P, Collantes-Estevez E. Evaluation of quality of life in patients with axial spondyloarthritis and its association with disease activity, functionality, mobility, and structural damage. Clin Rheumatol. 2018;37(6):1581–8.
34. Essers I, Ramiro S, Stolwijk C, Blaauw M, Landewe R, van der Heijde D, van den Bosch F, Dougados M, van Tubergen A. Do extra-articular manifestations influence outcome in ankylosing spondylitis? 12-year results from OASIS. Clin Exp Rheumatol. 2016;34(2):214–21.
35. Bussing A, Ostermann T, Neugebauer EA, Heusser P. Adaptive coping strategies in patients with chronic pain conditions and their interpretation of disease. BMC Public Health. 2010;10:507.
36. Fernandez O, Baumstarck-Barrau K, Simeoni MC, Auquier P, MusiQo Lsg. Patient characteristics and determinants of quality of life in an international population with multiple sclerosis: assessment using the MusiQoL and SF-36 questionnaires. Mult Scler. 2011;17(10):1238–49.
37. Parker PA, Baile WF, de Moor C, Cohen L. Psychosocial and demographic predictors of quality of life in a large sample of cancer patients. Psycho-Oncology. 2003;12(2):183–93.
38. Sarna L, Padilla G, Holmes C, Tashkin D, Brecht ML, Evangelista L. Quality of life of long-term survivors of non-small-cell lung cancer. J Clin Oncol. 2002; 20(13):2920–9.
39. Schunk M, Reitmeir P, Ruckert-Eheberg IM, Tamayo T, Schipf S, Meisinger C, Peters A, Scheidt-Nave C, Ellert U, Hartwig S, et al. Longitudinal change in health-related quality of life in people with prevalent and incident type 2 diabetes compared to diabetes-free controls. PLoS One. 2017;12(5): e0176895.
40. Rao Y, Xu X, Liu D, Reis C, Newman IM, Qin L, Sharma M, Shen J, Zhao Y. Health-related quality of life in patients with arthritis: a cross-sectional survey among middle-aged adults in Chongqing, China. Int J Environ Res Public Health. 2018;15(4):768.
41. Wang R, Wu C, Zhao Y, Yan X, Ma X, Wu M, Liu W, Gu Z, Zhao J, He J. Health related quality of life measured by SF-36: a population-based study in Shanghai, China. BMC Public Health. 2008;8:292.
42. Michael YL, Berkman LF, Colditz GA, Kawachi I. Living arrangements, social integration, and change in functional health status. Am J Epidemiol. 2001; 153(2):123–31.
43. Fossa SD, Hess SL, Dahl AA, Hjermstad MJ, Veenstra M. Stability of health-related quality of life in the Norwegian general population and impact of chronic morbidity in individuals with and without a cancer diagnosis. Acta Oncol. 2007;46(4):452–61.
44. Morck B, Pullerits R, Geijer M, Bremell T, Forsblad-d'Elia H. Infliximab dose reduction sustains the clinical treatment effect in active HLAB27 positive ankylosing spondylitis: a two-year pilot study. Mediat Inflamm. 2013;2013: 289845.
45. Revicki DA, Luo MP, Wordsworth P, Wong RL, Chen N, Davis JC Jr, Group AS. Adalimumab reduces pain, fatigue, and stiffness in patients with ankylosing spondylitis: results from the adalimumab trial evaluating long-term safety and efficacy for ankylosing spondylitis (ATLAS). J Rheumatol. 2008;35(7):1346–53.
46. Deodhar AA, Dougados M, Baeten DL, Cheng-Chung Wei J, Geusens P, Readie A, Richards HB, Martin R, Porter B. Effect of secukinumab on patient-reported outcomes in patients with active ankylosing spondylitis: a phase III randomized trial (MEASURE 1). Arthritis Rheumatol. 2016;68(12):2901–10.

10

Prevalence of peripheral and extra-articular disease in ankylosing spondylitis versus non-radiographic axial spondyloarthritis

Janneke J. de Winter[1], Leonieke J. van Mens[1], Désirée van der Heijde[2], Robert Landewé[1] and Dominique L. Baeten[1,3*]

Abstract

Background: Peripheral disease (arthritis, enthesitis and dactylitis) and extra-articular disease (uveitis, psoriasis and inflammatory bowel disease) is common in ankylosing spondylitis (AS) and non-radiographic axial spondyloarthritis (nr-axSpA). So far, however, summary data on the prevalence are lacking. The objective of this meta-analysis was to assess the prevalence of peripheral and extra-articular manifestations in ankylosing spondylitis (AS) and nr-axSpA.

Methods: We performed a systematic literature search to identify publications describing the prevalence of peripheral and extra-articular disease manifestations in patients with AS and nr-axSpA. We assessed the risk of bias and between-study heterogeneity, and extracted data. Pooled prevalence and prevalence differences were calculated.

Results: Eight studies comprising 2236 patients with AS and 1242 with nr-axSpA were included: 7 of the studies were longitudinal cohort studies. There was male predominance in AS (70.4 %, 95 % CI 64.4, 76.0 %) but not in nr-axSpA (46.8 %, 95 % CI 41.7, 51.9), which was independent of the prevalence of human leukocyte antigen (HLA)-B27. The prevalence of HLA-B27 was similar in AS (78.0 % (95 % CI 73.9, 81.9 %) and nr-axSpA (77.4 %, 95 % CI 68.9, 84.9 %)). The pooled prevalence of arthritis (29.7 % (95 % CI 22.4, 37.4 %) versus 27.9 % (95 % CI 16.0, 41.6 %)), enthesitis (28.8 % (95 % CI 2.6, 64.8) versus 35.4 % (95 % CI 6.1, 71.2)). dactylitis (6.0 % (95 % CI 4.7, 7.5 %) versus 6.0 % (95 % CI 1.9, 12.0 %)), psoriasis (10.2 % (95 % CI 7.5, 13.2 %) versus 10.9 % (95 % CI 9.1, 13.0 %)) and inflammatory bowel disease (4.1 % (95 % CI 2.3, 6.5 %) versus 6.4 % (95 % CI 3.6, 9.7 %)) were similar in AS and nr-axSpA. The pooled prevalence of uveitis was higher in AS (23.0 % (95 % CI 19.2, 27.1 %)) than in nr-axSpA (15.9 % (95 % CI 11.8, 20.4 %)).

Conclusion: Peripheral and extra-articular manifestations are equally prevalent in AS and nr-axSpA, except for uveitis, which is slightly more prevalent in AS. These data provide evidence for the largely equal nature of disease manifestations in nr-axSpA and AS.

Keywords: Spondyloarthritis, Axial spondyloarthritis, Ankylosing spondylitis, Non-radiographic axial spondyloarthritis, Peripheral manifestations, Extra-articular manifestations, Meta-analysis

Abbreviations: AS, ankylosing spondylitis; ASAS, Assessment of Spondyloarthritis International Society;

(Continued on next page)

* Correspondence: d.l.baeten@amc.uva.nl
[1]Department of Clinical Immunology and Rheumatology, Amsterdam Rheumatology and immunology Center, Academic Medical Center/University of Amsterdam, Meibergdreef 9, 1105, AZ, Amsterdam, The Netherlands
[3]Department of Experimental Immunology, Academic Medical Center/University of Amsterdam, Amsterdam, The Netherlands
Full list of author information is available at the end of the article

(Continued from previous page)
CENTRAL, Cochrane Central Register of Controlled Trials; CRP, C-reactive protein; DESIR, DEvenir des Spondylarthropathies Indifferenciées Récentes ; ESPAC, Erciyes SPondyloArthritis Cohort; ESSG, European Spondylarthropathy Study Group; GESPIC, GErman SPondyloarthritis Inception Cohort; HLA-B27, human leukocyte antigen-B27; IBD, inflammatory bowel disease; M-H, Mantel-Haenszel; mNYc, modified New York criteria; MORE, Methodological evaluation of Observational REsearch; MRI, magnetic resonance imaging; Nr-axSpA, non-radiographic axial spondyloarthritis; PICO, participants, intervention, control and outcome; PRISMA, Preferred Reporting Items for Systematic reviews and Meta-Analyses; PsA, psoriatic arthritis; SCQM, Swiss Clinical Quality Management; SI, sacroiliac; SpA, spondyloarthritis; SPACE, SPondyloArthritis Caught Early; TNF, tumor necrosis factor

Background

Spondyloarthritis (SpA) is a prevalent and potentially disabling form of chronic inflammatory arthritis, affecting 0.5–1.5 % of the Western population [1, 2]. SpA has classically been subdivided into several subtypes, including ankylosing spondylitis (AS), psoriatic arthritis (PsA), reactive arthritis, arthritis/spondylitis associated with inflammatory bowel disease (IBD), and undifferentiated SpA. Classification criteria for SpA have been developed by the Assessment of SpondyloArthritis International Society (ASAS), which classifies SpA as axial or peripheral SpA [3–5]. The axial SpA disease spectrum classifies patients as having either ankylosing spondylitis (AS) whether the modified New York criteria (mNYc) are fulfilled, or as having non-radiographic axial SpA (nr-axSpA) in the absence of definite sacroiliac (SI) joint changes on plain radiograph.

Whether nr-axSpA is a different form [6, 7] of AS, an early form [8–10] of (AS) or two manifestations in the same disease continuum [11–13] is still subject to debate. There are several reasons to assume that AS and nr-axSpA should be considered as the same disease. First, AS and nr-axSpA in general have similar clinical characteristics, especially when related to disease activity [9–11]. Patients with AS and nr-axSpA not only have similar levels of disease activity, they also have a similar clinical disease course in the absence of tumor necrosis factor (TNF)α inhibiting treatment, as shown by recent longitudinal results from the German Spondyloarthritis Inception Cohort (GESPIC) [14]. Second, patients with nr-axSpA respond similarly to TNFα inhibiting treatment [15–18]. Third, radiographic changes only appear after several years; therefore, the requirement for radiographic change clearly reduces the sensitivity of the mNYc. Not only is sensitivity of the mNYc rather limited, but several studies have shown that scoring of radiographs is subject to considerable inter-reader and intra-reader variability. Scoring by both trained readers and local rheumatologists/radiologists not only yields modest sensitivity and specificity at best, but also has only moderate agreement in the recognition of radiographic sacroiliitis [19, 20]. These limitations challenge the crucial role of radiographic scoring in the process of diagnosing AS. Magnetic resonance imaging (MRI) is increasingly being used to visualize inflammation in the SI joints, as active inflammatory lesions are evident on MRI before radiographic lesions are detected [13]. However, MRI also has limitations in terms of scoring agreement, sensitivity, specificity and costs.

On the other hand, AS is characterized by male predominance and a higher level of C-reactive protein (CRP) in comparison to nr-axSpA [9–11]. Other studies suggest that AS and nr-axSpA differ in their genetics, as in some studies human leukocyte antigen (HLA)-B27 carriage is higher in AS than in nr-axSpA [21, 22], whilst other studies suggest there is no difference in HLA-B27 carriage between the two [9, 23, 24].

Even though spinal inflammation and structural damage are the main features of axial SpA, many patients have concomitant peripheral disease (arthritis, enthesitis, dactylitis) and/or extra-articular disease (uveitis, IBD, psoriasis). In AS, previous studies have reported 18–58 % prevalence of arthritis [9, 11, 25–27], 34–74 % prevalence of enthesitis of [9, 25] and a 6–8 % prevalence of dactylitis [9, 26, 28] (reported at any time during the disease course). The reported prevalence of uveitis occurring at some point in time during the course of the disease varies from 22–37 % [25, 27, 29–31], and the prevalence of IBD is estimated at 4–16 % [27, 30–34] and the prevalence of psoriasis at 4–9 % [6, 27, 30, 31, 33, 34].

In contrast, the prevalence of peripheral and extra-articular disease manifestations in nr-axSpA remains less well-defined. Hypothesizing that AS and nr-axSpA reflect subsets of a single disease entity and have similar disease burden, we performed a meta-analysis of published studies of axial SpA in order to assess if the best available estimate of the prevalence of peripheral and extra-articular disease manifestations is similar in AS and nr-axSpA.

Methods

We conducted a literature search by database searching, citation searching, "pearl growing" [35] and reference list checking. We performed this systematic review and meta-analysis in accordance with the Preferred Reporting Items for Systematic reviews and Meta-Analyses (PRISMA) guidelines [36].

Search methods

One of the authors (JdW) performed a systematic literature search with the assistance of an experienced librarian (RS). We used the following electronic bibliographical databases: Medline, the Cochrane Central Register of Controlled Trials (CENTRAL) and The Cochrane Library on 1 October 2015 (see Additional file 1: Table S1 for participants, intervention, control and outcome (PICO) and search strategy). The search was performed without language restrictions. In order to retrieve additional references, we used Citation Pearl Growing [35]. Furthermore, primary and secondary references from retrieved publications were manually checked to identify additional studies.

One review author (JdW) screened each title and abstract and selected potentially eligible studies. Thereafter, two review authors (JdW, LvM) independently selected eligible articles according to predetermined selection criteria. If there was any doubt, the full-text article was read by the review authors. Consensus of inclusion was in all cases achieved by discussion. If multiple publications presented data from the same study population, only the publication with the largest sample size was included. Reviews were only included if they presented original data.

Selection criteria for studies

Studies were included in this meta-analysis if data on prevalence of peripheral and extra-articular disease manifestations in both AS and nr-axSpA were available. We included both longitudinal and cross-sectional studies. Randomized controlled trials and retrospective studies were not included to avoid selection bias and maximize the accuracy of the data. Reporting the prevalence of peripheral and extra-articular disease manifestations did not necessarily have to be the primary outcome of the study.

All patients with axSpA had to fulfill the ASAS axial SpA criteria as defined in 2009 or an equivalent if the study was conducted before 2009 [3] (a modified version of the European Spondylarthropathy Study Group (ESSG) criteria [37]). All patients with AS had to meet the mNY-criteria for AS [38]. All nr-axSpA patients had to fulfill the ASAS MRI criteria or the clinical arm of the ASAS criteria for axial SpA [4] (or an equivalent if the study was conducted before 2009).

SPondyloArthritis Caught Early (SPACE) cohort study

We added unpublished data to our meta-analysis from one prospective cohort study. The SPACE cohort was described in detail previously [23]. In short, the SPACE cohort is a longitudinal cohort of patients aged 16 years and older, with chronic back pain for at least 3 months but less than 2 years, and with onset before the age of 45 years. In this meta-analysis, we added data for all patients with AS and nr-axSpA included between January 2009 and 2014 at two of the participating centers (Academic Medical Center Amsterdam and the Leiden University Medical Center).

Data extraction and management

Two review authors (JdW, LvM) independently extracted data using a predesigned form. The following details were extracted whenever available: first author, name of the study, country, year of publication, study design, study characteristics, sample size, mean age of patients, male/female ratio, mean disease duration, HLA-B27 positivity and percentage of the cohort in which HLA-B27 was measured and the timing and prevalence of peripheral and extra-articular disease manifestations. Whenever data on certain peripheral or extra-articular disease manifestations were missing, we contacted the authors of the article concerned. Furthermore, we requested data on the distribution of male/female participants among HLA-B27-positive and HLA-B27-negative patients with AS and nr-axSpA.

Assessment of risk of bias

Two review authors (JdW, LvM) assessed the potential risk of bias in all of the included studies by using the Methodological evaluation of Observational REsearch (MORE) checklist [39], which we adapted to our research question. The MORE checklist includes parameters on reporting of statement of potential conflicts of interest, study funding, ethical approval, external validity (was the gold standard for the diagnosis of AS and nr-axSpA used? Was there (reporting on) sampling bias?), and internal validity (how and when was the prevalence of peripheral or extra-articular disease symptoms measured?).

Assessment of heterogeneity

First, we assessed qualitative heterogeneity across studies by comparing them according to predefined criteria. Second, we evaluated the degree of statistical heterogeneity and inconsistency by using the T_2, Chi^2 and I^2 statistics. Heterogeneity was considered significant at $P < 0.10$ [40]. I^2 values of 25, 50 and 75 % were considered to indicate low, moderate and high inconsistency, respectively [40]. We used a random effects model for studies that we considered sufficiently homogeneous to include in the meta-analysis, as we anticipated there would not be one true effect size for all studies, despite potential measured quantitative homogeneity [41].

Data synthesis

We pooled studies in a random-effects model using the Mantel-Haenszel method, which estimates the between-study variation by comparing the result of each study with a Mantel-Haenszel random-effect meta-analysis result. Data were calculated as pooled prevalence with the corresponding 95 % confidence interval (CI) and as the difference in pooled prevalence between AS and nr-axSpA, with the corresponding 95 % CI. We performed data analyses using MetaXL [42] in Microsoft Excel 2010 and Review Manager 5. Forest plots were produced for all analyses using Review Manager 5, and we adapted these to our specific needs (to show the difference in prevalence instead of the difference in risk).

Results

Search

The electronic database search identified 447 articles (Fig. 1). The use of citation pearl growing resulted in one additional article. After merging for duplicates and screening of the titles and abstracts, we completely reviewed 44 unique articles. One article reported retrospective data. One full-text article could not be retrieved. Five articles did not report symptoms of peripheral or extra-articular disease manifestations. In 25 articles, there was no clear differentiation between AS and nr-axSpA. Two articles did not use the ASAS and mNY criteria to classify axial SpA. Eight articles reported data on duplicate cohort studies. Finally, eight studies were included in the meta-analysis [6, 11, 23, 43–45].

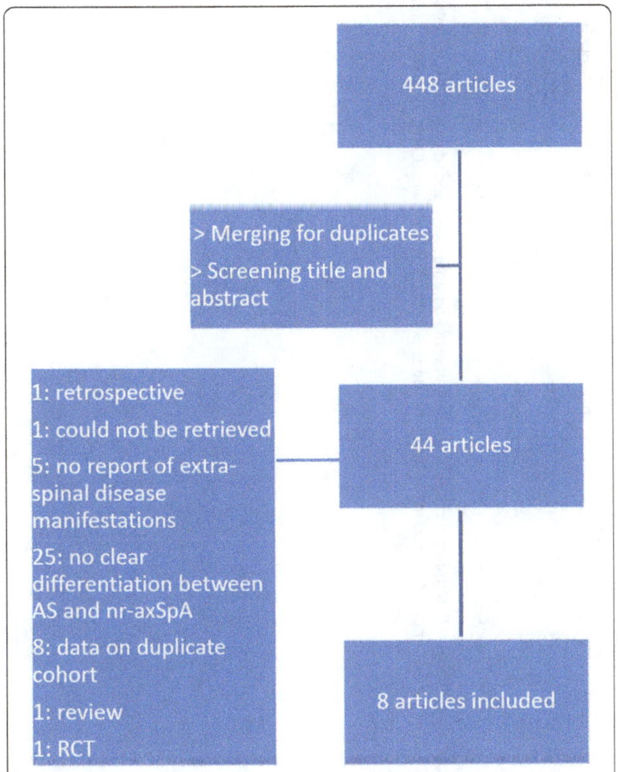

Fig. 1 Flow chart of included studies on prevalence of peripheral and extra-articular disease manifestations in non-radiographic axial spondyloarthritis and ankylosing spondylitis

Characteristics of the included studies

Eight studies fulfilled the inclusion criteria. The characteristics of the enrolled studies are summarized in Table 1. Seven out of eight studies were longitudinal SpA cohort studies. One study was a cross-sectional study of 100 consecutive patients attending outpatient clinics. In total, 3478 patients were included, of whom 2236 had AS and 1242 had nr-axSpA. Patients with AS fulfilled the mNY criteria in all studies. Patients with nr-axSpA fulfilled the ASAS criteria in six out of eight studies. Both GESPIC and Swiss Clinical Quality Management (SCQM) used the ASAS criteria with minor modifications, as patients were included before the development of the ASAS criteria.

The mean symptom duration varied from 1.2 ± 0.6 years in AS and 1.0 ± 0.7 year in nr-axSpA (Esperanza) to 17.7 ± 12.3 years in AS and 12.1 ± 8.5 years in nr-axSpA (Wallis). In pooled analysis the male prevalence of AS was 70.4 % (CI 64.4-76.0 %) and of nr-axSpA it was 46.8 % (CI 41.7, 51.9 %), resulting in a difference in pooled prevalence of 23.2 % (CI 15.3, 31.1 %). When we compared the male prevalence of AS and nr-axSpA among HLA-B27-positive and HLA-B27-negative patients, the difference in prevalence remained (24.2 % more male patients among patients with AS who were HLA-B27-positive (CI 15.1, 32.9 %) and 22.3 % more male patients among those with AS who were HLA-B27-negative (CI 14.4, 30.0 %)). The pooled prevalence of HLA-B27 did not differ in AS compared to nr-axSpA, with 78.0 % prevalence in AS (CI 73.9, 81.9 %) in AS compared to 77.4 % (CI 68.9, 84.9 %) in nr-axSpA.

All eight studies collected information about peripheral and extra-articular disease manifestations at baseline. Three out of eight studies (GESPIC, Kiltz and SPACE) reported patients who currently had, or had ever had, peripheral and extra-articular manifestations. Three studies only reported disease manifestations that had ever occurred (SCQM, Wallis and ESPAC) and two cohort studies reported only current disease manifestations (DESIR, Esperanza).

Risk of bias

All published studies (seven out of eight) were published in journals with an impact factor 3.5. The risk of bias summary for all studies is shown in Additional file 2: Table S2. In short, the risk of bias in all studies was considered sufficiently low to be included in this meta-analysis. General bias (role of funding, reporting on ethical approval, conflict of interest) was considered low in all eight studies. Internal validity was considered high in three out of eight studies (Esperanza, SCQM and SPACE) and intermediate in five out of eight studies. The source of the measure of prevalence of peripheral or extra-articular disease manifestations was reported in two of the eight studies (SCQM and SPACE).

Table 1 Characteristics of the eight included studies.

Name cohort or author	nr-axSpA *n*	AS *n*	Study design	Year of inclusion	Data collection	Maximum disease duration for inclusion, years	Mean symptom duration nr-axSpA, mean years (SD)	Mean symptom duration AS, mean years (SD)
GESPIC	226	236	Cohort	2000–2004	Baseline	AS: <10; nr-axSpA <5	2.6 (1.7)	5.2 (2.3)
Kiltz	44	56	Cross-sectional	Unknown	n.a.	No	9.4 (9.5)	12.8 (10.7)
DESIR	295	180	Cohort	2007–2010	Baseline	<3	1.5 (0.9)	1.6 (0.9)
SCQM	232	838	Cohort	2005–2011	Baseline	No	5.5 (1.8–13.7)[b]	12.7 (6.4–22.7)[b]
SPACE	58	23	Cohort	2009–2014	Baseline	<2	1.1 (0.6)	1.3 (0.7)
Esperanza	182	109	Cohort	2008–2011	Baseline	<2	1.0 (1.6)	1.2 (0.5)
Wallis	73	639	Cohort	2003–2012	Baseline	No	12.1 (8.5)[a]	17.7 (12.3)[a]
ESPAC	132	155	Cohort	2009–2014	Unknown	No	5.8 (5.5)	11.7 (7.7)

[a]Mean disease duration. [b]Median (interquartile range). *Nr-axSpA* non-radiographic axial spondyloarthritis, *AS* ankylosing spondylitis, *SD* standard deviation, *GESPIC* GErman SPondyloarthritis Inception Cohort, *n.a.* not applicable, *DESIR* Devenir des Spondylarthropathies Indifferenciées Récentes, *SCQM* Swiss Clinical Quality Management, *SPACE* SPondyloArthritis Caught Early, *ESPAC* Erciyes SPondyloArthritis

External validity was considered high in five out of eight studies (Esperanza, Kiltz, SCQM, SPACE and DESIR), intermediate in one out of eight studies (ESPAC) and low in two out of eight studies (GESPIC and Wallis).

Heterogeneity

When comparing all study characteristics as summarized in Table 1, all eight studies were homogeneous enough to include in the meta-analysis. Statistical heterogeneity was measured for each of the peripheral or extra-articular disease manifestations.

Meta-analysis

Peripheral arthritis

In pooled analysis the prevalence of current peripheral arthritis was 22.9 % (CI 5.7, 46.0 %) in AS and 25.2 % (CI 8.9, 45.7 %) in nr-axSpA, resulting in a difference in pooled prevalence of 0.7 % (CI −5.4, 6.7 %) favoring AS. Quantitative heterogeneity was not statistically significant and the level of inconsistency was moderate ($Chi^2 = 7.29$, $P = 0.12$, $Tau^2 = 0.00$, $I^2 = 45$ %). The pooled prevalence of a history of peripheral arthritis was 29.7 % (CI 22.4, 37.4 %) in AS and 27.9 % (CI 16.0, 41.6 %) in nr-axSpA, resulting in a difference in pooled prevalence of −3.8 % (CI −8.8, 1.1 %) favoring nr-axSpA (Fig. 2a). Quantitative heterogeneity was not statistically significant and the level of inconsistency was low ($Chi^2 = 1.25$, $P = 0.74$, $Tau^2 = 0.00$, $I^2 = 0$ %).

Enthesitis

In pooled analysis the prevalence of current enthesitis was 13.6 % (CI 1.8, 31.8 %) in AS and 19.5 % (CI 7.1, 35.7 %) in nr-axSpA, resulting in a difference in the pooled prevalence of −4.9 % (CI -10.9, 1.0 %) favoring nr-axSpA. Quantitative heterogeneity was statistically significant and the level of inconsistency was moderate ($Chi^2 = 11.37$, $P = 0.02$, $Tau^2 = 0.00$, $I^2 = 65$ %). The pooled prevalence of a history of enthesitis was 28.8 % (CI 2.6, 64.8 %) in AS and 35.4 % (CI 6.1, 71.2 %) in nr-axSpA, resulting in a difference in pooled prevalence of −5.4 % (CI -9.7, 0.0 %) favoring nr-axSpA (Fig. 2b). Quantitative heterogeneity was statistically significant and the level of inconsistency was moderate ($Chi^2 = 12.17$, $P = 0.03$, $Tau^2 = 0.00$, $I^2 = 34$ %).

Dactylitis

In pooled analysis the prevalence of current dactylitis was 5.6 % (CI 0.0, 16.2 %) in AS and 5.2 % (CI 0.4, 13.7 %) in nr-axSpA, resulting in a difference in pooled prevalence of −0.5 % (CI -2.6-1.6 %) favoring nr-axSpA. Quantitative heterogeneity was not statistically significant and the level of inconsistency was moderate ($Chi^2 = 3.31$, $P = 0.19$, $Tau^2 = 0.00$, $I^2 = 40$ %). The pooled prevalence of a history of dactylitis was 6.0 % (CI 4.7, 7.5 %) in AS and 6.0 % (CI 1.9, 12.0 %) in nr-axSpA, resulting in a pooled prevalence difference of −0.9 % (CI -6.7, 4.8 %) favoring nr-axSpA (Fig. 2c). Quantitative heterogeneity was statistically significant and the level of inconsistency was moderate ($Chi^2 = 7.37$, $P = 0.03$, $Tau^2 = 0.00$, $I^2 = 73$ %).

Uveitis

In pooled analysis the prevalence of current uveitis prevalence was 5.7 % (CI 1.4-12.2 %) in AS and 6.1 % (CI 2.8-10.5 %) in nr-axSpA, resulting in a difference in pooled prevalence of -0.3 % (CI -2.3-1.8 %) favoring nr-axSpA. Quantitative heterogeneity was not statistically significant and the level of inconsistency was low ($Chi^2 = 3.46$, $P = 0.48$, $Tau^2 = 0.00$, $I^2 = 0$ %). The pooled prevalence of a history of uveitis was 23.0 % (CI 19.2-27.1 %) in AS and 15.9 % (CI 11.8-20.4 %) in nr-axSpA, resulting in a difference in pooled prevalence of 6.2 % (CI 2.7, 9.6 %) favoring AS (Fig. 3a). Quantitative heterogeneity was statistically significant and the level of inconsistency was low ($Chi^2 = 5.94$, $P = 0.008$, $Tau^2 = 0.00$, $I^2 = 16$ %).

Psoriasis

In pooled analysis the prevalence of psoriasis was 10.2 % (CI 7.5, -13.2 %) in AS and 10.9 % (CI 9.1, 13.0 %) in nr-axSpA, resulting in a difference in pooled prevalence of −0.7 % (CI −2.9, -1.6 %) favoring nr-axSpA (Fig. 3b). Quantitative heterogeneity was not statistically significant and the level of inconsistency was low ($Chi^2 = 7.01$, $P = 0.43$, $Tau^2 = 0.00$, $I^2 = 0$ %).

Inflammatory bowel disease

Pooled analysis showed an IBD prevalence of 4.1 % (CI 2.3-6.5 %) in AS and 6.4 % (CI 3.6-9.7 %) in nr-axSpA, resulting in a pooled prevalence difference of 1.4 % (CI -0.1-2.9 %) favoring AS (Fig. 3c). Quantitative heterogeneity was not statistically significant and the level of inconsistency was low ($Chi^2 = 6.17$, $P = 0.52$, $Tau^2 = 0.00$, $I^2 = 0$ %).

Discussion

In this meta-analysis we have shown that peripheral disease (arthritis, enthesitis, dactylitis) and extra-articular disease (uveitis, psoriasis, inflammatory bowel disease) manifestations are frequent and, with the exception of a history of uveitis, equally prevalent in AS and nr-axSpA.

Our data on peripheral disease are consistent with earlier published data on peripheral disease in AS, with 18–58 % prevalence of arthritis [9, 11, 25–27], 34–74 % prevalence of enthesitis [9, 25] and 6–8 % prevalence of dactylitis [9, 26, 28] (all reported at any time during the disease). In one study by Vander Cruyssen et al. the

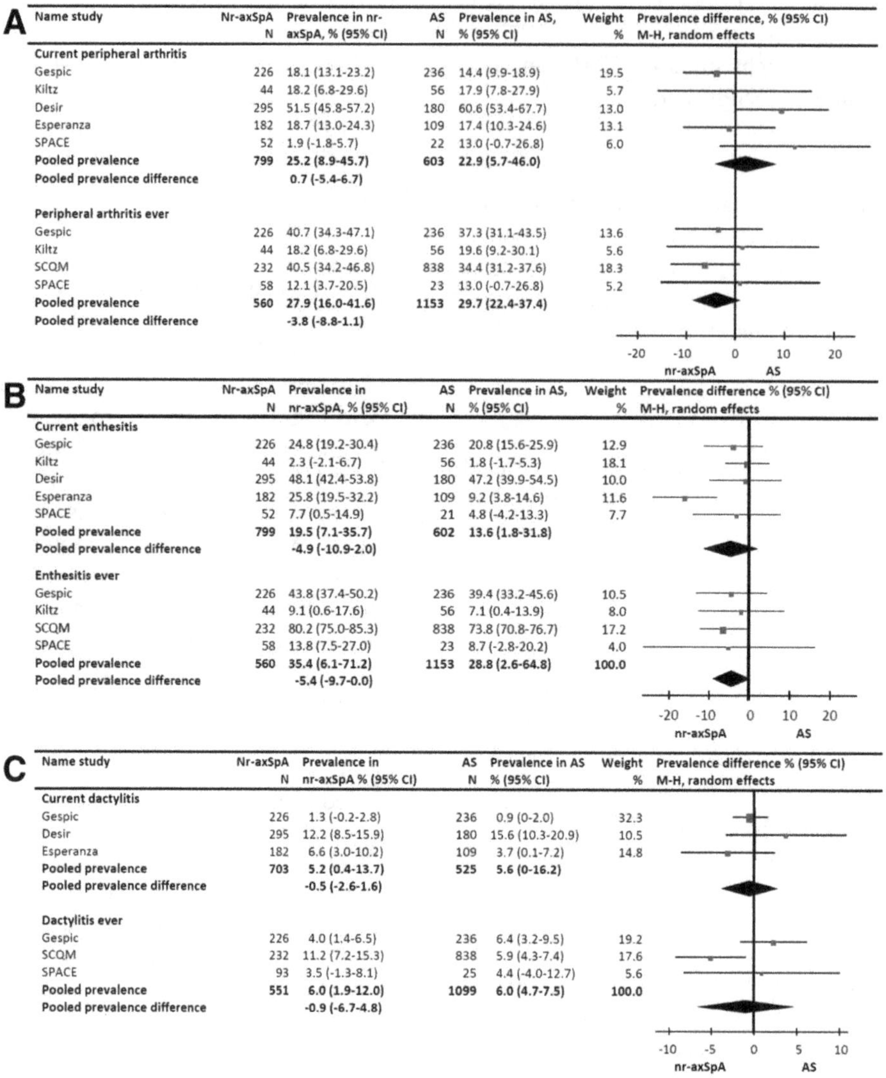

Fig. 2 Prevalence of peripheral manifestations in patients with ankylosing spondylitis and non-radiographic axial spondyloarthritis. **a** pooled prevalence difference of arthritis in patients with ankylosing spondylitis versus non-radiographic axial SpA. **b** pooled prevalence difference of enthesitis in patients with ankylosing spondylitis versus non-radiographic axial SpA. **c** pooled prevalence difference of dactylitis in patients with ankylosing spondylitis versus non-radiographic axial SpA. *GESPIC* GErman SPondyloarthritis Inception Cohort, *SCQM* Swiss Clinical Quality Management, *SPACE* SPondyloArthritis Caught Early, *M-H* Mantel-Haenszel

prevalence of arthritis (58 %) and enthesitis (50 %) (ever occurrence) was higher [25]. Longer mean symptom duration (11 years) and the retrospective reporting in this study may have caused this difference. Importantly, the prevalence of peripheral disease in AS was not reported as the primary outcome in any of the AS studies.

Our prevalence data for extra-articular disease were also in line with previous data on AS, showing 22–37 % prevalence of uveitis [25, 27, 29–31], 4–16 % prevalence of IBD [27, 30–34], and 4–9 % prevalence of psoriasis [6, 27, 30, 31, 33, 34], which all adds to the robustness of our aggregated estimates. The prevalence of uveitis in our study population was lower than in the meta-analyses of Stolwijk et al. and Zeboulon et al., who reported pooled prevalence of 25.8 % and 32.7 %, respectively [29, 30]. This might be caused by a higher mean disease duration (15.9 years in the meta-analysis of Stolwijk et al. and 17.7 years in the meta-analysis of Zeboulon et al.). Another explanation for this difference in prevalence is that both review studies also included clinical trials, enriched with patients with more active and severe disease.

When we compared patients with AS and nr-axSpA, HLA-B27 was equally prevalent in patients with nr-axSpA and AS. Because HLA-B27 is the main entry requirement for fulfilling the ASAS criteria for nr-axial SpA via the clinical arm, HLA-B27 might be artificially overrepresented in the nr-axSpA arm. However, the Esperanza

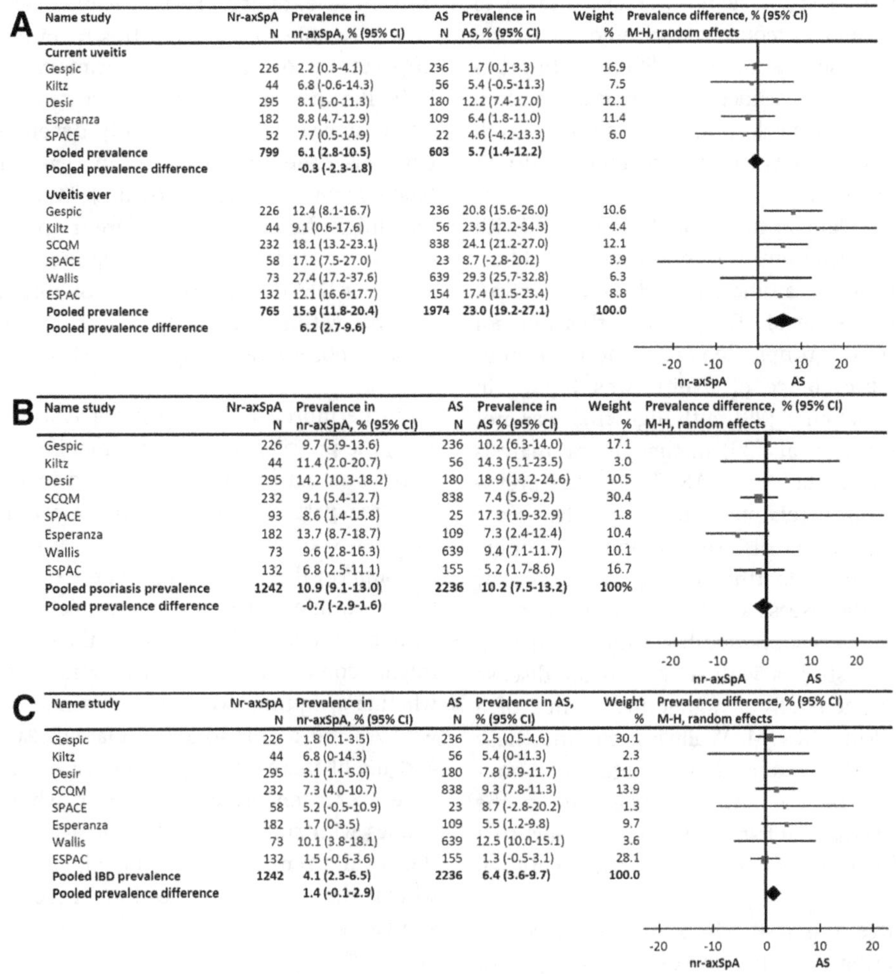

Fig. 3 Prevalence of extra-articular manifestations in patients with ankylosing spondylitis and non-radiographic axial spondyloarthritis. **a** pooled prevalence difference of uveitis in patients with ankylosing spondylitis versus non-radiographic axial SpA. **b** pooled prevalence difference of psoriasis in patients with ankylosing spondylitis versus non-radiographic axial SpA. **c** pooled prevalence difference of IBD in patients with ankylosing spondylitis versus non-radiographic axial SpA. *GESPIC* GErman SPondyloarthritis Inception Cohort, *SCQM* Swiss Clinical Quality Management, *SPACE* SPondyloArthritis Caught Early, *M-H* Mantel-Haenszel

cohort differentiated axSpA in AS and nr-axSpA in a clinical and imaging arm, enabling us to compare the HLA-B27 prevalence in both arms. There was no statistically significant difference in the prevalence of HLA-B27 in the imaging arm of nr-axSpA (where HLA-B27 is not required to fulfill the ASAS criteria) and in AS (58.3 % vs. 67.6 %, respectively) [44], providing evidence for equal HLA-B27 prevalence in nr-axSpA and AS.

Our data show that AS patients were more frequently male than nr-axSpA patients (23.2 % difference in prevalence). These results are in line with previous studies showing that male patients with axial SpA have more structural damage on radiographs than female patients [11, 46–48]. Because the mNY criteria require radiographic evidence of sacroiliitis, channeling of male patients occurs. For nr-axSpA, this channeling does not exist, which is reflected in the equal gender distribution in nr-axSpA.

Interestingly, when we subcategorized the study population in HLA-B27-positive and HLA-B27-negative patients with AS or nr-axSpA, the male predominance among patients with AS was the same in HLAB27-positive and HLAB27-negative patients, challenging the concept of AS as an HLA-B27-positive driven, predominantly male disease.

Our study data show that peripheral and extra-articular disease manifestations are, with the exception of uveitis, frequent and equally prevalent in AS and nr-axSpA. These data further support the concept of axial SpA being one disease continuum irrespective of the presence and extent of radiographic changes [11–13]. Two important conclusions can be drawn from this meta-analysis. First, peripheral and extra-articular disease manifestations significantly contribute to the burden of disease in axial SpA. These results are in contrast with the relatively limited contribution of peripheral and extra-articular disease to disease monitoring and outcome measurement in axial SpA. Second, these results show that differentiating between AS and nr-axSpA is artificial and should therefore be avoided, especially when selecting patients for research and treatment. These patients can best be combined into one group with axial SpA.

Uveitis is less prevalent in nr-axSpA than in AS (with a difference in the pooled prevalence of 6.2 %). This difference was not explained by a difference between nr-axSpA and AS in the prevalence of HLA-B27, as this did not differ between the two groups. Zeboulon and colleagues showed that the prevalence of uveitis was higher in HLA-B27-positive patients [29], although this was not confirmed by Stolwijk et al. [30] in their meta-analysis of extra-articular manifestations in AS. The higher prevalence of uveitis in AS in this meta-analysis might be explained by the longer mean disease duration (presuming that uveitis in axial spondyloarthritis does not necessarily occur at the start of the disease and thus needs time to develop). This hypothesis is supported by 1) the fact that in the included cohort studies with longer mean disease duration there was generally a higher prevalence of a history of uveitis (Kiltz, SCQM, Wallis): excluding those cohort studies from the meta-analysis resulted in a non-significant difference between AS and nr-axSpA in the prevalence of uveitis (data not shown) and 2) the fact that the prevalence of current uveitis did not differ between AS and nr-axSpA.

To our knowledge, this is the first meta-analysis systematically comparing AS with nr-axSpA. Strengths of the current study are the systematic approach in which we have chosen to include only studies that were designed to compare both disease entities, preferably in a prospective manner. Importantly, we have excluded clinical trials that included patients who were selected because of a higher activity and/or severity of their disease (which would have led to channeling bias).

This study has several limitations. First, summarizing the prevalence of peripheral and extra-articular disease manifestations was not the main objective of most of the primary studies included. This might influence the accuracy of reporting these disease manifestations (potential detection bias). Most studies did not report on how the different disease manifestations were measured. We should take into account that the prevalence of some of the disease manifestations that had ever occurred, were mainly obtained by collecting historic patient-reported information (recollection bias). However, the between-study inconsistency of most of the disease manifestations was only moderate (arthritis, enthesitis and dactylitis) or even low (uveitis, psoriasis, IBD), suggesting a significant level of agreement. Second, selection bias is another possible weakness of this meta-analysis and, more importantly, of the included primary studies. We hopefully limited the magnitude of selection bias in this meta-analysis by a thoroughly developed search strategy and other methods to increase finding accuracy (such as citation pearl growing). Within-study selection bias might be caused by different approaches to the inclusion of patients: early spondyloarthritis cohorts (such as DESIR and SPACE) possibly include different patients with shorter disease duration than are included in large observational SpA cohorts.

Furthermore, by applying the ASAS criteria for axial SpA, the prevalence of disease manifestations and characteristics might be artificially raised in nr-axSpA, because they are part of those classification criteria. The higher prevalence of uveitis in patients with AS, however, does not support this hypothesis. On the other hand, the longer mean duration of symptoms in patients with AS when compared to nr-axSpA in five of the eight included studies might confound the interpretation of the results of whether symptoms were ever present, which gives patients with AS more time to accumulate disease manifestations, and might increase the prevalence of manifestations that have ever been present. However, when we left out the studies with substantial differences in symptom duration, the results remained unchanged, except for uveitis, for which the difference no longer remained (data not shown).

Conclusions

This meta-analysis summarized the prevalence of peripheral or extra-articular disease in patients with AS and nr-axSpA. Awareness of the prevalent nature of these disease manifestations is important in the diagnostic process, both for treatment choices and for health-related quality of life. This meta-analysis provides evidence for the largely equal nature of disease manifestations in nr-axSpA and AS, which should have consequences for research and treatment strategies.

Acknowledgements

We acknowledge Sanne Jansen of Lorkeers, MD PhD at the University Medical Center Utrecht, for her assistance with the study design used in the meta-analysis. We acknowledge René Spijker, information retrieval specialist at the Academic Medical Center/University of Amsterdam for assistance with the development of the search strategy. We acknowledge Zineb Ez-Zaitouni, PhD student at the Leiden University Medical Center, for collecting the data for the SPACE cohort. We acknowledge Maxime Dougados and Anna Moltó (DESIR), Martin Rudwaleit (GESPIC), Adrian Ciurea (SCQM), Eva Tomero (Esperanza), Salih Özgöçmen (ESPAC) and Uta Kiltz (Kiltz et al) for providing additional data.

Funding
DB was supported by a VICI grant from The Netherlands Organization for Scientific Research (NWO), by an ERC grant and by a grant from the Dutch Arthritis Foundation (Reumafonds).

Authors' contributions
JdW: study conception and design, acquisition of data, analysis and interpretation of data, drafting the article and final approval of the version of the article to be published. LvM: acquisition of data, analysis and interpretation of data, revising the article and final approval of the version of the article to be published. DvdH: analysis and interpretation of data, revising the article and final approval of the version of the article to be published. RL: study conception and design, analysis and interpretation of data, revising the article and final approval of the version of the article to be published. DB: study conception and design, acquisition of data, analysis and interpretation of data, drafting the article, final approval of the version of the article to be published.

Competing interests
The authors declare that they have no competing interests.

Author details
[1]Department of Clinical Immunology and Rheumatology, Amsterdam Rheumatology and immunology Center, Academic Medical Center/University of Amsterdam, Meibergdreef 9, 1105, AZ, Amsterdam, The Netherlands. [2]Department of Rheumatology, Leiden University Medical Center, Leiden, The Netherlands. [3]Department of Experimental Immunology, Academic Medical Center/University of Amsterdam, Amsterdam, The Netherlands.

References

1. Dougados M, Baeten D. Spondyloarthritis. Lancet. 2011;377:2127–37.
2. Reveille JD, Witter JP, Weisman MH. Prevalence of axial spondylarthritis in the United States: estimates from a cross-sectional survey. Arthritis Care Res (Hoboken). 2012;64:905–10.
3. Rudwaleit M, Landewé R, van der Heijde D, Listing J, Brandt J, Braun J, et al. The development of Assessment of SpondyloArthritis international Society classification criteria for axial spondyloarthritis (part I): classification of paper patients by expert opinion including uncertainty appraisal. Ann Rheum Dis. 2009;68:770–6.
4. Rudwaleit M, van der Heijde D, Landewé R, Listing J, Akkoc N, Brandt J, et al. The development of Assessment of SpondyloArthritis international Society classification criteria for axial spondyloarthritis (part II): validation and final selection. Ann Rheum Dis. 2009;68:777–83.
5. Rudwaleit M, van der Heijde D, Landewé R, Akkoc N, Brandt J, Chou CT, et al. The Assessment of SpondyloArthritis International Society classification criteria for peripheral spondyloarthritis and for spondyloarthritis in general. Ann Rheum Dis. 2011;70:25–31.
6. Wallis D, Haroon N, Ayearst R, Carty A, Inman RD. Ankylosing spondylitis and nonradiographic axial spondyloarthritis: part of a common spectrum or distinct diseases? J Rheumatol. 2013;40:2038–41.
7. Robinson PC, Wordsworth BP, Reveille JD, Brown M. Axial spondyloarthritis: a new disease entity, not necessarily early ankylosing spondylitis. Ann Rheum Dis. 2013;72:162–4.
8. Huerta-Sil G, Casasola-Vargas JC, Londono JD, Rivas-Ruiz R, Chavez J, Pacheco-Tena C, et al. Low grade radiographic sacroiliitis as prognostic factor in patients with undifferentiated spondyloarthritis fulfilling diagnostic criteria for ankylosing spondylitis throughout follow up. Ann Rheum Dis. 2006;65:642–6.
9. Ciurea A, Scherer A, Exer P, Bernhard JJ, Dudler J, Beyeler B, et al. Tumor necrosis factor alpha inhibition in radiographic and nonradiographic axial spondyloarthritis: results from a large observational cohort. Arthritis Rheum. 2013;65:3096–106.
10. Kiltz U, Baraliakos X, Karakostas P, Igelmann M, Kalthoff L, Klink C, et al. Do patients with non-radiographic axial spondylarthritis differ from patients with ankylosing spondylitis? Arthritis Care Res (Hoboken). 2012;64:1415–22.
11. Rudwaleit M, Haibel H, Baraliakos X, Listing J, Märker-Hermann E, Zeidler H, et al. The early disease stage in axial spondylarthritis: results from the GErman SPondyloarthritis Inception Cohort. Arthritis Rheum. 2009;60:717–27.
12. Baeten D, Breban M, Lories R, Schett G, Sieper J. Are spondylarthritides related but distinct conditions or a single disease with a heterogeneous phenotype? Arthritis Rheum. 2013;65:12–20.
13. Rudwaleit M, Khan MA, Sieper J. Commentary: The challenge of diagnosis and classification in early ankylosing spondylitis: do we need new criteria? Arthritis Rheum. 2005;52:1000–8.
14. Poddubnyy D, Haibel H. Clinical course over two years in patients with early non-radiographic axial spondyloarthritis and ankylosing spondylitis without anti-tumour necrosis factor α treatment: results from the GErman SPondyloarthritis Inception Cohort (GESPIC). Arthritis Rheumatol. 2015;67:2369–75.
15. Sieper J, van der Heijde D, Dougados M, Mease PJ, Maksymowych WP, Brown M a, et al. Efficacy and safety of adalimumab in patients with non-radiographic axial spondyloarthritis: results of a randomised placebo-controlled trial (ABILITY-1). Ann Rheum Dis. 2012;72:815–822.
16. Song I-H, Weiß A, Hermann K-G a, Haibel H, Althoff CE, Poddubnyy D, et al. Similar response rates in patients with ankylosing spondylitis and non-radiographic axial spondyloarthritis after 1 year of treatment with etanercept: results from the ESTHER trial. Ann Rheum Dis. 2013;72:823–5.
17. Callhoff J, Sieper J, Weiß A, Zink A, Listing J. Efficacy of TNFα blockers in patients with ankylosing spondylitis and non-radiographic axial spondyloarthritis: a meta-analysis. Ann Rheum Dis. 2015;74:1241–8.
18. McCormick D, McKnight J, Pendleton a. Anti-TNF response rates in radiographic and non-radiographic axial spondyloarthropathy. Ann Rheum Dis. 2014;74:e21.
19. van den Berg R, Lenczner G, Feydy A, van der Heijde D, Reijnierse M, Saraux A, et al. Agreement between clinical practice and trained central reading in reading of sacroiliac joints on plain pelvic radiographs: results from the DESIR cohort. Arthritis Rheumatol. 2014;66:2403–11.
20. van Tubergen a, Heuft-Dorenbosch L, Schulpen G, Landewé R, Wijers R, van der Heijde D, et al. Radiographic assessment of sacroiliitis by radiologists and rheumatologists: does training improve quality? Ann Rheum Dis. 2003;62:519–25.
21. Sieper J, van der Heijde D, Dougados M, Mease PJ, Maksymowych WP, Brown MA, et al. Efficacy and safety of adalimumab in patients with non-radiographic axial spondyloarthritis: results of a randomised placebo-controlled trial (ABILITY-1). Ann Rheum Dis. 2013;72:815–22.
22. Haibel H, Rudwaleit M, Listing J, Heldmann F, Wong RL, Kupper H, et al. Efficacy of adalimumab in the treatment of axial spondylarthritis without radiographically defined sacroiliitis: results of a twelve-week randomized, double-blind, placebo-controlled trial followed by an open-label extension up to week fifty-two. Arthritis Rheum. 2008;58:1981–91.
23. van den Berg R, de Hooge M, van Gaalen F, Reijnierse M, Huizinga T, van der Heijde D. Percentage of patients with spondyloarthritis in patients referred because of chronic back pain and performance of classification criteria: experience from the SPondyloArthritis Caught Early (SPACE) cohort. Rheumatology (Oxford). 2013;52:1492–9.
24. Kiltz U, Baraliakos X, Karakostas P, Igelmann M, Kalthoff L, Klink C, et al. The degree of spinal inflammation is similar in patients with axial spondyloarthritis who report high or low levels of disease activity: a cohort study. Ann Rheum Dis. 2012;71:1207–11.
25. Vander Cruyssen B, Ribbens C, Boonen A, Mielants H, de Vlam K, Lenaerts J, et al. The epidemiology of ankylosing spondylitis and the commencement of anti-TNF therapy in daily rheumatology practice. Ann Rheum Dis. 2007;66:1072–7.
26. Paramarta JE, De Rycke L, Ambarus CA, Tak PP, Baeten D. Undifferentiated spondyloarthritis vs ankylosing spondylitis and psoriatic arthritis: a real-life prospective cohort study of clinical presentation and response to treatment. Rheumatology (Oxford). 2013;52:1873–8.
27. Heuft-Dorenbosch L, van Tubergen A, Spoorenberg A, Landewé R, Dougados M, Mielants H, et al. The influence of peripheral arthritis on disease activity in ankylosing spondylitis patients as measured with the Bath Ankylosing Spondylitis Disease Activity Index. Arthritis Rheum. 2004;51:154–9.
28. Pérez Alamino R, Maldonado Cocco J a, Citera G, Arturi P, Vazquez-Mellado J, Sampaio-Barros PD, et al. Differential features between primary ankylosing spondylitis and spondylitis associated with psoriasis and inflammatory bowel disease. J Rheumatol. 2011;38:1656–60.

29. Zeboulon N, Dougados M, Gossec L. Prevalence and characteristics of uveitis in the spondyloarthropathies: a systematic literature review. Ann Rheum Dis. 2008;67:955–9.
30. Stolwijk C, van Tubergen A, Castillo-Ortiz JD, Boonen A. Prevalence of extra-articular manifestations in patients with ankylosing spondylitis: a systematic review and meta-analysis. Ann Rheum Dis. 2013;74:65–73.
31. Exarchou S, Redlund-Johnell I, Karlsson M, Mellstrom D, Ohlsson C, Turesson C, et al. The prevalence of moderate to severe radiographic sacroiliitis and the correlation with health status in elderly Swedish men–the MrOS study. BMC Musculoskelet Disord. 2013;14:352.
32. Rudwaleit M, Baeten D. Ankylosing spondylitis and bowel disease. Best Pract Res Clin Rheumatol. 2006;20:451–71.
33. Essers I, Ramiro S, Stolwijk C, Blaauw M, Landewé R, van der Heijde D, et al. Characteristics associated with the presence and development of extra-articular manifestations in ankylosing spondylitis: 12-year results from OASIS. Rheumatology (Oxford). 2014;54:633–40.
34. Stolwijk C, Essers I, van Tubergen A, Boonen A, Bazelier MT, De Bruin ML, et al. The epidemiology of extra-articular manifestations in ankylosing spondylitis: a population-based matched cohort study. Ann Rheum Dis. 2014;74:1373–8.
35. Schlosser RW, Wendt O, Bhavnani S, Nail-Chiwetalu B. Use of information-seeking strategies for developing systematic reviews and engaging in evidence-based practice: the application of traditional and comprehensive Pearl Growing. A review. Int J Lang Commun Disord. 2006;41:567–82.
36. Moher D, Liberati A, Tetzlaff J, Altman DG. Preferred Reporting Items for Systematic reviews and Meta-Analyses: the PRISMA statement. J Clin Epidemiol. 2009;62:1006–12.
37. Dougados M, Van der Linden S, Juhlin R, Huitfeldt B, Amor B, Calin A, et al. The European Spondylarthropathy Study Group preliminary criteria for the classification of spondylarthropathy. Arthritis Rheum. 1991;34:1218–27.
38. Van der Linden S, Valkenburg H, Cats A. Evaluation of diagnostic criteria for ankylosing spondylitis. A proposal for modification of the New York criteria. Arthritis Rheumatol. 1984;27:361–8.
39. Shamliyan T a, Kane RL, Ansari MT, Raman G, Berkman ND, Grant M, et al. Development quality criteria to evaluate nontherapeutic studies of incidence, prevalence, or risk factors of chronic diseases: pilot study of new checklists. J Clin Epidemiol. 2011;64:637–57.
40. Higgins JPT, Thompson SG, Deeks JJ, Altman DG. Measuring inconsistency in meta-analyses. BMJ. 2003;327:557–60.
41. Borenstein M, Hedges L, Higgins J, Rothstein H. Introduction to meta-analysis. 2009.
42. Barendregt JJ, Doi S a, Lee YY, Norman RE, Vos T. Meta-analysis of prevalence. J Epidemiol Community Health. 2013;67:974–8.
43. Blachier M, Canouï-Poitrine F, Dougados M, Lethuaut A, Fautrel B, Ferkal S, et al. Factors associated with radiographic lesions in early axial spondyloarthritis. Results from the DESIR cohort. Rheumatology (Oxford). 2013;52:1686–93.
44. Hernández-sanz A, Fernández-carballido VNC, Montilla-morales C, Mulero-mendoza J, de Miguel E. Ankylosing spondylitis and non-radiographic spondyloarthritis: the same syndrome or different diseases? Analyses from Esperanza cohort. In: ACR annual meeting; 2014: Abstract number: 2604.
45. Kilic E, Kilic G, Akgul O, Ozgocmen S. Discriminant validity of the Ankylosing Spondylitis Disease Activity Score (ASDAS) in patients with non-radiographic axial spondyloarthritis and ankylosing spondylitis: a cohort study. Rheumatol Int. 2014;35:981–989.
46. Resnick D, Dwosh IL, Goergen TG, Shapiro RF, Utsinger PD, Wiesner KB, et al. Clinical and radiographic abnormalities in ankylosing spondylitis: a comparison of men and women. Radiology. 1976;119:293–7.
47. Gran JT, Husby G, Hordvik M, Stormer J, Romberg-Andersen O. Radiological changes in men and women with ankylosing spondylitis. Ann Rheum Dis. 1984;43:570–5.
48. Boyer GS, Templin DW, Bowler A, Lawrence RC, Heyse SP, Everett DF, et al. Spondyloarthropathy in the community: differences in severity and disease expression in Alaskan Eskimo men and women. J Rheumatol. 2000;27:170–6.

11

Chondrocyte activity is increased in psoriatic arthritis and axial spondyloarthritis

Natasja Stæhr Gudmann[1*], Heidi Lausten Munk[2], Anne Friesgaard Christensen[3], Leif Ejstrup[4], Grith Lykke Sørensen[5], Anne Gitte Loft[3,6], Morten Asser Karsdal[1], Anne-Christine Bay-Jensen[1], Yi He[1], Anne Sofie Siebuhr[1] and Peter Junker[2]

Abstract

Background: Psoriatic arthritis (PsA) and axial spondyloarthritis (axSpA) are chronic inflammatory rheumatic diseases with complex origins. Both are characterized by altered extracellular matrix remodeling in joints and entheses that results in destructive and osteochondral proliferative lesions. There is a need for biomarkers reflecting core disease pathways for diagnosis and disease mapping. Pro-C2 reflects mature cartilage collagen type IIB formation, while C-Col10 represents turnover of type X collagen, which is exclusively expressed by hypertrophic chondrocytes. The objectives of this study were to study cartilage metabolism in axSpA and PsA by assessing Pro-C2 and C-Col10 and to evaluate their diagnostic utility against a healthy reference population.

Methods: Patients with PsA ($n = 101$) or axSpA ($n = 110$) were recruited consecutively from three rheumatology outpatient clinics. Demographic and clinical disease measures were recorded. Pro-C2 and C-Col10 were quantified in serum by using newly developed and specific competitive enzyme-linked immunosorbent assays based on monoclonal antibodies. One-way analysis of variance and Tukey's multiple comparison tests were performed on log-transformed data. ROC curve analysis was carried out to evaluate their discriminative power.

Results: Pro-C2 levels in serum were significantly increased in both axSpA (median concentration 1.11 ng/ml, 0.67–1.64) and PsA (median concentration 1.03 ng/ml, 0.53–1.47) compared with healthy controls (median concentration 0.30 ng/ml, 0.16–0.41) ($p < 0.0001$). Pro-C2 did not differ according to treatment. C-Col10 was slightly but equally elevated in the PsA and axSpA groups vs. the control group, but it was significantly lower in patients with axSpA undergoing tumor necrosis factor-α inhibitor (TNFi) treatment. ROC curve analysis revealed AUCs of 0.85 (95 % CI 0.79–0.89) for axSpA and 0.81 (95 % CI 0.75–0.86) for PsA.

Conclusions: These findings indicate that cartilage collagen metabolism was enhanced in the axSpA and PsA groups compared with the healthy control group. The lower C-Col10 level in patients with axSpA undergoing TNFi treatment may reflect that hypertrophic chondrocytes in axSpA are targeted by TNFi. ROC curve analysis showed a diagnostic potential for Pro-C2 in axSpA and PsA.

Keywords: Spondyloarthritis, Psoriatic arthritis, Type II collagen, Type X collagen, Pro-C2, C-Col10

Background

The spondyloarthropathies (SpAs) are chronic inflammatory rheumatic diseases with shared as well as distinctive genetic and clinical features. Joint structural elements and entheses of the axial and peripheral skeleton are principal targets of the diseases [1], which are occasionally also manifested at extraskeletal sites (e.g., anterior uveitis, aortic valvulopathy, and apical lung fibrosis) [1, 2]. Both genetic and environmental factors are implicated in the disease course [3–5], and human leukocyte antigen (HLA)-B27 is overrepresented, occurring in up to 83 % of patients with axial involvement [6].

Disease presentation and progression in SpAs differ between individuals. If left untreated, many patients will experience spinal and peripheral joint deformities due to altered bone and cartilage turnover. Osteochondral proliferative lesions are hallmarks of axial and entheseal

* Correspondence: nsg@nordicbioscience.com
[1]Nordic Bioscience Biomarkers and Research, Herlev Hovedgade 207, Herlev 2730, Denmark

involvement [7]. Current treatments include nonsteroidal anti-inflammatory drugs, methotrexate, and biological agents such as tumor necrosis factor-α inhibitors (TNFi) [8]. Early intervention is recommended to prevent or slow the progression rate. However, early diagnosis is challenging because of a lack of pathognomonic features and/or laboratory tests, and the average diagnostic delay has been reported to be approximately 8–11 years [7]. In psoriatic arthritis (PsA), early diagnosis has been shown to significantly decrease morbidity and increase quality of life [9]. Thus, interest in developing sensitive and specific tools for diagnostic and prognostic purposes is increasing. The utility of several cartilage and bone biochemical markers has been assessed, particularly in osteoarthritis and rheumatoid arthritis, and also, although less intensively, in axial spondyloarthritis (axSpA) and PsA [10]. Thus, markers of cartilage formation (type II collagen [CII] [11]) and degradation (collagen type II cleavage [C2C] [11] and C-terminal telopeptide of type II collagen [CTX-II] [12]) have been shown to be elevated in axSpA and PsA. Similar findings have been reported recently with use of the regenerative collagen type IIA N-terminal propeptide (PIIANP) and matrix metalloproteinase-generated type II collagen degradation fragment (C2M) [13]. The Pro-C2 assay is the first laboratory tool for specific measurement of the N-terminal propeptide of the procollagen IIB splice variant (PIIBNP), which is the most prevalent collagen species in healthy adult cartilage. By contrast, previous candidate markers for type II collagen formation either do not segregate other variants such as CII [11], NPII [14], and PIINP [15] or are specific for PIIANP, which is expressed mainly during embryogenesis, fracture healing, and cartilage regeneration [16–18]. Additionally, C-Col10 is, to our knowledge, the first marker available for the assessment of type X collagen turnover, and so far it has been applied only to patients with osteoarthritis [19].

On the basis of these observations, we hypothesized that remodeling of mature collagen IIB and collagen X, a minor collagen species that is produced only by hypertrophic chondrocytes, is increased in axSpA and PsA. The aims of this study were (1) to study cartilage collagen metabolism in further detail using novel molecular markers for the synthesis and turnover of mature collagen IIB (Pro-C2) [20] and collagen X (C-Col10) [19] in well-characterized cohorts of patients with axSpA and PsA, and (2) to assess their diagnostic utility in comparison with healthy control subjects.

Methods

Study populations

Patients from three rheumatology centers in Southern Denmark were recruited from November 2011 through February 2014 (33–120 patients per center). The inclusion criteria and patient characteristics have previously been published [13]. In short, 110 patients with axSpA classified according to the Assessment of SpondyloArthritis international Society (ASAS) criteria [21, 22] and 101 patients with PsA fulfilling the Classification of Psoriatic Arthritis (CASPAR) criteria [23] were enrolled in the study. Sixteen of the patients fulfilled both the CASPAR and the ASAS criteria, and these patients were labeled as having PsA in this study. Exclusion criteria were age <18 years and age >75 years, past or present malignancy (except nonmalignant skin cancer), congestive cardiac disease (New York Heart Association classes III and IV), pulmonary disease (dyspnea at rest), serum creatinine above the upper limit of normal, serum concentration of alanine aminotransferase more than two times the upper limit of normal, infection with hepatitis B or hepatitis C virus, and/or presence of other chronic inflammatory diseases. The patient characteristics recorded included sex, body mass index (BMI), age, smoking habit, alcohol consumption, treatment, and HLA-B27 status. Disease measures recorded included 68 swollen joint count (68SJC), 68 tender joint count (68TJC), Spondyloarthritis Research Consortium of Canada enthesitis index, Health Assessment Questionnaire (HAQ), visual analogue scale (VAS; patient pain, patient global, patient fatigue, and physician global scores on a 0–10 scale), Bath Ankylosing Spondylitis Disease Activity Index (BASDAI), Disease Activity Score in 28 joints (DAS28), and Ankylosing Spondylitis Disease Activity Score (ASDAS). X-rays or magnetic resonance imaging (MRI) scans of sacroiliac joints of patients with axSpA and of patients with PsA with axial involvement were available when the disease was diagnosed, but they were not repeated in this study. Twelve patients with axSpA had ankylosis of the sacroiliac joints visualized on x-rays or MRI scans. Demographic data and disease parameters are summarized in Table 1. One hundred eighteen blood donors aged 20–65 years served as healthy control subjects. Blood samples were collected in plain tubes from subjects in nonfasting state. The samples were allowed to clot for 30–120 minutes and then centrifuged for 12 minutes at 2200 rpm. Serum samples were frozen at −80 °C until used for analysis.

Biomarker measurements

The Pro-C2 competitive enzyme-linked immunosorbent assay (ELISA) has been described previously by Gudmann et al. [20]. In short, 96-well streptavidin-coated plates (Roche Diagnostics, Risch-Rotkreuz, Switzerland) were coated with the biotinylated synthetic peptide Bio-QDVRQPG, dissolved in assay buffer (100 mM PBS, 1 % bovine serum albumin, 0.1 % Tween-20, 0.36 % 5-bromo-5-nitro-1,3-dioxane [Bronidox; BASF,

Table 1 Patient characteristics, disease measures, and serum levels of Pro-C2 and C-Col10

	axSpA (n = 110)	PsA (n = 101)	Control
Male sex, %	72 %	59 %	
Age, years	36.6 (35.3–38.0)	37.0 (35.6–38.5)	
BMI, kg/m^2	25.5 (24.8–26.3)	27.4 (26.2–28.5)	
Smoker, %	36 %	35 %	
HLA-B27 positive, %	87 %	20 %	
Disease duration, years	6.4 (5.4–7.5)	6.7 (5.6–7.8)	
VAS			
Patient global	34 (29–39)	39 (34–45)	
Patient pain	32 (27–37)	32 (27–37)	
Patient fatigue	40 (34–45)	43 (37–49)	
Physician global	4 [1–16]	3 [1–14]	
BASDAI	31 (26–35)	36 (31–41)	
BASFI	23 (19–27)	27 (22–32)	
BASMI	10 [0–20]	10 [0–10]	
ASDAS (CRP)	2.0 (1.8–2.3)	2.1 (1.9–2.4)	
Swollen joints, %	9 %	38 %	
hs-CRP, mg/dl	3 [1–7]	3 [1–9]	
Pro-C2, ng/ml	1.11 [0.67-1.64]	1.03 [0.53-1.47]	0.30 [0.16-0.41]
Col-X, ng/ml	0.45 [0.28-0.67]	0.42 [0.31-0.72]	0.33 [0.31-0.45]

Abbreviations: ASDAS Ankylosing Spondylitis Disease Activity Score, *axSpA* axial spondyloarthritis, *BASDAI* Bath Ankylosing Spondylitis Disease Activity Index, *BASFI* Bath Ankylosing Spondylitis Functional Index, *BASMI* Bath Ankylosing Spondylitis Metrology Index, *BMI* body mass index, *HLA-B27* human leukocyte antigen B27, *hs-CRP* high-sensitivity C-reactive protein, *PsA* psoriatic arthritis, *VAS* visual analogue scale
Data are presented as mean (95 % CI) for variables with a normal distribution and as median [25th–75th percentile range] for variables that were not normally distributed

Florham Park, NJ, USA], 8 % NaCl, pH 7.4), and incubated for 30 minutes at 20 °C. The peptide calibrator or sample in a quantity of 20 µl was added to appropriate wells, followed by 100 µl of antibody of the NB443-3-2-1 clone. The plates were then incubated for 2 h. Afterward, 100 µl of EnVision (Dako, Glostrup, Denmark) was added, and the plate was incubated for 1 h. Finally, 100 µl of 3,3′,5,5′-tetramethylbenzidine (TMB) (Kem-En-Tec Nordic, Taastrup, Denmark) was added, and the plate was incubated for 15 minutes at 20 °C in the dark. The C-Col10 ELISA method has been described in detail previously by He et al. [19]. Measurements were performed as follows: 100 µl of biotinylated peptide of the sequence SFSGFLVAPM was added to plates precoated with streptavidin (Roche Diagnostics) and incubated at 20 °C for 30 minutes. Standard or patient samples in a quantity of 20 µl was then added to the appropriate wells together with 100 µl of peroxidase-labeled antibody NB509-11G8 and incubated at 4 °C overnight with shaking. Afterward, 100 µl of TMB was added to each well of the plates and incubated in the dark at 20 °C for 15 minutes. All samples were measured in duplicate, and incubation steps included shaking at 300 rpm for both assays. After each incubation except the last one in which TMB was added, the plates were washed five times in washing buffer (20 mM Tris, 50 mM NaCl, pH 7.2). The TMB reaction was stopped by adding 100 µl of stopping solution (1 % H_2SO_4) and measured at 450 nm with 650 nm as the reference.

Statistics

All analyses were performed using MedCalc statistical software version 14.8.1 (2014 release; MedCalc Software bvba, Ostend, Belgium). Means were calculated for variables with a normal distribution, and medians were calculated for variables that were not normally distributed. Biomarker levels and parameters that did not meet the criteria for normal distribution were log-transformed. Normally distributed variables were compared using t tests, and one-way analysis of variance followed by Tukey's multiple comparisons test were applied for intergroup comparisons. Correlation analyses were performed by using Pearson's test. A p value ≤0.05 was considered statically significant. The discriminative power of the serum markers between healthy and diseased states was calculated by using ROC and expressed by the AUC. The Youden index was applied to determine the optimum sensitivity and specificity and the corresponding cutoff values.

Results

Patient demographics

Patient demographics and disease characteristics are presented in Table 1. Male sex was more common in both axSpA (72 %) and PsA (59 %) than in the control group (50 %). The clinical parameters are listed for patients, but they were not available for healthy blood donors.

Cartilage turnover is increased in axSpA and PsA

Pro-C2 was significantly increased in the axSpA and PsA groups compared with the healthy control group (Fig. 1a). Similarly, C-Col10 was significantly elevated in patients with PsA compared with healthy control subjects, and the same trend was observed in patients with axSpA (Fig. 1b). Of note, in patients with axSpA naïve to TNFi treatment (n = 34), C-Col10 was significantly higher in patients with axSpA than in TNFi-treated patients and healthy control subjects (p = 0.008). There was no significant difference in Pro-C2 or C-Col10 between the axSpA and PsA groups.

Pro-C2 associations

Pro-C2 correlated with ASDAS in the patients with axSpA naïve to disease-modifying antirheumatic drugs

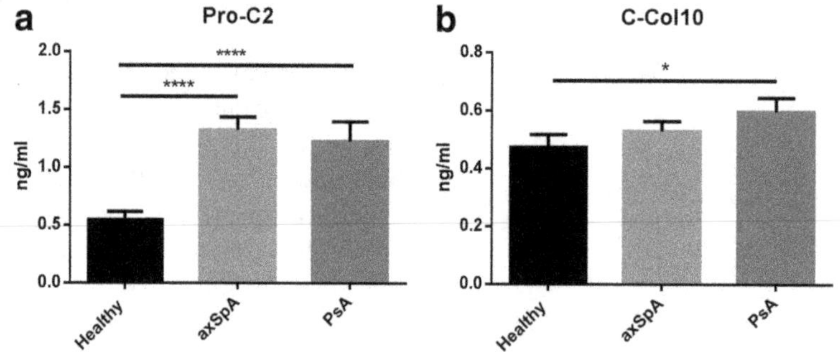

Fig. 1 a Pro-C2 was significantly increased in the axial spondyloarthritis (axSpA) and psoriatic arthritis (PsA) groups compared with the healthy control group. **b** C-Col 10 concentrations were slightly but significantly higher in the PsA group compared with the healthy control group. Error bars are shown as SEM. One-way analysis of variance was performed for intergroup comparisons. $^{*}p < 0.05$, $^{****}p < 0.0001$

(DMARDs). In treatment-naïve patients with PsA Pro-C2, there was a borderline correlation with age, BMI, and disease duration. Patients with axSpA currently being treated with synthetic and/or biological DMARDs had a significant correlation between Pro-C2 and HAQ and Bath Ankylosing Spondylitis Functional Index (BASFI). HAQ and Pro-C2 were also significantly correlated in currently treated patients with PsA (Table 2).

HLA-B27-positive patients with axSpA had significantly lower Pro-C2 levels than HLA-B27-negative patients ($p = 0.026$) (Fig. 2). In contrast, we found no statistically significant differences in Pro-C2 levels when we compared subjects according to smoking status ($p = 0.51$), male vs. female sex ($p = 0.46$), current treatment (neither biologics [$p = 0.50$] nor synthetic DMARDs [$p = 0.15$]), SJC28 ($p = 0.63$), or TJC28 ($p = 0.28$). We observed no significant differences in

Table 2 Pearson correlations between Pro-C2 levels in axial spondyloarthritis and psoriatic arthritis and clinical parameters

	axSpA				PsA			
	Total ($n = 110$)	Treatment-naïve ($n = 34$)	Currently treated, total ($n = 63$)	Previously treated ($n = 13$)	Total ($n = 101$)	Treatment-naïve ($n = 13$)	Currently treated, total ($n = 76$)	Previously treated ($n = 12$)
Age	ns	ns	ns	ns	ns	$r = -0.55$ $p = -0.051$	ns	ns
BMI	ns	ns	ns	ns	ns	$r = 0.60$ $p = 0.032$	ns	ns
Disease duration	ns	ns	ns	$r = 0.54$ $p = 0.030$	ns	$r = 0.55$ $p = 0.052$	ns	ns
ASDAS	ns	$r = 0.45$ $p = 0.008$	ns	ns	ns	ns	ns	ns
HAQ	ns	ns	$r = 0.47$ $p = 0.010$	ns	$r = -0.34$ $p = 0.004$	ns	$r = -0.35$ $p = 0.008$	ns
Sex	ns	ns	ns	ns	ns	ns	ns	ns
BASDAI	ns	ns	ns	ns	ns	ns	ns	ns
BASFI	ns	ns	$r = -0.30$ $p = 0.008$	ns	ns	ns	ns	ns
SJC68	ns	ns	ns	ns	ns	ns	ns	$r = -0.92$ $p = 0.0001$
TJC68	ns	ns	ns	ns	ns	ns	ns	$r = -0.89$ $p = 0.0003$

Abbreviations: ASDAS Ankylosing Spondylitis Disease Activity Score, *axSpA* axial spondyloarthritis, *BASDAI* Bath Ankylosing Spondylitis Disease Activity Index, *BASFI* Bath Ankylosing Spondylitis Functional Index, *BASMI* Bath Ankylosing Spondylitis Metrology Index, *BMI* body mass index, *HAQ* Health Assessment Questionnaire, *ns* not significant, *SJC68* 68 swollen joint count, *TJC68* 68 tender joint count

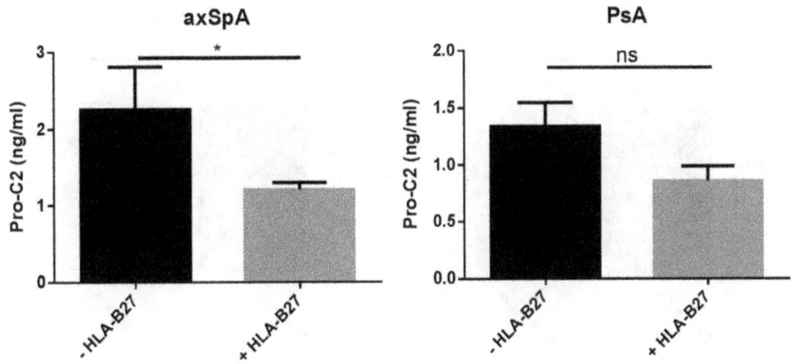

Fig. 2 Pro-C2 was significantly lower in patients with axial spondyloarthritis (axSpA) who were positive for the human leukocyte antigen (HLA)-B27 gene compared with the HLA-B27-negative patients. In patients with psoriatic arthritis (PsA), Pro-C2 did not differ significantly according to HLA-B27 status (p=0.31). Error bars are shown as SEM. Student's t test was applied to compare the two groups. *$p < 0.05$. *ns* not significant

Pro-C2 when we compared subjects according to HLA-B27 status in PsA ($p = 0.18$), and this applied to other clinical parameters as well (data not shown).

C-Col10 associations

In patients with axSpA who were naïve to treatment, a weak correlation was found between C-Col10 and disease duration and SJC68. In patients with axSpA currently receiving treatment (synthetic and/or biologic DMARDs), a correlation was found between sex and C-Col10. No correlation was found between type X collagen in serum and disease parameters in patients with PsA (Table 3).

C-Col10 levels were significantly lower in patients with axSpA who received or had previously received DMARD biologics ($p = 0.019$) than in those who did not, whereas treatment with a synthetic DMARD did not affect C-Col10 concentration ($p = 0.96$) (Fig. 3). This pattern did not apply to patients with PsA ($p = 0.34$). C-Col10 did not associate with sex, HLA-B27, SJC28, TJC28, or disease state as assessed using either DAS28, ASDAS, BASDAI, or BASFI in patients with axSpA or PsA (data not shown).

Discriminative power of Pro-C2 and C-Col10

The discriminating power between the healthy control, axSpA, and PsA groups was assessed by ROC analysis (Fig. 4). The AUCs of the healthy control group vs. disease groups were, for both biomarkers, approximately

Table 3 Pearson correlations between C-Col10 levels in axial spondyloarthritis and psoriatic arthritis and clinical parameters

	axSpA				PsA			
	Total ($n = 110$)	Treatment-naïve ($n = 34$)	Currently treated ($n = 63$)	Previously treated ($n = 13$)	Total ($n = 101$)	Treatment-naïve ($n = 13$)	Currently treated ($n = 76$)	Previously treated ($n = 12$)
Age	ns	ns	ns	ns	ns	ns	ns	ns
BMI	ns	ns	ns	ns	ns	ns	ns	ns
Disease duration	ns	$r = -0.38$ $p = 0.027$	ns	ns	ns	ns	ns	ns
ASDAS	ns	ns	ns	ns	ns	ns	ns	ns
Alcohol consumption	ns	ns	ns	$r = -0.60$ $p = 0.022$	ns	ns	ns	ns
HAQ	ns	ns	ns	ns	ns	ns	ns	ns
Sex	ns	ns	$r = 0.30$ $p = 0.021$	ns	ns	ns	ns	ns
BASDAI	ns	ns	ns	ns	ns	ns	ns	ns
SJC68	ns	$r = -0.36$ $p = -0.037$	ns	ns	ns	ns	ns	ns
TJC68	$r = -0.20$ $p = 0.043$	ns	ns	ns	ns	ns	ns	$r = -0.73$ $p = 0.011$

Abbreviations: ASDAS Ankylosing Spondylitis Disease Activity Score, *axSpA* axial spondyloarthritis, *BASDAI* Bath Ankylosing Spondylitis Disease Activity Index, *BMI* body mass index, *HAQ* Health Assessment Questionnaire, *ns* not significant, *PsA* psoriatic arthritis, *SJC68* 68 swollen joint count, *TJC68* 68 tender joint count

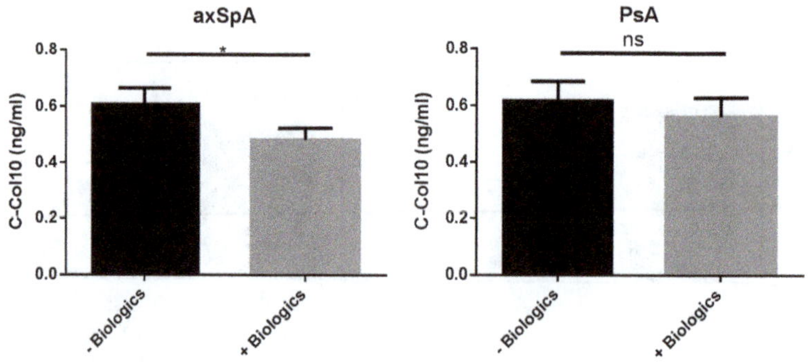

Fig. 3 C-Col10 was significantly higher in patients with axial spondyloarthritis (axSpA) naïve to biological treatment than in those currently or formerly treated with biologic DMARDs. The same trend was observed in patients with psoriatic arthritis (PsA), though it did not reach statistical significance. Error bars are shown as SEM. Student's *t* test was applied to compare the two groups. $^*p < 0.05$. *ns* not significant

the same for the two diseases. For Pro-C2, the healthy control group vs. the axSpA group had an AUC of 0.85 (95 % CI 0.79–0.89); for the healthy control group vs. the PsA group, the AUC was 0.81 (95 % CI 0.75–0.86) (see Table 4). For C-Col10, the AUC of the healthy control group vs. the disease groups was lower than that for Pro-C2 but approximately the same in the two disease groups. The AUC for the healthy control group vs. the axSpA group was 0.58 (95 % CI 0.51–0.65), and for the healthy control group vs. the PsA group it was 0.61 (95 % CI 0.54–0.67) (Table 4).

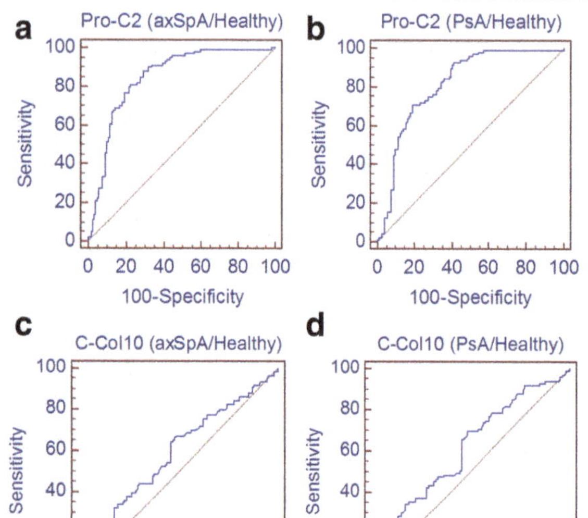

Fig. 4 ROC analysis of (**a**) Pro-C2 in the axial spondyloarthritis (axSpA) group vs. the healthy control group, (**b**) Pro-C2 in the psoriatic arthritis (PsA) group vs. the healthy control group, (**c**) C-Col10 levels in the axSpA group vs. the healthy control group, and (**d**) C-Col10 in the PsA group vs. the healthy control group

Discussion

Structural elements in joints and entheses are major disease targets in axSpA [24] and PsA [25]. Therefore, in the present study, we measured two recently developed cartilage biochemical markers—C-Col10 and Pro-C2—to study chondrocyte differentiation and mature cartilage collagen IIB formation in axSpA and PsA.

Pro-C2 concentrations were significantly elevated in both the axSpA and PsA groups compared with levels in control subjects. In addition, C-Col10 levels were slightly higher in both disease subsets than the levels in control subjects, although they reached statistical significance only in the PsA group. Pro-C2 correlated with ASDAS in untreated patients with axSpA and with HAQ and BASFI in TNFi-treated patients with axSpA. C-Col10 was weakly associated with SJC68. While Pro-C2 was not influenced by TNFi treatment, C-Col10 was lower in patients with axSpA currently or previously receiving biologics than in patients naïve to TNFi treatment. Good discrimination for Pro-C2 was seen for patients with axSpA and patients with PsA vs. healthy subjects.

Table 4 ROC analysis of ability of Pro-C2 and C-Col10 to differentiate between healthy control, psoriatic arthritis, and axial spondyloarthritis groups

	AUC (95 % CI)	Youden index	Sensitivity	Specificity
Pro-C2				
Healthy vs. axSpA	0.85 (0.79–0.89)	0.58	87.9	70.6
Healthy vs. PsA	0.81 (0.75–0.86)	0.51	92.7	58.8
axSpA vs. PsA	0.54 (0.47–0.61)	0.13	17.43	95.2
C-Col10				
Healthy vs. axSpA	0.58 (0.51–0.65)	0.18	67.0	51.4
Healthy vs. PsA	0.61 (0.54–0.67)	0.21	69.7	51.4
axSpA vs. PsA	0.52 (0.45–0.59)	0.11	94.5	16.8

axSpA axial spondyloarthritis, *PsA* psoriatic arthritis

Guidelines for treatment of axSpA and PsA rely mainly on clinical assessment of disease activity and progression [26, 27]. Thus, biologically plausible biomarkers may provide additional information regarding diagnosis and assessment of disease activity, and they may also help to guide treatment [28, 29]. We previously reported that type II collagen seromarkers differ between axSpA and PsA [13]. However, this report was based on the marker of mature collagen II (C2M) [30] and a marker of regenerative collagen II formation (PIIANP) [31]. In the present study, we wanted to extend these previous observations using Pro-C2, a marker of mature collagen synthesis, and C-Col10, a fragment of collagen X. Thus, Pro-C2 and PIIANP reflect the synthesis of two different splice variants of procollagen II. Type IIA procollagen is expressed mainly during embryogenesis [32] and has been found to be reexpressed in osteoarthritis [16]. The PIIANP splice variant is considered to represent a dedifferentiated version of type II collagen [31]. By contrast, collagen type IIB N-terminal propeptide (PIIBNP) is considered to be the only procollagen expressed during type II collagen formation in healthy adult cartilage [17]. Pro-C2 is specific for evaluation of the PIIBNP splice variant [20]. This allows for discrimination between structural type IIB vs. regenerative cartilage type IIA formation in healthy and diseased states. The present study shows that mature collagen II synthesis as reflected by Pro-C2 is increased in both axSpA and PsA, while our previous study showed that PIIANP was increased only in currently untreated patients with PsA and in treatment-naïve patients with axSpA compared with control subjects [13]. Notably, Pro-C2 was not affected by DMARD treatment in axSpA or PsA, while PIIANP was lower in treated than in untreated patients, probably reflecting suppression of a cartilage pathogenic pathway [13]. The increased on-treatment Pro-C2 levels likely reflect that mature cartilage collagen IIB synthesis is maintained despite drug treatment. The increased Pro-C2 levels correlated significantly with physical function scores but not with joint counts, which may reflect a mature chondrocyte response to altered mechanical influences on cartilage elicited by synovial and entheseal pathologies [33]. The lower Pro-C2 concentration in HLA-B27-positive patients with axSpA than in HLA-B27-negative patients suggests that the HLA-B27 gene is implicated in the regulation of type II collagen expression, as recently proposed for procollagen IIA in axSpA [13]. Our findings add to those described by Pedersen et al., who reported that the urinary excretion of CTX-II, a marker of collagen II degradation, was increased in axSpA but decreased during TNFi treatment [12]. Thus, the current increased Pro-C2 level may reflect an anabolic chondrocyte response to counterbalance increased collagen type II degradation in active disease.

By analogy with osteoarthritis, we hypothesized that C-Col10 levels would be increased in SpA as a marker of syndesmophyte outgrowth similar to osteophyte formation [21, 22, 34, 35]. Thus, C-Col10 was significantly increased in patients with PsA as compared with control subjects. The same trend was observed in axSpA, although it did not reach statistical significance. However, C-Col10 was significantly lower in patients with axSpA treated with biologic DMARDs than in those naïve to biological treatment, indicating that hypertrophic chondrocytes and collagen X expression are suppressed by TNFi. This response contrasts with Pro-C2, indicating that household collagen II formation is left unaffected by TNF-α inhibition, while potential cartilage osteochondral precursor collagen is suppressed. This observation and the association between C-Col10 and SJC lend support to the concept that chondrocyte hypertrophy and increased expression of type X collagen are implicated in the axSpA disease pathway. However, in a recent study, Bleil et al. [23] reported that chondrocyte hypertrophy was not present in the facet joints of patients with axSpA as assessed by immunohistochemistry. These authors studied cartilage from patients with advanced ankylosing spondylitis, in which the chondrocyte phenotype and distribution may be different from early active disease and therefore may have a different type X collagen expression profile. C-Col10 levels in osteoarthritis (OA) have previously been studied in patients stratified according to the Kellgren and Lawrence scoring system. In that study, C-Col10 was significantly elevated in patients with intermediate structural OA changes vs. patients with severe or no abnormalities [19]. However, the cartilage pathology of OA may differ from that of axSpA, and the patient populations were not comparable in terms of age, sex, or disease duration. Alternatively, the increased release of type X collagen fragments may originate from cartilage in areas other than the facet joints in patients with axSpA. However, the risk of concurrent osteoarthritis in the present patient populations is considered to be low because the median age was only around 35 years.

Some limitations of the present study should be considered. The cross-sectional design provides an opportunity to evaluate the biochemical disease profile at a specific time point, but it does not provide prognostic information. No updated x-rays or MRI scans were available. Since this is the first report on Pro-C2 in a clinical setting, it is uncertain how the present results compare with findings in other joint diseases. The strengths of this study are inclusion of two large and clinically well-characterized patient populations with axSpA and PsA and a large number of healthy control subjects. In addition, this is the first time that Pro-C2 and C-Col10 have been applied to axSpA and PsA.

Conclusions

This study presents a biochemical cartilage marker profile in two disease subsets within the spondyloarthropathy complex indicating the presence of hypertrophic and enhanced chondrocyte activity, particularly in active disease. While increased collagen IIB production was unaffected by TNFi treatment, type X collagen of hypertrophic chondrocytes was suppressed by these agents. This may indicate that the SpA-related type II collagen response of normal chondrocytes is preserved, while the collagen type X expression of cartilaginous and enthesopathic lesions is modified by TNFi. Prospective studies are needed to validate this concept.

Abbreviations

ASAS, Assessment of SpondyloArthritis international Society; ASDAS, Ankylosing Spondylitis Disease Activity Score; axSpA, axial spondyloarthritis; BASDAI, Bath Ankylosing Spondylitis Disease Activity Index; BASFI, Bath Ankylosing Spondylitis Functional Index; BASMI, Bath Ankylosing Spondylitis Metrology Index; BMI, body mass index; CASPAR, Classification of Psoriatic Arthritis; C2C, collagen type II cleavage; C2M, matrix metalloproteinase-generated type II collagen degradation fragment; CII, type II collagen; CRP, C-reactive protein; CTX-II, C-terminal telopeptide of type II collagen; DAS28, Disease Activity Score in 28 joints; DMARD, disease-modifying antirheumatic drug; ELISA, enzyme-linked immunosorbent assay; HAQ, Health Assessment Questionnaire; HLA-B27, human leukocyte antigen B27; hs-CRP, high-sensitivity C-reactive protein; MRI, magnetic resonance imaging; NPII, N-terminal procollagen type II; NPIIB, N-terminal propeptide of the procollagen IIB splice variant; ns, not significant; OA, osteoarthritis; PIIANP, collagen type IIA N-terminal propeptide; PIIBNP, collagen type IIB N-terminal propeptide; PIINP, collagen type II N-terminal propeptide; PsA, psoriatic arthritis; SJC68, 68 swollen joint count; SpA, spondyloarthropathy; TJC68, 68 tender joint count; TMB, 3,3′,5,5′-tetramethylbenzinidine; TNFi, tumor necrosis factor-α inhibitor; VAS, visual analogue scale

Acknowledgements

The authors are grateful to the study participants and the participating general practitioners.

Funding

This study was supported by research grants from the region of Southern Denmark and Department of Rheumatology C, Odense University Hospital, Odense, Denmark. The research leading to these results received partial funding from the European Union Seventh Framework Programme (FP7/2007-2013) under grant agreement 305815 and partial funding from the Danish Research Foundation (DFF under Act 2013).

Authors' contributions

All authors made substantial contributions to (1) the conception and design of the study, or acquisition of data, or analysis and interpretation of data; (2) the drafting of the manuscript or revising it critically for important intellectual content; and (3) final approval of the manuscript version to be submitted. NSG, HLM, ASS, and PJ conceived and designed the study. NSG, LE, AGL, and HLM acquired data. NSG, HLM, YH, AFC, MAK, ACBJ, ASS, GLS, and PJ analyzed and interpreted data. NSG, ASS, and PJ drafted the manuscript. NSG, HLM, YH, AFC, LE, GLS, AGL, ACBJ, MAK, ASS, and PJ revised the manuscript critically for important intellectual content. NSG, HLM, AFC, LE, GLS, AGL, ACBJ, YH, MAK, ASS, and PJ gave final approval of the manuscript version submitted for publication. NSG and PJ provided statistical expertise. HLM, PJ, ACBJ, and MAK obtained funding. NSG, ASS, and HLM collection and assembled data. NSG takes responsibility for the integrity of the work as a whole, from inception to the final version of the article.

Competing interests

NSG, MAK, YH, ACBJ, and ASS were employed at Nordic Bioscience while this study was conducted, and MAK holds stock in Nordic Bioscience. The other authors declare that they have no competing interests. The authors have no financial or personal relationships with other organizations or people that could potentially and inappropriately influence (bias) their work and conclusions.

Consent for publication

The authors received informed consent from the participants for data publication in an anonymized form.

Author details

[1]Nordic Bioscience Biomarkers and Research, Herlev Hovedgade 207, Herlev 2730, Denmark. [2]Department of Rheumatology, Odense University Hospital, Odense, Denmark. [3]Department of Rheumatology, Vejle Hospital, Vejle, Denmark. [4]Department of Rheumatology, Esbjerg Hospital, Esbjerg, Denmark. [5]Institute of Molecular Medicine, University of Southern Denmark, Odense, Denmark. [6]Department of Rheumatology, Aarhus University Hospital, Aarhus, Denmark.

References

1. Paramarta JE, Baeten D. Spondyloarthritis: from unifying concepts to improved treatment. Rheumatology (Oxford). 2014;53:1547–59.
2. Golder V, Schachna L. Ankylosing spondylitis: an update. Aust Fam Physician. 2013;42:780–4.
3. Khan MA. Update on spondyloarthropathies. Ann Intern Med. 2002;136:896–907.
4. Pedersen OB, Svendsen AJ, Ejstrup L, Skytthe A, Harris JR, Junker P. Ankylosing spondylitis in Danish and Norwegian twins: occurrence and the relative importance of genetic vs. environmental effectors in disease causation. Scand J Rheumatol. 2008;37:120–6.
5. Pedersen OB, Svendsen AJ, Ejstrup L, Skytthe A, Junker P. The occurrence of psoriatic arthritis in Denmark. Ann Rheum Dis. 2008;67:1422–6.
6. Londono J, Santos AM, Pena P, Calvo E, Espinosa LR, Reveille JD, et al. Analysis of HLA-B15 and HLA-B27 in spondyloarthritis with peripheral and axial clinical patterns. BMJ Open. 2015;5:e009092.
7. Garg N, van den Bosch F, Deodhar A. The concept of spondyloarthritis: where are we now? Best Pract Res Clin Rheumatol. 2014;28:663–72.
8. Braun J, Brandt J, Listing J, Rudwaleit M, Sieper J. Biologic therapies in the spondyloarthritis: new opportunities, new challenges. Curr Opin Rheumatol. 2003;15:394–407.
9. Lloyd P, Ryan C, Menter A. Psoriatic arthritis: an update. Arthritis. 2012;2012:176298.
10. Siebuhr AS, He Y, Gudmann NS, Gram A, Kjelgaard-Petersen CF, Qvist P, et al. Biomarkers of cartilage and surrounding joint tissue. Biomark Med. 2014; 8:713–31.
11. Kim TH, Stone M, Payne U, Zhang X, Ionescu M, Lobanok T, et al. Cartilage biomarkers in ankylosing spondylitis: relationship to clinical variables and treatment response. Arthritis Rheum. 2005;52:885–91.
12. Pedersen SJ, Sorensen IJ, Garnero P, Johansen JS, Madsen OR, Tvede N, et al. ASDAS, BASDAI and different treatment responses and their relation to biomarkers of inflammation, cartilage and bone turnover in patients with axial spondyloarthritis treated with TNFα inhibitors. Ann Rheum Dis. 2011;70:1375–81.
13. Munk HL, Gudmann NS, Christensen AF, Ejstrup L, Sorensen GL, Loft AG, et al. Cartilage collagen type II seromarker patterns in axial spondyloarthritis and psoriatic arthritis: associations with disease activity, smoking and HLA-B27. Rheumatol Int. 2016;36:541–9.
14. Nemirovskiy OV, Sunyer T, Aggarwal P, Abrams M, Hellio Le Graverand MP, Mathews WR. Discovery and development of the N-terminal procollagen type II (NPII) biomarker: a tool for measuring collagen type II synthesis. Osteoarthritis Cartilage. 2008;16:1494–500.
15. Olsen AK, Sondergaard BC, Byrjalsen I, Tanko LB, Christiansen C, Muller A, et al. Anabolic and catabolic function of chondrocyte ex vivo is reflected by the metabolic processing of type II collagen. Osteoarthritis Cartilage. 2007;15:335–42.

16. Aigner T, Zhu Y, Chansky HH, Matsen III FA, Maloney WJ, Sandell LJ. Reexpression of type IIA procollagen by adult articular chondrocytes in osteoarthritic cartilage. Arthritis Rheum. 1999;42:1443–50.
17. Sandell LJ, Morris N, Robbins JR, Goldring MB. Alternatively spliced type II procollagen mRNAs define distinct populations of cells during vertebral development: differential expression of the amino-propeptide. J Cell Biol. 1991;114:1307–19.
18. Garnero P, Ayral X, Rousseau JC, Christgau S, Sandell LJ, Dougados M, et al. Uncoupling of type II collagen synthesis and degradation predicts progression of joint damage in patients with knee osteoarthritis. Arthritis Rheum. 2002;46:2613–24.
19. He Y, Siebuhr AS, Brandt-Hansen NU, Wang J, Su D, Zheng Q, et al. Type X collagen levels are elevated in serum from human osteoarthritis patients and associated with biomarkers of cartilage degradation and inflammation. BMC Musculoskelet Disord. 2014;15:309.
20. Gudmann NS, Wang J, Hoielt S, Chen P, Siebuhr AS, He Y, et al. Cartilage turnover reflected by metabolic processing of type II collagen: a novel marker of anabolic function in chondrocytes. Int J Mol Sci. 2014;15:18789–803.
21. Ronneberger M, Schett G. Pathophysiology of spondyloarthritis. Curr Rheumatol Rep. 2011;13:416–20.
22. Lories RJ, Luyten FP, de Vlam K. Progress in spondylarthritis. Mechanisms of new bone formation in spondyloarthritis. Arthritis Res Ther. 2009;11:221.
23. Bleil J, Sieper J, Maier R, Schlichting U, Hempfing A, Syrbe U, et al. Cartilage in facet joints of patients with ankylosing spondylitis (AS) shows signs of cartilage degeneration rather than chondrocyte hypertrophy: implications for joint remodeling in AS. Arthritis Res Ther. 2015;17:170.
24. Resorlu M, Gokmen F, Resorlu H, Adam G, Akbal A, Cevizci S, et al. Association between apparent diffusion coefficient and intervertebral disc degeneration in patients with ankylosing spondylitis. Int J Clin Exp Med. 2015;8:1241–6.
25. Tan AL, McGonagle D. Psoriatic arthritis: correlation between imaging and pathology. Joint Bone Spine. 2010;77:206–11.
26. Gossec L, Smolen JS, Gaujoux-Viala C, Ash Z, Marzo-Ortega H, van der Heijde D, et al. European League Against Rheumatism recommendations for the management of psoriatic arthritis with pharmacological therapies. Ann Rheum Dis. 2012;71:4–12.
27. Smolen JS, Braun J, Dougados M, Emery P, Fitzgerald O, Helliwell P, et al. Treating spondyloarthritis, including ankylosing spondylitis and psoriatic arthritis, to target: recommendations of an international task force. Ann Rheum Dis. 2014;73:6–16.
28. Schett G. Erosive arthritis. Arthritis Res Ther. 2007;9 Suppl 1:S2.
29. Schett G. Osteoimmunology in rheumatic diseases. Arthritis Res Ther. 2009;11:210
30. Bay-Jensen AC, Liu Q, Byrjalsen I, Li Y, Wang J, Pedersen C, et al. Enzyme-linked immunosorbent assay (ELISAs) for metalloproteinase derived type II collagen neoepitope, CIIM—increased serum CIIM in subjects with severe radiographic osteoarthritis. Clin Biochem. 2011;44:423–9.
31. Rousseau JC, Sandell LJ, Delmas PD, Garnero P. Development and clinical application in arthritis of a new immunoassay for serum type IIA procollagen NH_2 propeptide. Methods Mol Med. 2004;101:25–37.
32. Zhu Y, McAlinden A, Sandell LJ. Type IIA procollagen in development of the human intervertebral disc: regulated expression of the NH_2-propeptide by enzymic processing reveals a unique developmental pathway. Dev Dyn. 2001;220:350–62.
33. Masi AT, Nair K, Andonian BJ, Prus KM, Kelly J, Sanchez JR, et al. Integrative structural biomechanical concepts of ankylosing spondylitis. Arthritis. 2011;2011:205904.
34. Tsang KY, Chan D, Cheah KS. Fate of growth plate hypertrophic chondrocytes: death or lineage extension? Dev Growth Differ. 2015;57:179–92.
35. Lories RJ, Haroon N. Bone formation in axial spondyloarthritis. Best Pract Res Clin Rheumatol. 2014;28:765–77.

12

Childhood hospitalisation with infections and later development of ankylosing spondylitis

Ulf Lindström[1*], Sofia Exarchou[2], Elisabeth Lie[3], Mats Dehlin[1], Helena Forsblad-d'Elia[4], Johan Askling[5] and Lennart Jacobsson[1]

Abstract

Background: The role of environmental exposures in the pathogenesis of ankylosing spondylitis (AS) remains unclear. In particular, two types of exposures have been suspected to play a role: mechanical stress and infections. The objective of this case-control study was to determine if childhood infections are associated with later development of AS.

Methods: The cases with AS were identified through the Swedish national outpatient specialised-care register, based on having been given at least one AS diagnosis in the register between 2001 and 2010. Five controls per case were identified in the Swedish population register, matched at the time-point of the index case's first spondyloarthritis diagnosis on sex, birth year, and county. All cases/controls matched prior to the age of 17 years were excluded, as well as all cases/controls given a diagnosis of reactive arthritis or juvenile arthritis at any time point, or any other diagnosis of a rheumatic disease, psoriasis, iridocyclitis, or inflammatory bowel disease before the time-point of matching. All events of hospitalisation with an infection before the age of 17 years were retrieved from the register, and categorised according to the focus of the infection. Odds ratios (ORs) and confidence intervals (CIs) were determined through conditional logistic regression analyses.

Results: Of the 2453 cases with AS and 10,257 controls, 17.4 % of the cases and 16.3 % of the controls had been hospitalised with an infection before the age of 17 years (OR 1.08, 95 % CI 0.96–1.22).
Appendicitis (1.5 % cases; 2.5 % controls; OR 0.59, 95 % CI 0.41–0.83), respiratory tract infections (cases 11.2 %; controls 9.2 %; OR 1.24, 95 % CI 1.07–1.44) and, in particular, tonsillitis (cases 3.7 %; controls 2.8 %; OR 1.31, 95 % CI 1.03–1.67) were associated with AS. There were no associations between AS and any other type of infection, and the point estimates were similar in several sensitivity analyses.

Conclusions: Childhood appendicitis was associated with a decreased risk, whereas respiratory tract infections were associated with an increased risk for later development of AS. These findings support a possible relationship between childhood infections and later development of AS, although the study is limited to infections resulting in inpatient care.

Keywords: Ankylosing spondylitis, Epidemiology, Infections, Spondyloarthritis

* Correspondence: ulf.lindstrom@gu.se
[1]Department of Rheumatology and Inflammation Research, Institute of Medicine, Sahlgrenska Academy, University of Gothenburg, Guldhedsgatan 10A, 405 30 Gothenburg, Sweden
Full list of author information is available at the end of the article

Background

An understanding of the genetic basis for ankylosing spondylitis (AS) is expanding rapidly. According to studies in twins, genetic factors, including human leukocyte antigen 27 (HLA-B27), are now thought to account for >90 % of the risk for AS [1]. In contrast, the role of environmental exposures in the aetiology of AS remains unclear. Whereas studies on twins and extended families do suggest that non-hereditary factors are likely to be involved in the pathogenesis, studies indicating a temporal relationship between environmental exposures and the development of AS are rare [2–4]. The two most prevailing theories suggest that onset of AS in genetically susceptible individuals may be triggered by either infections or by mechanical stress [5, 6], and sparse data also suggests an association with smoking [7].

Reactive arthritis, another spondyloarthritis (SpA) disease, is usually triggered by enteric or urogenital infections, but other infections, such as respiratory tract infections, can also trigger the disease onset [8–10]. Like AS, reactive arthritis is also strongly associated with HLA-B27 [11], suggesting a significant genetic overlap with AS. Similarly, in inflammatory bowel disease (IBD), enteric infections or alterations in gut flora have been implicated in the disease pathogenesis [12]. For example, in ulcerative colitis, a decreased risk for developing the disease, associated with prior appendicitis, has been described in several patient cohorts. IBD also shares a genetic overlap with AS, and while only a minority of patients with AS have a clinically overt IBD, the majority have been found to have a subclinical gut inflammation [13, 14]. The definitive role of this gut inflammation in SpA has not been determined, but it appears to share inflammatory pathways with the bone/joint inflammation [15]. Studies have also indicated differences in the gut flora between patients with AS and healthy controls, suggesting that gut dysbiosis may be involved in the disease pathogenesis [16], a finding further supported by SpA models in HLA-B27 transgenic rats, where animals reared in a germ-free environment fail to develop gut and joint inflammation [17]. In psoriasis, also related to the SpA disease group, tonsillitis, specifically with streptococci, is well known to trigger the guttate form, but is also suspected to play a role in exacerbations of plaque psoriasis [18].

In contrast to the growing data supporting a role for infections in the pathogenesis of other SpA and SpA-related diseases, no such relationship has been shown for AS, and attempts to link specific pathogens to the disease have either not been successful or not possible to replicate [16, 19, 20]. In this study, we compared the frequency of childhood infections at hospitalisation between cases later diagnosed with AS and matched population controls. Our hypothesis was that AS would be associated with childhood infections, and considering the similarities with reactive arthritis and inflammatory bowel disease, in particular with enteric and urogenital infections.

Methods

Setting

This is a case-control study based on four national registers in Sweden.

Data sources

The Patient Register was initiated in 1964 as a hospitalisation register, and was expanded in 2001 with an outpatient register for specialised care [21]. The registers are considered to have an overall high validity [21].

The Population Register contains demographic data for all residents in Sweden [22].

The Prescribed Drug Register was started in July 2005, and contains anatomical therapeutic chemical (ATC) codes and administrative data on all prescribed drugs dispensed in Sweden [23].

The Swedish Rheumatology Quality Register (SRQ) contains information on anti-rheumatic treatment in Sweden. The register coverage for patients treated with tumour necrosis factor alpha inhibitors (TNFi) is 85–90 % [24].

Study population

The AS cases were defined as having been given ≥1 diagnosis (according to the International Classification of Diseases (ICD)) of AS in the specialised care outpatient register between 2001 and 2010, being born in Sweden in 1964 or later, and having lived in Sweden at least up to the age of 17 years. The high validity of the AS diagnoses in the register has been described previously [25].

Five controls per case were retrieved from the population register, matched on sex, birth year, and county of birth, at the time of the index cases' first registered diagnosis of SpA, and with the same requirement of having lived in Sweden at least until the age of 17 years.

In order to minimise the risk for the cases and controls already having an inflammatory disorder before the age of 17 years, all cases receiving their first registered diagnosis of SpA before the age of 17 years, as well as all cases and controls given a diagnosis of juvenile arthritis or reactive arthritis at any time, or a diagnosis of any other rheumatic disease, IBD, psoriasis, or iridocyclitis before the time-point of the match were excluded (for ICD and ATC codes see Additional file 1).

Exposure data

For cases and controls, all ICD codes corresponding to an infection given at the time of discharge from inpatient care before the age of 17 years were identified. The data were categorised according to the primary focus of the infection and, as a supplement to enteric infections and respiratory tract infections, data for appendectomy and tonsillectomy were also collected. Data were also retrieved from the prescribed drugs register and the SRQ regarding use of immunosuppressive drugs and antibiotics in 2006–2011.

Statistics

Odds ratios (ORs) with 95 % confidence intervals (CIs) were computed for the association between the different infectious exposures and AS using simple conditional logistic regression.

SAS 9.4 was used for aggregation of data and SPSS 21 for statistical analysis.

Sensitivity analyses and stratification

Three a priori defined sensitivity analyses were performed. The first included only cases matched at an age of >26 years. The purpose of this analysis was to further separate the time period of exposure to the infections from the time-point of receiving the first SpA diagnosis, giving a minimum of a 10-year lag period between the exposures and the outcome, as recorded in the register.

The second included only cases treated with methotrexate, sulphasalazine, and/or TNFi, with the intention of probably selecting a more severe AS phenotype.

The third included only cases/controls matched in 2007–2011, excluding all cases and controls treated with immunosuppressive or cytostatic drugs, as well as specific drugs for IBD, during the year prior to matching. The purpose of this was to further eliminate possible cases and controls with an inflammatory disorder before the match. The limitation to cases matched after 2007 was due to the fact that the Prescribed Drug Register was started in July 2005. Comparisons of the frequencies of dispensed prescriptions of antibiotics in the year prior to match between cases and controls were also performed using Fisher's exact test.

An additional, fourth, post-hoc sensitivity analysis was also performed, excluding cases and controls with a diagnosis of IBD between the time-point of match and up until 2 years after the first AS diagnosis, the rationale for this being the previously described association between appendicitis and a lower risk for ulcerative colitis [26, 27].

Two stratified analyses were also performed; the first stratified on median age at first SpA diagnosis, and the second for median age at appendectomy and tonsillectomy. For the latter analysis, the procedures of appendectomy and tonsillectomy were chosen, rather than the codes for the corresponding infections/inflammations, in order to avoid cases and controls with multiple registered diagnoses at different ages. For the few cases and controls with more than one registered tonsillectomy procedure, the first was used for the analysis.

Results

Cases and controls

We identified 2453 cases with AS (64 % men) and 10,257 controls (mean 4.3 controls per case). Demographics, AS-related disease manifestations, and pharmacological treatment are shown in Table 1.

Table 1 Demographics, ankylosing spondylitis (AS)-related inflammatory diseases, and pharmacological treatment in cases and controls

Demographics	Cases (*n* = 2453)	Controls (*n* = 10,257)
Men, *n* (%)	1569 (64)	6587 (64)
Year of birth, median (min–max)	1971 (1964–1992)	1971 (1964–1992)
Age at first SpA-diagnosis (years), mean, SD (min–max)	30, 6.2 (17–46)	30, 6.2 (17–46)
AS-related inflammatory diseases[a]		
Iridocyclitis, *n* (%)	453 (19)	45 (0)
Inflammatory bowel disease, n (%)	102 (4)	37 (0)
Psoriasis, *n* (%)	122 (5)	79 (1)
Pharmacological treatment in 2011[b]		
NSAID, *n* (%)	1279 (52)	9 (0)
TNF inhibitor, *n* (%)	553 (23)	NA[c]
Methotrexate, *n* (%)	169 (7)	0
Sulphasalazine, *n* (%)	263 (11)	1 (0)

[a]AS-related inflammatory diseases are given as cumulative incidence until 2 years after first AS diagnosis for the cases and their matched controls

[b]Based on prescriptions in the prescribed drugs register during 2011, apart from the tumour necrosis factor alpha (TNF) inhibitor infliximab for which data were based on recorded treatment in the Swedish Rheumatology Quality Register (SRQ) during 2011

[c]Total TNF inhibitor exposure was not possible to determine for controls since treatment with infliximab for nonrheumatic diseases cannot be detected through either the prescribed drugs register or SRQ. The frequency of any subcutaneous TNF inhibitors for controls during 2011 was *n* = 2

NA Not available, *NSAID* nonsteroidal anti-inflammatory drug, *SpA* spondyloarthritis

Analyses

Of the AS cases, 426 (17.4 %) had a registered diagnosis of any infection at a time of hospitalisation before the age of 17 years, with the values for the controls being 1668 (16.3 %) (OR 1.08, 95 % CI 0.96–1.22). Figure 1 presents the numbers of exposed cases and controls for each category of infection, and the corresponding ORs.

Appendicitis (cases $n = 37$ (1.5 %) and controls $n = 260$ (2.5 %); OR 0.59, 95 % CI 0.41–0.83) and appendectomy (cases $n = 60$ (2.4 %) and controls $n = 336$ (3.3 %); OR 0.73, 95 % CI 0.55–0.97) were significantly associated with a decreased OR for AS. Respiratory tract infections (cases $n = 274$ (11.2 %) and controls $n = 941$ (9.2 %); OR 1.24, 95 % CI 1.07–1.44) and, in particular, tonsillectomy (cases $n = 82$ (3.3 %) and controls $n = 244$ (2.4 %); OR 1.38, 95 % CI 1.06–1.77) were associated with an increased OR for AS. For enteric infections overall and urogenital infections there were no associations.

For the group registered with both appendicitis and appendectomy (cases $n = 37$ (1.5 %) and controls $n = 254$ (2.5 %)) the OR was 0.60 (95 % CI 0.42–0.85), while for the group registered with only appendectomy but not appendicitis (cases $n = 23$ (0.9 %) and controls $n = 82$ (0.8 %)) the OR was 1.16 (95 % CI 0.73–1.86). For the group registered with both tonsillitis and tonsillectomy (cases $n = 74$ (3.0 %) and controls $n = 222$ (2.2 %)), the OR was 1.38 (95 % CI 1.04–1.78). For the respiratory tract infections, excluding tonsillectomy or tonsillitis (cases $n = 179$ (7.3 %) and controls $n = 636$ (6.2 %)), the OR was 1.20 (95 % CI 1.00–1.43).

The point estimates were of a similar direction and magnitude in all of the sensitivity analyses (Table 2). In the sensitivity analysis only including cases matched 2007–2011 there was no statistically significant difference in the proportions receiving prescriptions of antibiotics in the year prior to matching between cases and controls.

In the analysis stratified by median age at first SpA diagnosis (17–30 years versus 31–46 years) all point estimates were in the same direction and of similar magnitude as in the primary analysis, apart from tonsillitis and tonsillectomy which were stronger in the younger age-groups (age 17–30 years at first SpA diagnosis: tonsillitis, OR 1.15 (95 % CI 1.13–2.94), and tonsillectomy, OR 1.65 (95 % CI 1.21 to 2.26); age 31–46 years at first SpA diagnosis: tonsillitis, OR 0.97 (95 % CI 0.62–1.51), and tonsillectomy, OR 0.94 (95 % CI 0.59–1.51).

The median age for appendectomy was 12 years and for tonsillectomy 9 years (all procedures at an age above 16 years are disregarded). In the analysis stratifying on median age at appendectomy, a stronger association was observed in the age group 0–12 years (OR 0.61, 95 % CI 0.42–0.89) compared to age group 13–16 years (OR 0.95, 95 % CI 0.63–1.43). For tonsillectomy, the association was similar in the stratified age groups (age 0–9 years, OR 1.43 (95 % CI 1.01–2.02), and age 10–16 years, OR 1.35 (95 % CI 0.94–1.93).

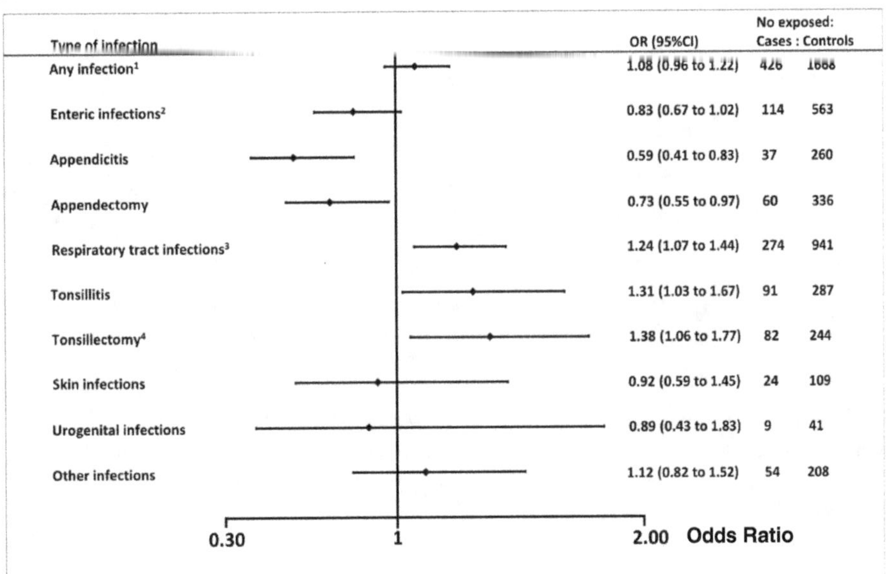

Fig. 1 Associations between childhood infections and a later diagnosis of ankylosing spondylitis. Based on a total of 2453 AS cases and 10,257 matched controls where exposure data to infections are based on registered events of an infection in inpatient care before the age of 17 years. [1]Including all infectious foci, but not the procedures appendectomy or tonsillectomy; [2]including appendicitis; [3]including tonsillitis; [4]also including adenoidectomy. *CI* confidence interval, *OR* odds ratio

Table 2 Sensitivity analyses of the associations between childhood infections and a later diagnosis of ankylosing spondylitis

Including only cases matched at an age of 27 years or older	Cases ($n = 1757$)	Controls ($n = 7305$)	OR	95 % CI
All infections[a]	258 (14.7)	964 (13.2)	1.13	0.97–1.32
Enteric[b]	74 (4.2)	333 (4.6)	0.91	0.70–1.19
Appendicitis	30 (1.7)	169 (2.3)	0.72	0.49–1.07
Appendectomy	46 (2.6)	234 (3.2)	0.82	0.59–1.13
Respiratory tract[c]	159 (9.0)	529 (7.2)	1.27	1.05–1.54
Tonsillitis	49 (2.8)	169 (2.3)	1.16	0.83–1.61
Tonsillectomy[d]	43 (2.4)	151 (2.1)	1.12	0.79–1.59
Skin	15 (0.9)	66 (0.9)	0.93	0.53–1.64
Urogenital tract	6 (0.3)	24 (0.3)	1.02	0.41–2.50
Other	35 (2.0)	113 (1.5)	1.34	0.91–1.97
Including only cases treated with methotrexate, sulphasalazine, and/or TNFi	Cases ($n = 794$)	Controls ($n = 3288$)	OR	95 % CI
All infections[a]	141 (17.8)	553 (16.8)	1.06	0.86–1.31
Enteric[b]	40 (5.0)	185 (5.6)	0.87	0.61–1.25
Appendicitis	12 (1.5)	85 (2.6)	0.58	0.31–1.06
Appendectomy	20 (2.5)	116 (3.5)	0.71	0.44–1.16
Respiratory tract[c]	93 (11.7)	329 (10.0)	1.20	0.93–1.54
Tonsillitis	34 (4.3)	96 (2.9)	1.48	0.98–2.24
Tonsillectomy[d]	27 (3.4)	78 (2.4)	1.42	0.90–2.24
Skin	12 (1.5)	38 (1.2)	1.37	0.71–2.66
Urogenital tract	1 (0.1)	16 (0.5)	0.28	0.037–2.10
Other	14 (1.8)	59 (1.8)	0.991	0.54–1.81
Including only cases matched 2007–2011 and excluding all with immunosuppressive or cytostatic treatment, as well as specific treatment for inflammatory bowel disease, 1 year prior to match	Cases ($n = 471$)	Controls ($n = 1836$)	OR	95 % CI
All infections[a]	96 (20.4)	329 (17.9)	1.16	0.89–1.52
Enteric[b]	26 (5.5)	102 (5.6)	0.92	0.59–1.45
Appendicitis	6 (1.3)	38 (2.1)	0.57	0.24–1.36
Appendectomy	11 (2.3)	48 (2.6)	0.84	0.43–1.63
Respiratory tract[c]	63 (13.4)	191 (10.4)	1.33	0.97–1.81
Tonsillitis	27 (5.7)	67 (3.6)	1.58	0.99–2.53
Tonsillectomy[d]	20 (4.2)	54 (2.9)	1.40	0.82–2.38
Skin	3 (0.6)	21 (1.1)	0.56	0.16–1.90
Urogenital tract	4 (0.8)	8 (0.4)	2.03	0.61–6.78
Other	14 (3.0)	45 (2.5)	1.29	0.70–2.40
Prescription of antibiotics 1 year prior to match	131 (27.8)	478 (26.0)	$p = 0.446$	
Excluding inflammatory bowel disease[e]	Cases ($n = 2307$)	Controls ($n = 9584$)	OR	95 % CI
All infections[a]	405 (17.6)	1555 (16.2)	1.10	0.97–1.25
Enteric[b]	108 (4.7)	528 (5.5)	0.84	0.67–1.04
Appendicitis	35 (1.5)	244 (2.5)	0.59	0.41–0.84
Appendectomy	56 (2.4)	312 (3.3)	0.74	0.55–0.98
Respiratory tract[c]	258 (11.2)	873 (9.1)	1.25	1.08–1.46

Table 2 Sensitivity analyses of the associations between childhood infections and a later diagnosis of ankylosing spondylitis *(Continued)*

Tonsillitis	87 (3.8)	257 (2.7)	1.37	1.07–1.77
Tonsillectomy[d]	78 (3.4)	219 (2.3)	1.42	1.09–1.85
Skin	23 (1.0)	102 (1.1)	0.94	0.59–1.49
Urogenital tract	9 (0.4)	40 (0.4)	0.90	0.44–1.86
Other	53 (2.3)	192 (2.0)	1.18	0.87–1.62

All values are shown as *n* (%)
Exposure data are based on registered events of an infection in inpatient care before the age of 17 years
[a]Including all infectious foci, but not the procedures appendectomy or tonsillectomy; [b]including appendicitis; [c]including tonsillitis; [d]also including adenoidectomy; [e]excluding all cases/controls with a diagnosis of ulcerative colitis, Crohns' disease, or any other non-infectious bowel inflammation (see Additional file 1) up until 2 years after the first AS diagnosis of the index case
CI confidence interval, *OR* odds ratio, *TNFi* tumour necrosis factor alfa inhibitors

Discussion

Principal findings

In this study we found that appendicitis in childhood was associated with a lower OR for AS, and that respiratory tract infections were associated with a weak increase in the OR, which was more pronounced for tonsillitis. Our initial hypothesis was that infections in general during childhood, particularly in the enteric and urogenital tracts, would be associated with an increased risk for later development of AS. However, our results did not indicate any such association with either infections in general, or specifically with enteric or urogenital tract infections.

Appendicitis has repeatedly been shown to have a protective association with ulcerative colitis, thought to be linked somehow to the inflammation itself rather than the appendectomy [26, 27]. In this study, the decreased OR observed for appendicitis remained much the same after exclusion of cases and controls with IBD, suggesting that the effect was not conveyed through IBD comorbidity. The point estimates for appendicitis and appendectomy were also conserved throughout the other sensitivity analyses, suggesting a robust effect. For respiratory tract infections, the OR also attained statistical significance; however, the magnitude of the effect was in fact similar to that of enteric infections and urogenital tract infections. The reason that the latter two did not meet statistical significance might be due to the relatively low frequency of these infections, implying that a larger number of cases and controls were needed for respiratory tract infections to reach statistical difference. This may suggest that the strength of the association between respiratory tract infections overall and the risk of developing AS is relatively weak. For tonsillitis and tonsillectomy, the increase in risk for development of AS was consistently stronger than for respiratory tract infections overall in all sensitivity analyses except when only including cases receiving a registered diagnosis of SpA after the age of 26 years.

There are several remarks to make concerning the possible biological interpretation of our findings. First, it is not possible to draw any conclusions concerning causality for the association found between different types of infections and later development of AS. Indeed, since the frequency for all types of infections was relatively low among both the cases and the controls, and the time span between the exposures and the outcome was long, such an effect may be biologically improbable. Still, it cannot be ruled out that the different infections during childhood could induce long-lasting immunological effects that may affect the disease onset in genetically predisposed individuals. If so, then it is also possible that repeated infections in the same individual may enforce such an effect, but the frequencies of readmissions with the same infection were too low to analyse in our study (data not shown). Second, we know that HLA is central to the function of the adaptive immune system, and that different HLA types have been shown to be associated with differences in the response to different pathogens; for example, HLA-B27 has been shown to be related to a higher chance for viral clearance in hepatitis C and a better prognosis in HIV [28, 29]. It is possible that the immune phenotype of AS, including HLA-B27, leading up to the development of AS also conveys a hitherto unknown increase in risk for respiratory tract infections and a decrease in risk for appendicitis. For appendicitis, a genetic component has been suggested but the inflammation is generally believed to be triggered by infections [30]. Third, it is also possible that the similar decrease in risk for both AS and ulcerative colitis, associated with appendicitis, is related to the connection between gut inflammation and AS. A fourth possibility is that appendicitis and respiratory tract infections, or the treatment of such, alters the gut flora, leading to a pathological imbalance between microbes and immune phenotype, which in turn affects the risk of developing AS [16]. In our stratified analysis, the association with appendicitis was stronger in the age group 0–12 years, which may suggest that the possible biological or immunological impact of the inflammation is of greater importance if occurring early in life.

Limitations

First, there may be an issue of reverse causality since the time point of disease onset for AS cannot be precisely determined from the healthcare registers used. We performed one sensitivity analysis in order to further separate the time period for exposures to infections from the time point of disease onset which resulted in similar point estimates, supporting the temporal order of the infections occurring prior to the AS onset. However, this temporal separation of exposures and disease onset also precludes the possibility of detecting any association between infections and AS onset that are close in time, as in the case of reactive arthritis. Second, we only have reliable data for infections diagnosed in inpatient care, reflecting more severe infections. This will underestimate the frequency of infections (e.g. enteric, respiratory, or urogenital) which are normally treated in outpatient care or not treated at all, and it cannot be assumed that the "tip of the iceberg" spectrum of infections that we detect are representative of all childhood infections. By contrast, appendicitis is routinely treated in inpatient care; hence, this result is unlikely to be biased by any selection with regard to exposure.

Strengths

First, this is the first study directly investigating the relationship between infections during childhood and later development of AS. Second, the high coverage of the national registers minimises selection bias, and our previous validation study of the AS diagnoses in the register support the validity and generalisability of the results [21, 25].

Conclusions and implications

Appendicitis during childhood was associated with a decreased risk for adult AS, whereas respiratory tract infections were associated with an increased risk. Further studies are required to determine if these associations are a result of the immune phenotype leading to AS, or whether the infections in fact alter the risk for AS. Such studies would preferably take into account HLA-B27 status, but also other risk genes and wider range of infectious exposures, not limiting the latter to infections at hospitalisation.

Abbreviations

AS: Ankylosing spondylitis; ATC: Anatomical therapeutic chemical; CI: Confidence interval; HLA-B27: Human leukocyte antigen 27; IBD: Inflammatory bowel disease; ICD: International Classification of Diseases; OR: Odds ratio; SpA: Spondyloarthritis; SRQ: Swedish Rheumatology Quality Register; TNFi: Tumour necrosis factor alpha inhibitors

Funding

Funding for the study was received from the following sources, which did not influence either the design of the study, the collection and analysis of the data, or the preparation of the manuscript: the Swedish Research Council, the Region Västra Götaland (ALF), the Stockholm County Council (ALF), the Swedish National Rheumatism Association, and the Swedish Foundation for Strategic Research. All authors state their complete independence from the funders with regard to this study.

Authors' contributions

All authors have contributed substantially in the process of completing this study and have had full access to the data. LJ and JA participated in the conception of the study. LJ, JA, HFd'E, MD, EL, UL, and SE participated in interpretation of data, and drafting and revising the manuscript. UL and LJ performed the analyses and aggregation of data. All authors read and approved the final manuscript.

Competing interests

EL has received personal fees from AbbVie, Bristol-Myers Squibb, Hospira, Pfizer, and UCB (outside the submitted work). JA and the ARTIS Study Group have or have had agreements with AstraZeneca, Pfizer, UCB, Roche, Merck, BMS, and Abbvie (outside the submitted work). UL, SE, MD, HFd'E, and LJ declare that they have no competing interests.

Author details

[1]Department of Rheumatology and Inflammation Research, Institute of Medicine, Sahlgrenska Academy, University of Gothenburg, Guldhedsgatan 10A, 405 30 Gothenburg, Sweden. [2]Section of Rheumatology, Department of Clinical Sciences, Lund University, 221 85 Lund, Sweden. [3]Diakonhjemmet Hospital, P.O. Box 23 Vinderen, 0319 Oslo, Norway. [4]Institution of Public Health and Clinical Medicine/Rheumatology, Umeå University, 901 87 Umeå, Sweden. [5]Rheumatology Unit & Clinical Epidemiology Unit, Department of Medicine Solna, Karolinska Institutet, Solna 171 76, Stockholm, Sweden.

References

1. Brown MA, Kenna T, Wordsworth BP. Genetics of ankylosing spondylitis—insights into pathogenesis. Nat Rev Rheumatol. 2015;12:81–91.
2. Brown MA, Kennedy LG, MacGregor AJ, Darke C, Duncan E, Shatford JL, et al. Susceptibility to ankylosing spondylitis in twins: the role of genes, HLA, and the environment. Arthritis Rheum. 1997;4010:1823–8.
3. Pedersen OB, Svendsen AJ, Ejstrup L, Skytthe A, Harris JR, Junker P. Ankylosing spondylitis in Danish and Norwegian twins: occurrence and the relative importance of genetic vs. environmental effectors in disease causation. Scand J Rheumatol. 2008;372:120–6.
4. Lindstrom U, Forsblad-d'Elia H, Askling J, Kristensen LE, Lie E, Exarchou S, et al. Perinatal characteristics, older siblings, and risk of ankylosing spondylitis: a case-control study based on national registers. Arthritis Res Ther. 2016;181:16.
5. Benjamin M, Toumi H, Suzuki D, Redman S, Emery P, McGonagle D. Microdamage and altered vascularity at the enthesis-bone interface provides an anatomic explanation for bone involvement in the HLA-B27-associated spondylarthritides and allied disorders. Arthritis Rheum. 2007;561:224–33.
6. Smith JA. Update on ankylosing spondylitis: current concepts in pathogenesis. Curr Allergy Asthma Rep. 2015;151:489.
7. Videm V, Cortes A, Thomas R, Brown MA. Current smoking is associated with incident ankylosing spondylitis—the HUNT population-based Norwegian health study. J Rheumatol. 2014;4110:2041–8.
8. Uotila T, Antonen J, Laine J, Kujansuu E, Haapala AM, Lumio J, et al. Reactive arthritis in a population exposed to an extensive waterborne gastroenteritis outbreak after sewage contamination in Pirkanmaa, Finland. Scand J Rheumatol. 2011;405:358–62.
9. Carter JD, Hudson AP. The evolving story of Chlamydia-induced reactive arthritis. Curr Opin Rheumatol. 2010;224:424–30.
10. Mackie SL, Keat A. Poststreptococcal reactive arthritis: what is it and how do we know? Rheumatology (Oxford). 2004;438:949–54.
11. Schiellerup P, Krogfelt KA, Locht H. A comparison of self-reported joint symptoms following infection with different enteric pathogens: effect of HLA-B27. J Rheumatol. 2008;353:480–7.
12. Frolkis A, Dieleman LA, Barkema HW, Panaccione R, Ghosh S, Fedorak RN, et al. Environment and the inflammatory bowel diseases. Can J Gastroenterol. 2013; 273:e18–24.

13. Klingberg E, Carlsten H, Hilme E, Hedberg M, Forsblad-d'Elia H. Calprotectin in ankylosing spondylitis—frequently elevated in feces, but normal in serum. Scand J Gastroenterol. 2012;474:435–44.
14. Van Praet L, Van den Bosch FE, Jacques P, Carron P, Jans L, Colman R, et al. Microscopic gut inflammation in axial spondyloarthritis: a multiparametric predictive model. Ann Rheum Dis. 2013;723:414–7.
15. Ciccia F, Guggino G, Rizzo A, Saieva L, Peralta S, Giardina A, et al. Type 3 innate lymphoid cells producing IL-17 and IL-22 are expanded in the gut, in the peripheral blood, synovial fluid and bone marrow of patients with ankylosing spondylitis. Ann Rheum Dis. 2015;749:1739–47.
16. Costello ME, Ciccia F, Willner D, Warrington N, Robinson PC, Gardiner B, et al. Intestinal dysbiosis in ankylosing spondylitis. Arthritis Rheumatol. 2014;67:686–691.
17. Taurog JD, Richardson JA, Croft JT, Simmons WA, Zhou M, Fernandez-Sueiro JL, et al. The germfree state prevents development of gut and joint inflammatory disease in HLA-B27 transgenic rats. J Exp Med. 1994;1806:2359–64.
18. Gudjonsson JE, Thorarinsson AM, Sigurgeirsson B, Kristinsson KG, Valdimarsson H. Streptococcal throat infections and exacerbation of chronic plaque psoriasis: a prospective study. Br J Dermatol. 2003;1493:530–4.
19. Ebringer R, Cooke D, Cawdell DR, Cowling P, Ebringer A. Ankylosing spondylitis: klebsiella and HL-A B27. Rheumatol Rehabil. 1977;163:190–6.
20. Stebbings S, Munro K, Simon MA, Tannock G, Highton J, Harmsen H, et al. Comparison of the faecal microflora of patients with ankylosing spondylitis and controls using molecular methods of analysis. Rheumatology (Oxford). 2002;4112:1395–401.
21. Ludvigsson JF, Andersson E, Ekbom A, Feychting M, Kim JL, Reuterwall C, et al. External review and validation of the Swedish national inpatient register. BMC Public Health. 2011;11:450.
22. Statistiska Centralbyrån (Statistics Sweden). http://www.scb.se/en_/. Accessed Apr 2016.
23. Wettermark B, Hammar N, Fored CM, Leimanis A, Otterblad Olausson P, Bergman U, et al. The new Swedish Prescribed Drug Register—opportunities for pharmacoepidemiological research and experience from the first six months. Pharmacoepidemiol Drug Saf. 2007;167:726–35.
24. Wadstrom H, Eriksson JK, Neovius M, Askling J. How good is the coverage and how accurate are exposure data in the Swedish Biologics Register (ARTIS)? Scand J Rheumatol. 2015;441:22–8.
25. Lindstrom U, Exarchou S, Sigurdardottir V, Sundstrom B, Askling J, Eriksson JK, et al. Validity of ankylosing spondylitis and undifferentiated spondyloarthritis diagnoses in the Swedish National Patient Register. Scand J Rheumatol. 2015;44:1–8.
26. Andersson RE, Olaison G, Tysk C, Ekbom A. Appendectomy and protection against ulcerative colitis. N Engl J Med. 2001;34411:808–14.
27. Frisch M, Pedersen BV, Andersson RE. Appendicitis, mesenteric lymphadenitis, and subsequent risk of ulcerative colitis: cohort studies in Sweden and Denmark. BMJ. 2009;338:b716.
28. Neumann-Haefelin C, McKiernan S, Ward S, Viazov S, Spangenberg HC, Killinger T, et al. Dominant influence of an HLA-B27 restricted CD8+ T cell response in mediating HCV clearance and evolution. Hepatology. 2006;433:563–72.
29. McNeil AJ, Yap PL, Gore SM, Brettle RP, McColl M, Wyld R, et al. Association of HLA types A1-B8-DR3 and B27 with rapid and slow progression of HIV disease. QJM. 1996;893:177–85.
30. Bhangu A, Soreide K, Di Saverio S, Assarsson JH, Drake FT. Acute appendicitis: modern understanding of pathogenesis, diagnosis, and management. Lancet. 2015;38610000:1278–87.

13

Clinical improvement and reduction in serum calprotectin levels after an intensive exercise programme for patients with ankylosing spondylitis and non-radiographic axial spondyloarthritis

Andrea Levitova[1,2], Hana Hulejova[1], Maja Spiritovic[1,2], Karel Pavelka[1], Ladislav Senolt[1] and Marketa Husakova[1*]

Abstract

Background: The efficacy of exercise therapy for ankylosing spondylitis (AS) is well-documented, but dearth of information is for non-radiographic axial spondyloarthritis (nr-axSpA).
Biomarkers like serum calprotectin, interleukins IL-6, IL-17 and tumour necrosis factor (TNF)-α may reflect the disease activity of axial spondyloarthritis (axSpA). In this study, we investigated clinical and laboratory parameters of both axSpA subgroups in response to intensive physical exercise.

Methods: Altogether, 46 patients with axSpA, characterised according to the Assessment of SpondyloArthritis International Society criteria as having nr-axSpA or AS underwent 6-month exercise programme. Clinical outcomes of disease activity, Bath AS Disease Activity Index (BASDAI), AS Disease Activity Index (ASDAS-CRP), mobility, Bath AS Metrology Index (BASMI) and function, Bath AS Functional Index (BASFI) were evaluated at baseline and at the end of the exercise programme. Serum IL-6 and IL-17, TNF-α and calprotectin were measured via ELISA. The clinical and laboratory data of 29 control axSpA patients were used for the evaluation of the results.

Results: In all axSpA patients, the ASDAS-CRP (2.10 ± 0.12 to 1.84 ± 0.11, p <0.01) and BASMI (1.28 ± 0.14 to 0.66 ± 0.84, p <0.0001) improved after 6 months of exercise therapy. There was a significant improvement in the ASDAS-CRP in the nr-axSpA subgroup (2.01 ± 0.19 to 1.73 ± 0.16, p <0.05) and in the BASMI in both, the nr-axSpA and the AS subgroups (1.09 ± 0.12 to 0.47 ± 0.08, p <0.0001 and 1.43 ± 0.24 to 0.82 ± 0.23, p <0.0001, respectively). Both, ASDAS-CRP and BASDAI, were significantly improved in the exercise axSpA group compared to the control axSpA group (mean -0.26 vs. -0.13 and -0.49 vs. 0.12, respectively, all p <0.05). Only calprotectin was significantly reduced after the exercise programme in nr-axSpA and AS patients (from 2379.0 ± 243.20 to 1779.0 ± 138.30 µg/mL and from 2430.0 ± 269.70 to 1816.0 ± 148.20 µg/mL, respectively, all p <0.01). The change in calprotectin was more profound in the axSpA intervention group (mean -604.56) than in the control axSpA (mean -149.28, p <0.05).

Conclusion: This study demonstrated similar efficacy for an intensive exercise programme in both nr-axSpA and AS patients. A significant decrease in serum calprotectin levels in both subgroups of axSpA patients after the exercise programme reflected an improvement in the disease activity and spinal mobility.

Keywords: Axial spondyloarthritis, Non-radiographic, Ankylosing spondylitis, Exercise programme, Disease activity, Calprotectin

* Correspondence: fojtikova05@gmail.com
[1]Department of Rheumatology, First Faculty of Medicine, Charles University and Rheumatology Institute, Prague, Czech Republic
Full list of author information is available at the end of the article

Background

Axial spondyloarthritis (axSpA) is thought to consist of two subtypes of one disease that share similar features, such as inflammatory back pain, peripheral arthritis, enthesitis, dactylitis, various extraarticular manifestations and a genetic background, which is evident in a common family history and HLA B27 positivity. The hallmarks of axSpA in particular are inflammation in the sacroiliac joints (SIJ) and in the tendons of the axial skeleton [1, 2].

The radiographic axSpA variant ankylosing spondylitis (AS) has been well-characterised by the modified New York criteria, which include evidence of typical bone changes on conventional radiographs of the SIJ [1]. The non-radiographic subgroup, nr-axSpA, on the other hand, can manifest as a spectrum of spondyloarthritic signs together with either human leukocyte antigen (HLA)-B27 positivity or inflammation of the SIJ, which can be detected by magnetic resonance imaging (MRI) but not by conventional radiography [2]. Although distinct differences, such as female-to-male ratio, impaired function, mobility and levels of C-reactive protein (CRP) distinguish AS from nr-axSpA, an analogous disease course and clinical activity are common to both subgroups, and nr-axSpA is considered to be an earlier stage of AS [3]. Similarly, an identical management approach to both subgroups of axSpA is proposed in the guidelines of the Assessment of SpondyloArthritis International Society (ASAS) [4].

Reduced disease activity and improved quality of life are the main treatment goals for patients with axSpA. Pharmacological agents, including non-steroidal anti-inflammatory drugs (NSAIDs) and tumour necrosis factor (TNF)-α inhibitors (TNFi), are efficacious in a majority of patients even though the effect of current treatment on structural progression remains unclear [5]. A combination of both pharmacological and non-pharmacological interventions such as physiotherapy and education, however, appears to be more effective in controlling the disease activity [6, 7] and periodic exercise ameliorates the effect of long-term AS on disability and deformity [8]. Current recommendations for AS exercise therapy focus not only on the modification of AS musculoskeletal sequelae but also on the secondary consequences of AS such as balance disturbances and cardiorespiratory abnormalities [7]. However, the efficacy of exercise therapy per se in patients with nr-axSpA has not yet been elucidated.

Disease activity and severity of axSpA are well-documented in a number of established indices, but only the AS Disease Activity Score (ASDAS) reflects inflammatory activity with entry values of CRP and patient-reported valuations [9]. Although increased CRP alone is not a specific condition of high AS disease activity and has only been found to be common in 40–50% of patients [10], they serve as a biomarker for the evaluation of inflammation in daily practice. Several other biomarkers, cytokines in particular, are purported to have a connection to disease activity and severity. Interleukins such as IL-6 and IL-17 and TNF-α are presumed to play an important role in axSpA pathogenesis due to the initiation and maintenance of inflammation [11–13]. In addition to the overproduction of IL-6 and TNF-α in SIJ tissues [11, 12], patients with greater disease activity were also found to have elevated circulating levels of IL-6, IL-17 and TNF-α [14, 15]. Similarly, calprotectin (S100A8/S100A9 heterodimer) is mainly produced by monocytes that infiltrate the inflamed synovium during spondyloarthritis [16], and elevated systemic levels reflect global autoimmune inflammation [17].

In this study, we carried out a 6-month exercise and education programme for patients who were suffering from both nr-axSpA and AS. We investigated the impact of intensive physical training on disease activity in the whole group and, in particular, on differences between the two defined subgroups. Variations in biomarker serum levels as affected by exercise were also evaluated.

Methods

Patients

AxSpA with exercise programme

A total of 46 patients with axSpA who were attending the Institute of Rheumatology in Prague were included in this study. All of the patients fulfilled the ASAS classification criteria for axSpA [2] and according to these criteria were characterised as having nr-axSpA (n = 23) or AS (n = 23). Patients in the nr-axSpA group had clinical signs and symptoms of SpA and were either positive for the HLA-B27 antigen and/or had inflammatory changes in the SIJ on MRI (73.9%) but no changes on radiography. All of the AS patients fulfilled the modified New York criteria for the diagnosis of AS, including the radiographic criterion [1]. Eight patients with AS with a longer disease duration (14.76 ± 2.17 and 9.50 ± 2.98 years since the first symptoms and diagnosis, respectively) had spinal involvement (25%), and fifteen patients with AS with shorter disease duration (11.93 ± 1.80 and 5.30 ± 1.26 years since the first symptoms and diagnosis, respectively) only had SIJ involvement. All of the patients with axSpA were fully or partially employed, mostly (95.7% of both nr-axSpA and AS) as "white-collar" workers [18]. The inclusion criteria for the study were stable disease and treatment for at least 6 months prior to baseline. During the entire study, transient changes in the dose of NSAIDs were allowed. Patients must not have received oral or intraarticular glucocorticoids during the study.

Control group - patients with axSpA with no intervention

The control group consisted of 29 age-matched and sex-matched patients with axSpA. Out of the control group,

15 subjects had nr-axSpA. All of the patients from the control group were selected retrospectively from the axSpA cohort in Prague, and the following parameters were required: dates of two medical examinations (marked as visits 1 and 2) that occurred concurrently with the ongoing study, stable disease activity and treatment for at least 6 weeks prior to visit 1, and no changes in pharmacological or other therapy between visits 1 and 2. In particular, subjects from the control group must not have undergone physical therapy, physical exercise or spa treatment for at least 6 weeks prior to baseline and between the two consecutive visits. Daily home exercise without any supervision and mobilisation techniques or massage was allowed. All of the control patients with axSpA were fully or partially employed, and the percentages of white-collar workers [18] were 93.4% for nr-axSpA and 85.7% for AS (not significantly different from groups with exercise).

Intervention

This was a 6-month single-centre study that started in September 2013. All of the subjects from the intervention group underwent outpatient group physiotherapy for 60 minutes twice a week and a daily home-based exercise programme. The absence of more than two consecutive sessions of outpatient physiotherapy excluded patients from further participation in the study. The supervised exercise unit was made up of three sections: warm-up at the beginning, the main part and cool-down at the end. During the warm-up, cardiorespiratory fitness methods were used. These methods focused on concentration, core strengthening and spinal traction. The following exercises were employed: spinal (rotatory) exercises developed by Cumpelik [19], an educational back school method [20] and McKenzie therapy [21], posture correction according to the Brügger concept [22], elements derived from pilates [23] and muscle stretching. The major part was dedicated to the practice of correct activation of deep core stabilisation and the precise involvement of muscles in motion and balance training, particularly using BOSU balls, which are an established method for the encouragement of abdominal muscle activity [24] as a tool for stretching, lumbar strengthening and hip-joint mobility [25]. The final part (cool-down) consisted of techniques of relaxation, breathing exercises and elements of yoga. Additionally, physiotherapy education for homework - practical training in postural correction exercises and motivation to change the daily routine was used at the end of the exercise unit.

Outcome measurements

Clinical

The clinical examination of signs of axSpA, including extraarticular manifestation, was carried out in all patients before and a few days (maximum 7 days) after the exercise programme termination. The measurement tools for disease activity and severity evaluation were the Bath AS Disease Activity Index (BASDAI) [26], Bath AS Functional Index (BASFI) [27], the 10 point Bath AS Metrology Index (BASMI) [28] and the AS Disease Activity Index (ASDAS)-CRP [9]. BASMI was rated by the same physiotherapist at the beginning and at the end of the exercise programme. In the control axSpA group, in which no intervention was performed, the disease activity was assessed using the BASDAI, BASFI and ASDAS-CRP in two consecutive visits after 6 months. The BASMI, however, was not available for this analysis.

Biomarkers

In the intervention group, serum sampling was carried out at baseline and at the end of the study on the same date as the clinical evaluation. Fasting blood samples were immediately centrifuged and stored at -80 °C and were removed before analysis, which was carried out on all intervention group samples simultaneously. In the axSpA control group, blood was withdrawn at each visit, and the samples were treated as above. CRP was measured with the immuno-turbidimetric test using a biochemical analyser (Olympus, model AU 400 Japan). IL-6, IL-17, TNF-α (RayBiotech, Inc., Norcross GA, USA) and calprotectin (Bühlmann Laboratories AG, Schőnenbuch, Switzerland) were analysed using a commercially available enzyme-linked immunosorbent assay (ELISA) according to the manufacturer`s protocols. All of the assays were run in duplicate. The inter-assay and intra-assay reliability of the IL-6 and IL-17 and TNF-α assays was <12% and <10%, respectively, and the inter-assay and intra-assay reliability of calprotectin was 5.8% and 4.3%, respectively. Absorbance was detected using the Sunrise ELISA reader (Tecan Group Ltd., Salzburg, Austria) with 450 nm as the primary wavelength. The sensitivity for IL-6, IL-17, TNF-α and calprotectin was determined to be 3 pg/mL, 80 pg/mL, 30 pg/mLl and 0.4 μg/mL, respectively.

Statistical analysis

The data are expressed as the means ± standard deviations. Qualitative variables were tested using the chi-squared or Fisher's exact test. Biomarker data were evaluated using the Friedman test. The variables at baseline and at the end of the exercise programme were analysed using the non-parametric Wilcoxon paired test. The differences between groups were analysed using the non-parametric unpaired test and the Mann-Whitney U test. Multiple comparisons were corrected using Monte Carlo exact significance testing. Ordinary least squares (OLS) regression models were used for predictive analysis. The Spearman correlation coefficient was used for correlation analysis. P values less than 0.05 were considered statistically significant. The SPSS (version 22) and GraphPad Prism 7 programmes were used for all analyses.

Results

Clinical characteristics of the cohort

A total of 40 patients with nr-axSpA (n = 18) or AS (n = 22) completed the exercise and educational programme. Six patients were excluded for the following reasons: current inflammatory bowel disease (IBD) in the nr-axSpA group, exacerbation of peripheral arthritis requiring a change in long-term therapy (AS group), and four patients who missed two or more consecutive sessions were also excluded (nr-axSpA group). At baseline, spondyloarthritic signs (HLA B27 positivity, extraarticular manifestation, hip involvement) and treatment were represented equally in both groups, and there was no significant difference in age, body mass index (BMI) or smoking history. Patients characterised as nr-axSpA, however, had significantly shorter disease duration since the occurrence of first symptoms and diagnosis (7.10 ± 2.19 versus 12.27 ± 1.42, p <0.001 and 1.81 ± 0.52 versus 5.84 ± 1.17, respectively, all p <0.05) and a trend of female predominance was observed (Table 1). During the exercise therapy, there were no significant differences in BMI, peripheral arthritis or the need to change long-term medication in either group. Similarly, the rate of exacerbation of the extraarticular manifestation was equal in the nr-axSpA and AS groups, and no patients developed clinical signs of colitis during the exercise therapy.

Patients in the control axSpA group used sulfasalazine more often than those in the intervention axSpA group (44.8% vs. 10.0%, $p < 0.05$), and more patients with AS in the intervention group had more frequent history of peripheral arthritis, but the exacerbation of peripheral arthritis was not different from the control group during the study (45.5% and 4.5% vs. 7.2% and 0%, $p < 0.05$ and not significant (ns), respectively). None of the patients from the control group had any clinical signs of colitis at baseline or after 6 months (data not shown). There were no significant differences in any other clinical parameters between the two groups (Additional file 1).

The intensive exercise intervention improved disease activity

In all of the patients with axSpA who were undergoing exercise therapy, the ASDAS-CRP score significantly decreased after 6 months of exercise (from 2.10 ± 0.12 to 1.84 ± 0.11, $p < 0.01$). Similarly, the BASMI values were also significantly lower at the end of the training programme compared to baseline (from 1.28 ± 0.14 to 0.66 ± 0.84, $p < 0.0001$) (Table 2). Additionally, there was a trend of a decline in the BASDAI ($p = 0.06$), but not in the BASFI, after 6 months of training (Table 2). The ASDAS-CRP score consists of four self-assessment questions, while the BASDAI score only reflects the patients' outcome reports. In further analyses, we focused on changes in patients' reports. For the ASDAS-CRP score, the following assessments decreased significantly: back pain (from 4.10 ± 0.34 to 2.97 ± 0.42, $p < 0.001$) and

Table 1 Demographic and clinical characteristics of patients with axSpA participating in exercise therapy

	All (n = 40)	AS (n = 22)	nr-axSpA (n = 18)	P value
Age, years	36.78 ± 1.09	36.91 ± 1.16	36.61 ± 2.03	ns
Gender (% female)	32.5	18.2	50.0	0.05
BMI at baseline	25.25 ± 0.44	25.51 ± 0.76	25.02 ± 0.50	ns
Disease duration since first symptoms (years)	9.94 ± 1.31	12.27 ± 1.42	7.10 ± 2.19	<0.001
Disease duration since diagnosis (years)	4.03 ± 0.75	5.84 ± 1.17	1.81 ± 0.52	<0.01
HLA-B27 positivity (%)	90.0	90.9	88.8	ns
History of uveitis/exacerbation (%)[a]	35.0/7.5	27.7/9.1	44.4/5.5	ns
History of peripheral arthritis/exacerbation (%)[a]	42.5/2.5	45.5/4.5	38.9/0	ns
Hip involvement (%)	17.5%	22.7%	11.1%	ns
Therapy - NSA (daily use/on demand) (%)	100 (27.5/72.5)	100 (18.2/81.8)	100 (38.9/61.1)	ns
NSA changes during exercise therapy/changes to daily use (%)	7.5/2.5	0/0	16.7/5.5	ns
Therapy - sulfasalazin (%)	10.0	4.5	16.6	ns
Therapy – biological agents (%)[b]	5.0	9.0	0	ns
Smokers ever/current	25.0/20.0	31.8/27.3	22.2/16.7	ns

[a]Exacerbations of uveitis/arthritis occurred during exercise intervention. No extraarticular signs other than uveitis were manifested. [b]Only tumour necrosis factor alpha inhibitors (TNFi) were used in long-term therapy for high disease activity. Statistical analysis: p value was calculated for comparison between the ankylosing spondylitis (AS) and the axial non-radiographic spondyloarthritis (nr-axSpA) group using either the Mann-Whitney test or chi-squared/Fisher's exact test. Data are characterised as mean ± standard deviation unless stated otherwise. *axSpA* axial spondyloarthritis, *BMI* body mass index, *NSA* non-steroidal antirheumatic drugs, *ns* not significant

Table 2 Clinical parameters and biomarker levels of axSpA at baseline and after 6 months of exercise therapy

	All axSpA (n = 40)			nr-axSpA (n = 18)			AS (n = 22)		
	Baseline	6 months	*P* value	Baseline	6 months	*P* value	Baseline	6 months	*P* value
ASDAS-CRP	2.10 ± 0.12	1.84 ± 0.11	<0.01	2.01 ± 0.19	1.73 ± 0.16	<0.05	2.17 ± 0.16	1.93 ± 0.15	ns
BASDAI	2.78 ± 0.31	2.30 ± 0.25	ns	2.98 ± 0.28	2.27 ± 0.41	ns	2.63 ± 0.35	2.31 ± 0.32	ns
BASFI	1.06 ± 0.16	1.01 ± 0.14	ns	1.23 ± 0.28	1.73 ± 0.16	ns	0.92 ± 0.17	0.93 ± 0.18	ns
BASMI	1.28 ± 0.14	0.66 ± 0.84	<0.0001	1.09 ± 0.12	0.47 ± 0.08	<0.0001	1.43 ± 0.24	0.82 ± 0.23	<0.0001
CRP (mg/l)	4.67 ± 0.89	3.86 ± 0.82	ns	2.10 ± 0.48	2.16 ± 0.56	ns	6.76 ± 1.45	5.24 ± 1.37	ns
IL-6 (pg/ml)	10.31 ± 3.93	10.07 ± 4.60	ns	14.78 ± 8.35	15.40 ± 9.79	ns	6.48 ± 1.46	5.51 ± 1.63	ns
IL-17 (pg/ml)	323.50 ± 57.06	401.50 ± 75.87	ns	349.20 ± 82.55	285.30 ± 72.73	ns	301.80 ± 80.57	499.30 ± 123.10	ns
TNF-α (pg/ml)	65.22 ± 12.30	56.89 ± 10.61	ns	55.87 ± 10.49	45.03 ± 6.76	ns	72.49 ± 20.45	62.12 ± 18.06	ns
Calprotectin (ng/ml)	2408.0 ± 183.30	1800.0 ± 101.90	<0.001	2379.0 ± 243.20	1779.0 ± 138.30	<0.01	2430.0 ± 269.70	1816.0 ± 148.20	<0.01

The statistical significance was determined as a *p* value < 0.05; the paired non parametric test (Wilcoxon) was used for analysis of baseline versus 6 month data for each group. All data are characterised as mean ± standard deviation. *axSpA* axial spondyloarthritis, *nr-axSpA* non-radiographic axial spondyloarthritis, *AS* ankylosing spondylitis, *ASDAS-CRP* AS disease activity score, *CRP* C-reactive protein, *BASDAI* Bath AS disease activity index, *BASFI* Bath AS functional index, *BASMI* Bath AS metrology index, *IL* interleukin, *TNF* tumour necrosis factor, *ns* not significant

patients global (from 3.70 ± 0.36 to 2.50 ± 0.42, $p < 0.05$). Only the responses to the first two BASDAI questions improved in patients with axSpA after the exercise intervention (from 37.90 ± 3.50 and 35.70 ± 4.21 to 28.10 ± 3.35 and 25.80 ± 3.15, respectively, $p < 0.05$ for both comparisons).

The measures of disease activity and severity (ASDAS-CRP, BASDAI, BASFI and BASMI) did not differ between groups at baseline or after 6 months of intervention. When all of the patients from the intervention cohort were divided into non radiographic and radiographic subgroups, the ASDAS-CRP decreased significantly in the nr-axSpA subgroup (from 2.01 ± 0.19 to 1.73 ± 0.16, $p < 0.05$) and non-significantly in the AS subgroup (from 2.17 ± 0.16 to 1.93 ± 0.15, p = 0.06). The BASMI score decreased after the intervention in both the nr-axSpA and AS subgroups (from 1.09 ± 0.12 to 0.47 ± 0.08 and from 1.43 ± 0.24 to 0.82 ± 0.23, respectively, $p < 0.0001$ for both comparisons) (Table 2). There were no significant differences between the two subgroups in the changes in ASDAS-CRP, BASDAI or BASMI over the exercise training (data not shown).

In the whole control group of patients with axSpA and both the nr-axSpA and AS subgroups without physical intervention, there were no significant changes in the ASDAS-CRP, BASDAI or BASFI scores between the two 6-month visits. The criterion "no change of therapy" was required to be included in this group, and this group served as a control group with stable disease. When we compared all three scores at visit 2 to the values of the BASDAI, BASFI and ASDAS-CRP of axSpA after physical intervention, no significant differences were found (see Additional file 1). However, when we looked for the ΔASDAS-CRP and ΔBASDAI, we found a significant decrease in both parameters in the axSpA exercise group (-0.26 and -0.49, respectively) compared to axSpA with no intervention (-0.13 and 0.12, respectively), both $p < 0.05$ (Table 3).

Calprotectin levels significantly decreased after exercise therapy in patients with axSpA

Overall, in the axSpA group, there was a significant difference ($p < 0.001$, Friedman test) in all biomarkers (CRP, IL-6, IL-17, TNF-α and calprotectin) at baseline and after 6 months of exercise therapy. However, of the biomarkers, only calprotectin significantly decreased in patients with axSpA during the study (from 2408.00 ± 183.30 to 1800.00 ± 101.90 μg/mL, $p < 0.001$) (Table 2).

There was a significant difference in CRP levels between the nr-axSpA and AS subgroups at baseline (2.10 ± 0.48 and 6.76 ± 1.45 mg/l, $p < 0.001$) and after the intervention (2.16 ± 0.56 and 5.24 ± 1.37 mg/l, $p < 0.05$), but the other biomarkers were comparable between both subgroups. On the other hand, CRP remained unchanged throughout the study, and only calprotectin significantly decreased after exercise therapy in both patients with nr-axSpA (from 2379.0 ± 243.20 to 1779.0 ± 138.3 μg/mL, p < 0.01) and in pPatients with AS (from 2430.0 ± 269.7 to 1816.0 ± 148.2 μg/mL, $p < 0.01$) (Table 2).

To exclude variation in calprotectin levels over time, an analysis of calprotectin levels in the control axSpA group with no intervention was performed.

Baseline calprotectin levels in the control axSpA (2749.0 ± 225.8), nr-axSpA (2514.0 ± 303.1) and AS (3001.0 ± 334.8) groups were similar to the intervention group and remained unchanged after 6 months in all axSpA (2579.0 ± 267.9), nr-axSpA (2324.0 ± 381.8) and AS (2852.0 ± 375.2) groups (data not shown). When the calprotectin levels at visit 2 in the control axSpA group were compared to the calprotectin levels in the axSpA group after the intervention (see previous), the

Table 3 Comparison of the changes in disease activity scores and biomarkers levels within 6 months in the axSpA groups with and without exercise intervention

	All axSpA			nr-axSpA			AS		
	Exercise group (n = 40)	Without exercise (n = 29)	*P* value	Exercise group (n = 18)	Without exercise (n = 15)	*P* value	Exercise group (n = 22)	Without exercise (n = 14)	*P* value
Δ ASDAS-CRP	*-0.26* (0.58)	-0.13 (0.77)	<0.05	*-0.29* (0.44)	*0.03* (0.84)	ns	*-0.24* (0.68)	*-0.13* (0.72)	ns
Δ BASDAI	*-0.49* (1.40)	*0.12* (1.40)	<0.05	*-0.70* (1.48)	*0.42* (1.22)	ns	*-0.32* (1.34)	*0.12* (1.22)	ns
Δ CRP	*-0.81* (4.67)	*-0.33* (9.70)	ns	*0.06* (1.94)	*1.94* (12.20)	ns	*-1.52* (6.02)	*-2.76* (5.49)	ns
Δ Calprotectin	*-604.56* (1042.80)	*-149.28* (1255.70)	<0.05	*-5[illegible]9.42* (824.00)	*-190.33* (1180.60)	ns	*-608.68* (1211.20)	*-149.28* (1255.70)	ns

Statistical analysis: the comparison of the mean of changes in all parameters was performed using the non-parametric Mann-Whitney *U* test. The multiple comparisons were corrected using Monte Carlo exact significance testing. All data are characterised as mean and (standard deviation). *axSpA* axial spondyloarthritis, *nr-axSpA* non-radiographic axial spondyloarthritis, *AS* ankylosing spondylitis, *ASDAS-CRP* AS disease activity score, *CRP* C-reactive protein, *BASDAI* Bath AS disease activity index, Δ changes in the scores/biomarkers values, *ns* not significant calprotectin levels were lower in all intervention groups (axSpA, nr-axSpA and AS, $p < 0.05$, ns and $p < 0.05$, respectively). The changes in calprotectin levels were significantly and consistently lower in the axSpA exercise group than the axSpA control (mean -604.56 vs. mean -149.28, $p < 0.05$), see Table 3.

Next, we studied whether improvements in disease activity and severity measures (ΔASDAS-CRP, ΔBASDAI, ΔBASFI and ΔCRP) were associated with changes in calprotectin levels over time. Using linear regression analysis, we found a positive association between changes in CRP and calprotectin over 6 months. Change in CRP of one unit resulted in an increase in calprotectin of 68 units (regression coefficient 67.99, $p < 0.01$) (Additional file 2). This effect was found in all groups independent of exercise intervention or subgroup characterisation. Moreover, in all patients with axSpA irrespective of exercise therapy, changes in calprotectin positively correlated with the changes in CRP ($\rho = 0.360$, $p < 0.01$) and ASDAS-CRP improvement ($\rho = 0.285$, $p < 0.05$) (data not shown).

The other biomarkers modestly reflected changes in scores for disease activity and mobility after exercise therapy

In all axSpA groups and in both the nr-axSpA and AS subgroups, we found positive correlation between ΔASDAS-CRP and ΔCRP (Table 4). Of the other cytokines, only ΔTNF-α positively reflected improvement in the clinical variables of ASDAS-CRP and BASMI, particularly in the nr-axSpA group (Table 4). This finding was supported by the linear regression model, in which only the effect of ΔTNF-α on the ΔASDAS-CRP and ΔBASMI was demonstrated in the nr-axSpA (regression coefficient 0.010 and 0.004, respectively, all $p < 0.05$, data not shown). On the other hand, there were no relationships between the selected biomarkers and ΔBASDAI (data not shown).

Discussion

This study demonstrates for the first time the clinical effectiveness of intensive exercise therapy for both radiographic and non-radiographic forms of axSpA. Although the outcomes may be affected by several limitations, we suggest that there was a positive effect on mobility and clinical activity. In addition, it appears that the reduction in serum calprotectin might be related to the improved clinical outcome in patients with axSpA.

The recent recommendations of rehabilitation for patients with axSpA suggest that complex physical activities may be used to maintain good clinical status [7]. The general endocrine, immune and metabolic changes that occur during physical activities might, however, be stressful, and the effects of exercise on patients with early stages of axSpA have not yet been examined. In this study, during the exercise intervention, disease activity, as measured by the ASDAS-CRP and BASDAI, significantly improved over time in subgroups of patients with both radiographic and non-radiographic axSpA, which is in agreement with previous studies that have demonstrated improved disease activity after exercise in patients with AS [6, 23, 29–31]. Moreover, there was no difference in extraarticular or articular exacerbations in either axSpA subgroup, and our clinical data may support the efficacy and safety of physical therapy not only in patients with AS but also in patients with nr-axSpA.

The first limitation of this study is the relatively small number of patients in each subgroup and the inclusion of patients with stable disease only. However, the small number reflects the real situation that is present in daily clinical practice and the need to adjust the exercise programme for patients with unstable disease as needed. A second limitation might be the occupational history - most of the patients with axSpA who participated in this study were working in white-collar professions. Recently, Ramiro et al. demonstrated greater radiographic progression in "blue-collar" workers within 2 years, and this occupational feature could amplify the effect of ASDAS-CRP on disease progression [32]. In light of this finding, the evaluation of the safety and efficacy of physical therapy in blue-collar workers with axSpA or those who perform additional physical activities such as sport, requires larger future studies. The next limitation may be the absence of imaging of the inflammatory signs in the SIJ prior to and after exercise therapy. Recent data from the DESIR cohort suggest a relationship between inflammation of the SIJ as detected on MRI and the ASDAS score in male patients [33]. Thus, it can be suggested that improvement in clinical disease activity after exercise therapy can be associated with the amelioration of inflammatory lesions in the SIJ in patients with axSpA. Further studies should be performed to elucidate this hypothesis.

After physical therapy, mobility was improved in both in patients with nr-axSpA and those with AS. However, our axSpA control group was selected retrospectively, and the BASMI data were excluded from the analysis; thus, the change in BASMI cannot be compared. In patients with AS, the efficacy of supervised and home-based exercise on mobility is well-demonstrated [29–31], and a positive effect on BASMI after 24 weeks of an exercise programme has been identified in TNFi-naive patients with AS [34] and in those on TNFi treatment [6, 35]. Our study demonstrated for the first time the same benefit of exercise therapy on spinal mobility in patients with nr-axSpA and patients with AS. Although mobility scores in patients with AS are generally worse than in patients with nr-axSpA [10, 36, 37], given that 10–12% of patients with nr-axSpA progress to develop

Table 4 Correlations between the clinical variables and laboratory markers in axSpA with exercise therapy

		Δ BASMI	Δ ASDAS-CRP	CRP baseline	IL-6 baseline	IL-17 baseline	TNF-α baseline	Δ CRP	Δ IL-6	Δ IL-17	Δ TNF-α
Δ BASMI	ρ	1	0.271	-0.017	0.236	-0.027	-0.311	0.003	-0.058	-0.049	0.417
All (n = 40)	ρ	.	ns	ns	ns	ns	0.09	ns	ns	ns	$p < 0.05$
Δ ASDAS-CRP	ρ	0.271	1	-0.231	0.391	-0.131	-0.02	0.406	-0.205	0.035	0.377
All (n = 40)	ρ	ns	.	ns	p < 0.05	ns	ns	$p < 0.001$	ns	ns	$p < 0.05$
Δ BASMI	ρ	1	0.774	-0.596	0.441	-0.230	-0.477	-0.098	-0.213	0.010	0.563
nr-axSpA (n = 18)	ρ	.	$p < 0.001$	$p < 0.01$	ns	ns	ns	ns	ns	ns	$p < 0.05$
Δ ASDAS-CRP	ρ	0.774	1	-0.187	0.388	0.028	-0.351	0.437	-0.249	-0.074	0.636
nr-axSpA (n = 18)	ρ	p < 0.001	.	ns	ns	ns	ns	$p < 0.05$	ns	ns	$p < 0.05$
Δ BASMI	ρ	1	0.007	0.233	0.099	0.217	-0.143	0.123	0.158	-0.110	0.273
AS (n = 22)	ρ	.	ns	ns	ns	ns	ns	ns	ns	ns	ns
Δ ASDAS-CRP	ρ	0.007	1	-0.328	0.356	-0.266	0.102	0.395	-0.147	0.154	0.186
AS (n = 22)	ρ	ns	.	ns	ns	ns	ns	$p < 0.05$	ns	ns	ns

Statistical analysis: correlation analyses were performed by Spearman correlation (ρ). Statistical significance was determined as $p < 0.05$. *axSpA* axial spondyloarthritis, *nr-axSpA* non-radiographic axial spondyloarthritis, *AS* ankylosing spondylitis, *ASDAS-CRP* AS disease activity score, *BASMI* Bath AS metrology index, *CRP* C-reactive protein, *IL* interleukin, *TNF* tumour necrosis factor, Δ changes of the scores/biomarkers values, *ns* not significant the form of the disease that is radiographically evident [10, 38], it seems appropriate to maintain mobility in the best form possible. In our group, the BASMI scores were similar in both groups at baseline and after exercise therapy - this distinction could be confirmed by a lower BASMI value in patients with AS (1.46 at baseline) compared to registries (2.84 and 2.0) [10, 36] and was probably due to the characterisation of patients with AS who were motivated by the training programme. However, there was no follow up after the end of the exercise programme, and thus, we were unable to demonstrate any long-term positive effects on the BASMI in the nr-axSpA or AS cohorts. Therefore, studies with longer follow-up periods are required in further research.

Increased serum calprotectin has been demonstrated in patients with other immune-mediated diseases, such as rheumatoid arthritis (RA) or psoriatic arthritis [39, 40], and in patients with AS [17, 41, 42] and nr-axSpA [41]. Serum calprotectin in patients with AS appears not to be influenced by medications such as NSAIDs or sulphasalazine [41, 43] and tends to be elevated in patients with AS with active peripheral arthritis [42]. In our study, baseline serum calprotectin was similar in patients with AS who were or were not on the exercise programme, although patients with AS who were not receivingexercise therapy had a more frequent history of peripheral arthritis.

To the best of our knowledge, we are the first to show a significant decrease in serum calprotectin after intensive physiotherapy in both nr-axSpA and patients with AS. As we have not studied the effect of this exercise programme on serum calprotectin in healthy individuals, we cannot be sure if this is a disease-specific effect or if the same might also occur in healthy subjects. Although skeletal muscles express calprotectin mRNA after contractions [44] and calprotectin plasma levels increase immediately and one hour after aerobic exercise in healthy individuals [45], there is no long-term effect of muscle contraction on systemic calprotectin. Kanda et al. performed a study in nine healthy volunteers who performed one-leg calf-raise exercises that included repetitive muscle contractions and found no significant differences in plasma or urine levels of IL-6, TNF-α and calprotectin immediately after and 96 hours after the exercise [46]. Similarly, Acar et al. recently found only a slight decrease in calprotectin levels in healthy subjects 8 weeks after they completed an exercise programme [47]. In agreement with our study, in patients with RA, the calprotectin levels decreased significantly and reflected improved disease activity and a decline in CRP [47].

In our study, the decrease in serum calprotectin levels was evident in both axSpA subgroups compared to control subjects with axSpA who underwent no exercise therapy. Interestingly, the synergistic effect of the decline in serum calprotectin and clinical improvement was found in two pharmacological studies in patients with AS, using TNFi (infliximab) [48] and anti-IL-17 (secukinumab) [49] treatments. However, in our study, regression analysis showed only a slight influence of exercise on serum calprotectin in patients with axSpA. This finding might be due to the small sample size. The regression analysis, on the other hand, supports the relationships between serum CRP and calprotectin, and those between ASDAS-CRP improvement and changes in calprotectin. Out of many biomarkers, serum calprotectin might represent a valuable tool for the assessment of disease activity improvement in patients with axSpA. In agreement with Turina et al. [48], our data also suggest that serum calprotectin may be a useful biomarker that reflects clinical improvement even in CRP-negative patients.

Calprotectin likely plays a role in axSpA pathogenesis and in the disease course. De Rycke et al. demonstrated 10-fold higher calprotectin in inflamed synovium than in serum [16]. Furthermore, the number of synovial monocytes and granulocytes that release calprotectin rapidly decreases after TNFi treatment in patients with peripheral SpA [50]. Recent data from the GESPIC cohort indicate that elevated serum calprotectin is an independent predictor of disease progression and syndesmophyte formation [51]. The precise immune mechanisms that occur in the inflamed joints during exercise are still unclear, but pharmacological studies suggest that decreased calprotectin serum levels might reflect local inflammation and possibly new bone formation [48–50]. However, larger studies based on registries and long-term observations are needed to evaluate the effect of physiotherapy on calprotectin and axSpA outcomes.

A possible limitation of our study is the absence of faecal calprotectin analysis. Faecal calprotectin has been shown to be elevated in patients with AS and SpA [41, 52], especially in patients with intestinal inflammatory changes [41] and in NSAID users [52]. Only 10% of patients with SpA develop IBD during the disease course [53], but 25–69% of patients without clinical IBD symptoms may have microscopic intestinal inflammation [43]. In our study, one patient was excluded due to a diagnosis of IBD, but none of the other participants underwent ileocolonoscopy because of a lack of clinical symptoms. Although the increased CRP and serum calprotectin appear to be predictive markers for intestinal involvement in SpA [41] and faecal calprotectin is a well-known marker of IBD activity [54], there is no correlation between serum and faecal calprotectin [41, 55]. A beneficial effect of mild exercise on the course of IBD has been suggested [56], but the relationship between intestinal inflammation and axSpA disease activity and progression in respect to physical activity requires further research.

Finally, in the evaluation of biomarkers after physical activity, we should bear in mind that exercise is a complex process that may lead to the release of mediators that influence metabolic, immune and neuroendocrine pathways. In relation to strenuous exercise, cytokines such as IL-6, IL-1 receptor antagonist, TNF-α and others are released over time [57] and regulate hormone, adaptive and innate immune cell activity. In the present study, interestingly, the changes in TNF-α correlated positively with the improvement in ASDAS-CRP and with the improvement in the mobility score but only in the nr-axSpA subgroup. There were no significant differences in calprotectin serum levels between patients with AS and those with nr-axSpA. We suggest that patients with axSpA who are in the early phase of the disease might respond to exercise differently from those with long-term disease duration and with different states of inflammation. It is well-known that both patients with nr-axSpA and those with AS respond positively to TNFi treatment [58]. Although the serum levels of TNF-α may not clearly reflect AS disease activity [59], it can be speculated that a decrease in TNF-α levels might serve as a biomarker of milder disease activity. In our study the levels of IL-17 increased, albeit not significantly, in the AS group. In healthy male subjects, physical activity such as high and mild-to-moderate training have not been shown to influence serum IL-17a [60], but another study in duathlon athletes suggests a potential role of the IL-17 axis in muscle damage after prolonged training [61]. On the other hand, women with multiple sclerosis were found to have lower levels of systemic IL-17 and a lower inflammatory status after an 8-week exercise programme [62]. The pivotal role of the IL-17 axis in axSpA pathogenesis has been suggested, and inhibition of IL-17 has recently been demonstrated to be safe and effective for AS treatment [49, 63]. In light of this, the variation in serum IL-17 after exercise therapy in the nr-axSpA and the AS group requires confirmation in further studies.

Conclusion

In conclusion, this is the first study to show that exercise therapy is beneficial for both radiographic and non-radiographic subgroups of axSpA. In addition to better mobility, disease activity improved after an intensive exercise programme. This suggests that exercise should be an essential aspect of the axSpA treatment strategy, particularly in the early phases of the disease. In addition, a decrease in serum calprotectin levels reflected improvement in disease activity in both axSpA subgroups. Larger studies are needed to confirm our results.

Additional files

Additional file 1: Demographic and clinical characteristics of patients with axSpA not on exercise therapy compared to patients with axSpA participating in the exercise intervention. Clinical and demographic data of control patients with axSpA are presented. Comparisons between control nr-axSpA and patients with AS and comparisons between patients with axSpA undergoing exercise therapy to control patients with axSpA with no intervention are included. (PDF 139 kb)

Additional file 2: The dependence of the change in calprotectin levels on the changes in clinical and laboratory parameters. This table presents the regression model of the dependent variable Δcalprotectin and the independent variables of clinical and laboratory parameters. Only ΔCRP significantly influenced Δcalprotectin. (PDF 198 kb)

Abbreviations

AS: ankylosing spondylitis; ASAS: Assessment of SpondyloArthritis International Society; ASDAS: ankylosing spondylitis disease activity score; axSpA: axial spondyloarthritis; BASDAI: Bath Ankylosing Spondylitis Disease Activity Index; BASFI: Bath Ankylosing Spondylitis Functional Index; BASMI: Bath Ankylosing Spondylitis Metrology Index; BMI: body mass index; CRP: C-reactive protein; ELISA: enzyme-linked immunosorbent assay; IBD: inflammatory bowel disease; IL: interleukin; MRI: magnetic resonance imaging; nr-axSpA: non-radiographic axial spondyloarthritis; ns: not significant; NSAIDs: non-steroidal anti-inflammatory drugs; SIJ: sacroiliac joints; TNFi: tumour necrosis factor (TNF)-α inhibitors; TNF-α: tumour necrosis factor-α

Acknowledgements

The authors would like to thank Mrs Jitka Smékalová for technical assistance during the laboratory analyses and Dr Petr Fučík for statistical analysis and consultation.

Funding

This study has been supported by the Project for Conceptual Development for the institution of Ministry of Health Czech Republic - Institute of Rheumatology (number 023728), by SVV for FTVS UK (number 2016-260346), GAUK (number 214615) and PRVOUK (number P38).

Authors' contributions

All of the authors participated in drafting the article or revising it critically for important intellectual content, and all of the authors approved the final version to be published. Study design: AL and MH. Clinical assessments: AL, MS, KP and MH. Exercise therapy: AL and MS. Laboratory analysis: HH. Clinical assessments and database of the control group: MH and KP. Analysis and interpretation of the data: AL, HH, KP, MH and LS.

Competing interests

All authors declare that they have no competing interests.

Ethical approval and consent to participate

Patients with axSpA undergoing the intervention: all patients signed informed consent to participate in whole exercise programme and to provide blood samples for laboratory analysis. The informed consent was approved by the local Ethics Committee of the Institute of Rheumatology, Prague, Czech Republic. The institutional Review Board of Institute of Rheumatology, Prague, Czech Republic, approved the entire study protocol. Patients with axSpA without intervention: all of the patients signed informed consent to be included in the clinical and laboratory database, which uses analyses for scientific purposes. They agreed with the new laboratory analyses of material in the serum bank if required. The informed consent of this project was approved by the local Ethics Committee of the Institute of

Rheumatology, Prague, Czech Republic. The establishment of the clinical and laboratory database was approved by the Institutional Review Board of the Institute of Rheumatology, Prague, Czech Republic. In this manuscript, there are no individual patient data.

Author details

[1]Department of Rheumatology, First Faculty of Medicine, Charles University and Rheumatology Institute, Prague, Czech Republic. [2]Charles University, Faculty of Physical Education and Sport, Prague, Czech Republic.

References

1. Van der Linden S, Valkenburg HA, Cats A. Evaluation of diagnostic criteria for ankylosing spondylitis. A proposal for modification of the New York criteria. Arthritis Rheum. 1984;27:361–8.
2. Sieper J, Rudwaleit M, Baraliakos X, Brandt J, Braun J, Burgos-Vargas R, Dougados M, Hermann KG, Landewé R, Maksymowych W, van der Heijde D. The Assessment of SpondyloArthritis international Society (ASAS) handbook: a guide to assess spondyloarthritis. Ann Rheum Dis. 2009;68:ii1–ii44. doi:10.1136/ard.2008.104018.
3. Baraliakos X, Braun J. Non-radiographic axial spondyloarthritis and ankylosing spondylitis: what are the similarities and differences? RMD Open. 2015;1:e000053. doi:10.1136/rmdopen-2015-000053.
4. Braun J, van den Berg R, Baraliakos X, Boehm H, Burgos-Vargas R, Collantes-Estevez E, Dagfinrud H, Dijkmans B, Dougados M, Emery P, Geher P, Hammoudeh M, Inman RD, Jongkees M, Khan MA, Kiltz U, Kvien T, Leirisalo-Repo M, Maksymowych WP, Olivieri I, Pavelka K, Sieper J, Stanislawska-Biernat E, Wendling D, Ozgocmen S, van Drogen C, van Royen B, van der Heijde D. 2010 update of ASAS/EULAR recommendations for the management of ankylosing spondylitis. Ann Rheum Dis. 2011;70:596–904. doi:10.1136/ard.2011.151027.
5. Sieper J, Poddubnyy D. New evidence on the management of spondyloarthritis. Nat Rev Rheumatol. 2016;12:282–95. doi:10.1038/nrrheum.2016.42.
6. Liang H, Li WR, Zhang H, Tian X, Wei W, Wang CM. Concurrent intervention with exercise and stabilized tumor necrosis factor inhibitor therapy reduced the disease activity in patients with ankylosing spondylitis: a meta-analysis. Medicine (Baltimore). 2015;94:e2254. doi:10.1097/MD.0000000000002254.
7. Millner JR, Barron JS, Beinke KM, Butterworth RH, Chasle BE, Dutton LJ, Lewington MA, Lim EG, Morley TB, O'Reilly JE, Pickering KA, Winzenberg T, Zochling J. Exercise for ankylosing spondylitis: an evidence-based consensus statement. Semin Arthritis Rheum. 2016;45:411–27. doi:10.1016/j.semarthrit.2015.08.003.
8. Nghiem FT, Donohue JP. Rehabilitation in ankylosing spondylitis. Curr Opin Rheumatol. 2008;20:203–7. doi:10.1097/BOR.0b013e3282f56868.
9. Van der Heijde D, Lie E, Kvien TK, Sieper J, Van den Bosch F, Listing J, Braun J, Landewé R, Assessment of SpondyloArthritis international Society (ASAS). ASDAS, a highly discriminatory ASAS-endorsed disease activity score in patients with ankylosing spondylitis. Ann Rheum Dis. 2009;68:1811–8. doi:10.1136/ard.2008.100826.
10. Rudwaleit M, Haibel H, Baraliakos X, Listing J, Märker-Hermann E, Zeidler H, Braun J, Sieper J. The early disease stage in axial spondyloarthritis: results from the German Spondyloarthritis Inception Cohort. Arthritis Rheum. 2009;60:717–27. doi:10.1002/art.24483.
11. François RJ, Neure L, Sieper J, Braun J. Immunohistological examination of open sacroiliac biopsies of patients with ankylosing spondylitis: detection of tumour necrosis factor alpha in two patients with early disease and transforming growth factor beta in three more advanced cases. Ann Rheum Dis. 2006;65:713–20.
12. Braun J, Bollow M, Neure L, Seipelt E, Seyrekbasan F, Herbst H, Eggens U, Distler A, Sieper J. Use of immunohistologic and in situ hybridization techniques in the examination of sacroiliac joint biopsy specimens from patients with ankylosing spondylitis. Arthritis Rheum. 1995;38:499–505.
13. Gaffen SL, Jain R, Garg AV, Cua DJ. The IL-23-IL-17 immune axis: from mechanisms to therapeutic testing. Nat Rev Immunol. 2014;14:585–600. doi:10.1038/nri3707.
14. Gratacós J, Collado A, Filella X, Sanmartí R, Cañete J, Llena J, Molina R, Ballesta A, Muñoz-Gómez J. Serum cytokines (IL-6, TNF-alpha, IL-1 beta and IFN-gamma) in ankylosing spondylitis: a close correlation between serum IL-6 and disease activity and severity. Br J Rheumatol. 1994;33:927–31.
15. Mei Y, Pan F, Gao J, Ge R, Duan Z, Zeng Z, Liao F, Xia G, Wang S, Xu S, Xu J, Zhang L, Ye D. Increased serum IL-17 and IL-23 in the patient with ankylosing spondylitis. Clin Rheumatol. 2011;30:269–73. doi:10.1007/s10067-010-1647-4.
16. De Rycke L, Baeten D, Foell D, Kruithof E, Veys EM, Roth J, De Keyser F. Differential expression and response to anti-TNFalpha treatment of infiltrating versus resident tissue macrophage subsets in autoimmune arthritis. J Pathol. 2005;206:17–27.
17. Oktayoglu P, Bozkurt M, Mete N, Caglayan M, Em S, Nas K. Elevated serum levels of calprotectin (myeloid-related protein 8/14) in patients with ankylosing spondylitis and its association with disease activity and quality of life. J Investig Med. 2014;62:880–4. doi:10.1097/JIM.0000000000000095.
18. Schreuder KJ, Roelen CA, Koopmans PC, Groothoff JW. Job demands and health complaints in white and blue collar workers. Work. 2008;31:425–32.
19. Cumpelik J, Vele F. Yoga-Based Training for Spinal Stability. In: Liebenson C, editor. Rehabilitation of Spine. A Practitioners Manual. Philadelphia: Lippincott Williams and Wilkins; 2006.
20. Poquet N, Lin CW, Heymans MW, van Tulder MW, Esmail R, Koes BW, Maher CG. Back schools for acute and subacute non-specific low-back pain. Cochrane Database Syst Rev. 2016. doi:10.1002/14651858.
21. McKenzie R, May S. The lumbar spine: Mechanical Diagnosis & Therapy. New Zealand: Spinal Publications; 2003.
22. Brügger A. Gesunde Körperhaltung im Alltag. Stuttgart: G. F. Verlag; 1990.
23. Altan L, Korkmaz N, Dizdar M, Yurtkuran M. Effect of Pilates training on people with ankylosing spondylitis. Rheumatol Int. 2012;32:2093–9. doi:10.1007/s00296-011-1932-9.
24. Saeterbakken AH, Andersen V, Jansson J, Kvellestad AC, Fimland MS. Effects of BOSU ball(s) during sit-ups with body weight and added resistance on core muscle activation. J Strength Cond Res. 2014;28:3515–22. doi:10.1519/JSC.0000000000000565.
25. Emilio EJ, Hita-Contreras F, Jimenez-Lara PM, Latorre-Román P, Martinez-Amat A. The association of flexibility, balance, and lumbar strength with balance ability: risk of falls in older adults. J Sports Sci Med. 2014;13:349–57.
26. Garrett S, Jenkinson T, Kennedy LG, Whitelock H, Gaisford P, Calin A. A new approach to defining disease status in ankylosing spondylitis: the Bath Ankylosing Spondylitis Disease Activity Index. J Rheumatol. 1994;21:2286–91.
27. Calin A, Garrett S, Whitelock H, Kennedy LG, O'Hea J, Mallorie P, Jenkinson T. A new approach to defining functional ability in ankylosing spondylitis: the development of the Bath Ankylosing spondylitis Functional Index. J Rheumatol. 1994;21:2281–5.
28. Jenkinson TR, Mallorie PA, Whitelock HC, Kennedy LG, Garrett SL, Calin A. Defining spinal mobility in ankylosing spondylitis (AS). The Bath AS Metrology Index. J Rheumatol. 1994;21:1694–8.
29. Karapolat H, Akkoc Y, Sari I, Eyigor S, Akar S, Kirazli Y, Akkoc N. Comparison of group-based exercise versus home-based exercise in patients with ankylosing spondylitis: effects on Bath Ankylosing Spondylitis Indices, quality of life and depression. Clin Rheumatol. 2008;27:695–700.
30. Kraag G, Stokes B, Groh J, Helewa A, Goldsmith C. The effects of comprehensive home physiotherapy and supervision on patients with ankylosing spondylitis-a randomized controlled trial. J Rheumatol. 1990;17:228–33.
31. Rosu MO, Topa I, Chirieac R, Ancuta C. Effects of pilates, McKenzie and Heckscher training on disease activity, spinal motility and pulmonary function in patients with ankylosing spondylitis: a randomized controlled trial. Rheumatol Int. 2014;34:367–72. doi:10.1007/s00296-013-2869-y.
32. Ramiro S, Landewé R, van Tubergen A, Boonen A, Stolwijk C, Dougados M, van den Bosch F, van der Heijde D. Lifestyle factors may modify the effect of disease activity on radiographic progression in patients with ankylosing spondylitis: a longitudinal analysis. RMD Open. 2015;1:e000153. doi:10.1136/rmdopen-2015-000153.
33. Navarro-Compán V, Ramiro S, Landewé R, Dougados M, Miceli-Richard C, Richette P, van der Heijde D. Disease activity is longitudinally related to sacroiliac inflammation on MRI in male patients with axial spondyloarthritis: 2-years of the DESIR cohort. Ann Rheum Dis. 2016;75:874–8. doi:10.1136/annrheumdis-2015-207786.
34. Rosu OM, Ancuta C. McKenzie training in patients with early stages of ankylosing spondylitis: results of a 24-week controlled study. Eur J Phys Rehabil Med. 2015;51:261–8.
35. Masiero SBL, Pigatto M, Lo Nigro A, Ramonda R, Punzi L. Rehabilitation treatment in patients with ankylosing spondylitis stabilized with tumour necrosis factor inhibitor therapy: a randomized controlled trial. J Rheumatol. 2011;38:1335–42. doi:10.3899/jrheum.100987.

36. Wallis D, Haroon N, Ayerst R, Carty A, Imman RD. Ankylosing spondylitis and nonradiographic axial spondyloarthritis: part of a common spectrum or distinct diseases? J Rheumatol. 2013;40:2038–41. doi:10.3899/jrheum.130588.
37. Kiltz U, Baraliakos X, Karakostas P, Igelmann M, Kalthoff L, Klink C, Krause D, Schmitz-Bortz E, Flörecke M, Bollow M, Braun J. Do patients with non-radiographic axial spondyloarthritis differ from patients with ankylosing spondylitis? Arthritis Care Res (Hoboken). 2012;64:1415–22. doi:10.1002/acr.21688.
38. Poddubnyy D, Rudwaleit M, Haibel H, Listing J, Märker-Hermann E, Zeidler H, Braun J, Sieper J. Rates and predictors of radiographic sacroiliitis progression over 2 years in patients with axial spondyloarthritis. Ann Rheum Dis. 2011;70:1369–74. doi:10.1136/ard.2010.145995.
39. Hansson C, Eriksson C, Alenius GM. S-calprotectin (S100A8/S100A9): a potential marker of inflammation in patients with psoriatic arthritis. J Immunol Res. 2014;2014:696415. doi:10.1155/2014/696415.
40. Andrés Cerezo L, Mann H, Pecha O, Pleštilová L, Pavelka K, Vencovský J, Senolt L. Decreases in serum levels of S100A8/9 (calprotectin) correlate with improvements in total swollen joint count in patients with recent-onset rheumatoid arthritis. Arthritis Res Ther. 2011;13:R122. doi:10.1186/ar3426.
41. Cypers H, Varkas G, Beeckman S, Debusschere K, Vogl T, Roth J, Drennan MB, Lavic M, Foell D, Cuvelier CA, De Vos M, Delanghe J, van den Bosch F, Elewaut D. Elevated calprotectin levels reveal bowel inflammation in spondyloarthritis. Ann Rheum Dis. 2016;75:1357–62. doi:10.1136/annrheumdis-2015-208025.
42. Gupta L, Bhattacharya S, Agarwal V, Aggarwal A. Elevated levels of serum MRP8/14 in ankylosing spondylitis: associated with peripheral arthritis and active disease. Clin Rheumatol, 2016; in print. doi:10.1007/s10067-016-3448-x.
43. Ciccia F, Rizzo A, Triolo G. Subclinical gut inflammation in ankylosing spondylitis. Curr Opin Rheumatol. 2016;28:89–96.
44. Mortensen OH, Andersen K, Fischer C, Nielsen AR, Nielsen S, Åkerström T, Aastrøm MB, Borup R, Pedersen BK. Calprotectin is released from human skeletal muscle tissue during exercise. J Physiol. 2008;586:3551–62. doi:10.1113/jphysiol.2008.153551.
45. Maharaj A, Slusher AL, Zourdos MC, Whitehurst M, Fico BG, Huang CJ. Association of calprotectin with leukocyte chemotactic and inflammatory mediators following acute aerobic exercise. Appl Physiol Nutr Metab. 2016;41:83–7. doi:10.1139/apnm-2015-0385.
46. Kanda K, Sugama K, Hayashida H, Sakuma J, Kawakami Y, Miura S, Yoshioka H, Mori Y, Suzuki K. Eccentric exercise-induced delayed-onset muscle soreness and changes in markers of muscle damage and inflammation. Exerc Immunol Rev. 2013;19:72–85.
47. Acar A, Guzel S, Sarifakioglu B, Guzel EC, Guzelant AY, Karadag C, Kiziler L. Calprotectin levels in patients with rheumatoid arthritis to assess and association with exercise treatment. Clin Rheumatol. 2016;35:2685–92.
48. Turina MC, Yeremenko N, Paramarta JE, De Rycke L, Baeten D. Calprotectin (S100A8/9) as serum biomarker for clinical response in proof-of-concept trials in axial and peripheral spondyloarthritis. Arthritis Res Ther. 2014;16:413. doi:10.1186/s13075-014-0413-4.
49. Baeten D, Baraliakos X, Braun J, Sieper J, Emery P, van der Heijde D, McInnes I, van Laar JM, Landewé R, Wordsworth P, Wollenhaupt J, Kellner H, Paramarta J, Wei J, Brachat A, Bek S, Laurent D, Li Y, Wang YA, Bertolino AP, Gsteiger S, Wright AM, Hueber W. Anti-interleukin-17A monoclonal antibody secukinumab in treatment of ankylosing spondylitis: a randomised, double-blind, placebo-controlled trial. Lancet. 2013;382:1705–13. doi:10.1016/S0140-6736(13)61134-4.
50. Kruithof E, De Rycke L, Vandooren B, De Keyser F, FitzGerald O, McInnes I, Tak PP, Bresnihan B, Veys EM, Baeten D, OMERACT Special Interest Group on Synovial Analysis in Clinical Trials. Identification of synovial biomarkers of response to experimental treatment in early-phase clinical trials in spondylarthritis. Arthritis Rheum. 2006;6:1795–804.
51. Turina MC, Sieper J, Yeremenko N, Conrad K, Haibel H, Rudwaleit M, Baeten D, Poddubnyy D. Calprotectin serum levels is an independent marker for radiographic spinal progression in axial spondyloarthritis. Ann Rheum Dis. 2014;73:1746–8. doi:10.1136/annrheumdis-2014-205506.
52. Klingberg E, Carlsten H, Hilme E, Hedberg M, Forsblad-D´elia H. Calprotectin in ankylosing spondylitis – frequently elevated in feces, but normal in serum. Scan J Gastroenterol. 2012;47:435–44. doi:10.3109/00365521.2011.648953.
53. Smale S, Natt RS, Orchard TR, Russel AS, Bjarnason I. Inflammatory bowel disease and spondyloarthropathy. Arthritis Rheum. 2001;44:2728–36. doi:10.1002/1529-0131(200112)44:12<2728::AID-ART459>3.0.CO;2-8.
54. Meuwis MA, Vernier-Massouille G, Grimaud JC, Bouhnik Y, Laharie D, Piver E, Seidel L, Colombel JF, Louis E, GETAID (Groupe d'Étude Thérapeutique Des Affections Inflammatoires Digestives). Serum calprotectin as a biomarker for Crohn's disease. J Crohns Colitis. 2013;7:e678–83. doi:10.1016/j.crohns.2013.06.008.
55. Boschetti G, Garnero P, Moussata D, Cuerq C, Préaudat C, Duclaux-Loras R, Mialon A, Drai J, Flourié B, Nancey S. Accuracies of serum and fecal S100 proteins (calprotectin and calgranulin C) to predict the response to TNF antagonists in patients with Crohn's disease. Inflamm Bowel Dis. 2015;21:331–6. doi:10.1097/MIB.0000000000000273.
56. Bilski J, Mazur-Bialy A, Brzozowski B, Magierowski M, Zahradnik-Bilska J, Wójcik D, Magierowska K, Kwiecien S, Mach T, Brzozowski T. Can exercise affect the course of inflammatory bowel disease? Experimental and clinical evidence. Pharmacol Rep. 2016;68:827–36. doi:10.1016/j.pharep.2016.04.009.
57. Mathur N, Pedersen BK. Exercise as a mean to control low-grade systemic inflammation. Mediators Inflamm. 2008;2008:109502. doi:10.1155/2008/109502.
58. Wallman JK, Kapetanovic MC, Petersson IF, Geborek P, Kristensen LE. Comparison of non-radiographic axial spondyloarthritis and ankylosing spondylitis patients—baseline characteristics, treatment adherence, and development of clinical variables during three years of anti-TNF therapy in clinical practice. Arthritis Res Ther. 2015;17:378. doi:10.1186/s13075-015-0897-6.
59. Schulz M, Dotzlaw H, Neeck G. Ankylosing spondylitis and rheumatoid arthritis: serum levels of TNF-α and its soluble receptors during the course of therapy with etanercept and infliximab. Biomed Res Int. 2014;2014:675108. doi:10.1155/2014/675108.
60. Dorneles GP, Haddad DO, Fagundes VO, Vargas BK, Kloecker A, Romão PR, Peres A. High intensity interval exercise decreases IL-8 and enhances the immunomodulatory cytokine interleukin-10 in lean and overweight-obese individuals. Cytokine. 2016;77:1–9. doi:10.1016/j.cyto.2015.10.003.
61. Sugama K, Suzuki K, Yoshitani K, Shiraishi K, Kometani T. IL-17, neutrophil activation and muscle damage following endurance exercise. Exerc Immunol Rev. 2012;18:116–27.
62. Golzari Z, Shabkhiz F, Soudi S, Kordi MR, Hashemi SM. Combined exercise training reduces IFN-γ and IL-17 levels in the plasma and the supernatant of peripheral blood mononuclear cells in women with multiple sclerosis. Int Immunopharmacol. 2010;10:1415–9. doi:10.1016/j.intimp.2010.08.008.
63. Baeten D, Sieper J, Braun J, Baraliakos X, Dougados M, Emery P, Deodhar A, Porter B, Martin R, Andersson M, Mpofu S, Richards HB, MEASURE 1 Study Group.; MEASURE 2 Study Group. Secukinumab, an interleukin-17A inhibitor, in ankylosing spondylitis. N Engl J Med. 2015;373:2534–48. doi:10.1056/NEJMoa1505066.

14

Genome-wide DNA methylation profile analysis identifies differentially methylated loci associated with ankylosis spondylitis

Jiangcan Hao[1], Yang Liu[2], Jiawen Xu[3], Wenyu Wang[1], Yan Wen[1], Awen He[1], Qianrui Fan[1], Xiong Guo[1] and Feng Zhang[1*]

Abstract

Background: Ankylosing spondylitis (AS) is a chronic rheumatic and autoimmune disease. Little is known about the potential role of DNA methylation in the pathogenesis of AS. This study was undertaken to explore the potential role of DNA methylation in the genetic mechanism of AS.

Methods: In this study, we compared the genome-wide DNA methylation profiles of peripheral blood mononuclear cells (PBMCs) between five AS patients and five healthy subjects, using the Illumina Infinium HumanMethylation450 BeadChip. Quantitative real-time reverse transcription-polymerase chain reaction (qRT-PCR) was performed to validate the relevance of the identified differentially methylated genes for AS, using another independent sample of five AS patients and five healthy subjects.

Results: Compared with healthy controls, we detected 1915 differentially methylated CpG sites mapped to 1214 genes. The HLA-DQB1 gene achieved the most significant signal (cg14323910, adjusted $P = 1.84 \times 10^{-6}$, β difference = 0.5634) for AS. Additionally, the CpG site cg04777551 of *HLA-DQB1* presented a suggestive association with AS (adjusted $P = 1.46 \times 10^{-3}$, β difference = 0.3594). qRT-PCR observed that the mRNA expression level of *HLA-DQB1* in AS PBMCs was significantly lower than that in healthy control PBMCs (ratio = 0.48 ± 0.10, $P < 0.001$). Gene Ontology (GO) and KEGG pathway enrichment analysis of differentially methylated genes identified four GO terms and 10 pathways for AS, functionally related to antigen dynamics and function.

Conclusions: Our results demonstrated the altered DNA methylation profile of AS and implicated HLA-DQB1 in the development of AS.

Keywords: Ankylosing spondylitis, Methylation, *HLA-DQB1*

Background

Ankylosing spondylitis (AS) is a chronic rheumatic and autoimmune disease, mainly damaging the axial skeleton, spine, and sacroiliac joints [1]. AS leads to the imbalance between bone resorption and bone formation, ultimately resulting in ligamentous ossifications and vertebral joint fusion [2]. AS usually starts before 30 years of age, manifested as chronic pain and stiffness of the low back. With age, loss of spinal mobility and chest expansion, extension of the lumbar spine becomes evident [3, 4], resulting in severe disability in AS patients [1]. It was reported that AS affects between 0.5 and 14 per 100,000 people every year [5].

Previous studies have demonstrated that AS is an inheritable disease with over 90% of AS risk determined by genetic factors [6]. HLA-B27 is a well-known susceptibility gene of AS. Approximately 95% of AS patients express the HLA-B27 genotype [7–9]. However, less than 5% of HLA-B27-positive individuals develop AS. Twin and family studies have suggested that HLA-B27 accounts for less than 40% of the overall risk of AS [7–9]. In addition, tumor necrosis factor was implicated in the genetic mechanism of AS with limited genetic effect [10]. The missing heritability of

* Correspondence: fzhxjtu@xjtu.edu.cn
[1]Key Laboratory of Trace Elements and Endemc Diseases of National Health and Family Planning Commission, School of Public Health, Health Science Center, Xi'an Jiaotong University, Xi'an, People's Republic of China

AS suggests unknown genetic factors that contribute to the development of AS.

DNA methylation is an important epigenetic mechanism, playing an important role in gene expression regulation [11–13]. Extensive studies have demonstrated dysfunction of methylation in the development of multiple rheumatic and autoimmune diseases [14, 15]. Genome-wide DNA methylation profile comparative studies are a powerful tool for interrogating methylation changes associated with disease status. However, to the best of our knowledge, although some studies of abnormal methylated loci in AS patients have been conducted [16, 17], no genome-wide DNA methylation profiling of AS has so far been conducted. Little is known about the potential role of DNA methylation in the genetic mechanism of AS, limiting our efforts to clarify the pathogenesis and develop effective treatments for AS.

In this study, we first performed a genome-wide DNA methylation profile comparative analysis of peripheral blood mononuclear cells (PBMCs) between five AS patients and five healthy controls. Quantitative real-time reverse transcription-polymerase chain reaction (qRT-PCR) was then conducted to validate the relevance of the identified differentially methylated genes with AS using another independent sample of five AS patients and five healthy controls.

Methods

Human subjects

Genetically unrelated male AS patients were recruited randomly from Xi'an 451 Hospital, Xi'an No.5 Hospital, and the Second Affiliated Hospital of Xi'an Jiaotong University in Xi'an city of Shaanxi province in China. All AS patients were diagnosed clinically and radiologically according to the modified New York criteria [18] by two AS experts. Specific for this study, 10 AS patients with bilateral grade 4 sacroiliitis and syndesmophytes were selected randomly from the recruited AS patients and used for genome-wide DNA methylation profile analysis and the qRT-PCR validation experiment, respectively (Table 1 and Fig. 1). Ten age-matched healthy males were recruited from Xi'an city as healthy control samples (Table 1). Clinical data for each participant were recorded by nurse-administered questionnaire, including self-reported ethnicity, lifestyle characteristics, health status, and family and medical histories. All study subjects are Chinese Han people. All patients were receiving only NSAIDs in the previous 3 months. Subjects with genetic bone diseases, cartilage diseases, rheumatic and autoimmune diseases, and undergoing biologic treatments were excluded from this study.

Table 1 Basic characteristics of the study subjects

Group	Ankylosing spondylitis		Healthy controls	
	Age (years)	Gender	Age (years)	Gender
Methylation chip				
1	22	Male	23	Male
2	25	Male	23	Male
3	27	Male	25	Male
4	31	Male	30	Male
5	31	Male	34	Male
qRT-PCR				
1	42	Male	32	Male
2	28	Male	29	Male
3	30	Male	32	Male
4	30	Male	31	Male
5	27	Male	25	Male

qRT-PCR quantitative real-time reverse transcription-polymerase chain reaction

Monocyte derivation, DNA extraction, and quality control

Five milliliters of peripheral blood was drawn from each participant. Following the manufacturer's recommended procedure, blood specimens were diluted with phosphate-buffered saline (PBS), laid with Lymphocyte Separation Medium (TBD Sciences), and centrifuged under 2500 rpm/min for 15 min to separate PBMCs. DNA was extracted from PBMCs using the TIANamp Blood DNA Kit (TIGEN Inc., China). The quality and concentration of extracted DNA were determined by NanoDrop ND-1000 Spectrophotometer (Thermo Fisher Scientific Inc., USA). The DNA specimens with A260/280 values varying from 1.8 to 2.0 were used in this study.

Genome-wide DNA methylation profiling

Genome-wide DNA methylation profiling of PBMCs was conducted using the Illumina Infinium HumanMethylation450 BeadChip according to the manufacturer's standard procedure. Briefly, bisulfite treatment of 500 ng DNA specimens was performed by the EZ DNA Methylation Kit (Zymo Research, USA). The bisulfite-converted DNA specimens were then amplified, hybridized to a HumanMethylation450 array, stained, and washed. The raw image intensities of the hybridized arrays were scanned using an iScan SQ scanner (iScan System; Illumina). The obtained raw image intensity data were processed by GenomeStudio software (Illumina). The percentage of methylated cytosine at a given CpG locus was expressed as a β value, varying from 0 (completely unmethylated) to 1 (completely methylated).

Statistical analysis

The correlations of study samples were first evaluated by calculating the Pearson correlation coefficients of β

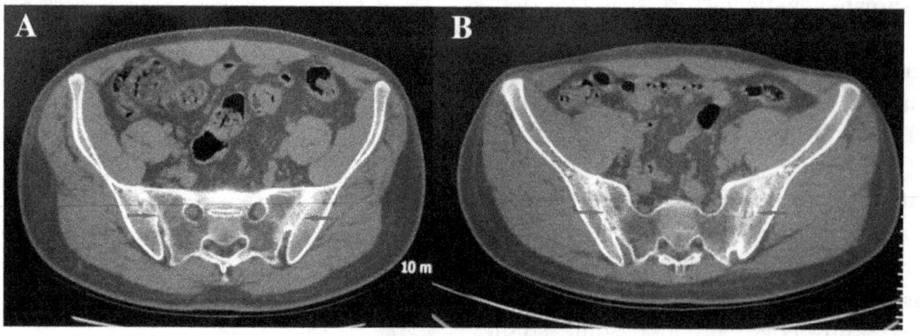

Fig. 1 Radiograph of two representative ankylosis spondylitis patients with bilateral grade 4 sacroiliitis: **a** male, 28 years old; **b** male, 25 years old

values. The Empirical Bayes moderated t test of the limma package from Bioconductor was used to compare the methylation profile difference between the AS group and the healthy control group. The Benjamini–Hochberg method was used to obtain an adjusted P value for each CpG locus. For quality control, the CpG sites with missing values or detection $P > 0.05$ in more than 90% of specimens were eliminated. The CpG sites with both adjusted $P < 0.05$ and $|\beta \text{ difference}| > 0.20$ were identified as significantly differentially methylated loci.

Gene Ontology and pathway enrichment analysis

Gene Ontology (GO) and pathway enrichment analysis were conducted by DAVID (http://david.abcc.ncifcrf.gov/) with all genes and pathways available on the Illumina Infinium HumanMethylation450 platform as the background to identify the cellular processes and canonical pathways that were enriched in the identified differentially methylated genes. Molecular function (MF), cellular component (CC), and biologic process (BP) were considered for GO enrichment analysis. For pathway enrichment analysis, we employed all 192 KEGG (http://www.genome.jp/kegg/) biopathways in this study. The GO terms and pathways were considered significantly enriched with FDR-adjusted $P < 0.05$.

qRT-PCR validation

qRT-PCR was conducted to validate the relevance of identified differentially methylated genes for AS using an independent sample (Table 1). Total RNA was isolated from PBMCs using the TRIZOL kit (Invitrogen 15596-026). The quality and purity of the isolated total RNA were examined by NanoDrop ND-1000 Spectrophotometer (Thermo Fisher Scientific Inc.). A total of 100 ng of RNA was reverse-transcribed to complementary DNA (cDNA) using TaKaRa PrimeScript™RT Master Mix (Takara Bio Inc., Japan). The quality and concentration of cDNA were determined by NanoDrop ND-1000 Spectrophotometer (Thermo Fisher Scientific Inc.). The cDNA specimens with A260/280 values varying from 1.8 to 2.0 were used in this study. All primers were supplied by TaKaRa. The forward and reverse primers of *HLA-DQB1* are 5′-GGTGGGCAGAGGAGGTAGAA-3′ and 5′-ACAGCACTCACCAAACCAGAAG-3′, respectively. Samples were run in triplicate using TaKaRa SYBR Premix® Ex Taq™ II (Tli RNaseH Plus). Glyceraldehyde-3-phosphate dehydrogenase (GAPDH) was assayed simultaneously by qRT-PCR as an endogenous invariant control. Relative differences in mRNA expression level between AS patients and healthy controls were determined using the $^{\Delta\Delta}C_t$ method as described previously [19].

Results

Identifying differentially methylated loci

Pearson correlation analysis results for methylation β values of all study subjects are presented in Additional file 1: Figure S1. Additional file 2: Figure S2 shows the two-way hierarchical cluster analysis results for genome-wide methylation profiles.

A total of 473,685 CpG sites passing the quality control procedure were analyzed in this study. Compared with healthy controls, we detected 1915 differentially methylated CpGs, including 1611 hypermethylated loci and 304 hypomethylated loci, in AS PBMCs. The 1915 differentially methylated loci were mapped to 1214 genes, including 1045 hypermethylated genes and 169 hypomethylated genes (Additional file 3: Table S1). Across the whole genome, the CpG locus cg14323910 located on the *HLA-DQB1* gene was the most significant for AS (adjusted $P = 1.84 \times 10^{-6}$, β difference = 0.5634). Additionally, the cg04777551 locus of *HLA-DQB1* presented a suggestive association with AS (adjusted $P = 1.46 \times 10^{-3}$, β difference = 0.3594).

GO and pathway enrichment analysis

We identified four GO terms significantly enriched in the differentially methylated genes, functionally related to antigen dynamics and function (Table 2). As presented in Table 3, pathway enrichment analysis detected 10 significant pathways for AS, such as antigen processing and presentation ($P = 1.76 \times 10^{-3}$), intestinal immune

Table 2 GO enrichment analysis results of differentially methylated genes between AS patients and healthy controls

GO ID	Description	Genes	*P* value
GO:0002504	Antigen processing and presentation of peptide or polysaccharide antigen via MHC class II	*HLA-DMB, HLA-DOA, HLA-DOB, HLA-DPB1, HLA-DQA1, HLA-DQB1*	1.11×10^{-5}
GO:0042605	Peptide antigen binding	*DHCR24, HLA-A, HLA-B, HLA-C, HLA-DQB1, HLA-DRB1, HLA-H, MAML1, SLC7A5*	5.14×10^{-6}
GO:0042613	MHC class II protein complex	*HLA-DMB, HLA-DOA, HLA-DOB, HLA-DPB1, HLA-DQA1, HLA-DQB1, HLA-DRB1*	7.97×10^{-6}
GO:0071556	Integral to lumenal side of endoplasmic reticulum membrane	*CALR, HLA-A, HLA-B, HLA-C, HLA-DPB1, HLA-DQA1, HLA-DQB1, HLA-DRB1*	8.79×10^{-5}

GO Gene Ontology, *AS* ankylosing spondylitis

network for IgA production ($P = 1.94 \times 10^{-4}$), and autoimmune thyroid disease ($P = 3.93 \times 10^{-5}$).

qRT-PCR validation

To further assess the functional relevance of the identified *HLA-DQB1* gene for AS, we compared the mRNA expression levels of *HLA-DQB1* in PBMCs between five AS patients and five healthy controls. The mRNA expression level of *HLA-DQB1* in AS patients was significantly lower than that in healthy controls. The average expression ratio of *HLA-DQB1* was 0.48 ± 0.10 (mean ± SD) ($P < 0.001$).

Discussion

In this study, we observed a significant difference in DNA methylation profiles of PBMCs between AS patients and healthy control subjects, suggesting the implication of methylation in the development of AS. We also identified the significantly hypermethylated *HLA-DQB1* gene in AS PBMCs. qRT-PCR further observed significant downregulation of *HLA-DQB1* mRNA in AS PBMCs compared with healthy controls, supporting the functional relevance of *HLA-DQB1* for AS.

One of the important findings of this study is that the *HLA-DQB1* gene is involved in the development of AS. Human leukocyte antigen (HLA) genes are highly polymorphic gene clusters responsible for the regulation of the immune system in humans [20–24]. *HLA-DQB1* belongs to the HLA class II molecules, which are involved in activating immune responses and recognizing self or foreign antigens [25]. *HLA-DQB1* plays a central role in the immune system by presenting peptides derived from extracellular proteins [26]. The highly polymorphic amino acid chains of DQB1 are capable of forming the peptide binding groove that presents antigen to $CD4^+$ T-helper cells [27], and controlling the immune response [28, 29]. Previous studies reported that *HLA-DQB1* was associated with radiographic severity in AS [30, 31]. The different alleles of *HLA-DQB1* were also associated with the age of AS onset [31]. In addition, *HLA-DQB1* was closely associated with multiple autoimmune-related diseases [28, 29], such as multiple sclerosis [28] and type I diabetes [32]. Based on previous and present study results, it is reasonable to infer that the aberrant expression of *HLA-DQB1* due to DNA hypermethylation contributed to the development of AS. Further biological studies are warranted to confirm our findings and clarify the potential mechanism of *HLA-DQB1* involved in the pathogenesis of AS.

We found that the identified differentially methylated regions tended to be located in the genes functionally related to immune-related dynamics and function. The GO and pathway enrichment analysis of differentially

Table 3 KEGG pathway enrichment analysis results of differentially methylated genes between AS patients and healthy controls

KEGG ID	Description	DMG	*P* value
hsa05332	Graft-versus-host disease	11	2.31×10^{-5}
hsa05320	Autoimmune thyroid disease	11	3.93×10^{-5}
hsa04940	Type I diabetes mellitus	11	5.05×10^{-5}
hsa05310	Asthma	9	5.19×10^{-5}
hsa05330	Allograft rejection	10	6.19×10^{-5}
hsa04672	Intestinal immune network for IgA production	11	1.94×10^{-4}
hsa04920	Adipocytokine signaling pathway	13	4.47×10^{-4}
hsa04514	Cell adhesion molecules	19	8.84×10^{-4}
hsa04612	Antigen processing and presentation	12	1.76×10^{-3}
hsa05416	Viral myocarditis	12	1.76×10^{-3}

AS ankylosing spondylitis, *KEGG* Kyoto Encyclopedia of Genes and Genomes, *DMG* differentially methylated genes methylated genes further revealed connections between the differentially methylated regions and the enrichment of immune-related genes. For instance, both GO and pathway enrichment analysis results support the implication of dysfunction of antigen processing and presentation (hsa04920) in the development of AS. Antigen processing and presentation is mainly mediated by HLA class I molecules. Zhu et al. [33] found that antigen processing and presentation is significantly associated with AS. As a high polymorphic member of HLA class I molecules, the important role of HLA-B27 in the pathogenesis of AS has been well documented. Briefly, *HLA-B27* binds unique peptides of microbial or self-origin (antigen) and presents them to $CD8^{+}$ T cells. Large multifunctional proteases and transporters associated with antigen presentation act as chaperones for peptide transport. Antigen peptides generated by proteasomal degradation can be further subjected to amino peptidase-mediated trimming before reaching the optimal size for HLA class I binding [34, 35]. The *HLA-C* of HLA class I molecules has also been confirmed to be associated with AS [36]. More interestingly, we found that the intestinal immune network for IgA production pathway (hsa04672), the autoimmune thyroid disease pathway (hsa05320), and the asthma pathway (hsa05310) were associated with AS in this study. Previous studies have observed the coexistence of abnormal IgA levels and AS [37, 38]. Compared with general populations, higher prevalence of autoimmune thyroid disease and asthma in AS patients have been reported by previous studies [39, 40].

There were some limitations in this study. First, we used five AS patients and five healthy controls as the study samples for DNA methylation profiling. This was a relatively small sample, which may lead to loss of statistical power caused by potential selection bias. Using another independent sample of five AS patients and five healthy controls, qRT-PCR was conducted to validate the functional relevance of the hypermethylated *HLA-DQB1* gene with AS. qRT-PCR observed significant downregulation of *HLA-DQB1* in AS patients, supporting the accuracy of the DNA methylation profile analysis results. Further biological studies are warranted to confirm our findings and clarify the molecular mechanism of *HLA-DQB1* involved in the development of AS. Second, it should be noted that AS patients usually underwent NSAID treatments. Because of the need for clinical AS treatments, it is difficult to exclude the possible impact of NSAIDs on DNA methylation in this study. Further biological studies are warranted to confirm our findings.

Conclusions

We conducted a genome-wide DNA methylation profile comparative study and observed significant difference in DNA methylation profiles between AS patients and healthy subjects. We also reported a set of differentially methylated genes and identified *HLA-DQB1* involved in the development of AS. This study provides novel clues for clarifying the genetic mechanism as well as identifying biomarkers for AS.

Additional files

Additional file 1: Figure S1. Showing Pearson correlation coefficient plot of the genome-wide DNA methylation study results. *X* axis, average β values in cases; *Y* axis, average β values in controls. (JPEG 104 kb)

Additional file 2: Figure S2. Showing two-way hierarchical cluster analysis results of study samples and DNA methylation profiles. (JPEG 1170 kb)

Additional file 3: Table S1. Presenting significantly differentially methylated CpG sites between AS patients and healthy controls. (XLSX 167 kb)

Additional file 4: Presents genome-wide DNA methylation microarray data. (CSV 244140 kb)

Abbreviations

AS: Ankylosing spondylitis; FDR: False discovery rate; GO: Gene Ontology; PBMC: Peripheral blood mononuclear cell; PBS: Phosphate-buffered saline; qRT-PCR: Quantitative real-time reverse transcription-polymerase chain reaction

Acknowledgements

Not applicable.

Funding

The study was supported by National Natural Scientific Fund of China (81472925, 81673112), the Technology Research and Development Program of in Shaanxi Province of China (2013KJXX-51), and the Fundamental Research Funds for the Central Universities.

Authors' contributions

FZ takes responsibility for the integrity of the work as a whole, from inception to the finished manuscript. FZ and XG were responsible for conception and design. JCH, YL, JWX, YW, and AWH were responsible for collection and analysis of data. JCH, WYW, and FZ were responsible for interpretation of the data. JCH, YL, JWX, YW, WYW, AWH, QRF, XG, and FZ were responsible for drafting, revising and final approval of the manuscript.

Authors' information

Not applicable.

Competing interests

The authors declare that they have no competing interests.

Author details

[1]Key Laboratory of Trace Elements and Endemc Diseases of National Health and Family Planning Commission, School of Public Health, Health Science Center, Xi'an Jiaotong University, Xi'an, People's Republic of China. [2]Xi'an No.5 Hospital, Xi'an, People's Republic of China. [3]Department of Clinical Medicine, Health Science Center, Xi'an Jiaotong University, Xi'an, People's Republic of China.

References

1. Seregin SS, Rastall DP, Evnouchidou I, Aylsworth CF, Quiroga D, Kamal RP, Godbehere-Roosa S, Blum CF, York IA, Stratikos E, et al. Endoplasmic reticulum aminopeptidase-1 alleles associated with increased risk of ankylosing spondylitis reduce HLA-B27 mediated presentation of multiple antigens. Autoimmunity. 2013;46(8):497–508.
2. Schett G. Bone formation versus bone resorption in ankylosing spondylitis. Adv Exp Med Biol. 2009;649:114–21.
3. El Tecle NE, Abode-Iyamah KO, Hitchon PW, Dahdaleh NS. Management of spinal fractures in patients with ankylosing spondylitis. Clin Neurol Neurosurg. 2015;139:177–82.
4. Feldtkeller E, Khan MA, van der Heijde D, van der Linden S, Braun J. Age at disease onset and diagnosis delay in HLA-B27 negative vs. positive patients with ankylosing spondylitis. Rheumatol Int. 2003;23(2):61–6.
5. Braun J, Bollow M, Remlinger G, Eggens U, Rudwaleit M, Distler A, Sieper J. Prevalence of spondylarthropathies in HLA-B27 positive and negative blood donors. Arthritis Rheum. 1998;41(1):58–67.
6. Reveille JD. The genetic basis of ankylosing spondylitis. Curr Opin Rheumatol. 2006;18(4):332–41.
7. Brown MA, Kennedy LG, MacGregor AJ, Darke C, Duncan E, Shatford JL, Taylor A, Calin A, Wordsworth P. Susceptibility to ankylosing spondylitis in twins: the role of genes, HLA, and the environment. Arthritis Rheum. 1997;40(10):1823–8.
8. Hamersma J, Cardon LR, Bradbury L, Brophy S, van der Horst-Bruinsma I, Calin A, Brown MA. Is disease severity in ankylosing spondylitis genetically determined? Arthritis Rheum. 2001;44(6):1396–400.
9. Brophy S, Hickey S, Menon A, Taylor G, Bradbury L, Hamersma J, Brown M, Calin A. Concordance of disease severity among family members with ankylosing spondylitis? J Rheumatol. 2004;31(9):1775–8.
10. Wright PB, McEntegart A, McCarey D, McInnes IB, Siebert S, Milling SW. Ankylosing spondylitis patients display altered dendritic cell and T cell populations that implicate pathogenic roles for the IL-23 cytokine axis and intestinal inflammation. Rheumatology (Oxford). 2016;55(1):120–32.
11. Levin HL, Moran JV. Dynamic interactions between transposable elements and their hosts. Nat Rev Genet. 2011;12(9):615–27.
12. Jaenisch R, Bird A. Epigenetic regulation of gene expression: how the genome integrates intrinsic and environmental signals. Nat Genet. 2003;33(Suppl):245–54.
13. Peters J. The role of genomic imprinting in biology and disease: an expanding view. Nat Rev Genet. 2014;15(8):517–30.
14. Glossop JR, Emes RD, Nixon NB, Haworth KE, Packham JC, Dawes PT, Fryer AA, Mattey DL, Farrell WE. Genome-wide DNA methylation profiling in rheumatoid arthritis identifies disease-associated methylation changes that are distinct to individual T- and B-lymphocyte populations. Epigenetics. 2014;9(9):1228–37.
15. de la Rica L, Urquiza JM, Gomez-Cabrero D, Islam AB, Lopez-Bigas N, Tegner J, Toes RE, Ballestar E. Identification of novel markers in rheumatoid arthritis through integrated analysis of DNA methylation and microRNA expression. J Autoimmun. 2013;41:6–16.
16. Aslani S, Mahmoudi M, Garshasbi M, Jamshidi AR, Karami J, Nicknam MH. Evaluation of DNMT1 gene expression profile and methylation of its promoter region in patients with ankylosing spondylitis. Clin Rheumatol. 2016;35(11):2723–31.
17. Lai NS, Chou JL, Chen GCW, Liu SQ, Lu MC, Chan MWY. Association between cytokines and methylation of SOCS-1 in serum of patients with ankylosing spondylitis. Mol Biol Rep. 2014;41(6):3773–80.
18. van der Linden S, Valkenburg HA, Cats A. Evaluation of diagnostic criteria for ankylosing spondylitis. A proposal for modification of the New York criteria. Arthritis Rheum. 1984;27(4):361–8.
19. Ciccia F, Rizzo A, Guggino G, Cavazza A, Alessandro R, Maugeri R, Cannizzaro A, Boiardi L, Iacopino DG, Salvarani C, et al. Difference in the expression of IL-9 and IL-17 correlates with different histological pattern of vascular wall injury in giant cell arteritis. Rheumatology (Oxford). 2015;54(9):1596–604.
20. Repiska V, Shawkatova I, Bohmer D, Hatzibougias D, Sisovsky V, Danihel L. Gestational choriocarcinoma analyzed by polymerase chain reaction amplification of polymorphic VNTR and human leukocyte antigen regions. Int J Gynaecol Obstet. 2010;110(2):152–4.
21. Andreoni A, Bondani M, Nardo L. Time-resolved FRET method for typing polymorphic alleles of the human leukocyte antigen system by using a single DNA probe. Photochem Photobiol Sci. 2009;8(8):1202–6.
22. Schroeder S, Reck M, Hoeft A, Stuber F. Analysis of two human leukocyte antigen-linked polymorphic heat shock protein 70 genes in patients with severe sepsis. Crit Care Med. 1999;27(7):1265–70.
23. Huang W, Connor E, Rosa TD, Muir A, Schatz D, Silverstein J, Crockett S, She JX, Maclaren NK. Although DR3-DQB1*0201 may be associated with multiple component diseases of the autoimmune polyglandular syndromes, the human leukocyte antigen DR4-DQB1*0302 haplotype is implicated only in beta-cell autoimmunity. J Clin Endocrinol Metab. 1996;81(7):2559–63.
24. Huh KB, Lee HC, Kim HM, Lee HR, Hong CS, Lee SY, Choi HJ, Park K, Kim CK. Human leukocyte antigen (HLA) in Korean patients with autoimmune thyroid diseases. Korean J Intern Med. 1986;1(2):243–8.
25. Luppi P, Licata A, Haluszczak C, Rudert WA, Trucco G, McGowan Jr FX, Finegold D, Boyle GJ, Trucco M. Analysis of TCR Vbeta repertoire and cytokine gene expression in patients with idiopathic dilated cardiomyopathy. J Autoimmun. 2001;16(1):3–13.
26. Veijola R, Reijonen H, Vahasalo P, Sabbah E, Kulmala P, Ilonen J, Akerblom HK, Knip M. HLA-DQB1-defined genetic susceptibility, beta cell autoimmunity, and metabolic characteristics in familial and nonfamilial insulin-dependent diabetes mellitus. Childhood Diabetes in Finland (DiMe) Study Group. J Clin Invest. 1996;98(11):2489–95.
27. Watts C. The exogenous pathway for antigen presentation on major histocompatibility complex class II and CD1 molecules. Nat Immunol. 2004;5(7):685–92.
28. Kollaee A, Ghaffarpor M, Ghlichnia HA, Ghaffari SH, Zamani M. The influence of the HLA-DRB1 and HLA-DQB1 allele heterogeneity on disease risk and severity in Iranian patients with multiple sclerosis. Int J Immunogenet. 2012;39(5):414–22.
29. Gashimova AD, Sokolov AI, Nikol'skaia GV, Gapparov MM. Changes in lipid metabolism and renewal of sialic acids in the composition of glycoproteins of adipose tissue during carbohydrate loading. Vopr Med Khim. 1989;35(1):114–8.
30. Ward MM, Hendrey MR, Malley JD, Learch TJ, Davis Jr JC, Reveille JD, Weisman MH. Clinical and immunogenetic prognostic factors for radiographic severity in ankylosing spondylitis. Arthritis Rheum. 2009;61(7):859–66.
31. Pimentel-Santos FM, Matos M, Ligeiro D, Mourao AF, Ribeiro C, Costa J, Santos H, Barcelos A, Pinto P, Cruz M, et al. HLA alleles and HLA-B27 haplotypes associated with susceptibility and severity of ankylosing spondylitis in a Portuguese population. Tissue Antigens. 2013;82(6):374–9.
32. Beretta L, Rueda B, Marchini M, Santaniello A, Simeon CP, Fonollosa V, Caronni M, Rios-Fernandez R, Carreira P, Rodriguez-Rodriguez L, et al. Analysis of class II human leucocyte antigens in Italian and Spanish systemic sclerosis. Rheumatology (Oxford). 2012;51(1):52–9.
33. Zhu ZQ, Tang JS, Cao XJ. Transcriptome network analysis reveals potential candidate genes for ankylosing spondylitis. Eur Rev Med Pharmacol Sci. 2013;17(23):3178–85.
34. Kim TH, Uhm WS, Inman RD. Pathogenesis of ankylosing spondylitis and reactive arthritis. Curr Opin Rheumatol. 2005;17(4):400–5.
35. Chou CT. Factors affecting the pathogenesis of ankylosing spondylitis. Chin Med J. 2001;114(2):211–2.
36. Kim K, Bang SY, Lee S, Lee HS, Shim SC, Kang YM, Suh CH, Sun C, Nath SK, Bae SC, et al. An HLA-C amino-acid variant in addition to HLA-B*27 confers risk for ankylosing spondylitis in the Korean population. Arthritis Res Ther. 2015;17:342.
37. Zambrano-Zaragoza JF, de Jesus Duran-Avelar M, Rodriguez-Ocampo AN, Garcia-Latorre E, Burgos-Vargas R, Dominguez-Lopez ML, Pena-Virgen S, Vibanco-Perez N. The 30-kDa band from Salmonella typhimurium: IgM, IgA and IgG antibody response in patients with ankylosing spondylitis. Rheumatology (Oxford). 2009;48(7):748–54.
38. Stergiouli I, Tsifetaki N, Voulgari PV, Kosta P, Argyropoulou MI, Drosos AA. Ankylosing spondylitis and IgA deficiency. Joint Bone Spine. 2009;76(1):110–1.
39. Emmungil H, Erdogan M, Kalfa M, Karabulut G, Kocanaogullari H, Inal V, Aksu K, Oksel F, Kabasakal Y, Keser G. Autoimmune thyroid disease in ankylosing spondylitis. Clin Rheumatol. 2014;33(7):955–61.
40. Shen TC, Lin CL, Wei CC, Chen CH, Tu CY, Hsia TC, Shih CM, Hsu WH, Sung FC. The risk of asthma in patients with ankylosing spondylitis: a population-based cohort study. PLoS One. 2015;10(2):e0116608.

15

Serum levels of leptin and high molecular weight adiponectin are inversely associated with radiographic spinal progression in patients with ankylosing spondylitis: results from the ENRADAS trial

Agnes Hartl[1], Joachim Sieper[1], Uta Syrbe[1], Joachim Listing[2], Kay-Geert Hermann[3], Martin Rudwaleit[4] and Denis Poddubnyy[1,2*]

Abstract

Background: Previous research indicates a role of adipokines in inflammation and osteogenesis. Hence adipokines might also have a pathophysiological role in inflammation and new bone formation in patients with ankylosing spondylitis (AS). The aim of this study was to investigate the role of adipokine serum levels as predictors of radiographic spinal progression in patients with AS.

Methods: A total of 120 patients with definite AS who completed a 2-year follow up in the ENRADAS trial were included in the current study. Radiographic spinal progression was defined as: (1) worsening of the modified Stoke Ankylosing Spondylitis spine (mSASSS) score by ≥2 points and/or (2) new syndesmophyte formation or progression of existing syndesmophytes after 2 years. Serum levels of adipokines (adiponectin (APN) and its high molecular weight form (HMW-APN), chemerin, leptin, lipocalin-2, omentin, resistin, visfatin) were measured using enzyme-linked immunosorbent assays.

Results: There was a significant association between radiographic spinal progression and both leptin and HMW-APN. Baseline serum levels of both adipokines were lower in patients who showed radiographic spinal progression after 2 years. This association was especially evident in men; they had generally lower leptin and HMW-APN serum levels as compared to women. The inverse association between adipokines and radiographic spinal progression was confirmed in the logistic regression analysis: the odds ratios (OR) for the outcome "no mSASSS progression ≥2 points" were 1.16 (95% CI 1.03 to 1.29) and 1.17 (95% CI 0.99 to 1.38), for leptin and HMW-APN, respectively; for "no syndesmophyte formation/progression" the respective OR were 1.29 (95% CI 1.11 to 1.50) and 1.18 (95% CI 0.98 to 1.42), adjusted for the presence of syndesmophytes at baseline, C-reactive protein at baseline, sex, body mass index (BMI), non-steroidal anti-inflammatory drugs intake score over 2 years, and smoking status at baseline.

(Continued on next page)

* Correspondence: denis.poddubnyy@charite.de
[1]Department of Gastroenterology, Infectiology and Rheumatology, Charité Universitätsmedizin Berlin, Hindenburgdamm 30, 12203 Berlin, Germany
[2]German Rheumatism Research Centre, Charitéplatz 1, 10117 Berlin, Germany
Full list of author information is available at the end of the article

(Continued from previous page)

Conclusion: Serum leptin and HMW-APN predict protection from spinal radiographic progression in patients with AS. Women generally have higher leptin and HMW-APN serum levels that might explain why they have less structural damage in the spine as compared to male patients with AS.

Keywords: Axial spondyloarthritis, Ankylosing spondylitis, Leptin, Adiponectin, Adipokine, Radiographic progression, Syndesmophytes

Background

Ankylosing spondylitis (AS) is a chronic inflammatory disease belonging to a family of spondyloarthritides (SpA), which is characterized by inflammation in the pelvis and the spine with subsequent new bone formation that might lead to partial or total ankylosis of the spine. New bone formation in the spine, and particularly development of specific bony bridges between the vertebral bodies, is usually assessed on spinal radiographs and is referred to as radiographic spinal progression. It has been shown in the past that radiographic spinal progression and disease activity are two main determinants of spinal mobility and functional status in AS [1–3]. However, there is substantial individual variation in the radiographic spinal progression rates in AS [4, 5]. It has been shown that baseline syndesmophytes [4, 5], inflammatory activity as assessed by C-reactive protein (CRP), by the Ankylosing Spondylitis Disease Activity Score (ASDAS), or by the presence of inflammatory changes on magnetic resonance imaging (MRI) [6–12], and cigarette smoking [13] are factors associated with more rapid radiographic spinal progression. Further, several biomarkers in the blood were found to be positively associated with new bone formation in the spine: the already mentioned CRP [7], matrix-metalloproteinase-3 [14], vascular endothelial growth factor [15], calprotectin [16], and the adipokine, visfatin [17]. Some biomarkers, such as sclerostin [18] and dickkopf 1 [19], have been associated with radiographic spinal progression, suggesting that these molecules might have a protective effect.

Identification of biomarkers related to the development of structural damage in AS helps not only to predict progression (there are currently no proven therapeutic options to retard progression; however, this might, change in the near future), but it also helps us to better understand disease mechanisms. For instance, until now, the reason why men with AS develop more structural damage in the axial skeleton than women has not been explained [5, 20].

Adipokines are biologically active substances, which are synthesized and released by fat tissue. They have a wide range of regulatory functions not only in energy metabolism, but also in inflammation and osteogenesis [21, 22]. The role of adipokines in the development of inflammation and new bone formation in AS, however, is as yet unclear. The aim of the present study was to investigate the association between adipokine serum levels and radiographic spinal progression in patients with AS.

Methods

Patients

Altogether 120 patients from the trial, Effects of NSAIDs on Radiographic Damage in AS (ENRADAS), who completed the study per protocol and for whom serum was available, were included in the analysis. Serum samples were not available for two patients who completed the study per protocol, and these patients were excluded, therefore, from the current study. Baseline characteristics of the 120 patients included in this analysis are shown in Table 1. The design of the ENRADAS trial has been described in detail elsewhere [23]. Briefly, ENRADAS was a prospective, randomized, controlled trial aimed at investigation of the influence of non-steroidal

Table 1 Baseline characteristics of the included patients from the ENRADAS trial

Parameter	All patients (n = 120)	Continuous (n = 61)	On demand (n = 59)
Age, years	42.9 ± 10.3	40.7 ± 9.7	45.1 ± 10.4
Male patients, *n* (%)	82 (68.3)	43 (70.5)	39 (66.1)
Symptom duration, years	14.8 ± 12.2	12.8 ± 11.4	16.9 ± 12.7
HLA-B27 positive, *n* (%)	108 (90)	54 (88.5)	54 (91.5)
ASDAS-CRP	2.8 ± 0.7	2.7 ± 0.7	2.8 ± 0.7
BASDAI, points NRS (0–10)	4.2 ± 1.5	4.1 ± 1.5	4.2 ± 1.5
BASFI, points NRS (0–10)	3.3 ± 2.2	2.9 ± 2.1	3.7 ± 2.2
CRP, mg/L	10.3 ± 12.1	7.9 ± 7.4	12.6 ± 15.2
CRP > 5 mg/L, *n* (%)	68 (57.1)	33 (55)	35 (59.3)
BASMI, points (0–10)	2.6 ± 2.2	2.2 ± 2.1	3.0 ± 2.3
mSASSS, points	13.8 ± 17.2	11.1 ± 15.6	16.6 ± 18.4
Patients with syndesmophytes at baseline, *n* (%)	68 (56.7)	32 (52.5)	36 (61.0)
BMI, kg/m^2	27.2 ± 5.3	27.3 ± 5.2	27.2 ± 5.4

Characteristics are presented as mean ± standard deviation unless indicated otherwise. *ASDAS* Ankylosing Spondylitis Disease Activity Score, *BASDAI* Bath Ankylosing Spondylitis Disease Activity Index, *BASFI* Bath Ankylosing Spondylitis Functional Index, *BASMI* Bath Ankylosing Spondylitis Metrology Index, *BMI* body mass index, *CRP* C-reactive protein, *mSASSS* modified Stoke Ankylosing Spondylitis Spine Score anti-inflammatory drugs (NSAIDs) on radiographic spinal progression in patients with AS. Patients were randomly assigned to treatment with diclofenac either continuously or on demand for a period of 2 years. Other NSAIDs in the same equivalent dose were allowed in patients with diclofenac intolerability; however, about 2/3 of the patients remained on diclofenac until the end of year 2. Tumor necrosis factor (TNF)α blockers were not allowed in the trial. There was no difference in radiographic spinal progression between patients who took NSAIDs continuously and those who took them on demand, justifying the decision to pool both treatment groups.

Assessment of radiographic spinal progression

Radiographs of the lumbar and cervical spine (lateral projection) were obtained at baseline and after a period of 2 years. Radiographs were centrally collected, digitized, anonymized, and subsequently scored by two experienced and calibrated readers (KGH and DP) in a randomly selected and concealed order according to the modified Stoke Ankylosing Spondylitis Spine Score (mSASSS) system [24]. The mean mSASSS was calculated from the two readers' scores. Radiographic spinal progression was defined as: (1) mSASSS worsening by ≥2 points after 2 years, and/or (2) development of at least one new syndesmophyte or progression of two single syndesmophytes into a bridging syndesmophyte, in the opinion of both readers after 2 years.

Measurement of adipokine serum levels

Adipokine serum levels were measured at baseline and after 2 years of follow up (week 100) using commercially available enzyme linked immunosorbent assays (ELISA). The following adipokines were selected based on data from the available literature [25, 26] indicating a possible association with bone metabolism and/or inflammation: adiponectin (APN) (BioVendor - Research and Diagnostic Products, Czech Republic) and its high molecular weight form (HMW-APN) (R&D Systems, MN, USA), chemerin (BioVendor - Research and Diagnostic Products), leptin (Invitrogen, CA, USA) lipocalin-2 (R&D Systems), omentin (BioVendor - Research and Diagnostic Products), resistin (Adipogen International, Switzerland), and visfatin (Adipogen International).

Statistical analysis

First, we analyzed differences in the mean adipokine serum levels between groups with and without radiographic spinal progression (Mann-Whitney *U* test). Adipokines with significantly different baseline serum levels in progressors and non-progressors were further analyzed. Since adipokines are mainly produced by adipose tissue and their serum levels correlate with body mass index (BMI) [25–27], the values were corrected for BMI by calculating an adipokine/BMI ratio that was used in the analysis in addition to the measured serum levels. Further, an HMW-APN/APN ratio reflecting a proportion of a more biologically active form of APN in the total APN [28] was calculated and included in the analysis. For the analysis of the influences of the treatment arm on the change in serum levels of adipokines, we performed the non-parametric Wilcoxon test on the paired measures, and an analysis of covariance (ANCOVA) with adjustment for the baseline adipokine levels. Receiver operating characteristic (ROC) analysis was performed to evaluate the adipokines as predictors of radiographic spinal progression. The association between serum adipokines and radiographic spinal progression was further explored in the logistic regression analysis. The parameter estimates were adjusted for the presence of syndesmophytes at baseline, baseline CRP, sex, BMI (for crude adipokine serum levels and the HMW-APN/APN ratio), NSAID intake score over 2 years, and smoking status at baseline. A p value <0.05 was considered to be statistically significant.

Results

A total of 29 patients had radiographic progression defined as mSASSS worsening by ≥2 points after 2 years; 25 patients had syndesmophyte formation/progression. The intraclass correlation coefficient (ICC) between the two readers of the X-rays was good: the ICC was 0.96 for baseline and 0.95 for year-2 X-rays; the ICC for change in the mSASSS was 0.50 [23].

Adipokine serum levels in patients with and without radiographic spinal progression are presented in Table 2. There were significant differences between progressors and non-progressors in the baseline serum levels of leptin and HMW-APN (and to a further extent in the HMW-APN/APN ratio). Therefore, these adipokines were included in the subsequent analysis.

HMW-APN serum levels did not differ between the two treatment arms (NSAIDs continuously vs. on demand) at baseline and after 2 years of follow up; there was, however, a difference in the leptin levels at baseline (but not at year 2): 13.6 ± 13.2 ng/mL in the continuous intake group vs. 15.5 ± 12.6 ng/mL in the on-demand group, $p = 0.046$. Overall, there was an increase in the leptin level after 2 years in both treatment groups (continuous vs. on-demand NSAIDs); this was statistically significant in the continuous treatment group only: increase of 13.6 ± 13.2 ng/ml to 15.6 ± 15.6 ng/mL, $p = 0.002$. However, in the ANCOVA, there was no statistically significant difference in the change in the leptin serum level: increase of 2.0 ± 4.84 ng/mL in the continuous vs. 1.26 ± 7.43 ng/mL in the on-demand group, $p = 0.405$, adjusted for baseline leptin. Further, there was no

Table 2 Levels of adipokines in patients with AS with and without radiographic spinal progression after 2 years

Adipokine	mSASSS progression ≥2 points (n = 29)	No mSASSS progression ≥2 points (n = 91)	P^a	Syndesmophyte formation/ progression (n = 25)	No new syndesmophyte formation/progression (n = 95)	P^a
Baseline						
Leptin, ng/mL	10.5 ± 9.0	16.4 ± 13.7	0.003	10.2 ± 9.6	16.2 ± 13.4	0.003
APN, μg/mL	10.1 ± 4.8	10.7 ± 4.4	0.366	9.5 ± 3.7	10.8 ± 4.6	0.210
HMW-APN, μg/mL	4.95 ± 3.52	6.35 ± 4.15	0.045	4.53 ± 2.86	6.40 ± 4.22	0.026
Lipocalin-2, ng/mL	308.4 ± 424.8	197.1 ± 188.8	0.668	257.9 ± 361.3	215.1 ± 238.9	0.851
Chemerin, ng/mL	211.5 ± 54.2	222.6 ± 53.6	0.356	223.4 ± 57.8	219 ± 52.9	0.831
Omentin, ng/mL	455.1 ± 168.3	425.8 ± 131.7	0.477	477.8 ± 164.7	421 ± 132.8	0.122
Resistin, ng/mL	37.7 ± 27.9	30.4 ± 25.3	0.098	35.6 ± 25.4	31.3 ± 26.2	0.161
Visfatin, ng/mL	44.7 ± 80.3	42.2 ± 58.9	0.484	39.98 ± 83.4	43.4 ± 58.7	0.151
Year 2						
Leptin, ng/mL	13.4 ± 12.8	17.5 ± 16.0	0.044	11.7 ± 9.8	17.7 ± 16.3	0.032
APN, μg/mL	9.1 ± 3.8	11.0 ± 5.9	0.129	8.6 ± 3.6	11.1 ± 5.8	0.029
HMW-APN, μg/mL	5.06 ± 3.31	5.99 ± 3.88	0.185	4.55 ± 2.8	6.08 ± 3.92	0.071
Lipocalin-2, ng/mL	235 ± 229.3	273 ± 311.1	0.762	194.7 ± 160.3	281.8 ± 316.7	0.613
Chemerin, ng/mL	216.2 ± 60.3	213 ± 56.7	0.990	218 ± 61.9	212.6 ± 56.4	0.893
Omentin, ng/mL	444.7 ± 133.6	426.4 ± 134.6	0.359	452 ± 139.9	425.3 ± 132.6	0.268
Resistin, ng/mL	47.4 ± 84.3	62.4 ± 204.8	0.332	49.8 ± 91	61.1 ± 200.4	0.500
Visfatin, ng/mL	43.6 ± 70	42.6 ± 62.3	0.627	43.9 ± 75.2	42.6 ± 61.2	0.499

AS ankylosing spondylitis, *APN* adiponectin, *HMW-APN* high molecular weight adiponectin, *mSASSS* modified Stoke Ankylosing Spondylitis Spine Score.
[a]Mann-Whitney *U* test

significant association between change in leptin and HMW-APN (or the BMI-corrected values) over 2 years and radiographic spinal progression. Treatment had no effect on the levels of other adipokines.

There was no evidence of association between radiographic spinal progression and BMI in this patient population: BMI at baseline was 26.9 ± 4.1 kg/m^2 vs. 27.4 ± 5.6 kg/m^2 in patients with and without mSASSS worsening by ≥2 points, respectively, $p = 0.93$, and 28.1 ± 6.6 kg/m^2 vs. 27.1 ± 4.9 kg/m^2 in patients with and without syndesmophytes formation respectively, $p = 0.58$.

There was no meaningful correlation between leptin and HMW-APN serum levels, and no correlation with serum CRP. In the ROC analysis, baseline serum leptin, the leptin/BMI ratio, serum HMW-APN, the HMW-APN/BMI ratio, and the HMW-APN/APN ratio were good predictors of no mSASSS progression ≥2 points and of no syndesmophyte formation/progression (Fig. 1). Leptin and the leptin/BMI ratio was generally a slightly better predictor as compared to HMW-APN.

Remarkably, male patients with AS had significantly lower levels of leptin and HMW-APN (and BMI-adjusted values and HMW-APN/APN ratio) compared to women (Table 3). In the analysis stratified by sex, the association between lower leptin and HMW-APN levels and radiographic spinal progression was evident in men only (Table 4). Furthermore, women had significantly lower mSASSS at baseline and after 2 years of follow up compared to men (7.9 ± 12.6 vs. 16.2 ± 18.2, respectively, $p = 0.015$ at baseline and 8.6 ± 12.9 vs. 17.4 ± 19.0, respectively, $p = 0.011$ after 2 years of follow up).

We further explored an association between leptin or HMW-APN and radiographic spinal progression in the logistic regression analysis (Table 5). Serum leptin and the leptin/BMI ratio were significantly inversely associated with radiographic spinal progression; this remained significant after adjusting for factors considered as confounders. The same trend was observed for HMW-APN (crude and BMI-adjusted levels), but this was not statistically significant. However, the HMW-APN/APN ratio was inversely associated with radiographic spinal progression in the logistic regression analysis (Table 5). Similar to the data presented in Table 4, the association between serum adipokines levels and radiographic spinal progression was evident in men but not in women when analyzed separately (Table 6).

Discussion

In the current study we investigated the association between serum adipokines and radiographic spinal progression in patients with AS. We report for the first time that baseline leptin and HMW-APN serum levels, and to a further extent the HMW-APN/APN ratio were inversely associated with (i.e., predicted protection against)

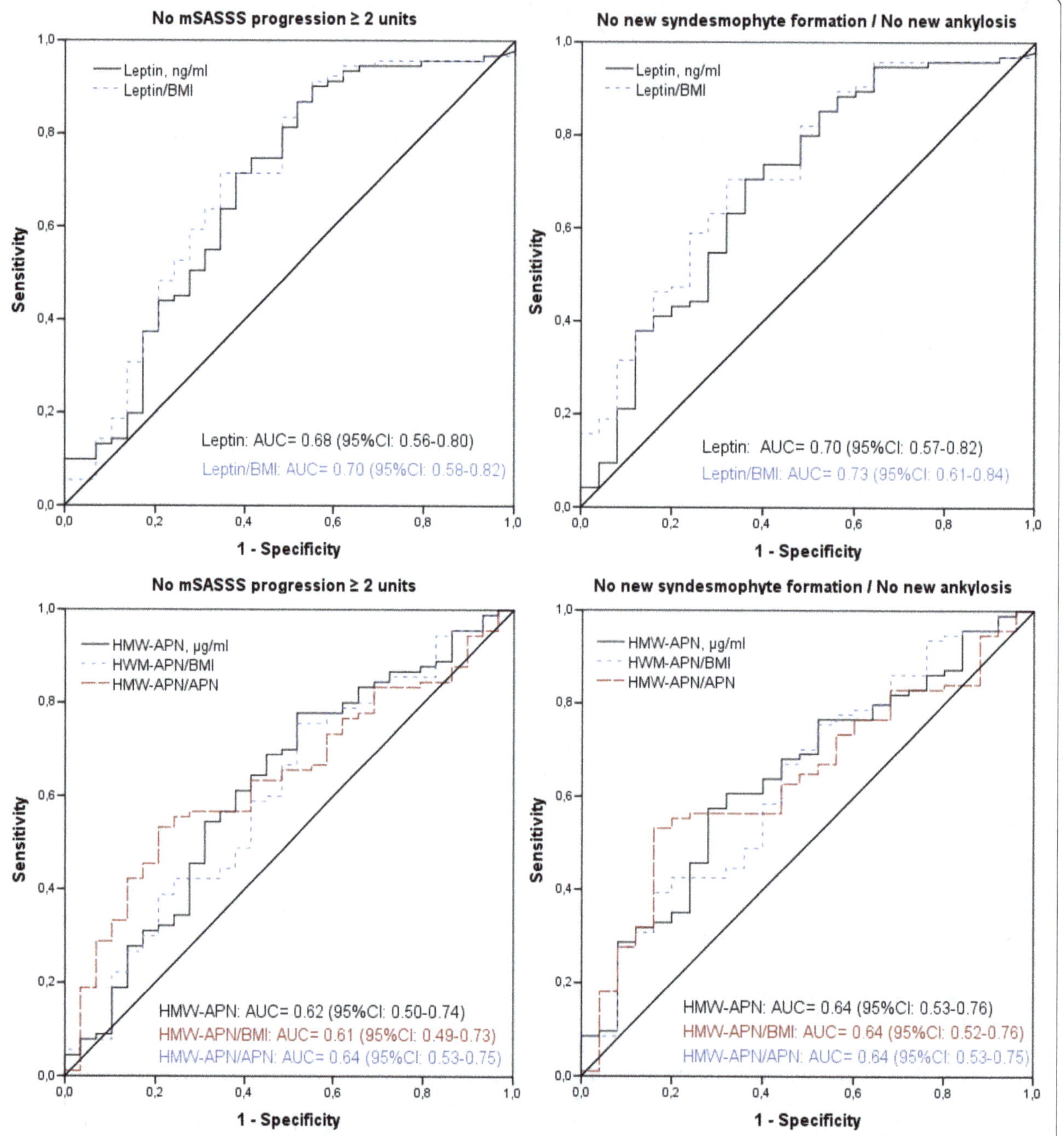

Fig. 1 Receiver operating characteristic analysis: association between leptin and high molecular weight adiponectin (*HMW-APN*) serum levels and radiographic spinal progression after 2 years. Baseline serum levels of leptin and HMW-APN shown as crude values and as values corrected for body mass index and adiponectin (only HMW-APN). *mSASSS* modified Stoke Ankylosing Spondylitis Spine Score, *AUC* area under the curve

radiographic spinal progression. Initially, we investigated eight adipokines and only those with evidence suggesting an association with radiographic progression were entered the main analysis. We have chosen the homogeneous population of the ENRADAS trial consisting of patients with advanced AS. The lack of differences in radiographic spinal progression between the study arms justified pooling both groups of patients (treated with NSAIDs continuously or on demand). However, due to some change in the leptin level over 2 years that was especially evident in the continuous treatment group, the parameter estimates in the regression analysis were adjusted for NSAID intake.

In the study population, leptin and HMW-APN levels were higher in female patients with AS compared to male patients, even after adjustment for BMI. At the

Table 3 Sex-related differences in serum leptin and high molecular weight adiponectin at baseline

	Males (n = 82)	Females (n = 38)	P[a]
Leptin, ng/mL	10.6 ± 6.9	24.4 ± 17.3	<0.001
Leptin/BMI	0.37 ± 0.19	0.84 ± 0.47	<0.001
HMW-APN, µg/mL	5.07 ± 3.06	8.04 ± 5.07	<0.001
HMW-APN/BMI	0.19 ± 0.13	0.32 ± 0.23	0.001
HMW-APN/APN	0.52 ± 0.23	0.61 ± 0.22	0.020

APN adiponectin, *HMW-APN* high molecular weight adiponectin, *BMI* body mass index. [a]Mann-Whitney *U* test

same time, there was no association between BMI and radiographic spinal progression. There are data on gender-dependent differences in adipokine levels in the general population [29, 30]. In one study, leptin and APN levels were higher in women than in men independent of BMI or waist-to-hip ratio [29], while in another study such an association was shown for leptin, but not for adiponectin [30]. Similarly, differences in adipokine levels between male and female patients have also been described in patients with AS [17, 31]. Such an association between sex and adipokine levels is especially interesting in the context of the current study, since the women in our study also had significantly lower mSASSS scores than men. It has been shown several times that female patients with AS develop new bone formation to a lesser extent than male patients with AS [5, 20]. Therefore, we can speculate that leptin and HMW-APN might be biomarkers (or even pathophysiological factors) linking gender with radiographic spinal progression in patients with AS.

Remarkably, in the analyses stratified by sex, an association between adipokines and radiographic spinal progression was evident in male patients only. On the one hand, the absence of association between serum adipokine and radiographic spinal progression in female patients could be related to the smaller sample size and a small number of progressors in the female group. On the other hand, female patients had generally higher levels of leptin and adiponectin in comparison to male patients, suggesting that in female patients who progressed after 2 years, there could have been other factors playing a part.

In our previous study involving patients from the German Spondyloarthropathy Inception Cohort (GESPIC) cohort, who had early axial SpA, we found a positive association between visfatin and radiographic spinal progression; leptin and HMW-APN were not investigated [17]. In the current study, we found only a trend for such an association for visfatin that might be related to the differences in disease duration in the GESPIC (early disease) and ENRADAS (rather advanced disease) studies or to the test system used.

Until now, serum adipokines and their relationship to clinical or radiographic parameters in AS have only been investigated in a few small trials. In some studies, leptin serum was found to be lower in patients with AS compared to healthy controls [32–34], but in others there were either no differences or even higher leptin serum

Table 4 Baseline serum leptin and HMW-APN in relation to radiographic spinal progression after 2 years

	All patients (n = 120)			Male patients (n = 82)			Female patients (n = 38)		
Outcome: mSASSS progression ≥2 points after 2 years									
	Progressors (n = 29)	Non-progressors (n = 91)	p[a]	Progressors (n = 22)	Non-progressors (n = 60)	p[a]	Progressors (n = 7)	Non-progressors (n = 31)	p[a]
Leptin, ng/mL	10.5 ± 9.0	16.4 ± 13.7	0.003	7.0 ± 4.7	11.9 ± 7.1	0.001	21.7 ± 10.5	25.0 ± 18.6	0.96
Leptin/BMI	0.38 ± 0.31	0.57 ± 0.38	0.001	0.25 ± 0.14	0.42 ± 0.19	<0.001	0.78 ± 0.35	0.86 ± 0.49	0.84
HMW-APN, µg/mL	4.95 ± 3.52	6.35 ± 4.15	0.045	3.93 ± 2.56	5.49 ± 3.15	0.018	8.16 ± 4.37	8.02 ± 5.27	0.75
HMW-APN/BMI	0.19 ± 0.14	0.25 ± 0.19	0.089	0.15 ± 0.11	0.21 ± 0.13	0.052	0.32 ± 0.18	0.33 ± 0.24	0.84
HMW-APN/APN	0.47 ± 0.19	0.57 ± 0.23	0.024	0.42 ± 0.14	0.56 ± 0.24	0.033	0.62 ± 0.25	0.60 ± 0.22	0.82
Outcome: syndesmophyte formation/progression after 2 years									
	Progressors (n = 25)	Non-progressors (n = 95)	p[a]	Progressors (n = 21)	Non-progressors (n = 61)	p[a]	Progressors (n = 4)	Non-progressors (n = 34)	p[a]
Leptin, ng/mL	10.2 ± 9.6	16.2 ± 13.4	0.003	9.0 ± 9.1	11.1 ± 5.9	0.018	16.4 ± 10.9	25.3 ± 17.8	0.27
Leptin/BMI	0.33 ± 0.22	0.57 ± 0.39	0.001	0.29 ± 0.19	0.40 ± 0.18	0.006	0.56 ± 0.23	0.88 ± 0.48	0.13
HMW-APN, µg/mL	4.53 ± 2.86	6.4 ± 4.22	0.026	4.1 ± 2.58	5.4 ± 3.17	0.075	6.8 ± 3.6	8.2 ± 5.23	0.85
HMW-APN/BMI	0.18 ± 0.13	0.25 ± 0.19	0.035	0.16 ± 0.11	0.21 ± 0.13	0.081	0.28 ± 0.18	0.33 ± 0.24	0.81
HMW-APN/APN	0.46 ± 0.2	0.57 ± 0.23	0.033	0.42 ± 0.15	0.55 ± 0.24	0.057	0.68 ± 0.32	0.60 ± 0.21	0.81

APN adiponectin, *HMW-APN* high molecular weight adiponectin, *BMI* body mass index, *mSASSS* modified Stoke Ankylosing Spondylitis Spine Score. [a]Mann-Whitney *U* test

Table 5 Analysis of the association of leptin and HMW-APN with radiographic spinal progression after 2 years

	OR unadjusted	95% CI	OR adjusted[a]	95% CI
Outcome: no mSASSS progression after 2 years (logistic regression)				
Leptin, ng/mL	1.06	1.003 to 1.12	1.16	1.03 to 1.29
Leptin/BMI	9.20	1.44 to 58.7	28.7	2.24 to 367.7
HMW-APN, µg/mL	1.12	0.98 to 1.27	1.17	0.99 to 1.38
HMW-APN/BMI	9.68	0.48 to 196.2	10.7	0.35 to 320.6
HMW-APN/APN	10.81	1.25 to 93.5	22.2	1.57 to 313.1
Outcome: no syndesmophyte formation/progression after 2 years (logistic regression)				
Leptin, ng/mL	1.07	1.002 to 1.14	1.29	1.11 to 1.50
Leptin/BMI	36.5	3.29 to 404.5	131.9	4.78 to 3638
HMW-APN, µg/mL	1.18	1.01 to 1.39	1.18	0.98 to 1.42
HMW-APN/BMI	34.3	0.89 to 1319	23.8	0.41 to 1382
HMW-APN/APN	10.9	1.11 to 106.3	10.8	0.74 to 156.1

[a]Adjusted for the presence of syndesmophytes at baseline, C-reactive protein at baseline, sex, non-steroidal anti-inflammatory drugs intake score over 2 years, and smoking status at baseline. Models with leptin, HMW-APN and HMW-APN/APN ratio were additionally adjusted for body mass index (BMI). *APN* adiponectin, *CI* confidence interval, *HMW-APN* high molecular weight adiponectin, *mSASSS* modified Stoke Ankylosing Spondylitis Spine Score, *OR* odds ratio

levels in patients with AS [35–37]. A meta-analysis from Mei et al, which included eight studies that had compared leptin levels in patients with AS with those in healthy controls, came to the conclusion that there are no significant differences in leptin levels in patients with AS vs. controls [38]. Differences in serum APN (including the HMW isoform) have also not been identified at group level in patients with AS and healthy controls [17, 32, 34]. However, in one study serum APN was higher in male patients with AS versus healthy controls, and at the same time there was almost no correlation between leptin or APN and inflammatory activity, and anti-inflammatory treatment (anti-TNF-α) did not have an effect on serum leptin and APN [35].

Data on the association between structural damage in the spine and leptin in AS are very limited. In one study, higher serum leptin was positively associated with the presence of syndesmophytes in a cross-sectional analysis; however, no prospective data were reported [36]. In the aforementioned study of patients with early axial SpA, APN was only numerically higher in non-progressors, but the HMW isoform was not investigated [17].

What are the possible mechanisms linking leptin and adiponectin with radiographic spinal progression in AS? Adipokines are known to be involved in the regulation of immune processes, displaying both pro-inflammatory and anti-inflammatory effects, and in bone metabolism that explains their possible relationship with the pathophysiology of chronic inflammatory conditions such as rheumatoid arthritis or AS [21, 22, 39]. Our current observation of a protective effect of leptin and APN (especially its HMW isoform) against radiographic spinal progression in AS can probably be best explained by the effects of both molecules on the process of osteogenesis, since there is no association between adipokines and inflammatory activity as measured by CRP.

Many studies have previously assessed the part played by leptin in bone metabolism; however, published data show both positive and negative effects of leptin on bone formation [40]. Two main regulatory pathways are currently discussed. One targets the central nervous system, the other one acts through peripheral regulation [41]. The peripheral effect is based on a rather direct interaction of leptin with several bone cell types. For instance, leptin enhances new bone formation through interaction with bone marrow stem cells, which can either differentiate into osteoblasts or into adipocytes. It promotes differentiation and growth of osteoblasts and enhances bone mineralization [42–44]. Furthermore, leptin administered peripherally can inhibit formation of human osteoclasts [44, 45].

In contrast, a central regulatory effect of leptin on bone metabolism is rather anti-osteoproliferative. It has been shown that bone loss could be induced in leptin-deficient mice through an intracerebrovascular infusion of leptin [46], indicating a role of leptin as a hormone which induces pathways of the sympathetic nervous system (SNS) through the ventromedial hypothalamus (VMH), which then results in bone loss. Further studies have confirmed this theory [47, 48]. The available evidence indicates that leptin binds to its receptors on neurons of the VMH, which then activate a signal pathway from the VMH to osteoblasts via β2 adrenergic receptors of the SNS.

Table 6 Analysis of association of leptin and HMW-APN with radiographic spinal progression stratified by sex

	OR unadjusted	95% CI	OR adjusted[a]	95% CI
Men (n = 82)				
Outcome: no mSASSS progression ≥2 points after 2 years (logistic regression)				
Leptin, ng/mL	1.20	1.06 to 1.36	1.45	1.18 to 1.78
Leptin/BMI	725.2	15.4 to 34099	4818.9	33.3 to 698123
HMW-APN µg/mL	1.25	1.002 to 1.57	1.35	1.04 to 1.75
HMW-APN/BMI	81.8	0.53 to 12683	186.4	0.63 to 54915
HMW-APN/APN	40.5	2.01 to 813.9	173.6	4.03 to 7479
Outcome: no syndesmophyte formation/progression after 2 years (logistic regression)				
Leptin, ng/mL	1.06	0.97 to 1.16	1.34	1.11 to 1.62
Leptin/BMI	54.5	1.99 to 1491	241.8	3.51 to 16651
HMW-APN, µg/mL	1.20	0.97 to 1.48	1.21	0.95 to 1.53
HMW-APN/BMI	55.3	0.37 to 8262	77.9	0.32 to 19249
HMW-APN/APN	31.5	1.60 to 621.5	55.6	1.56 to 1973
Women (n = 38)				
Outcome: no mSASSS progression ≥2 points after 2 years (logistic regression)				
Leptin, ng/mL	1.01	0.96 to 1.07	1.04	0.95 to 1.14
Leptin/BMI	1.53	0.21 to 11.29	1.67	0.15 to 18.8
HMW-APN, µg/mL	0.99	0.85 to 1.17	1.04	0.85 to 1.27
HMW-APN/BMI	1.22	0.03 to 48.9	3.03	0.05 to 196.9
HMW-APN/APN	0.69	0.02 to 30.4	0.47	0.003 to 68.6
Outcome: no syndesmophyte formation/progression after 2 years (logistic regression)				
Leptin, ng/mL	1.05	0.95 to 1.16	1.17	0.90 to 1.51
Leptin/BMI	20.5	0.23 to 1872	18.7	0.06 to 5989
HMW-APN, µg/mL	1.07	0.83 to 1.38	1.13	0.84 to 1.51
HMW-APN/BMI	3.48	0.02 to 738.3	14.8	0.03 to 7869
HMW-APN/APN	0.15	0.001 to 21.4	0.15	0.0004 to 59.5

[a]Adjusted for the presence of syndesmophytes at baseline, C reactive protein at baseline, non steroidal anti inflammatory drugs intake score over two years, and smoking status at baseline. Models with leptin, high molecular weight adiponectin (HMW-APN) and HMW-APN/adiponectin (APN) ratio were additionally adjusted for body mass index (BMI). *CI* confidence interval, *mSASSS* modified Stoke Ankylosing Spondylitis Spine Score, *OR* odds ratio

Through the signals of the SNS two cascades in osteoblasts are activated leading to increased osteoclast formation and decreased osteoblast differentiation [41].

Hamrick et al. proved in 2004 that the effects of leptin on the skeleton differ between skeletal regions. Comparing leptin-deficient obese mice (ob/ob) with lean mice they found that ob/ob mice had significantly reduced femoral bone mineral density (BMD), bone mineral content (BMC), cortical thickness and trabecular bone volume compared to lean mice. On the other hand, they found ob/ob mice to have higher BMC, BMD and trabecular bone volume in the lumbar spine than the lean mice. Hence, their study suggests that leptin regulates bone metabolism differently according to the location within the skeleton [49]. Martin et al. found in 2007 that there could be a bimodal threshold response to serum leptin levels, meaning that slight increases in leptin might initially stimulate bone formation, while higher leptin levels inhibit bone formation [50].

Thus, leptin might have contradictory effects on bone metabolism that also depend on the localization of the bone. We hypothesize that in patients with AS a higher level of leptin has protective properties against radiographic spinal progression mainly via the central pathway with inhibition of excessive new bone formation.

As for APN, different effects on bone metabolism have been discovered as well, yielding similarly conflicting results. APN was found to be expressed in osteoblasts along with its receptors and to stimulate their proliferation and differentiation, for example, through enhancement of the expression of bone morphogenetic protein 2 (BMP-2) [51–53]. Additionally, APN was found to be able to suppress osteoclastogenesis and promote osteoblastogenesis [54]. However, APN is also able to indirectly activate osteoclasts by stimulating receptor activator of nuclear factor kappa-B (NFκB) ligand (RANKL) and inhibiting osteoprotegerin (OPG) production in osteoblasts, which are known to be essential stimulators of osteoclastogenesis [55].

An inverse relationship between APN and BMD was found in vivo in a number of studies [39] indicating that APN might have predominantly catabolic effects on bone. In line with this, the meta-analysis of Biver et al., which included 59 studies of healthy male and female patients who were evaluated for BMD or fracture risk and adipokines, showed that APN seems to be the most important adipokine that is negatively associated with BMD [56].

There are two main circulating isoforms of APN in the blood stream: one low molecular weight (LMW) hexamer and the HMW multimer [28, 57]. Previous data suggest that HMW-APN might be the predominantly active isoform and that the HMW-APN/APN ratio might be an important determinant of the metabolic effects of the hormone [28]. The importance of the HMW-APN/APN ratio was also confirmed in another study, in which the ratio was a better predictor of insulin resistance and metabolic syndrome than total plasma APN [58]. In line with these data, we found that HMW-APN (and to a further extent the HMW-APN/APN ratio) was inversely associated with radiographic spinal progression in AS, and the association between radiographic progression and HMW-APN was better than that between radiographic progression and total APN.

Our study has limitations. First, this was an analysis based on a population of a randomized controlled trial. Although we corrected our analysis for differences in the intervention, we cannot completely exclude bias resulting from treatment. Further, only relatively few women were included in this trial, which made the interpretation of the subgroup analysis results difficult in this population. Also, no fat mass measurement was performed in the ENRADAS trial beyond BMI calculation. Finally, since no biologic agents were allowed in the ENRADAS trial it is currently unclear whether leptin and HMW-APN might also have protective effects against radiographic spinal progression in patients treated with anti-TNF or anti-interleukin-17 drugs. Therefore, an independent validation of our results is highly desirable not only in patients treated with NSAIDs but also in patients undergoing biologic treatment. Despite a significant association with radiographic spinal progression, leptin or HMW-APN alone would not be sufficient for identification of patients at high (or low) risk of radiographic spinal progression. However, these biomarkers seem to be good candidates for inclusion in multi-parameter predictive models for estimation of the risk of radiographic spinal progression in AS.

Conclusion

Serum levels of leptin and HMW-APN are inversely associated with radiographic spinal progression in patients with AS. Current data on the role of adipokines in bone metabolism indicates that leptin and HMW-APN might not only be markers but also true pathophysiological factors influencing new bone formation in AS. Female patients with AS have a higher level of leptin and APN, which might play a natural protective role against radiographic spinal progression in AS, explaining the generally lower prevalence of extended new bone formation in the spine in female patients with AS.

Abbreviations

ANCOVA: Analysis of covariance; APN: Adiponectin; AS: Ankylosing spondylitis; ASDAS: Ankylosing Spondylitis Disease Activity Score; BMC: Bone mineral content; BMD: Bone mineral density; BMI: Body mass index; BMP-2: Bone morphogenetic protein 2; CRP: C-reactive protein; ELISA: Enzyme-linked immunosorbent assays; ENRADAS: Effects of NSAIDs on radiographic damage in AS; GESPIC: German spondyloarthropathy inception cohort; HMW-APN: High molecular weight adiponectin; LMW: Low molecular weight; MRI: Magnetic resonance imaging; mSASSS: Modified Stoke Ankylosing Spondylitis spine score; NFκB: Nuclear factor kappa B; NSAIDs: Non-steroidal anti-inflammatory drugs; OPG: Osteoprotegerin; RANKL: Receptor activator of NFκB ligand; ROC: Receiver operating characteristic; SNS: Sympathetic nervous system; SpA: Spondyloarthritides; TNF: Tumor necrosis factor; VMH: Ventromedial hypothalamus

Acknowledgements

We would like to thank the participating patients and study centers: PD Dr. J. Brandt-Jürgens, Berlin; Prof. Dr. J. Braun, Herne; Dr. K. Karberg, Berlin; Dr. S. Jacki, Tübingen; Dr. N. Rinaldi, Ulm; Prof. K. Manger, Bamberg; Dr. W. Ochs, Bayreuth; Prof. H. Kellner, München; Dr. K-H. Göttl, Passau; Dr. R. Dockhorn, Weener; Dr. U. Schoo, Rheine; Dr. F. Heldmann, Herne; Dr. D. Pick, Grafschaft Bad Neuenahr-Ahrweiler; Dr. A. Gräßler, Pirna; Dr. C. Kühne, Haldensleben, Dr. F. Mielke, Berlin, Dr. T. Schneider-Stiebler, Wismar, Prof. C. Kneitz, Rostock. We thank Dr. In-Ho Song who was actively involved in the preparation and the initial phase of the study. Special thanks to Renate Lies and Beate Buss who coordinated the trial. We would also like to thank the external members of the Data and Safety Monitoring Board (DSMB) Prof. Désirée van der Heijde, Leiden, The Netherlands, Prof. Bernhard Manger, Erlangen, Germany, and Dr. Wolfgang Bolten, Wiesbaden, for their expert advice. We further appreciate the data management and statistical support from Dr. Johanna Callhoff. Finally, we would like to thank Torsten Karge (Clinical Guideline Service, Hamburg, Germany) for establishing the scoring interface for the reading of images.

Funding

This ENRADAS trial was funded by the German Ministry of Education and Research (Bundesministerium für Bildung und Forschung - BMBF), grant number: FKZ 01KG0801. The biomarker analysis was conducted as a part of METARTHROS (grant number FKZ 01EC1407A) and ArthroMark (FKZ 01EC1401A) projects funded by BMBF; additional support was obtained from the clinical research unit (CRU) of the Berlin Institute of Health (BIH). The initial study drug diclofenac was provided by Novartis as a donation.

Authors' contributions

AH: design of the adipokine substudy, acquisition of data, statistical analysis and interpretation of the results, and drafting the manuscript. JS, MR: conception and design of the ENRADAS study, data acquisition, analysis and interpretation of the data, and revising the manuscript. US: data acquisition, analysis and interpretation of the data, and revising of the manuscript. JL:

conception and design of the ENRADAS study, analysis and interpretation of the data, and revising the manuscript. KGH: data acquisition, analysis and interpretation of the data, and revising the manuscript. DP: conception and design of the adipokine substudy, data acquisition, analysis and interpretation of the data, and drafting the manuscript. The final version of the manuscript to be published was approved by all authors.

Competing interests

The authors declare no competing interests. The study drug diclofenac was provided by Novartis, but Novartis did not have any influence on the design, conduct and analysis of the trial.

Author details

[1]Department of Gastroenterology, Infectiology and Rheumatology, Charité Universitätsmedizin Berlin, Hindenburgdamm 30, 12203 Berlin, Germany. [2]German Rheumatism Research Centre, Charitéplatz 1, 10117 Berlin, Germany. [3]Department of Radiology, Charité Universitätsmedizin Berlin, Charitéplatz 1, 10117 Berlin, Germany. [4]Klinikum Bielefeld Rosenhöhe, An der Rosenhöhe 27, 33647 Bielefeld, Germany.

References

1. van Tubergen A, Ramiro S, van der Heijde D, Dougados M, Mielants H, Landewe R. Development of new syndesmophytes and bridges in ankylosing spondylitis and their predictors: a longitudinal study. Ann Rheum Dis. 2012;71(4):518–23.
2. Landewe R, Dougados M, Mielants H, van der Tempel H, van der Heijde D. Physical function in ankylosing spondylitis is independently determined by both disease activity and radiographic damage of the spine. Ann Rheum Dis. 2009;68(6):863–7.
3. Machado P, Landewe R, Braun J, Hermann KG, Baker D, van der Heijde D. Both structural damage and inflammation of the spine contribute to impairment of spinal mobility in patients with ankylosing spondylitis. Ann Rheum Dis. 2010;69(8):1465–70.
4. Baraliakos X, Listing J, von der Recke A, Braun J. The natural course of radiographic progression in ankylosing spondylitis–evidence for major individual variations in a large proportion of patients. J Rheumatol. 2009; 36(5):997–1002.
5. Ramiro S, Stolwijk C, van Tubergen A, van der Heijde D, Dougados M, van den Bosch F, et al. Evolution of radiographic damage in ankylosing spondylitis: a 12 year prospective follow-up of the OASIS study. Ann Rheum Dis. 2015;74(1):52–9.
6. Ramiro S, van der Heijde D, van Tubergen A, Stolwijk C, Dougados M, van den Bosch F, et al. Higher disease activity leads to more structural damage in the spine in ankylosing spondylitis: 12-year longitudinal data from the OASIS cohort. Ann Rheum Dis. 2014;73(8):1455–61.
7. Poddubnyy D, Haibel H, Listing J, Marker-Hermann E, Zeidler H, Braun J, et al. Baseline radiographic damage, elevated acute-phase reactant levels, and cigarette smoking status predict spinal radiographic progression in early axial spondylarthritis. Arthritis Rheum. 2012;64(5):1388–98.
8. Poddubnyy D, Protopopov M, Haibel H, Braun J, Rudwaleit M, Sieper J. High disease activity according to the Ankylosing Spondylitis Disease Activity Score is associated with accelerated radiographic spinal progression in patients with early axial spondyloarthritis: results from the GErman SPondyloarthritis Inception Cohort. Ann Rheum Dis. 2016; 75(12):2114–8.
9. Baraliakos X, Listing J, Rudwaleit M, Sieper J, Braun J. The relationship between inflammation and new bone formation in patients with ankylosing spondylitis. Arthritis Res Ther. 2008;10(5):R104.
10. van der Heijde D, Machado P, Braun J, Hermann KG, Baraliakos X, Hsu B, et al. MRI inflammation at the vertebral unit only marginally predicts new syndesmophyte formation: a multilevel analysis in patients with ankylosing spondylitis. Ann Rheum Dis. 2012;71(3):369–73.
11. Baraliakos X, Heldmann F, Callhoff J, Listing J, Appelboom T, Brandt J, et al. Which spinal lesions are associated with new bone formation in patients with ankylosing spondylitis treated with anti-TNF agents? A long-term observational study using MRI and conventional radiography. Ann Rheum Dis. 2014;73(10):1819–25.
12. Machado PM, Baraliakos X, van der Heijde D, Braun J, Landewe R. MRI vertebral corner inflammation followed by fat deposition is the strongest contributor to the development of new bone at the same vertebral corner: a multilevel longitudinal analysis in patients with ankylosing spondylitis. Ann Rheum Dis. 2016;75(8):1486–93.
13. Poddubnyy D, Haibel H, Listing J, Marker-Hermann E, Zeidler H, Braun J, et al. Cigarette smoking has a dose-dependent impact on progression of structural damage in the spine in patients with axial spondyloarthritis: results from the GErman SPondyloarthritis Inception Cohort (GESPIC). Ann Rheum Dis. 2013;72(8):1430–2.
14. Maksymowych WP, Landewe R, Conner-Spady B, Dougados M, Mielants H, van der Tempel H, et al. Serum matrix metalloproteinase 3 is an independent predictor of structural damage progression in patients with ankylosing spondylitis. Arthritis Rheum. 2007;56(6): 1846–53.
15. Poddubnyy D, Conrad K, Haibel H, Syrbe U, Appel H, Braun J, et al. Elevated serum level of the vascular endothelial growth factor predicts radiographic spinal progression in patients with axial spondyloarthritis. Ann Rheum Dis. 2014;73(12):2137–43.
16. Turina MC, Sieper J, Yeremenko N, Conrad K, Haibel H, Rudwaleit M, et al. Calprotectin serum level is an independent marker for radiographic spinal progression in axial spondyloarthritis. Ann Rheum Dis. 2014;73(9):1746–8.
17. Syrbe U, Callhoff J, Conrad K, Poddubnyy D, Haibel H, Junker S, et al. Serum adipokine levels in patients with ankylosing spondylitis and their relationship to clinical parameters and radiographic spinal progression. Arthritis Rheumatol. 2015;67(3):678–85.
18. Appel H, Ruiz-Heiland G, Listing J, Zwerina J, Herrmann M, Mueller R, et al. Altered skeletal expression of sclerostin and its link to radiographic progression in ankylosing spondylitis. Arthritis Rheum. 2009;60(11):3257–62.
19. Heiland GR, Appel H, Poddubnyy D, Zwerina J, Hueber A, Haibel H, et al. High level of functional dickkopf-1 predicts protection from syndesmophyte formation in patients with ankylosing spondylitis. Ann Rheum Dis. 2012; 71(4):572–4.
20. Feldtkeller E, Bruckel J, Khan MA. Scientific contributions of ankylosing spondylitis patient advocacy groups. Curr Opin Rheumatol. 2000;12(4): 239–47.
21. Ouchi N, Parker JL, Lugus JJ, Walsh K. Adipokines in inflammation and metabolic disease. Nat Rev Immunol. 2011;11(2):85–97.
22. Neumann E, Junker S, Schett G, Frommer K, Muller-Ladner U. Adipokines in bone disease. Nat Rev Rheumatol. 2016;12(5):296–302.
23. Sieper J, Listing J, Poddubnyy D, Song IH, Hermann KG, Callhoff J, et al. Effect of continuous versus on-demand treatment of ankylosing spondylitis with diclofenac over 2 years on radiographic progression of the spine: results from a randomised multicentre trial (ENRADAS). Ann Rheum Dis. 2016;75(8):1438–43.
24. Creemers MC, Franssen MJ, van't Hof MA, Gribnau FW, van de Putte LB, van Riel PL. Assessment of outcome in ankylosing spondylitis: an extended radiographic scoring system. Ann Rheum Dis. 2005;64(1):127–9.
25. Abella V, Scotece M, Conde J, Lopez V, Lazzaro V, Pino J, et al. Adipokines, Metabolic Syndrome and Rheumatic Diseases. J Immunol Res. 2014;2014:343746.
26. Neumann E, Frommer KW, Vasile M, Muller-Ladner U. Adipocytokines as driving forces in rheumatoid arthritis and related inflammatory diseases? Arthritis Rheum. 2011;63(5):1159–69.
27. Wang Y, Lam KS, Kraegen EW, Sweeney G, Zhang J, Tso AW, et al. Lipocalin-2 is an inflammatory marker closely associated with obesity, insulin resistance, and hyperglycemia in humans. Clin Chem. 2007;53(1):34–41.
28. Pajvani UB, Hawkins M, Combs TP, Rajala MW, Doebber T, Berger JP, et al. Complex distribution, not absolute amount of adiponectin, correlates with thiazolidinedione-mediated improvement in insulin sensitivity. J Biol Chem. 2004;279(13):12152–62.
29. Andreasson AN, Unden AL, Elofsson S, Brismar K. Leptin and adiponectin: distribution and associations with cardiovascular risk factors in men and women of the general population. Am J Hum Biol. 2012;24(5):595–601.
30. Lew J, Sanghavi M, Ayers CR, McGuire DK, Omland T, Atzler D, et al. Sex-based differences in cardiometabolic biomarkers. Circulation. 2017; 135(6):544–55.

31. Miranda-Filloy JA, Lopez-Mejias R, Genre F, Carnero-Lopez B, Ochoa R. Diaz de Teran T, et al. Leptin and visfatin serum levels in non-diabetic ankylosing spondylitis patients undergoing TNF-alpha antagonist therapy. Clin Exp Rheumatol. 2013;31(4):538–45.
32. Toussirot E, Streit G, Nguyen NU, Dumoulin G, Le Huede G, Saas P, et al. Adipose tissue, serum adipokines, and ghrelin in patients with ankylosing spondylitis. Metabolism. 2007;56(10):1383–9.
33. Sari I, Demir T, Kozaci LD, Akar S, Kavak T, Birlik M, et al. Body composition, insulin, and leptin levels in patients with ankylosing spondylitis. Clin Rheumatol. 2007;26(9):1427–32.
34. Toussirot E, Grandclement E, Gaugler B, Michel F, Wendling D, Saas P, et al. Serum adipokines and adipose tissue distribution in rheumatoid arthritis and ankylosing spondylitis.A comparative study. Front Immunol. 2013;4:453.
35. Derdemezis CS, Filippatos TD, Voulgari PV, Tselepis AD, Drosos AA, Kiortsis DN. Leptin and adiponectin levels in patients with ankylosing spondylitis. The effect of infliximab treatment. Clin Exp Rheumatol. 2010;28(6):880–3.
36. Kim KJ, Kim JY, Park SJ, Yoon H, Yoon CH, Kim WU, et al. Serum leptin levels are associated with the presence of syndesmophytes in male patients with ankylosing spondylitis. Clin Rheumatol. 2012;31(8):1231–8.
37. Park MC, Lee SW, Choi ST, Park YB, Lee SK. Serum leptin levels correlate with interleukin-6 levels and disease activity in patients with ankylosing spondylitis. Scand J Rheumatol. 2007;36(2):101–6.
38. Mei YJ, Wang P, Chen LJ, Li ZJ. Plasma/serum leptin levels in patients with ankylosing spondylitis: a systematic review and meta-analysis. Arch Med Res. 2016;47(2):111–7.
39. Scotece M, Conde J, Abella V, Lopez V, Pino J, Lago F, et al. Bone metabolism and adipokines: are there perspectives for bone diseases drug discovery? Expert opinion on drug discovery. May. 2014;24:1–13.
40. Vadacca M, Margiotta DP, Navarini L, Afeltra A. Leptin in immuno-rheumatological diseases. Cell Mol Immunol. 2011;8(3):203–12.
41. Chen XX, Yang T. Roles of leptin in bone metabolism and bone diseases. J Bone Miner Metab. 2015;33(5):474–85.
42. Thomas T, Gori F, Khosla S, Jensen MD, Burguera B, Riggs BL. Leptin acts on human marrow stromal cells to enhance differentiation to osteoblasts and to inhibit differentiation to adipocytes. Endocrinology. 1999;140(4):1630–8.
43. Reseland JE, Syversen U, Bakke I, Qvigstad G, Eide LG, Hjertner O, et al. Leptin is expressed in and secreted from primary cultures of human osteoblasts and promotes bone mineralization. J Bone Miner Res. 2001; 16(8):1426–33.
44. Gordeladze JO, Drevon CA, Syversen U, Reseland JE. Leptin stimulates human osteoblastic cell proliferation, de novo collagen synthesis, and mineralization: Impact on differentiation markers, apoptosis, and osteoclastic signaling. J Cell Biochem. 2002;85(4):825–36.
45. Holloway WR, Collier FM, Aitken CJ, Myers DE, Hodge JM, Malakellis M, et al. Leptin inhibits osteoclast generation. J Bone Miner Res. 2002;17(2): 200–9.
46. Ducy P, Amling M, Takeda S, Priemel M, Schilling AF, Beil FT, et al. Leptin inhibits bone formation through a hypothalamic relay: a central control of bone mass. Cell. 2000;100(2):197–207.
47. Takeda S, Elefteriou F, Levasseur R, Liu X, Zhao L, Parker KL, et al. Leptin regulates bone formation via the sympathetic nervous system. Cell. 2002; 111(3):305–17.
48. Elefteriou F, Ahn JD, Takeda S, Starbuck M, Yang X, Liu X, et al. Leptin regulation of bone resorption by the sympathetic nervous system and CART. Nature. 2005;434(7032):514–20.
49. Hamrick MW, Pennington C, Newton D, Xie D, Isales C. Leptin deficiency produces contrasting phenotypes in bones of the limb and spine. Bone. 2004;34(3):376–83.
50. Martin A, David V, Malaval L, Lafage-Proust MH, Vico L, Thomas T. Opposite effects of leptin on bone metabolism: a dose-dependent balance related to energy intake and insulin-like growth factor-I pathway. Endocrinology. 2007; 148(7):3419–25.
51. Berner HS, Lyngstadaas SP, Spahr A, Monjo M, Thommesen L, Drevon CA, et al. Adiponectin and its receptors are expressed in bone-forming cells. Bone. 2004;35(4):842–9.
52. Luo XH, Guo LJ, Yuan LQ, Xie H, Zhou HD, Wu XP, et al. Adiponectin stimulates human osteoblasts proliferation and differentiation via the MAPK signaling pathway. Exp Cell Res. 2005;309(1):99–109.
53. Huang CY, Lee CY, Chen MY, Tsai HC, Hsu HC, Tang CH. Adiponectin increases BMP-2 expression in osteoblasts via AdipoR receptor signaling pathway. J Cell Physiol. 2010;224(2):475–83.
54. Oshima K, Nampei A, Matsuda M, Iwaki M, Fukuhara A, Hashimoto J, et al. Adiponectin increases bone mass by suppressing osteoclast and activating osteoblast. Biochem Biophys Res Commun. 2005;331(2):520–6.
55. Luo XH, Guo LJ, Xie H, Yuan LQ, Wu XP, Zhou HD, et al. Adiponectin stimulates RANKL and inhibits OPG expression in human osteoblasts through the MAPK signaling pathway. J Bone Miner Res. 2006;21(10): 1648–56.
56. Biver E, Salliot C, Combescure C, Gossec L, Hardouin P, Legroux-Gerot I, et al. Influence of adipokines and ghrelin on bone mineral density and fracture risk: a systematic review and meta-analysis. J Clin Endocrinol Metab. 2011; 96(9):2703–13.
57. Şodi R, Hazell MJ, Durham BH, Rees C, Ranganath LR, Fraser WD. The circulating concentration and ratio of total and high molecular weight adiponectin in post-menopausal women with and without osteoporosis and its association with body mass index and biochemical markers of bone metabolism. Clin Biochem. 2009;42(13-14):1375–80.
58. Hara K, Horikoshi M, Yamauchi T, Yago H, Miyazaki O, Ebinuma H, et al. Measurement of the high-molecular weight form of adiponectin in plasma is useful for the prediction of insulin resistance and metabolic syndrome. Diabetes Care. 2006;29(6):1357–62.

16

Serum biomarkers and changes in clinical/MRI evidence of golimumab-treated patients with ankylosing spondylitis: results of the randomized, placebo-controlled GO-RAISE study

Robert D. Inman[1,2*], Xenofon Baraliakos[3], Kay-Geert A. Hermann[4], Jürgen Braun[3], Atul Deodhar[5], Désirée van der Heijde[6], Stephen Xu[7] and Benjamin Hsu[8]

Abstract

Background: In the present study, we evaluated relationships between serum biomarkers and clinical/magnetic resonance imaging (MRI) findings in golimumab-treated patients with ankylosing spondylitis.

Methods: In the GO-RAISE study, 356 patients with ankylosing spondylitis randomly received either placebo ($n = 78$) or golimumab 50 mg or 100 mg ($n = 278$) injections every 4 weeks through week 24 (placebo-controlled); patients continuing GO-RAISE received golimumab through week 252. Up to 139/125 patients had sera collected for biomarkers/serial spine MRI scans (sagittal plane, 1.5-T scanner). Two blinded readers employed modified ankylosing spondylitis spine magnetic resonance imaging score for activity (ASspiMRI-a) and ankylosing spondylitis spine magnetic resonance imaging score for chronicity. Spearman correlations (r_s) were assessed between serum biomarkers ($n = 73$) and Bath Ankylosing Spondylitis Disease Activity Index (BASDAI), C-reactive-protein (CRP)-based Ankylosing Spondylitis Disease Activity Score (ASDAS), modified Stokes Ankylosing Spondylitis Spine Score (mSASSS), and ASspiMRI scores. Serum biomarkers predicting postbaseline spinal fatty lesion development and inflammation were analyzed by logistic regression.

Results: Significant, moderately strong correlations were observed between baseline inflammatory markers interleukin (IL)-6, intracellular adhesion molecule-1, complement component 3 (C3), CRP, haptoglobin, and serum amyloid-P and baseline ASDAS ($r_s = 0.39$–0.66, $p \leq 0.01$). Only baseline leptin significantly correlated with ASDAS improvement at week 104 ($r_s = 0.55$, $p = 0.040$), and only baseline IL-6 significantly predicted mSASSS week 104 change ($\beta = 0.236$, SE $= 0.073$, $p = 0.002$, model $R^2 = 0.093$). By logistic regression, baseline leptin, C3, and tissue inhibitor of metalloproteinase (TIMP)-1 correlated with new fatty lesions per spinal MRI at week 14 and week 104 (both $p < 0.01$). Changes in serum C3 levels at week 4 ($r_s = 0.55$, $p = 0.001$) and week 14 ($r_s = 0.49$, $p = 0.040$) significantly correlated with BASDAI improvement at week 14. Baseline IL-6 and TIMP-1 ($r_s = -0.63$, -0.67; $p < 0.05$) and reductions at week 4 in IL-6 ($r_s = 0.61$, $p < 0.05$) and C3 ($r_s = 0.72$; $p < 0.05$) significantly correlated with week 14 ASspiMRI-a improvement.

(Continued on next page)

* Correspondence: robert.inman@uhn.ca
[1]Department of Immunology, University of Toronto, Toronto, ON, Canada
[2]Department of Medicine, University of Toronto, Toronto, ON, Canada
Full list of author information is available at the end of the article

(Continued from previous page)

Conclusions: Extensive serum biomarker multiparametric analyses in golimumab-treated patients with ankylosing spondylitis demonstrated few correlations with disease activity or MRI changes; IL-6 weakly correlated with radiographic progression.

Keywords: ASDAS, Biologic, Monoclonal antibody, MRI, TNF inhibitor

Background

Magnetic resonance imaging (MRI) is now an established outcome instrument in the assessment of treatment for ankylosing spondylitis (AS), based on results of randomized, placebo-controlled studies. Such studies have shown that MRI can provide an objective assessment of response to tumor necrosis factor (TNF) inhibition in patients with AS [1, 2].

In the GO-RAISE trial of golimumab in AS (ClinicalTrials.gov identifier: NCT00265083), patients with active AS showed significant improvement in signs and symptoms after treatment with golimumab [3] that were maintained through 2 years [4]. In the MRI substudy of GO-RAISE, golimumab significantly reduced MRI-detected spinal inflammation, and these observed improvements correlated with improvement in signs and symptoms of disease [5]. Data from observational studies suggest that long-term treatment with TNF antagonists, especially if started early, may inhibit radiographic progression [6]. In another study, a clear causal relationship between the level of inflammation as assessed by the Ankylosing Spondylitis Disease Activity Score (ASDAS) and radiographic progression has been established [7]. Moreover, a moderate relationship between spinal inflammation detected by MRI and syndesmophyte formation has been proven [8–11]. Therefore, we conducted additional analyses of data from the GO-RAISE trial to further assess potential relationships between serum biomarkers of inflammation and clinical measures of disease activity, as well as with spinal inflammation and fatty lesions detected by MRI.

Methods

Patients and study design

The details of the GO-RAISE study have been described previously [3, 4]. The protocol was reviewed and approved by the institutional review board or independent ethics committee at each site of this multicenter trial. (See Acknowledgements section below for further details.) All patients provided written informed consent. The study was conducted at 57 sites in the United States, Canada, Europe, and Asia. The MRI substudy was conducted at ten sites with the capability and willingness to participate. All patients enrolled at participating substudy sites were included in the MRI substudy.

GO-RAISE patients were adults with definite AS (for ≥3 months) according to modified New York criteria, a Bath Ankylosing Spondylitis Disease Activity Index (BASDAI) score ≥4 (0- to 10-point scale), a total back pain score ≥4 on a visual analogue scale (0- to 10-cm scale), and an inadequate response to current or previous nonsteroidal anti-inflammatory drugs (NSAIDs). Patients were randomly assigned in a 1:1.8:1.8 ratio to receive subcutaneous injections every 4 weeks of placebo, golimumab 50 mg, or golimumab 100 mg. Randomization was stratified by investigational site and screening C-reactive protein (CRP) concentration. Patients were allowed to continue stable doses of methotrexate, sulfasalazine, hydroxychloroquine, corticosteroids, and NSAIDs throughout study participation.

At week 16, patients who achieved <20% improvement from baseline in both the total back pain and morning stiffness scores entered into double-blinded early escape, such that patients in the placebo group received golimumab 50 mg, patients in the golimumab 50 mg group received 100 mg, and patients in the golimumab 100-mg group had no change to their study therapy. The placebo-controlled portion of the study ended at week 24, following which all patients who had been receiving placebo injections crossed over to receive golimumab 50 mg. Injections continued to be administered subcutaneously every 4 weeks through week 252, and the last study assessments for the period covered by the current analyses were at week 208.

Biomarker evaluations

Serum samples collected at weeks 0, 4, and 14 of the GO-RAISE trial were tested by Rules Based Medicine (Austin, TX, USA) and Pacific Biomarkers (Seattle, WA, USA) for selected markers using Luminex (Luminex, Austin, TX, USA) and enzyme-linked immunoassay platforms, respectively. The extensive list of candidate biomarkers implicated from previous studies (Additional file 1: Table S1) [12] was selected for correlation analyses with imaging and clinical endpoints, including leptin, interleukin (IL)-6, tissue inhibitor of metalloproteinase (TIMP)-1, complement component 3 (C3), intracellular adhesion molecule (ICAM)-1, CRP, haptoglobin, and serum amyloid-P.

Disease activity and progression evaluations

Clinical assessments of disease activity included the BASDAI [13] and the ASDAS employing CRP [14] determined at weeks 0, 14, and 104. MRI was employed to assess inflammation and structural changes in the spine. Serial spine 1.5-T MRI scans of the cervical, thoracic, and lumbar spine regions in the sagittal plane were acquired at baseline, week 14, and week 104 [5]. Two qualified readers who were blinded to treatment information, patient identity, and chronology of the images independently scored each sequence using modified versions of the ankylosing spondylitis spine magnetic resonance imaging score for activity (ASspiMRI-a) and the Ankylosing spondylitis spine magnetic resonance imaging score for chronicity (ASspiMRI-c) [15, 16]. ASspiMRI-a scoring of each vertebral unit (VU) was previously described [5]. For the modified ASspiMRI-c score, each VU was scored as follows: 0 (normal, no lesions), 1 (minor fatty degeneration), 2 (much fatty degeneration), 3 (one or two syndesmophytes), 4 (more than two syndesmophytes), 5 (vertebral bridging with <25% of disc length and/or bridging of one side), or 6 (vertebral fusion with >25% of disc length and/or bridging of both sides). If a fatty lesion was present in a VU scored 3–6, it was noted. Lateral view radiographs of the cervical and lumbar spine regions were obtained at weeks 0, 104, and 208 and scored by two trained readers blinded to treatment group and chronology using the modified Stokes Ankylosing Spondylitis Spine Score (mSASSS) method [17], as described previously [18].

Data analysis

All analyses of MRI data collected through week 104 employed observed data; missing data were not imputed. Of the unique serum biomarkers tested in this trial, 73 had <80% of values below the lower limit of quantitation at baseline and are included in the analyses described herein (Additional file 1: Table S1).

A total of 4940 analyses were performed to determine Spearman correlation coefficients describing relationships between serum biomarkers at weeks 0, 4, and 14 and subsequent efficacy endpoints, including ASDAS, BASDAI, ASspiMRI-a, ASspiMRI-c (all determined at weeks 0, 14, and 104), and mSASSS (determined at weeks 0, 104, and 208). Correlations at baseline were assessed on the basis of all patients, whereas those at follow-up time points were assessed according to randomized treatment groups (placebo versus golimumab). For all postbaseline assessments, changes from baseline in biomarkers were used. Only correlations found to be statistically significant after Bonferroni multiplicity-of-testing adjustment are reported herein.

Relationships between four biomarker levels (IL-6, leptin, TIMP-1, and C3) and changes from baseline to week 104 in mSASSS were also assessed using a generalized linear model. In this model, mSASSS scores were adjusted for VUs with fat indicated via ASspiMRI-c score at baseline, because the presence of fatty lesions on MRI images is a known contributor to radiographic (mSASSS) progression [19, 20] and because these markers affect adipocytes.

Logistic regression analyses were also conducted to assess the influence of baseline and earlier (week 14) changes in biomarker levels on the development of new fatty lesions on a patient level (yes or no, i.e., not detected by MRI at baseline but detected at week 14 or week 104). In such analyses, all patients were combined, with no adjustment for treatment group or multiplicity of testing. The resulting odds ratios and 95% confidence intervals were determined.

Results

Patient analysis

One hundred thirty-nine patients had serum biomarker data, and 98 of these patients at 10 sites with MRI capability participated in the GO-RAISE MRI substudy. The vast majority of randomized patients (299 [84.0%] of 356) had pre- and posttreatment data obtained for the GO-RAISE radiographic substudy. Of these, up to 139 patients had sera collected for biomarker evaluations, and up to 125 underwent spine MRI scans. As reported previously, the demographic and baseline characteristics for the MRI substudy patients were generally consistent with those of the overall GO-RAISE patient population [5].

Correlations between baseline biomarker levels and baseline disease activity

At baseline among all patients with serum biomarker assessments ($n = 98–139$), significant and moderately strong correlations were observed between ASDAS and levels of the following serum biomarkers of inflammation: IL-6, ICAM-1, haptoglobin, serum amyloid-P, and C3 ($r_s = 0.39–0.59$, all $p \leq 0.01$) (Table 1). As would be expected, ASDAS correlated with CRP ($r_s = 0.66$, $p = 0.00$) (Table 1). With respect to baseline serum markers and baseline spinal inflammation (ASspiMRI-a score) or structural lesions (ASspiMRI-c score), no significant correlations were observed.

Correlations between baseline biomarker levels and subsequent changes in measures of disease activity, radiographic progression, and spinal inflammation

Baseline leptin level was the only significant biomarker correlated with ASDAS clinical improvement at week 104 of golimumab treatment ($r_s = 0.55$, $p = 0.040$). Higher baseline levels of IL-6 ($r_s = -0.63$, $p = 0.009$) and TIMP-1 ($r_s = -0.67$, $p = 0.044$), but not baseline CRP,

Table 1 Correlations between baseline serum biomarker levels and baseline ASDAS

	Baseline ASDAS Spearman correlation coefficient (r_s)		
Baseline serum biomarker	Patients (*n*)	r_s	Bonferroni-adjusted *p* value
IL-6	132	0.59	0.000
ICAM-1	139	0.39	0.011
C3	98	0.53	0.000
CRP	98	0.66	0.000
Haptoglobin	98	0.46	0.010
Serum amyloid-P	98	0.50	0.001

Abbreviations: ASDAS Ankylosing Spondylitis Disease Activity Score employing C-reactive protein, *CRP* C-reactive protein, *C3* Complement component 3, *ICAM-1* Intracellular adhesion molecule-1, *IL* Interleukin

significantly correlated with subsequent improvement in ASspiMRI-a score (i.e., greater reduction) from baseline to week 14 of golimumab treatment (Table 2). All other correlations tested between baseline biomarkers and subsequent changes in measures of disease activity or spinal inflammation yielded insignificant relationships.

Using a generalized linear model to assess the ability of baseline serum leptin, C3, TIMP-1, and IL-6 levels to predict subsequent change in mSASSS, only baseline serum IL-6 levels were found to significantly predict change in mSASSS at week 104 ($\beta = 0.236$, SE = 0.073, $p = 0.002$, model $R^2 = 0.093$; data not shown). Results of logistic regression analyses indicated that baseline levels of inflammatory and metabolic markers leptin, C3, and TIMP-1 were statistically significant factors in the development of new fatty lesions in the spine at both week 14 and week 104 of golimumab treatment. Change from baseline to week 14 in TIMP-1 also significantly factored into the development of fatty lesions at week 104 (Table 3). Whereas most of these predictive relationships were very weak, those between higher baseline C3 levels and the seven- to eightfold lower risk of subsequent fatty lesion development were of note.

Results of a separate generalized linear model used to evaluate potential interactions between biomarkers and baseline patient characteristics show that IL-6, leptin, TIMP-1, and C3 influenced mSASSS progression independently of demographic factors of age, sex, and human leukocyte antigen B27 positivity (data not shown).

Table 2 Significant correlations between serum biomarkers and Ankylosing Spondylitis Disease Activity Score, Bath Ankylosing Spondylitis Disease Activity Index, and ankylosing spondylitis spine magnetic resonance imaging score for activity changes among golimumab-treated patients

Serum biomarker, time, number of golimumab-treated patients	Spearman correlation coefficient (r_s); Bonferroni-adjusted *p*-value with respective outcome
	Change in ASDAS from baseline to week 104
Leptin	
Baseline, $n = 58$	0.55; 0.040
	Change in BASDAI from baseline to week 14
C3	
Change from baseline to week 4, $n = 76$	0.55; 0.001
Change from baseline to week 14, $n = 76$	0.49; 0.040
	Change in ASspiMRI-a score from baseline to week 14
IL-6	
Baseline, $n = 48$	−0.63; 0.009
Change from baseline to week 4, $n = 48$	0.61; 0.022
Change from baseline to week 14, $n = 48$	0.59; 0.043
TIMP-1	
Baseline, $n = 35$	−0.67; 0.044
C3	
Change from baseline to week 4, $n = 35$	0.72; 0.005

Abbreviations: ASDAS Ankylosing Spondylitis Disease Activity Score employing C-reactive protein, *ASspiMRI-a* Ankylosing spondylitis spine magnetic resonance imaging score for activity, *BASDAI* Bath Ankylosing Spondylitis Disease Activity Index, *C3* Complement component 3, *IL* Interleukin, *TIMP-1* Tissue inhibitor of metalloproteinase-1

Correlations between posttreatment biomarker levels and posttreatment measures of disease activity and spine inflammation

Reductions in C3 observed from baseline to week 4 ($r_s = 0.55$, $p = 0.001$) and week 14 ($r_s = 0.49$, $p = 0.040$) significantly correlated with improvement from baseline to week 14 in the BASDAI score. Similarly, improvement from baseline to week 4 in serum IL-6 ($r_s = 0.61$, $p = 0.022$) and C3 ($r_s = 0.72$, $p = 0.005$) levels, as well as improvement from baseline to week 14 in serum IL-6 levels ($r_s = 0.59$, $p = 0.043$), correlated significantly with improvement in ASspiMRI-a scores from baseline to week 14 of golimumab treatment (Table 2). All other correlations tested between posttreatment biomarker levels and posttreatment measures of disease activity or spinal inflammation yielded insignificant relationships.

Discussion

The search for serum biomarkers of prognostic utility in AS reflects, in part, the need for objective measures of disease activity and response to treatment, as well as the unresolved issues of pathogenesis in the disease. The

Table 3 Logistic regression analysis of serum biomarkers and fatty lesion development visualized by magnetic resonance imaging

	Fatty lesion development, odds ratio (95% confidence interval); p value	
Serum biomarker, time	Week 14 ($n = 125$)	Week 104 ($n = 117$)
Leptin		
Baseline	0.92 (0.87–0.98); $p = 0.005$	0.86 (0.78–0.95); $p = 0.004$
C3		
Baseline	0.13 (0.04–0.44); $p = 0.001$	0.15 (0.04–0.61); $p = 0.008$
TIMP-1		
Baseline	1.02 (1.01–1.03); $p = 0.005$	1.02 (1.01–1.04); $p = 0.001$
Change from baseline to week 14	0.98 (0.97–1.00); $p = 0.030$	0.96 (0.94–0.98); $p = 0.000$

Abbreviations: C3 Complement component 3, *TIMP-1* Tissue inhibitor of metalloproteinase-1

structured nature of a randomized controlled trial provides more clinical uniformity in treatment regimen and outcome measures than is possible in real-world observational studies. In the present study, significant and moderately strong correlations were observed between ASDAS and levels of IL-6, ICAM-1, haptoglobin, serum amyloid-P, and C3. As expected, similar results were observed for CRP. These correlations suggest possible roles for these biomarkers in AS-related inflammation. Baseline serum IL-6 and TIMP-1, as well as reductions in IL-6 and C3, correlated with reduction in ASspiMRI-a scores. Of note, ASDAS has been shown to correlate well with ASspiMRI-a scores, and weakly with BASDAI change, among golimumab-treated patients with AS [5].

Decreases in TIMP-1 at week 14 correlated with fatty lesion development at weeks 14 and 104. The biological basis of local inflammation being associated with reparative processes in spine and local inflammation being reflected as new fatty lesions have yet to be defined, and TIMP-1 would be a candidate factor for future studies. Previously described predictors, such as insulin, matrix metalloproteinase-3, vascular endothelial growth factor, or bone resorption markers, did not significantly correlate with clinical or imaging outcomes.

Fatty lesion development (fat metaplasia) is thought to reflect postinflammation "repair" and may be a precursor of new bone formation. When assessed by logistic regression, baseline levels of inflammatory and metabolic markers leptin, C3, and TIMP-1 were statistically significant factors in the risk of development of new fatty lesions in the spine at both week 14 and week 104 of golimumab treatment, but only the relationship between higher baseline C3 levels and a seven- to eightfold decreased risk of subsequent fatty lesion development offers potential clinical utility. Both leptin and C3, the precursor of C3adesArg acylation-stimulating protein, are involved in triglyceride uptake into adipocytes and homeostasis of adipose tissue. Deficiency of leptin is associated with lipodystrophy and resistance to obesity, whereas increased C3 is linked to increased central obesity and insulin resistance [21]. Furthermore, inflammatory cytokines such as TNF-α and IL-6 stimulate production of leptin and C3, and decreased levels of the receptor for C3adesArg, C5L2 [21, 22]. Together with these properties of leptin and C3, our finding that increased baseline levels of leptin and C3 were correlated with decreased risk of vertebral fatty lesion development suggests that these are key regulators of local adipogenesis within bone tissue in AS. Although Li and colleagues also demonstrated underexpression of C3 in patients with AS ($n = 6$) relative to healthy volunteers ($n = 6$) in a preliminary search for disease-associated proteins in the sera of patients with AS [23], additional studies are needed to confirm these findings.

Limitations

A limitation of the present study is the large number of analytes, which precludes analyses such as principal component analysis or supervised cluster analysis. To guard against identifying a false-positive relationship between the large number of analytes assessed and disease activity outcomes, we employed the Bonferroni correction in the statistical modeling to account for multiplicity of testing. The crossover to active anti-TNF agent after a relatively short placebo period complicates interpretation of "placebo group" imaging data at weeks 104 and 208. These analyses are also limited by the fact that golimumab doses were combined and not assessed individually; however, given that no dose-response relationship was observed between golimumab 50 mg and 100 mg when analyzed by randomized groups at week 104 [4], the doses were combined to maximize the patient numbers in the golimumab arm. Despite this approach, there remained few patients on whom to base correlation analyses for radiographic progression and development of fatty lesions. This is an unresolved issue and should be the focus of future research in this field. Additionally, IL-6 levels can be influenced by therapeutic corticosteroid use via suppression of endogenous cortisol levels [24, 25] and also by visceral fat secretion [26]; our analyses did not adjust for these potential confounders in assessing relationships between IL-6 and MRI-detected spinal inflammation and clinical measures of disease activity.

Conclusions

An extensive serum biomarker analysis in golimumab-treated patients with AS demonstrated that few biomarkers

showed correlation with disease activity or MRI changes in multiparametric analysis. Although IL-6 weakly correlated with radiographic progression, other biomarkers found in prior studies to be significantly associated with AS imaging changes were not confirmed.

Abbreviations

AS: Ankylosing spondylitis; ASDAS: Ankylosing Spondylitis Disease Activity Score; ASspiMRI-a: Ankylosing spondylitis spine magnetic resonance imaging score for activity; ASspiMRI-c: Ankylosing spondylitis spine magnetic resonance imaging score for chronicity; BASDAI: Bath Ankylosing Spondylitis Disease Activity Index; C3: Complement component 3; CRP: C-reactive protein; ICAM-1: Intracellular adhesion molecule-1; IL: Interleukin; MRI: Magnetic resonance imaging; mSASSS: Modified Stokes Ankylosing Spondylitis Spine Score; NSAID: Nonsteroidal anti-inflammatory drug; r_S: Spearman correlation coefficient; TIMP-1: Tissue inhibitor of metalloproteinase-1; TNF: Tumor necrosis factor; VU: Vertebral unit

Acknowledgements

The authors thank the patients, the investigators, and the study personnel who made this trial possible. The authors also thank Michelle Perate, MS, and Mary Whitman, PhD, of Janssen Scientific Affairs, LLC, who helped prepare and submit the manuscript. The authors also thank the following institutional review boards/ethics committees: China Medical University Hospital Instituted Review of Board 9 F, Taichung, Taiwan, Republic of China; Comité de Protection des Personnes Ile-de-France III, Hôpital Tarnier-Cochin 89, Paris, France; Commissie Medische ethiek van de Universitaire Ziekenhuizen KU Leuven/U.Z. Gasthuisberg, Leuven, Belgium; Ethikkommission der ärztekammer Westfalen-Lippe und der Medizinischen Fakultät der WWU Münster, Münster, Germany; Human Experiment and Ethics Committee, Kaohsiung Medical University Hospital, Kaohsiung, Taiwan, Republic of China; HUS Helsingin ja Uudenmaan sairaanhoitopiiri, Medisiininen eettinen toimikunta, Biomedicum Helsinki, HUS, Finland; Institutional Review Board, Biomedical Research Institute, Seoul National University Hospital, Jongro-gu, Seoul, South Korea; Institutional Review Board, Dong-A University Hospital Clinical Research Center, Seo-Gu, Busan, South Korea; Institutional Review Board, Guro Hospital, Korea University Medical Center, Guro-Gu, Seoul, South Korea; Institutional Review Board, Hanyang University Hospital, Sungdong-Ku, Seoul, South Korea; Institutional Review Board, Pusan National University Hospital, Seo-Gu, Busan, South Korea; Institutional Review Board, Seoul St. Mary's Hospital/The Catholic University of Korea, Seocho-gu, Seoul, South Korea; Joint Institutional Review Board. No. 201, Taipei, Taiwan, Republic of China; METC azM/UM Maastricht, Maastricht, The Netherlands; and Western Institutional Review Board, Olympia, WA, USA.

Funding

This study was funded by Janssen Research & Development, LLC, and Merck/Schering-Plough.

Authors' contributions

RDI made substantial intellectual contributions to the study conception and data interpretation, helped draft and revise the manuscript for important intellectual content, approved the final version to be published, and agreed to be accountable for all aspects of the work. XB made substantial intellectual contributions to the study conception and data interpretation, revised the manuscript for important intellectual content, approved the final version to be published, and agreed to be accountable for all aspects of the work. KGAH made substantial intellectual contributions to the study conception and data interpretation, revised the manuscript for important intellectual content, approved the final version to be published, and agreed to be accountable for all aspects of the work. JB made substantial intellectual contributions to the study conception and data interpretation, revised the manuscript for important intellectual content, approved the final version to be published, and agreed to be accountable for all aspects of the work. AD made substantial intellectual contributions to the study conception and data interpretation, revised the manuscript for important intellectual content, approved the final version to be published, and agreed to be accountable for all aspects of the work. DvdH made substantial intellectual contributions to the study conception and data interpretation, revised the manuscript for important intellectual content, approved the final version to be published, and agreed to be accountable for all aspects of the work. SX made substantial intellectual contributions to the data analysis and interpretation, helped to draft and revise the manuscript for important intellectual content, approved the final version to be published, and agreed to be accountable for all aspects of the work. BH made substantial intellectual contributions to the study conception and design, data acquisition, and data analysis/interpretation; helped to draft and revise the manuscript for important intellectual content; approved the final version to be published; and agreed to be accountable for all aspects of the work. All authors read and approved the final manuscript.

Competing interests

No nonfinancial conflicts of interest exist for any authors. RDI has received consulting fees from Janssen, Merck, AbbVie, Amgen, and UCB. XB has received honoraria for talks and serving on advisory boards as well as grants for studies from AbbVie, Amgen, Janssen Research & Development, MSD (Schering-Plough), Novartis, Pfizer (Wyeth), and UCB. KGAH has received honoraria for educational lectures from Abbott, Janssen Research & Development, MSD (Schering-Plough), Pfizer (Wyeth), and UCB. JB has received honoraria for talks and serving on advisory boards as well as grants for studies from Celltrion, Amgen, Abbott, Roche, Bristol-Myers Squibb, Janssen, Novartis, Pfizer (Wyeth), MSD (Schering-Plough), Sanofi-Aventis, and UCB. AD has received research grants and has served on the advisory boards of AbbVie, Amgen, Janssen, Pfizer, Novartis, and UCB. These potential conflicts of interest have been reviewed and managed by Oregon Health & Science University. DvdH has received consulting fees from AbbVie, Amgen, AstraZeneca, Augurex, Bristol-Myers Squibb, Celgene, Chugai Pharmaceutical Co., Covagen, Daiichi Sankyo, Eli Lilly, Galapagos, GSK, Janssen Biologics, Merck, Novartis, Novo Nordisk, Otsuka, Pfizer, Roche, Sanofi-Aventis, UCB, and Vertex, and is director of imaging rheumatology, Leiden University Medical Center. SX and BH are employees of Janssen Research & Development, LLC

Author details

[1]Department of Immunology, University of Toronto, Toronto, ON, Canada. [2]Department of Medicine, University of Toronto, Toronto, ON, Canada. [3]Department of Rheumatology, Rheumazentrum Ruhrgebiet Herne, Ruhr-University Bochum, Herne, Germany. [4]Department of Radiology, Charité Medical School, Berlin, Germany. [5]Division of Arthritis & Rheumatic Diseases, Oregon Health & Science University, Portland, OR, USA. [6]Department of Rheumatology, Leiden University Medical Center, Leiden, The Netherlands. [7]Department of Biostatistics, Janssen Research & Development, LLC, Spring House, PA, USA. [8]Department of Immunology, Janssen Research & Development, LLC, Spring House, PA, USA.

References

1. Braun J, Landewé R, Hermann KG, Han J, Yan S, Williamson P, et al. Major reduction in spinal inflammation in patients with ankylosing spondylitis after treatment with infliximab: results of a multicenter, randomized, double-blind, placebo-controlled magnetic resonance imaging study. Arthritis Rheum. 2006;54:1646–52.
2. Lambert RG, Salonen D, Rahman P, Inman RD, Wong RL, Einstein SG, et al. Adalimumab significantly reduces both spinal and sacroiliac joint inflammation in patients with ankylosing spondylitis: a multicenter, randomized, double-blind, placebo-controlled study. Arthritis Rheum. 2007;56:4005–14.
3. Inman RD, Davis Jr JC, van der Heijde D, Diekman L, Sieper J, Kim SI, et al. Efficacy and safety of golimumab in patients with ankylosing spondylitis:

results of a randomized, double-blind, placebo-controlled, phase III trial. Arthritis Rheum. 2008;58:3402–12.

4. Braun J, Deodhar A, Inman RD, van der Heijde D, Mack M, Xu S, et al. Golimumab administered subcutaneously every 4 weeks in ankylosing spondylitis: 104-week results of the GO-RAISE study. Ann Rheum Dis. 2012;71:661–7.
5. Braun J, Baraliakos X, Hermann KG, van der Heijde D, Inman RD, Deodhar AA, et al. Golimumab reduces spinal inflammation in ankylosing spondylitis: MRI results of the randomised, placebo-controlled GO-RAISE study. Ann Rheum Dis. 2012;71:878–84.
6. Haroon N, Inman RD, Learch TJ, Weisman MH, Lee M, Rahbar MH, et al. The impact of tumor necrosis factor inhibitors on radiographic progression in ankylosing spondylitis. Arthritis Rheum. 2013;65:2645–54.
7. Ramiro S, van der Heijde D, van Tubergen A, Stolwijk C, Dougados M, van den Bosch F, et al. Higher disease activity leads to more structural damage in the spine in ankylosing spondylitis: 12-year longitudinal data from the OASIS cohort. Ann Rheum Dis. 2014;73:1455–61.
8. Baraliakos X, Listing J, Rudwaleit M, Sieper J, Braun J. The relationship between inflammation and new bone formation in patients with ankylosing spondylitis. Arthritis Res Ther. 2008;10:R104.
9. Maksymowych WP, Chiowchanwisawakit P, Clare T, Pedersen SJ, Østergaard M, Lambert RG. Inflammatory lesions of the spine on magnetic resonance imaging predict the development of new syndesmophytes in ankylosing spondylitis: evidence of a relationship between inflammation and new bone formation. Arthritis Rheum. 2009;60:93–102.
10. Rudwaleit M, Jurik AG, Hermann KG, Landewé R, van der Heijde D, Baraliakos X, et al. Defining active sacroiliitis on magnetic resonance imaging (MRI) for classification of axial spondyloarthritis: a consensual approach by the ASAS/OMERACT MRI group. Ann Rheum Dis. 2009;68:1520–7.
11. van der Heijde D, Machado P, Braun J, Hermann KG, Baraliakos X, Hsu B, et al. MRI inflammation at the vertebral unit only marginally predicts new syndesmophyte formation: a multilevel analysis in patients with ankylosing spondylitis. Ann Rheum Dis. 2012;71:369–73.
12. Wagner C, Visvanathan S, Braun J, van der Heijde D, Deodhar A, Hsu B, et al. Serum markers associated with clinical improvement in patients with ankylosing spondylitis treated with golimumab. Ann Rheum Dis. 2012;71:674–80.
13. Garrett S, Jenkinson T, Kennedy LG, Whitelock H, Gaisford P, Calin A. A new approach to defining disease status in ankylosing spondylitis: the Bath Ankylosing Spondylitis Disease Activity Index. J Rheumatol. 1994;21:2286–91.
14. van der Heijde D, Lie E, Kvien TK, Sieper J, Van den Bosch F, Listing J, et al. ASDAS, a highly discriminatory ASAS-endorsed disease activity score in patients with ankylosing spondylitis. Ann Rheum Dis. 2009;68:1811–8.
15. Braun J, Baraliakos X, Golder W, Brandt J, Rudwaleit M, Listing J, et al. Magnetic resonance imaging examinations of the spine in patients with ankylosing spondylitis, before and after successful therapy with infliximab: evaluation of a new scoring system. Arthritis Rheum. 2003;48:1126–36.
16. Baraliakos X, Landewé R, Hermann KG, Listing J, Golder W, Brandt J, et al. Inflammation in ankylosing spondylitis: a systematic description of the extent and frequency of acute spinal changes using magnetic resonance imaging. Ann Rheum Dis. 2005;64:730–4.
17. Creemers MCW. Franssen MJAM, van 't Hof MA, Gribnau FWJ, van de Putte LBA, van Riel PLCM. Assessment of outcome in ankylosing spondylitis: an extended radiographic scoring system Ann Rheum Dis. 2005;64:127–9.
18. Braun J, Baraliakos X, Hermann KG, Deodhar A, van der Heijde D, Inman R, et al. The effect of two golimumab doses on radiographic progression in ankylosing spondylitis: results through 4 years of the GO-RAISE trial. Ann Rheum Dis. 2014;73:1107–13.
19. Chiowchanwisawakit P, Lambert RG, Conner-Spady B, Maksymowych WP. Focal fat lesions at vertebral corners on magnetic resonance imaging predict the development of new syndesmophytes in ankylosing spondylitis. Arthritis Rheum. 2011;63:2215–25.
20. Baraliakos X, Heldmann F, Callhoff J, Listing J, Appelboom T, Brandt J, et al. Which spinal lesions are associated with new bone formation in patients with ankylosing spondylitis treated with anti-TNF agents? A long-term observational study using MRI and conventional radiography. Ann Rheum Dis. 2014;73:1819–25.
21. Cianflone K, Xia Z, Chen LY. Critical review of acylation-stimulating protein physiology in humans and rodents. Biochim Biophys Acta. 2003;1609:127–43.
22. MacLaren R, Kalant D, Cianflone K. The ASP receptor C5L2 is regulated by metabolic hormones associated with insulin resistance. Biochem Cell Biol. 2007;85:11–21.
23. Li T, Huang Z, Zheng B, Liao Z, Zhao L, Gu J. Serum disease-associated proteins of ankylosing spondylitis: results of a preliminary study by comparative proteomics. Clin Exp Rheumatol. 2010;28:201–7.
24. Kirwan JR, Clarke L, Hunt LP, Perry MG, Straub RH, Jessop DS. Effect of novel therapeutic glucocorticoids on circadian rhythms of hormones and cytokines in rheumatoid arthritis. Ann N Y Acad Sci. 2010;1193:127–33.
25. Spies CM, Straub RH, Cutolo M, Buttgereit F. Circadian rhythms in rheumatology - a glucocorticoid perspective. Arthritis Res Ther. 2014;16 Suppl 2:S3.
26. Pellegrinelli V, Rouault C, Rodriguez-Cuenca S, Albert V, Edom-Vovard F, Vidal-Puig A, et al. Human adipocytes induce inflammation and atrophy in muscle cells during obesity. Diabetes. 2015;64:3121–34.

17

Comparison of non-radiographic axial spondyloarthritis and ankylosing spondylitis patients–baseline characteristics, treatment adherence, and development of clinical variables during three years of anti-TNF therapy in clinical practice

Johan K. Wallman[1,4*], Meliha C. Kapetanovic[1], Ingemar F. Petersson[1,2], Pierre Geborek[1] and Lars Erik Kristensen[1,3]

Abstract

Background: The relationship between non-radiographic axial spondyloarthritis (nr-axSpA) and ankylosing spondylitis (AS) is currently debated. Using observational data from the South Swedish Arthritis Treatment Group register, we thus aimed to compare clinical development and treatment adherence between nr-axSpA and AS patients during three years of anti-TNF (tumor necrosis factor) therapy in clinical practice, and to explore the impact of inflammatory activity measured by CRP (C-reactive protein) at treatment initiation.

Methods: Nr-axSpA and AS patients (n = 86/238) in southern Sweden, commencing anti-TNF therapy 1999-2011, were followed during three years. Anti-TNF cessation was defined as stopping therapy, without restarting another anti-TNF agent within three months. Differences in the three year developments of patient's visual analogue scale (VAS) scores for global health and pain, EuroQol 5-Dimensions utility, evaluator's global disease activity assessment, CRP, and ESR (erythrocyte sedimentation rate) were assessed by repeated ANOVA. Anti-TNF adherence was compared by Log rank test and Cox regression. In a subanalysis, the same outcomes were studied after splitting both groups into patients with/without baseline CRP elevation.

Results: Nr-axSpA patients were more often female and had lower acute phase reactants at baseline. Apart from CRP, which remained lower in the nr-axSpA group throughout follow-up ($p = 0.004$), no between-group differences were detected regarding clinical developments ($p > 0.1$ for all comparisons) or anti-TNF adherence (hazard ratio: 1.1 (95 % CI 0.7 to 1.8) for the nr-axSpA vs. AS group) during three years. Elevated baseline CRP was similarly associated with superior clinical outcomes and treatment adherence in both groups.

Conclusions: With the exception of constantly lower CRP levels in the nr-axSpA group, three years anti-TNF therapy resulted in similar clinical outcomes and treatment adherence in nr-axSpA and AS patients, thus strengthening the hypothesis that these diagnoses represent different aspects/phases of the same disease.

Keywords: Spondyloarthritis, Axial spondyloarthritis, Non-radiographic axial spondyloarthritis, Ankylosing spondylitis, Anti-TNF, Treatment outcome, Medication adherence, C-reactive protein

* Correspondence: johan.81.karlsson@gmail.com

[1]Section of Rheumatology, Department of Clinical Sciences Lund, Lund University, Lund, Sweden

[4]Reumatologiska kliniken, Skånes Universitetssjukhus Lund, Kioskgatan 3, 22185 Lund, Sweden

Full list of author information is available at the end of the article

Background

Spondyloarthritis (SpA) comprises a range of rheumatic disorders - ankylosing spondylitis (AS), undifferentiated SpA, psoriatic arthritis, arthritis related to inflammatory bowel disease, reactive arthritis, and a juvenile form - sharing common clinical features, extraarticular manifestations, and a genetic association with the type 1 major histocompatibility complex HLA-B27. Typical musculoskeletal symptoms are divided into peripheral (arthritis, enthesitis, dactylitis) or axial (sacroiliitis, spondylitis) disease, of which patients may suffer from either or both. AS, the classical form of axial SpA, is defined by structural damage of the sacroiliac joints on conventional radiographs [1]. Many patients, however, display similar axial symptoms and signs of active sacroiliitis on magnetic resonance imaging (MRI) in the absence of such radiographic changes [2], entailing a risk of delayed or missed diagnosis. Thus, in 2009, the Assessment of SpondyloArthritis International Society (ASAS) developed novel classification criteria for axial SpA, encompassing patients both with (AS) and without radiographic sacroiliitis - the latter phenotype thereby formally characterized as non-radiographic axial SpA (nr-axSpA) [3].

Since then a number of studies have compared subjects with nr-axSpA and AS, finding similar levels of disease activity, overall physical impairment, and health-related quality of life (HRQoL), while the nr-axSpA patients are more often female, have shorter mean disease duration, and display lower levels of acute phase reactants and less spinal immobility [2, 4–10]. The observation that 10–12 % of nr-axSpA patients progress to develop AS within 2 years, strengthens the hypothesis that the two entities represent different aspects/phases of a common pathology [9, 11].

Current treatment guidelines for axial manifestations of SpA, including both AS and nr-axSpA, recommend the use of anti-TNF (tumor necrosis factor) agents in cases of insufficient response or intolerance to non-steroidal anti-inflammatory drugs (NSAIDs), as conventional disease-modifying anti-rheumatic drugs (DMARDs) have not been shown to be effective in this situation [12–14]. The efficacy of anti-TNF treatment in nr-axSpA has been shown to be similar to that in AS, at least in patients with objective signs of inflammation, such as elevation of C-reactive protein (CRP) or inflammatory lesions seen on MRI at baseline [5, 9, 15, 16].

While acknowledging these important previous findings, the overall evidence base concerned with nr-axSpA remains fairly limited, and results should be confirmed in further cohorts. Data on long-term efficacy and adherence to anti-TNF therapy in nr-axSpA is also largely absent. In light of this, we thus applied observational data from southern Sweden, aiming to compare baseline characteristics, anti-TNF adherence, and development of clinical variables during three years of anti-TNF therapy between nr-axSpA and AS patients treated in clinical practice.

Methods

Patients

Since the late 1990s, patients with chronic arthritis treated with biologic DMARDs in southern Sweden have been monitored in the observational SSATG (South Swedish Arthritis Treatment Group) register, involving 12 rheumatology centers [17]. For the present study, bio-naive patients (≥15 years) with nr-axSpA (n = 86) or AS (n = 238), commencing anti-TNF treatment between 1999 and 2011, were retrieved from the SSATG register and compared for baseline characteristics and clinical development during 3 years of anti-TNF therapy. AS patients had a clinical diagnosis according to treating rheumatologists, which in a previous SSATG validation study corresponded to at least 90 % fulfillment of the modified New York criteria (the remaining patients had either incomplete or missing information in their medical records, unabling a validation of the AS diagnosis) [1, 18]. The included nr-axSpA patients were all followed at the central SSATG university clinic in Lund/Malmö, did not have a clinical diagnosis of psoriatic arthritis, and - based on data collected on initiation of anti-TNF therapy - fulfilled the ASAS classification criteria for axial spondyloarthritis, without having skin psoriasis or radiographic sacroiliitis on conventional radiographs (48 and 38 patients, respectively, according to the imaging and clinical arms) [3]. In Sweden, anti-TNF agents were often used to treat patients with this undifferentiated, axial SpA phenotype even before it was formally characterized by ASAS in 2009, explaining the earlier anti-TNF therapy start dates of some patients (31 of 86 nr-axSpA patients commencing anti-TNF therapy prior to 2009).

Treatment

Anti-TNF therapy was started due to high disease activity and inadequate response or intolerance to one or more NSAIDs. Treatment decisions were taken by the responsible rheumatologists, and no formal disease activity level was required for initiation of anti-TNF therapy. Indications in both nr-axSpA and AS were, however, supported by guidelines when they began to emerge [12, 19], with the non-mandatory Swedish guidelines recommending a Bath ankylosing spondylitis disease activity index (BASDAI) score ≥4 during ≥4 weeks and previous treatment attempts with ≥2 NSAIDs during >3 months in total before starting anti-TNF therapy in both conditions [14]. Administration intervals and dosing of etanercept, adalimumab, golimumab, and certolizumab pegol were in general as recommended by the manufacturers. Infliximab was started at 3 mg/kg at weeks 0, 2, 6, and then every 8 weeks, although in cases of insufficient response, dose increments were allowed in steps of 100 mg to a maximum of 500 mg every 4–8 weeks. Facing adverse events, inefficacy, or other causes, decisions to discontinue anti-TNF therapy altogether or switch to another agent were left to the responsible rheumatologists according to clinical practice.

Patients could receive NSAIDs, low dose oral glucocorticoids, intra-articular glucocorticoid injections, and conventional DMARDs both prior to and during the study period according to clinical practice - the latter mainly applied in patients with peripheral arthritis.

Follow up and study outcomes

At the start of anti-TNF therapy, demographic data, disease characteristics (allowing for disease classification as outlined above), and information on past and present treatments were reported according to a structured protocol. [17] Patients were followed for 3 years, with scheduled visits at baseline, 3, 6, 12, 24, and 36 months of follow up. At each visit, disease activity was measured by patient's visual analog scales (VAS) for global health and pain (VAS global and VAS pain), evaluator's global assessment on a 5-grade Likert scale (Evaluator's global), and acute phase reactants (erythrocyte sedimentation rate (ESR) and CRP), while HRQoL was estimated as EuroQol 5-Dimensions (EQ-5D) utility, a metric anchored at 1 (full health) and 0 (death), applying the standard British EQ-5D preference set [20, 21]. Use of the BASDAI and Bath ankylosing spondylitis functional index (BASFI) were also recommended [22, 23], although not mandatory within the SSATG during the study period, leading to numbers of missing data values that were too high for meaningful analysis beyond the presentation of baseline values.

Thus, the primary outcomes of the present study were between-group differences (nr-axSpA vs. AS) in the developments of VAS pain, VAS global, Evaluator's global, ESR, CRP, and EQ-5D during 3 years from the start of anti-TNF treatment. Adherence to anti-TNF therapy was also compared as a secondary outcome. For this analysis, switches between anti-TNF therapies occurring within 3 months were allowed and regarded as continuous treatment, whereas anti-TNF cessation was defined as discontinuing one treatment course without starting another within 3 months.

Statistics

Baseline characteristics in the nr-axSpA and AS patients were compared by chi square (χ^2) or Fisher's exact test for categorical variables and the Mann–Whitney U test for continuous variables. Whether the two groups differed in the development of clinical parameters during 3 years of anti-TNF therapy were assessed by repeated analysis of variance (ANOVA), including all study time points and adjusting for sex, age, disease duration, presence of peripheral arthritis (yes/no), and baseline CRP (the latter excluded from analyses of ESR and CRP development). In the main analysis, last observation carried forward (LOCF) was applied to impute missing data, as well as from anti-TNF cessation (without restarting anti-TNF therapy within 3 months) in order to exclude potential effects of later treatments. For EQ-5D, due to a relatively high proportion of missing data, missing values at baseline (n(nr-axSpA/AS) = 40/60) and 3 months (n(nr-axSpA/AS) = 46/81) were first imputed by group-wise linear regression models with sex, age, disease duration, peripheral arthritis status (yes/no), VAS global, VAS pain, evaluator's global, and health assessment questionnaire (HAQ) scores at the respective time points as covariates [24]. Repeated ANOVA restricted to observed data from patients remaining on anti-TNF treatment was also conducted for sensitivity analysis.

Adherence to anti-TNF therapy was compared by Kaplan-Meier curves and the log rank test, and Cox proportional hazards regression, adjusting for age, sex, disease duration, presence of peripheral arthritis, and baseline CRP, was also applied to derive a between-group hazard ratio.

As a sub-analysis, we then split both patient groups into subjects with (CRP >3.0 mg/l; % (nr-axSpA/AS) = 58/81) or without CRP elevation at baseline, and compared anti-TNF adherence and developments of VAS global, VAS pain, EQ-5D, and evaluatior's global between the two subgroups within each diagnosis. Statistics were as described above, although limited to analyses of LOCF imputed data and excluding adjustments for baseline CRP. Finally, anti-TNF adherence of all four subgroups were compared by the log rank test.

Ethics, consent and permissions

Ethical approval for the SSATG register study has been granted by the Regional Ethics Committee at Lund University, and informed consent was given orally by all patients before SSATG enrolment. Due to its quality control character, the SSATG register is part of the legislative documentation demanded in Sweden, and hence no specific ethical approval was required for the present study.

Results

Baseline characteristics

Patients with nr-axSpA were significantly younger and had a shorter mean disease duration and fewer previous and ongoing conventional DMARDs than their counterparts with AS (Table 1). The male predominance was also less pronounced in the nr-axSpA group. For disease

Table 1 Patient characteristics at initiation of anti-TNF therapy

Baseline characteristics	nr-axSpA, n = 86	AS, n = 238	*P* value[a]
Male sex, n (%)	53 (62)	180 (76)	0.013
Age, years	38 (13)	43 (12)	<0.001
Disease duration, years	9 (9)	16 (12)	<0.001
Peripheral arthritis, n (%)	39 (45)	118 (50)	0.501
VAS global, mm	60 (19)	61 (22)	0.313
VAS pain, mm	60 (22)	62 (22)	0.292
Evaluator's global, score 0–4	1.7 (0.6)	2.0 (0.7)	0.001
BASDAI score	5.3 (1.7)	5.4 (1.9)	0.727
BASFI score	4.1 (2.3)	4.3 (2.1)	0.503
ESR, mm/h	23 (21)	28 (23)	0.026
CRP, mg/l	10 (13)	23 (26)	<0.001
Elevated CRP, n (%)[b]	47 (58)	177 (81)	<0.001
EQ-5D (UK)			0.381
Mean (SD)	0.43 (0.32)	0.45 (0.33)	
Median (IQR; range)	0.59 (0.64; −0.22 to 0.80)	0.62 (1.3; −0.48 to 0.80)	
Concomitant DMARD (%)	29 (34)	150 (63)	<0.001
Previous DMARDs (n)	0.8 (0.9)	1.5 (1.0)	<0.001
First anti-TNF agent used, n (%)			<0.001[c]
Infliximab	19 (22)	112 (47)	
Etanercept	37 (43)	89 (37)	
Adalimumab	20 (23)	37 (16)	
Golimumab	7 (8)	0 (0)	
Certolizumab pegol	3 (4)	0 (0)	

Mean (SD) if not otherwise stated. Missing data in the non-radiographic axial spondyloarthritis (*nr-axSpA*)/ankylosing spondylitis (*AS*) groups, n (%) as follows: Disease duration 1(1)/0(0); visual analog scale (*VAS*) global 7(8)/24(10); VAS pain 7(8)/24(10); Evaluator's global 2(2)/18(8); Bath ankylosing spondylitis disease activity index (*BASDAI*) 36(42)/105(44); Bath ankylosing spondylitis functional index (*BASFI*) 35(41)/108(45); erythrocyte sedimentation rate (*ESR*) 4(5)/19(8); C-reactive protein (*CRP*) 5(6)/20(8); EuroQ ol 5-Dimensions (*EQ-5D*) 40(47)/60(25); Concomitant disease-modifying anti-rheumatic drug (DMARD) 1(1)/1(0.4). [a]$\chi 2$ for categorical and Mann–Whitney *U* test for continuous variables. [b]CRP >3.0 mg/l. [c]Fisher's exact test

activity all patient-reported outcomes were similar between the two groups at initiation of anti-TNF therapy, whereas the more objective measures - evaluator's global, ESR and CRP - were significantly higher among the AS patients.

Development during anti-TNF therapy

Following anti-TNF initiation, mean values of VAS global, VAS pain, EQ-5D utility, Evaluator's global, ESR, and CRP improved rapidly in both nr-axSpA and AS patients, and within 3 to 6 months had reached a plateau, which was then sustained throughout the 3 years of follow up (Fig. 1 and Additional file 1: Figure S1). By repeated ANOVA, regardless of analyzing imputed (Fig. 1) or observed (Additional file 1: Figure S1) data, no between-group differences were seen in the 3-year developments of VAS global, VAS pain, EQ-5D utility, or Evaluator's global assessment (p >0.1 for all comparisons). Point estimate means of ESR and CRP remained higher in the AS patients throughout follow up. For CRP, this between-group difference in the 3-year pattern was statistically significant when analyzing imputed data ($p = 0.004$), while it was only borderline significant in the observed data analysis ($p = 0.06$). ESR development did not differ significantly by either method (p >0.1 for both analyses).

Adherence to anti-TNF therapy

After three years of follow up, the proportions of patients with nr-axSpA (n = 60; 70 %) and AS (n = 183; 77 %) remaining on anti-TNF therapy did not differ significantly (Fig. 2; log rank test, $p = 0.2$, Cox proportional hazard ratio 1.1 (95 % CI 0.7 to 1.8) for the nr-axSpA as compared to the AS group). Male sex and higher baseline CRP levels were significantly associated with better treatment adherence.

Of the 60 nr-axSpA patients adhering to therapy at 3 years, 46 were still receiving their first anti-TNF agent, 11 had switched treatment once, and 3 had switched treatment twice within 3 months. The corresponding

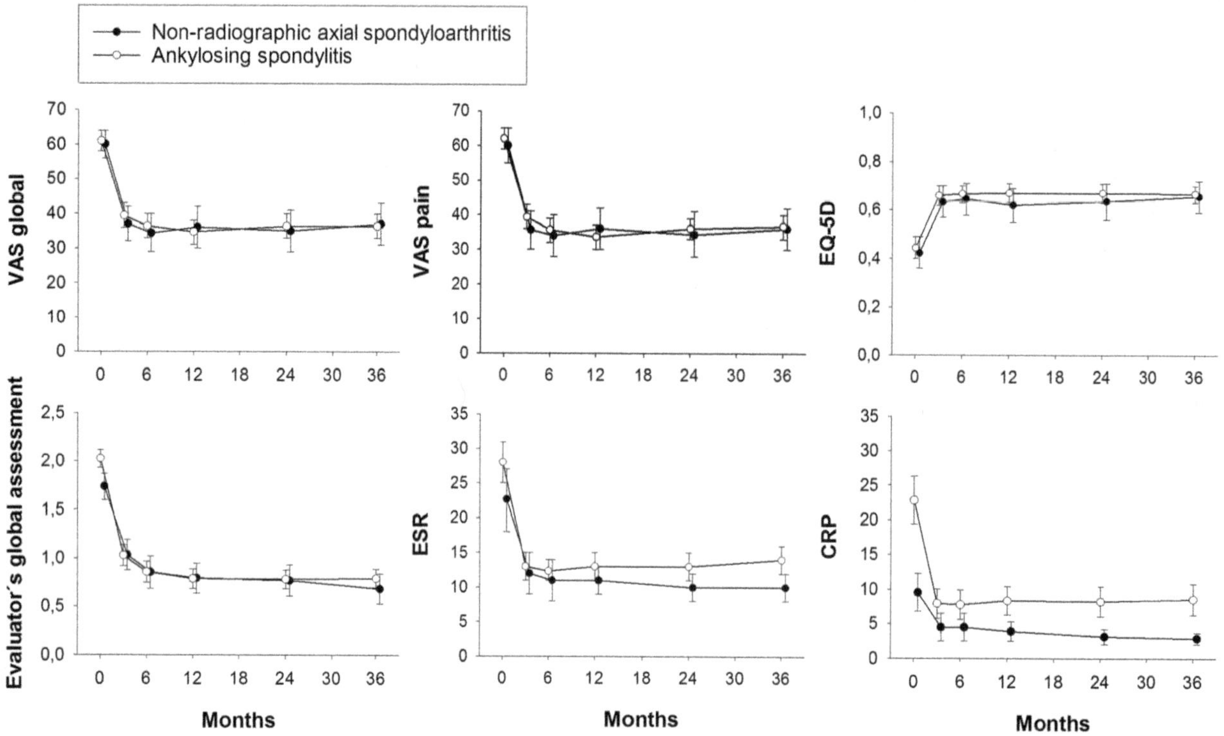

Fig. 1 Clinical developments during three years of anti-TNF therapy. Mean (95 % CI) developments in visual analog scale (*VAS*) global, VAS pain, EuroQol 5-Dimensions (*EQ-5D*) utility, Evaluator's global assessment of disease activity, erythrocyte sedimentation rate (*ESR*), and C-reactive protein (*CRP*) in the non-radiographic axial spondyloarthritis and ankylosing spondylitis groups over time, using last observation carried forward imputed data

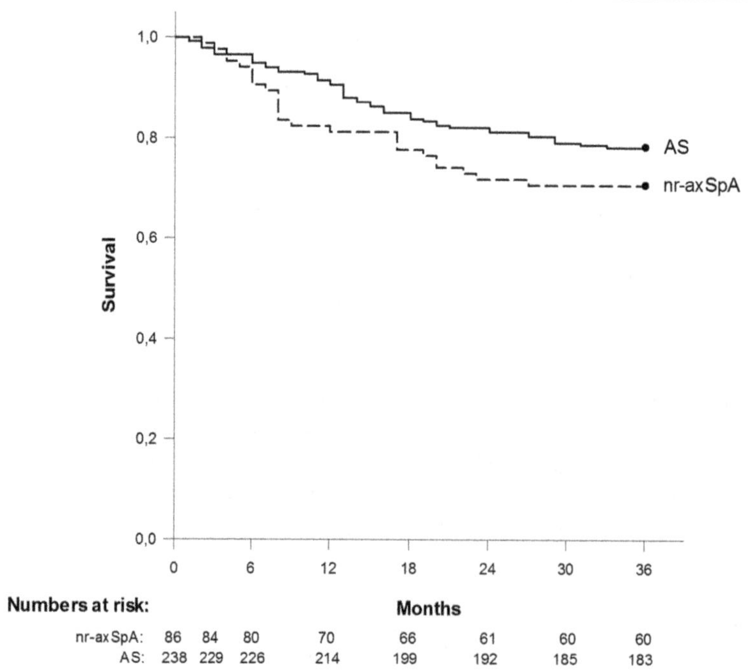

Fig. 2 Adherence to anti-TNF therapy. Kaplan-Meier survival curves from initiation of anti-TNF therapy, showing adherence to anti-TNF treatment in the non-radiographic axial spondyloarthritis (*nr-axSpA*) and ankylosing spondylitis (*AS*) groups, respectively. Cessation of anti-TNF therapy was defined as stopping therapy without restarting another anti-TNF agent within 3 months. Numbers of patients still on anti-TNF treatment at the respective time points are shown below the graph

figures in the AS group were 155, 24, and 4 patients, respectively. Of the 26 nr-axSpA and 55 AS patients ceasing anti-TNF therapy prior to 3 years, 6 and 7 patients, respectively, did so after having switched treatment once within 3 months, and 2 additional AS patients quit treatment after having switched anti-TNF agents twice.

When only focusing on the first anti-TNF agent used, the adherence rate over 3 years was better in the AS group when analyzed by the log rank test ($p = 0.04$). By Cox regression analysis, however, no significant between-group difference was observed (hazard ratio 1.3 (95 % CI 0.9 to 1.9), whereas male sex and higher

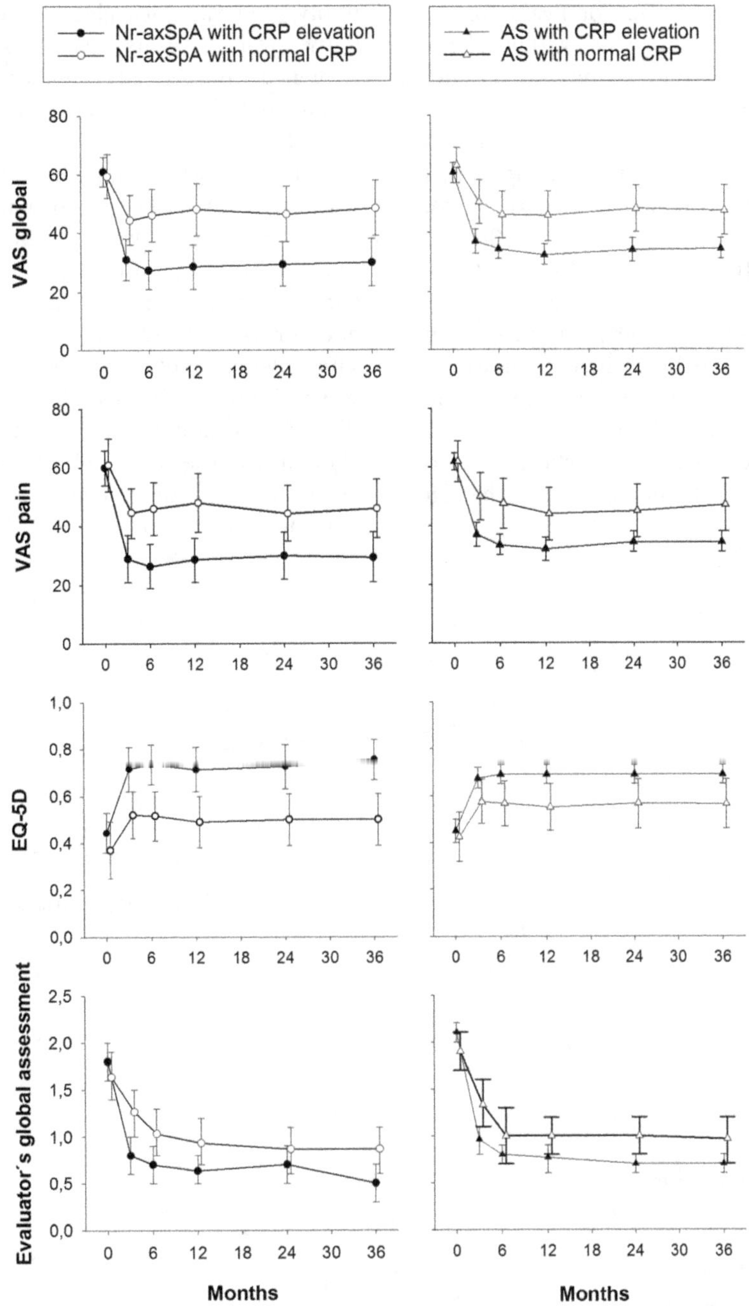

Fig. 3 Clinical developments according to C-reactive protein (*CRP*) status at baseline. Mean (95 % CI) developments in visual analog scale (*VAS*) global, VAS pain, EuroQ ol 5-Dimensions (*EQ-5D*) utility, and Evaluator's global assessment of disease activity during 3 years of anti-TNF therapy in patients with non-radiographic axial spondyloarthritis (*nr-axSpA*) and ankylosing spondylitis (*AS*), who had CRP elevation (CRP >3.0 mg/l) or did not have CRP elevation (CRP ≤3.0 mg/l) at baseline

baseline CRP again significantly predicted superior treatment retention.

Baseline CRP sub-analysis

Among both nr-axSpA and AS patients, significantly larger improvements were seen on repeated ANOVA in VAS global, VAS pain, and EQ-5D utility scores among subjects with elevated CRP at baseline (p <0.05 for all comparisons; Fig. 3). For Evaluator's global assessment, this was also true within the nr-axSpA group, while it was only borderline significant among AS patients ($p = 0.06$).

Likewise, anti-TNF adherence during 3 years of follow up was also significantly superior among both nr-axSpA and AS patients with increased CRP at baseline (Fig. 4; nr-axSpA: log rank test, p <0.001; Cox proportional hazard ratio 0.2 (95 % CI 0.1 to 0.6) for patients with CRP elevation, as compared to those without; AS: log rank test, $p = 0.006$, Cox proportional hazard ratio 0.5 (0.3 to 0.9)). When comparing all four subgroups, drug survival did not differ significantly between nr-axSpA and AS patients either with, or without CRP elevation at baseline, whereas the two CRP-positive subgroups both outperformed the CRP-negative groups.

Discussion

Main findings

In this study, comparing outcomes of anti-TNF therapy in patients with nr-axSpA and AS treated in clinical practice, despite baseline characteristics indicating more longstanding and objectively more severe disease in the AS group, no between-group differences were observed in adherence to anti-TNF therapy, or in developments of VAS global, VAS pain, EQ-5D utility, or Evaluator's global assessment of disease activity over 3 years. Mean ESR and CRP levels remained numerically higher in the AS group throughout follow up, although only significantly so for CRP.

Moreover, when splitting patients according to CRP status at baseline (normal vs. elevated), similar outcome patterns were again observed in the two groups, with significantly better treatment adherence and improvements in clinical variables among both nr-axSpA and AS patients with CRP elevation. The diversion of anti-TNF adherence curves observed between the overall nr-axSpA and AS groups (Fig. 2), although non-significant, were thus explained by the relatively large proportion of nr-axSpA patients displaying normal CRP at treatment initiation.

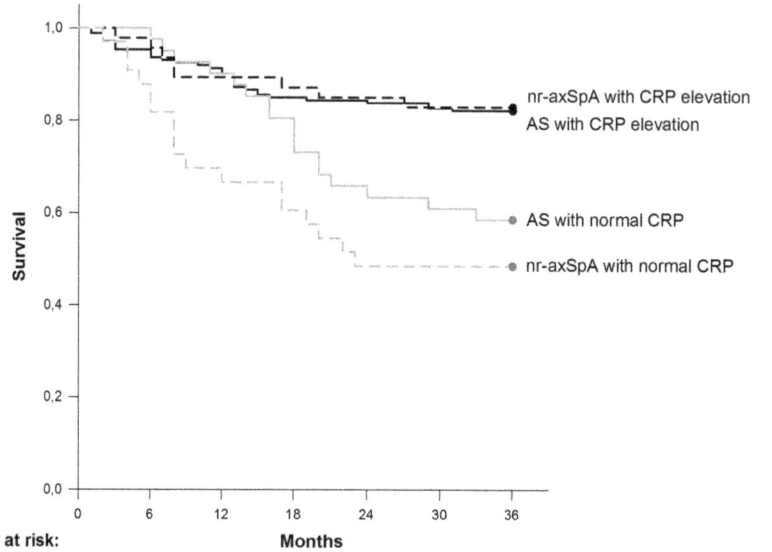

Numbers at risk:

	0		6	12	18	24	30	36
nr-axSpA with CRP elevation:	47	47	46	42	41	40	39	39
AS with CRP elevation:	177	169	166	159	148	147	144	143
nr-axSpA with normal CRP:	34	32	29	23	20	16	16	16
AS with normal CRP:	41	41	41	37	33	27	25	24

Fig. 4 Adherence to anti-TNF therapy according to C-reactive protein (*CRP*) status at baseline. Kaplan-Meier survival curves from initiation of anti-TNF therapy, showing adherence to anti-TNF treatment in patients with non-radiographic axial spondyloarthritis (*nr-axSpA*) and ankylosing spondylitis (*AS*) who had CRP elevation (CRP >3.0 mg/l) or did not have CRP elevation (CRP ≤3.0 mg/l) at baseline. Cessation of anti-TNF therapy was defined as stopping therapy, without restarting another anti-TNF agent within 3 months. Numbers of patients still on anti-TNF treatment at the respective time points are shown below the graph

Previous research

The present comparison of baseline characteristics mainly confirm previous findings, with more female patients and lower levels of acute phase reactants in the nr-axSpA group, whereas no differences were seen in patient-reported disease activity, function, or HRQoL [2, 4–8, 25]. The observed differences in age (absent from most prior comparisons) and disease duration (present in most prior comparisons) should be interpreted with caution, because this was not an inception cohort. The larger proportions of patients with baseline CRP elevation in our study than in most former studies may be due to varying cutoff levels and inclusion criteria, but the intergroup relation remained similar to those previously reported [2, 4–6, 25]. Although the relationship between nr-axSpA and AS remains fiercely debated, there is some evidence that male sex and CRP elevation may predict the development of radiographic changes [9]. According to this hypothesis, in particular women with low levels of inflammation may thus remain in the non-radiographic stage for many years (perhaps lifelong), thereby potentially explaining both the baseline differences seen at the group level and the relatively long mean disease duration observed in the nr-axSpA cohorts of this (9 years) and other studies.

The mean baseline BASDAI, BASFI, and VAS global scores in our cohort are all in the lower ranges of those reported in randomized controlled trials (RCTs) of anti-TNF therapy in nr-axSpA and AS [26–32]. Reasons for this are likely to reside in the observational setting of our study, without strict inclusion criteria or any mandatory requirement based on disease activity, to start anti-TNF therapy. The between-group differences in the first anti-TNF agent used (Table 1) reflect the earlier approval of this treatment indication in AS. Although no head-to-head studies have been performed, there is no evidence to support a difference in efficacy of the various TNF inhibitors on manifestations of axial or peripheral SpA [13, 33].

Direct comparisons of the effects of anti-TNF therapy in patients with nr-axSpA and AS have hitherto been published from two RCTs and one observational cohort [5, 15, 16, 25, 34]. In line with the current results, these studies have demonstrated similar treatment response rates in both groups, at least in the presence of comparable signs of inflammation at baseline, such as elevation of CRP or inflammatory lesions seen on MRI - both identified as predictors of anti-TNF response in patients with nr-axSpA [30–32, 35], and in AS [36–41]. A recent meta-analysis, assessing all available RCT evidence, also came to a similar conclusion, with comparable greater anti-TNF therapy effect sizes over placebo in both diagnoses when adjusting for publication year as a proxy of disease severity (as early AS trials enrolled patients with more longstanding disease) [26]. In terms of effects on HRQoL, developments in the EQ-5D during anti-TNF treatment of patients with nr-axSpA and AS have not been previously compared, although the available 2-year Short Form 36 and AS quality of life data also point to comparable HRQoL gains in both groups [16]. Contrasting with the present results, in the RCT by Song et al., no difference was observed between the nr-axSpA and AS groups in development of CRP [34]. Inclusion in that trial, however, required the presence of inflammatory lesions seen on MRI, and as opposed to most other comparisons [2, 5, 7, 25], mean CRP levels also did not differ at baseline.

Apart from a previous report from our group, finding inflammatory sacroiliitis lesions on MRI to predict better drug survival of a first TNF inhibitor in nr-axSpA [42], data on anti-TNF adherence in this diagnosis remain sparse. In contrast to our findings, based on retrospective data, Wallis et al. reported indications of worse adherence to anti-TNF therapy among patients with nr-axSpA as compared to AS [7], but prospectively conducted comparisons are still lacking. In line with the present results, however, male sex and CRP elevation at baseline have been shown to predict better adherence to anti-TNF therapy in patients with AS [43, 44].

In view of the relatively worse outcomes among both patient groups without CRP elevation, it may be hypothezised that in some of these subjects comorbidity in the form of chronic widespread pain (CWP) was falsely interpreted as spondyloarthritis activity, thus contributing to the decision to start anti-TNF therapy but not responding to this treatment. On the contrary, in patients with more active SpA - as reflected, for example, by CRP elevation - a certain improvement with anti-TNF therapy would be expected regardless of the presence of concomitant CWP or not. While the clinical arm of the ASAS axial SpA classification criteria has met with repeated concern that it may falsely classify CWP patients as having spondyloarthritis [45, 46], in a recent study presented in abstract form, no patients with primary fibromyalgia did indeed meet these criteria [47]. On the contrary, however, around 15 % of both AS and nr-axSpA patients also fulfilled criteria for fibromyalgia, and other studies have likewise reported a prevalence of concurrent fibromyalgia in AS at around 10–15 % [48, 49]. Furthermore, patient-reported SpA measures are known to differentiate poorly between symptoms related to SpA or CWP [48], with generally worse outcomes among patients with such comorbidity [49, 50], and poorer adherence to anti-TNF therapy was also recently reported in SpA patients with concurrent fibromyalgia [50].

Strengths and limitations

The relatively long follow up (3 years) and the opportunity to compare outcomes of anti-TNF therapy in patients with nr-axSpA and AS treated in clinical practice within the same observational setting, comprise major strengths of the present study. To our knowledge, a direct comparison of adherence to anti-TNF therapy in patients with these diagnoses based on prospectively collected data has been performed here for the first time. Furthermore, the available data on EQ-5D developments during anti-TNF therapy in patients with nr-axSpA was previously limited to 1-year results from a single study [30].

In terms of limitations, the open, observational setting entails inherent risks of bias in patient selection, assignment of treatment, and collection of clinical data. Moreover, the relatively high proportion of missing data for some outcomes is another frequent problem in observational studies, and for this reason the results of the main analysis are presented based on both imputed and observed data. On the other hand, the observational SSATG setting also implies that patient inclusion will not be restricted by any predefined level of disease activity, by rigid treatment guidelines or economical aspects, but rather will reflect clinical practice. At the same time, all patients were indeed selected for anti-TNF therapy, and results are thus not necessarily generalizable to the nr-axSpA and AS populations at large. The generalizability in nr-axSpA is also compromised by the exclusion of patients with a clinical diagnosis of psoriatic arthritis. For certainty of the diagnoses in our cohort, high validity for AS diagnoses has previously been demonstrated within the SSATG register, while review of the medical records confirmed that all included nr-axSpA patients fulfilled the ASAS classification criteria for axial disease without fulfilling the modified New York criteria. This said, however, a certain misclassification between the two diagnoses cannot be entirely ruled out [51]. Finally, due to their non-mandatory status within the SSATG during the study period, the lack of SpA-specific outcome measures such as BASDAI and BASFI beyond the baseline values is a main drawback of the present study. Based on the limited data available, however, developments in BASDAI closely resembled those of the presented patient-reported outcomes, whereas this was less apparent for BASFI, although the numbers of observations were small.

Conclusions

In this comparison of patients with nr-axSpA and AS in southern Sweden receiving anti-TNF therapy during 3 years in clinical practice, many similarities, and only a few differences were observed. Patients with nr-axSpA were more often female and had less elevation of acute phase reactants at baseline, with CRP levels remaining significantly lower than in the AS group throughout follow up. In spite of this, patient-reported measures of disease activity and HRQoL did not differ at baseline and followed nearly identical trajectories in both groups during the 3 years of follow up. Furthermore, no between-group difference was detected in adherence to anti-TNF therapy, and CRP elevation at baseline was similarly associated with superior clinical outcomes and anti-TNF treatment persistence in both groups. Overall, the current results thus seem to strengthen the prevailing hypothesis that nr-axSpA and AS represent different aspects/phases of the same underlying disease.

Abbreviations

ANOVA: analysis of variance; AS: ankylosing spondylitis; ASAS: Assessment of SpondyloArthritis International Society; BASDAI: Bath ankylosing spondylitis disease activity index; BASFI: Bath ankylosing spondylitis functional index; CI: confidence interval; CRP: C-reactive protein; CWP: chronic widespread pain; DMARD: disease-modifying anti-rheumatic drug; EQ-5D: EuroQol 5-Dimensions; ESR: erythrocyte sedimentation rate; HAQ: Health Assessment Questionnaire; HLA: human leukocyte antigen; HRQoL: health-related quality of life; IQR: interquartile range; LOCF: last observation carried forward; MRI: magnetic resonance imaging; nr-axSpA: non-radiographic axial spondyloarthritis; NSAID: non-steroidal anti-inflammatory drug; RCT: randomized controlled trial; SD: standard deviation; SpA: spondyloarthritis; SSATG: South Swedish Arthritis Treatment Group; TNF: tumor necrosis factor; UK: United Kingdom; VAS: visual analog scale.

Competing interests

IFP has received fees for speaking from Pfizer, UCB, and AbbVie. LEK has received consultancy fees and fees for speaking from Pfizer, UCB, AbbVie, BMS, and MSD. The remaining authors declare no conflict of interest.

Authors' contributions

JKW made substantial contributions to study conception and design, to data acquisition, analysis and interpretation of data, and drafted the manuscript. MCK, IFP and PG made substantial contributions to data acquisition, analysis and interpretation of data, and revised the manuscript critically for important intellectual content. LEK made substantial contributions to study conception and design, to data acquisition, analysis and interpretation of data, and helped draft the manuscript. All authors read and approved the final manuscript.

Acknowledgements

We are indebted to all patients, colleagues, and staff involved in the SSATG register study.
This work was supported by Region Skåne, Lund University Hospital, the Swedish Research Council, the Faculty of Medicine at Lund University, Österlund and Kock Foundations, the Swedish Rheumatism Association, King Gustav V 80-year fund, and the Oak Foundation. The sponsors had no role in study design, data collection, data analysis, data interpretation, or writing of the report.

Author details

[1]Section of Rheumatology, Department of Clinical Sciences Lund, Lund University, Lund, Sweden. [2]Section of Orthopedics, Department of Clinical Sciences Lund, Lund University, Lund, Sweden. [3]The Parker Institute, Department of Rheumatology, Copenhagen University Hospital,

Frederiksberg and Bispebjerg, Denmark. [4]Reumatologiska kliniken, Skånes Universitetssjukhus Lund, Kioskgatan 3, 22185 Lund, Sweden.

References

1. van der Linden S, Valkenburg HA, Cats A. Evaluation of diagnostic criteria for ankylosing spondylitis. A proposal for modification of the New York criteria. Arthritis Rheum. 1984;27:361–8.
2. Rudwaleit M, Haibel H, Baraliakos X, Listing J, Marker-Hermann E, Zeidler H, et al. The early disease stage in axial spondylarthritis: results from the German Spondyloarthritis Inception Cohort. Arthritis Rheum. 2009;60:717–27.
3. Rudwaleit M, van der Heijde D, Landewe R, Listing J, Akkoc N, Brandt J, et al. The development of Assessment of SpondyloArthritis international Society classification criteria for axial spondyloarthritis (part II): validation and final selection. Ann Rheum Dis. 2009;68:777–83.
4. Kiltz U, Baraliakos X, Karakostas P, Igelmann M, Kalthoff L, Klink C, et al. Do patients with non-radiographic axial spondylarthritis differ from patients with ankylosing spondylitis? Arthritis Care Res (Hoboken). 2012;64:1415–22.
5. Ciurea A, Scherer A, Exer P, Bernhard J, Dudler J, Beyeler B, et al. Tumor necrosis factor alpha inhibition in radiographic and nonradiographic axial spondyloarthritis: results from a large observational cohort. Arthritis Rheum. 2013;65:3096–106.
6. van den Berg R, de Hooge M, van Gaalen F, Reijnierse M, Huizinga T, van der Heijde D. Percentage of patients with spondyloarthritis in patients referred because of chronic back pain and performance of classification criteria: experience from the Spondyloarthritis Caught Early (SPACE) cohort. Rheumatology (Oxford). 2013;52:1492–9.
7. Wallis D, Haroon N, Ayearst R, Carty A, Inman RD. Ankylosing spondylitis and nonradiographic axial spondyloarthritis: part of a common spectrum or distinct diseases? J Rheumatol. 2013;40:2038–41.
8. Blachier M, Canoui-Poitrine F, Dougados M, Lethuaut A, Fautrel B, Ferkal S, et al. Factors associated with radiographic lesions in early axial spondyloarthritis. Results from the DESIR cohort. Rheumatology (Oxford). 2013;52:1686–93.
9. Poddubnyy D, Sieper J. Similarities and differences between nonradiographic and radiographic axial spondyloarthritis: a clinical, epidemiological and therapeutic assessment. Curr Opin Rheumatol. 2014;26: 377–83.
10. Boonen A, Sieper J, van der Heijde D, Dougados M, Bukowski JF, Valluri S, et al. The burden of non-radiographic axial spondyloarthritis. Semin Arthritis Rheum. 2015;44:556–62.
11. Poddubnyy D, Rudwaleit M, Haibel H, Listing J, Marker-Hermann E, Zeidler H, et al. Rates and predictors of radiographic sacroiliitis progression over 2 years in patients with axial spondyloarthritis. Ann Rheum Dis. 2011;70: 1369–74.
12. van der Heijde D, Sieper J, Maksymowych WP, Dougados M, Burgos-Vargas R, Landewe R, et al. 2010 Update of the international ASAS recommendations for the use of anti-TNF agents in patients with axial spondyloarthritis. Ann Rheum Dis. 2011;70:905–8.
13. Braun J, van den Berg R, Baraliakos X, Boehm H, Burgos-Vargas R, Collantes-Estevez E, et al. 2010 update of the ASAS/EULAR recommendations for the management of ankylosing spondylitis. Ann Rheum Dis. 2011;70:896–904.
14. Svensk Reumatologisk Förening. Riktlinjer för läkemedelsbehandling vid ankyloserande spondylit och psoriasisartrit (mars-2015). http://svenskreumatologi.se/sites/default /files/Riktlinjer_AS_PsoA_2015.pdf. Accessed 9 Nov 2015.
15. Song IH, Weiss A, Hermann KG, Haibel H, Althoff CE, Poddubnyy D, et al. Similar response rates in patients with ankylosing spondylitis and non-radiographic axial spondyloarthritis after 1 year of treatment with etanercept: results from the ESTHER trial. Ann Rheum Dis. 2013;72: 823–5.
16. Sieper J, Landewe R, Rudwaleit M, van der Heijde D, Dougados M, Mease PJ, et al. Effect of Certolizumab Pegol Over Ninety-Six Weeks in Patients With Axial Spondyloarthritis: Results from a Phase III Randomized Trial. Arthritis Rheumatol. 2015;67:668–77.
17. Geborek P, Crnkic M, Petersson IF, Saxne T. Etanercept, infliximab, and leflunomide in established rheumatoid arthritis: clinical experience using a structured follow up programme in southern Sweden. Ann Rheum Dis. 2002;61:793–8.
18. Kristensen LE, Petersson IF, Geborek P, Joud A, Saxne T, Jacobsson LT, et al. Sick leave in patients with ankylosing spondylitis before and after anti-TNF therapy: a population-based cohort study. Rheumatology (Oxford). 2012;51: 243–9.
19. Braun J, Davis J, Dougados M, Sieper J, van der Linden S, van der Heijde D, et al. First update of the international ASAS consensus statement for the use of anti-TNF agents in patients with ankylosing spondylitis. Ann Rheum Dis. 2006;65:316–20.
20. Brooks R. EuroQol: the current state of play. Health Policy. 1996;37:53–72.
21. Dolan P. Modeling valuations for EuroQol health states. Med Care. 1997;35: 1095–108.
22. Garrett S, Jenkinson T, Kennedy LG, Whitelock H, Gaisford P, Calin A. A new approach to defining disease status in ankylosing spondylitis: the Bath Ankylosing Spondylitis Disease Activity Index. J Rheumatol. 1994;21:2286–91.
23. Calin A, Garrett S, Whitelock H, Kennedy LG, O'Hea J, Mallorie P, et al. A new approach to defining functional ability in ankylosing spondylitis: the development of the Bath Ankylosing Spondylitis Functional Index. J Rheumatol. 1994;21:2281–5.
24. Fries JF, Spitz PW, Young DY. The dimensions of health outcomes: the health assessment questionnaire, disability and pain scales. J Rheumatol. 1982;9:789–93.
25. Landewe R, Braun J, Deodhar A, Dougados M, Maksymowych WP, Mease PJ, et al. Efficacy of certolizumab pegol on signs and symptoms of axial spondyloarthritis including ankylosing spondylitis: 24-week results of a double-blind randomised placebo-controlled Phase 3 study. Ann Rheum Dis. 2014;73:39–47.
26. Callhoff J, Sieper J, Weiss A, Zink A, Listing J. Efficacy of TNFalpha blockers in patients with ankylosing spondylitis and non-radiographic axial spondyloarthritis: a meta-analysis. Ann Rheum Dis. 2015;74:1241–8.
27. Braun J, Brandt J, Listing J, Zink A, Alten R, Golder W, et al. Treatment of active ankylosing spondylitis with infliximab: a randomised controlled multicentre trial. Lancet. 2002;359:1187–93.
28. Davis Jr JC, Van Der Heijde D, Braun J, Dougados M, Cush J, Clegg DO, et al. Recombinant human tumor necrosis factor receptor (etanercept) for treating ankylosing spondylitis: a randomized, controlled trial. Arthritis Rheum. 2003;48:3230–6.
29. van der Heijde D, Kivitz A, Schiff MH, Sieper J, Dijkmans BA, Braun J, et al. Efficacy and safety of adalimumab in patients with ankylosing spondylitis: results of a multicenter, randomized, double-blind, placebo-controlled trial. Arthritis Rheum. 2006;54:2136–46.
30. Haibel H, Rudwaleit M, Listing J, Heldmann F, Wong RL, Kupper H, et al. Efficacy of adalimumab in the treatment of axial spondylarthritis without radiographically defined sacroiliitis: results of a twelve-week randomized, double-blind, placebo-controlled trial followed by an open-label extension up to week fifty-two. Arthritis Rheum. 2008;58:1981–91.
31. Sieper J, van der Heijde D, Dougados M, Mease PJ, Maksymowych WP, Brown MA, et al. Efficacy and safety of adalimumab in patients with non-radiographic axial spondyloarthritis: results of a randomised placebo-controlled trial (ABILITY-1). Ann Rheum Dis. 2013;72:815–22.
32. Dougados M, van der Heijde D, Sieper J, Braun J, Maksymowych WP, Citera G, et al. Symptomatic efficacy of etanercept and its effects on objective signs of inflammation in early nonradiographic axial spondyloarthritis: a multicenter, randomized, double-blind, placebo-controlled trial. Arthritis Rheumatol. 2014;66:2091–102.
33. McLeod C, Bagust A, Boland A, Dagenais P, Dickson R, Dundar Y, et al. Adalimumab, etanercept and infliximab for the treatment of ankylosing spondylitis: a systematic review and economic evaluation. Health Technol Assess. 2007;11:1–158. iii-iv.
34. Song IH, Hermann KG, Haibel H, Althoff CE, Poddubnyy D, Listing J, et al. Consistently Good clinical response in patients with early axial spondyloarthritis after 3 years of continuous treatment with etanercept: longterm data of the ESTHER trial. J Rheumatol. 2014;41:2034–40.
35. Barkham N, Keen HI, Coates LC, O'Connor P, Hensor E, Fraser AD, et al. Clinical and imaging efficacy of infliximab in HLA-B27-Positive patients with magnetic resonance imaging-determined early sacroiliitis. Arthritis Rheum. 2009;60:946–54.
36. Rudwaleit M, Listing J, Brandt J, Braun J, Sieper J. Prediction of a major clinical response (BASDAI 50) to tumour necrosis factor alpha blockers in ankylosing spondylitis. Ann Rheum Dis. 2004;63:665–70.

37. Stone MA, Payne U, Pacheco-Tena C, Inman RD. Cytokine correlates of clinical response patterns to infliximab treatment of ankylosing spondylitis. Ann Rheum Dis. 2004;63:84–7.
38. Rudwaleit M, Schwarzlose S, Hilgert ES, Listing J, Braun J, Sieper J. MRI in predicting a major clinical response to anti-tumour necrosis factor treatment in ankylosing spondylitis. Ann Rheum Dis. 2008;67:1276–81.
39. Rudwaleit M, Claudepierre P, Wordsworth P, Cortina EL, Sieper J, Kron M, et al. Effectiveness, safety, and predictors of good clinical response in 1250 patients treated with adalimumab for active ankylosing spondylitis. J Rheumatol. 2009;36:801–8.
40. Lord PA, Farragher TM, Lunt M, Watson KD, Symmons DP, Hyrich KL, et al. Predictors of response to anti-TNF therapy in ankylosing spondylitis: results from the British Society for Rheumatology Biologics Register. Rheumatology (Oxford). 2010;49:563–70.
41. Vastesaeger N, van der Heijde D, Inman RD, Wang Y, Deodhar A, Hsu B, et al. Predicting the outcome of ankylosing spondylitis therapy. Ann Rheum Dis. 2011;70:973–81.
42. Gulfe A, Kapetanovic MC, Kristensen LE. Efficacy and drug survival of anti-tumour necrosis factor-alpha therapies in patients with non-radiographic axial spondyloarthritis: an observational cohort study from Southern Sweden. Scand J Rheumatol. 2014;43:493–7.
43. Kristensen LE, Karlsson JA, Englund M, Petersson IF, Saxne T, Geborek P. Presence of peripheral arthritis and male sex predicting continuation of anti-tumor necrosis factor therapy in ankylosing spondylitis: an observational prospective cohort study from the South Swedish Arthritis Treatment Group Register. Arthritis Care Res (Hoboken). 2010;62:1362–9.
44. Luc M, Gossec L, Ruyssen-Witrand A, Salliot C, Duclos M, Guignard S, et al. C-reactive protein predicts tumor necrosis factor-alpha blocker retention rate in axial ankylosing spondylitis. J Rheumatol. 2007;34:2078–81.
45. Tournadre A, Pereira B, Lhoste A, Dubost JJ, Ristori JM, Claudepierre P, et al. Differences between women and men with recent-onset axial spondyloarthritis: results from a prospective multicenter French cohort. Arthritis Care Res (Hoboken). 2013;65:1482–9.
46. Braun J, Baraliakos X, Kiltz U, Heldmann F, Sieper J. Classification and diagnosis of axial spondyloarthritis–what is the clinically relevant difference? J Rheumatol. 2015;42:31–8.
47. Baraliakos X, Regel A, Kiltz U, Kiefer D, Menne H-J, Dybowski F, et al. Patients with fibromyalgia (FM) do not fulfill classification criteria for axial spondyloarthritis (axSpA) but patients with axSpA may fulfill classification criteria for FM. Ann Rheum Dis. 2015;74 Suppl 2:80. doi:10.1136/annrheumdis-2015-eular.5965.
48. Salaffi F, De Angelis R, Carotti M, Gutierrez M, Sarzi-Puttini P, Atzeni F. Fibromyalgia in patients with axial spondyloarthritis: epidemiological profile and effect on measures of disease activity. Rheumatol Int. 2014;34:1103–10.
49. Haliloglu S, Carlioglu A, Akdeniz D, Karaaslan Y, Kosar A. Fibromyalgia in patients with other rheumatic diseases: prevalence and relationship with disease activity. Rheumatol Int. 2014;34:1275–80.
50. Bello Vega N, Béal C, Etcheto A, Dougados M, Molto A. How fibromyalgia impacts clinical and treatment aspects in spondyloarthritis patients: results of the Fispa study. Ann Rheum Dis. 2015;74 Suppl 2:506–7. doi:10.1136/annrheumdis-2015-eular.2831.
51. U.S. Food and Drug Administration. Arthritis advisory committee meeting July 23, 2013. sBLA 125057/323: adalimumab for the treatment of Active non-radiographic axial spondyloarthritis in adults with objective signs of inflammation by elevated c-reactive protein (CRP) or magnetic resonance imaging (MRI), who have had an inadequate response to, or are intolerant to, a nonsteroidal anti-inflammatory drug. http://www.fda.gov/downloads/AdvisoryCommittees/CommitteesMeetingMaterials/Drugs/ArthritisAdvisoryCommittee/UCM361563.pdf. Accessed 21 Nov 2015.

18

Comparable long-term efficacy, as assessed by patient-reported outcomes, safety and pharmacokinetics, of CT-P13 and reference infliximab in patients with ankylosing spondylitis: 54-week results from the randomized, parallel-group PLANETAS study

Won Park[1], Dae Hyun Yoo[2*], Janusz Jaworski[3], Jan Brzezicki[4], Andriy Gnylorybov[5], Vladimir Kadinov[6], Irmgadt Goecke Sariego[7], Carlos Abud-Mendoza[8], William Jose Otero Escalante[9], Seong Wook Kang[10], Daina Andersone[11], Francisco Blanco[12], Seung Suh Hong[13], Sun Hee Lee[13] and Jürgen Braun[14*]

Abstract

Background: CT-P13 (Remsima®, Inflectra®) is a biosimilar of the infliximab reference product (RP; Remicade®) and is approved in Europe and elsewhere, mostly for the same indications as RP. The aim of this study was to compare the 54-week efficacy, immunogenicity, pharmacokinetics (PK) and safety of CT-P13 with RP in patients with ankylosing spondylitis (AS), with a focus on patient-reported outcomes (PROs).

Methods: This was a multinational, double-blind, parallel-group study in patients with active AS. Participants were randomized (1:1) to receive CT-P13 (5 mg/kg) or RP (5 mg/kg) at weeks 0, 2, 6 and then every 8 weeks up to week 54. To assess responses, standardized assessment tools were used with an intention-to-treat analysis of observed data. Anti-drug antibodies (ADAs), PK parameters, and safety outcomes were also assessed.

Results: Of 250 randomized patients (n = 125 per group), 210 (84.0 %) completed 54 weeks of treatment, with similar completion rates between groups. At week 54, Assessment of Spondylo Arthritis international Society (ASAS)20 response, ASAS40 response and ASAS partial remission were comparable between treatment groups. Changes from baseline in PROs such as mean Bath Ankylosing Spondylitis Disease Activity Index (BASDAI; CT-P13 −3.1 versus RP −2.8), Bath Ankylosing Spondylitis Functional Index (BASFI; −2.9 versus −2.7), and Short Form Health Survey (SF-36) scores (9.26 versus 10.13 for physical component summary; 7.30 versus 6.54 for mental component summary) were similar between treatment groups. At 54 weeks, 19.5 % and 23.0 % of patients receiving CT-P13 and RP, respectively, had ADAs. All observed PK parameters of CT-P13 and RP, including maximum and minimum serum concentrations, were similar through 54 weeks. The influence of ADAs on PK was similar in the two treatment groups. Most adverse events were mild or moderate in severity. There was no notable difference between treatment groups in the incidence of adverse events, serious adverse events, infections and infusion-related reactions.

(Continued on next page)

* Correspondence: dhyoo@hanyang.ac.kr; juergen.braun@elisabethgruppe.de
[2]Hanyang University Hospital, Seoul, Republic of Korea
[14]Rheumazentrum Ruhrgebiet, Herne, Germany

(Continued from previous page)

Conclusions: CT-P13 and RP have highly comparable efficacy (including PROs) and PK up to week 54. Over a 1-year period, CT-P13 was well tolerated and displayed a safety profile comparable to RP; no differences in immunogenicity were observed.

Keywords: Biosimilar, CT-P13, Infliximab, Ankylosing spondylitis, Efficacy, Immunogenicity, Pharmacokinetics, Safety, ASAS, Clinical trial

Background

Infliximab is a human-murine chimeric monoclonal antibody directed against tumor necrosis factor (TNF). Originator infliximab (Remicade®; hereafter referred to as the reference product (RP)) was the first TNF antagonist proven to be efficacious in patients with ankylosing spondylitis (AS) [1, 2], and is now regarded as an important component of AS care [3, 4]. However, the costs of infliximab RP and other originator biologics are often high, placing considerable financial burden on healthcare systems and, in many countries, restricting patient access [5, 6]. As a result, the development of biosimilar drugs has garnered considerable interest as many originator biologics have reached or are close to patent expiry. A biosimilar may be defined as 'a biotherapeutic product that is similar in terms of quality, safety and efficacy to an already licensed reference biotherapeutic product' [7]. Due to their assumed lower price, biosimilars have the potential to reduce costs and increase patient access and drug therapy adherence.

CT-P13 (Remsima®, Inflectra®) is a biosimilar of RP produced in the same murine hybridoma cell line as RP and approved in Europe and elsewhere for the same indications. CT-P13 and RP are identical in amino acid sequence, pharmaceutical form, strength, composition, and route of administration [8, 9]. Secondary and tertiary structures of CT-P13 and RP are highly comparable to each other, although not identical. Both drugs bind to known infliximab ligands and receptors (e.g., TNF, Fcγ and C1q) with similar affinity, while neither bind to lymphotoxin. In vitro studies have shown that CT-P13 and RP possess equivalent TNF neutralization activity, apoptotic activity, complement-dependent cytotoxicity and antibody-dependent cellular toxicity [8, 9].

Biosimilar guidelines in Europe and the US state that demonstration of clinical comparability between a biosimilar and its innovator requires completion of comparator clinical trials assessing pharmacokinetics (PK), efficacy and safety [10, 11]. Efficacy equivalence of CT-P13 and RP was established in the PLANETRA (Programme evaLuating the Autoimmune disease iNvEstigational drug cT-p13 in Rheumatoid Arthritis) study [12]. Another study called PLANETAS (Programme evaLuating the Autoimmune disease iNvEstigational drug cT-p13 in AS patients) was conducted to assess PK equivalence and comparability of efficacy and safety in patients with AS. The primary analysis of PLANETAS was performed at week 30 of the study [13]. That analysis showed that the primary endpoint of the study—PK equivalence of CT-P13 and RP as assessed by steady state area under the serum concentration curve (AUC) and maximum serum concentration (C_{max}) between weeks 22 and 30—was met. Efficacy and safety findings up to week 30 were also similar in the patients with AS.

In order to compare the extended efficacy, immunogenicity, PK and safety of CT-P13 and RP in patients with AS, PLANETAS continued up to 54 weeks (plus a subsequent off-dose period of 8 weeks). Here, we report the results of the study at week 54.

Methods

Study methods have been reported in detail previously [13].

Patients

AS patients aged 18–75 years meeting the 1984 modified New York classification criteria [14] for ≥3 months prior to screening, with Bath Ankylosing Spondylitis Disease Activity Index (BASDAI) score of ≥4 (range 0–10) and a visual analogue scale score for spinal pain of ≥4 (range 0–10) were eligible for the PLANETAS study. Patients were permitted to receive both oral glucocorticoids (equivalent to ≤10 mg daily prednisolone) and nonsteroidal anti-inflammatory drugs, if they had received a stable dose for ≥4 weeks prior to screening.

Study design and treatment

This randomized, double-blind, parallel-group study (ClinicalTrials.gov identifier: NCT01220518) was conducted in 46 centers in 10 countries. Patients were randomly assigned in a 1:1 ratio to receive CT-P13 (CELLTRION Inc, Incheon, Republic of Korea) or RP (Janssen Biotech Inc, Horsham, Pennsylvania, USA), at a dose of 5 mg/kg via 2-hour intravenous infusion at weeks 0, 2 and 6, and then every 8 weeks thereafter up to week 54. Antihistamines were provided prior to infusion at the investigator's discretion. The overall randomization code was broken for regulatory reporting purposes once the database up to week 30 had been finalized for analysis [13]. However, the study remained blinded to the investigators and patients up to week 54.

The study was carried out according to the principles of the Declaration of Helsinki and International Conference on Harmonisation good clinical practice guidelines. The study was approved by the relevant independent ethics committees (see Acknowledgements). All patients provided written informed consent.

Study endpoints and assessments

Efficacy was assessed at baseline and weeks 14, 30 and 54. Efficacy endpoints included: patient-reported outcomes (PROs), including BASDAI, the Bath Ankylosing Spondylitis Functional Index (BASFI), and the Short Form (36) Health Survey (SF-36); the proportion of patients achieving clinical response according to Assessment of Spondyloarthritis international Society (ASAS)20 and ASAS40 criteria; the proportion of patients with ASAS partial remission; changes from baseline in Ankylosing Spondylitis Disease Activity Score (ASDAS)-C-reactive protein (CRP), Bath Ankylosing Spondylitis Metrology Index (BASMI) and chest expansion.

The proportion of patients who tested positive for anti-drug antibodies (ADAs) was assessed at baseline and weeks 14, 30 and 54 using an electrochemiluminescent immunoassay method, as previously reported [13]. The neutralizing activity of ADAs was also assessed by a flow-through immunoassay method utilizing the Gyros Immunoassay platform (Gyros AB, Sweden). Primary PK endpoints included the area under the concentration time curve over the dosing interval, at steady state between week 22 and week 30 (AUC_{τ}) and the observed maximum serum concentration at steady state between week 22 and week 30 ($C_{max,ss}$). Secondary assessments included C_{max} and minimum concentration (C_{min}) immediately before the next infusion up to week 54. Blood samples were collected immediately before each treatment, at the end of each infusion, and 60 minutes post-infusion. PK analyses were performed using a flow-through immunoassay platform (Gyros AB, Sweden). The influence of ADA titer level on primary PK endpoints was assessed with a low, medium and high ADA titer based on tertile grouping of the data.

Regarding safety, adverse events (AEs) were assessed from enrollment and up to 8 weeks after last study treatment. A treatment-emergent AE (TEAE) was defined as any event not present before exposure to study treatment or an event that worsened in intensity or frequency after exposure to study treatment. Other safety assessments included vital signs monitoring, physical examination, clinical laboratory analyses, and tuberculosis (TB) monitoring. An AE of latent TB was reported if a patient had a positive result on interferon-γ release assay after a negative result at baseline together with a negative result on chest X-ray examination. Patients were monitored for infusion-related reactions, including hypersensitivity and anaphylactic reaction.

In a series of subgroup analyses, the impact of ADA status on efficacy, PK and safety was determined. For subanalysis of ASAS20 response, ADA status was determined at week 54. For C_{max} subanalysis, a non-visit-based approach was adopted to evaluate the incidence of patients who developed ADAs up to and including week 54. In subgroup analysis of infusion-related reactions, patients were grouped according to their seroconversion status, which was defined as positive if the patient had a negative ADA test followed by a positive ADA test at a subsequent visit; all other patients who provided at least one ADA test result were included in the non-seroconverted group.

Statistical analyses

Statistical analyses were performed using Version 9.1.3 of SAS software (SAS Institute, Inc, Cary, North Carolina, USA). All efficacy analyses were performed by intention-to-treat, using the 'missing equals excluded' (MEX) approach. The proportion of patients achieving clinical response (ASAS20/ASAS40) was analyzed by a logistic regression model, with treatment group as a fixed effect and the stratification factors (region and baseline BASDAI score) as covariates. Treatment effect was estimated by calculating the odds ratio (OR) and 95 % confidence interval (CI). Other efficacy endpoints were analyzed using descriptive statistics.

For PK analyses, serum drug concentrations were summarized using quantitative descriptive statistics by actual treatment group, visit and time point. The PK population included patients who received at least the first five doses of study treatment, had sufficient blood concentration data to facilitate the calculation of PK parameters, and had no major protocol deviations. The safety population included all patients who received at least one (full or partial) dose of CT-P13 or RP during any dosing period.

Sensitivity analyses of ASAS response data were conducted using a last observation carried forward (LOCF) approach to compare the full-set analysis (LOCF) with the complete-case analysis (MEX).

Results

Patient disposition and baseline characteristics

Overall, 250 patients were randomly assigned to study treatment (n = 125 in each group; Fig. 1). A total of 210 patients completed 54 weeks of treatment (n = 106 (84.8 %) and 104 (83.2 %) in the CT-P13 and RP groups, respectively). The most common reason for discontinuation was AEs (n = 13 (10.4 %) and 10 (8.0 %), respectively) in each group.

Baseline patient demographics and disease characteristics are shown in Table 1. In both the CT-P13 and RP

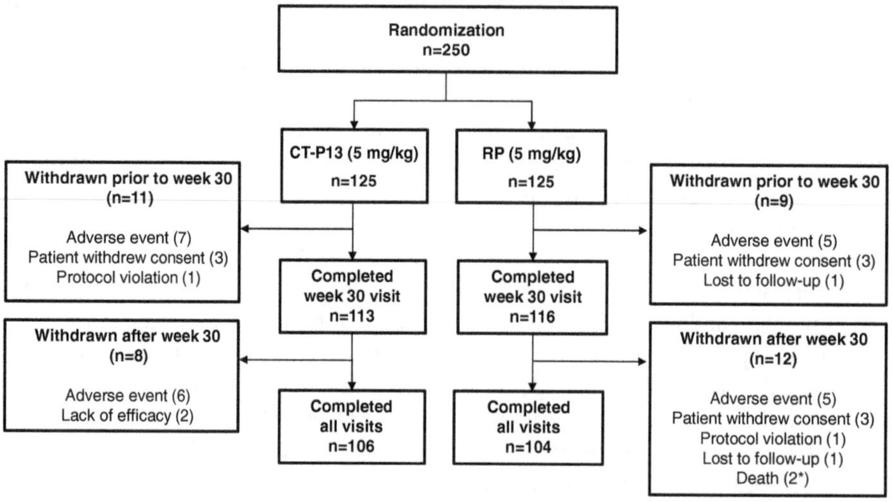

Fig. 1 Flowchart of patient disposition. A total of 250 eligible patients were randomized into the CT-P13 group (n = 125) or RP group (n = 125) to receive 5 mg/kg of CT-P13 or RP, respectively. All 250 randomly assigned patients were included in the intention-to-treat population. *One patient randomly assigned to RP received at least one dose of CT-P13 unintentionally. *RP* reference product (i.e., reference infliximab)

groups the majority of patients were male (n = 99 (79.2 %) and n = 103 (82.4 %), respectively), and median age was 38 years in both groups (range 18–69 years). Baseline scores for efficacy assessments, including PROs, were similar between groups.

Efficacy

Efficacy was similar between both treatment groups, as measured by all efficacy endpoints. The proportion of patients achieving clinical response according to ASAS20 and ASAS40 criteria at weeks 14, 30 and 54 was similar between the CT-P13 and RP groups, as were ASAS partial remission rates (Fig. 2a). Logistic regression indicated no difference in ASAS20 responses between CT-P13 and RP at week 54 (0.89 (0.50, 1.59)). Similarly, there was no difference between CT-P13 and RP for ASAS40 responses at week 54 (1.26 (0.73, 2.15)). Sensitivity analyses of ASAS response rates using the full-set (LOCF) population also showed no differences between CT-P13 and RP (Fig. 2b). In a subgroup analysis performed according to ADA status, the proportion of ADA-negative patients achieving ASAS20 at week 54 was 72.3 % in the CT-P13 group and 73.1 % in the RP group. In comparison, 47.8 % and 60.0 % of ADA-positive patients in the CT-P13 and RP groups, respectively, achieved ASAS20 at week 54.

ASDAS-CRP score (mean ± standard deviation (SD)) at baseline (3.8 ± 0.8 and 3.9 ± 1.1 in the CT-P13 and RP groups, respectively) and the mean change from baseline were similar in the CT-P13 and RP groups at week 54 (−1.7 ± 1.3 and −1.7 ± 1.3).

In terms of PROs, baseline scores of BASDAI and BASFI were similar between groups, and the scores decreased from baseline up to week 54 to a similar extent in both the CT-P13 and RP groups (mean ± SD BASDAI scores at baseline: 6.7 ± 1.4 versus 6.6 ± 1.6 in the CT-P13 and RP groups, respectively; change from baseline BASDAI scores: −2.9 ± 2.2 versus −2.8 ± 2.1 (week 14), −3.0 ± 2.2 versus −2.7 ± 2.2 (week 30) and −3.1 ± 2.3 versus −2.8 ± 2.2 (week 54); BASFI scores at baseline: 6.2 ± 1.9 versus 6.2 ± 2.2; change from baseline BASFI scores: −2.5 ± 2.1 versus −2.5 ± 2.2 (week 14), −2.6 ± 2.2 versus −2.5 ± 2.2 (week 30) and −2.9 ± 2.3 versus −2.7 ± 2.1 (week 54)) (Fig. 3a and b). Regarding the SF-36 quality of life questionnaire, scores were similar between CT-P13 and RP groups for all components of the questionnaire at baseline and weeks 14, 30 and 54. Mean SF-36 score increased from baseline to week 54 in both groups. For the physical component summary (Fig. 3c), the mean ± SD scores at baseline were 33.4 ± 6.7 and 32.2 ± 6.8, and at week 54 were 42.4 ± 8.6 and 42.2 ± 9.0 with CT-P13 and RP, respectively. For the mental component summary (Fig. 3d), the mean scores at baseline were 38.1 ± 10.3 and 37.5 ± 11.2, and at week 54 were 44.9 ± 10.9 and 44.9 ± 11.0 with CT-P13 and RP, respectively. In the CT-P13 and RP groups, respectively, mean change from baseline to week 54 was 9.26 and 10.13 for the physical component summary and 7.30 and 6.54 for the mental component summary.

Mean ± SD BASMI scores and chest expansion (cm) at baseline were 4.0 ± 2.1 versus 4.1 ± 2.1, and 3.2 ± 1.3 versus 2.9 ± 1.3 in the CT-P13 and RP groups, respectively. Mean change from baseline values were similar in the CT-P13 and RP groups (week 14: −0.7 ± 1.2 versus −0.7 ± 1.4; week 30: −1.0 ± 1.4 versus −0.9 ± 1.4; week 54: −1.1 ± 1.5 versus −0.9 ± 1.6 for BASMI (Fig. 3e); week 14: 0.4 ± 1.0

Table 1 Baseline patient demographics and disease characteristics

Characteristic	CT-P13 5 mg/kg (n = 125)	RP 5 mg/kg (n = 125)	Total (n = 250)
Age, years	38.0 (18–69)	38.0 (18–66)	38.0 (18–69)
Gender, no. (%)			
Male	99 (79.2)	103 (82.4)	202 (80.8)
Female	26 (20.8)	22 (17.6)	48 (19.2)
Ethnicity, no. (%)			
Caucasian	97 (77.6)	92 (73.6)	189 (75.6)
Asian	16 (12.8)	13 (10.4)	29 (11.6)
Other	12 (9.6)	20 (16.0)	32 (12.8)
Height, cm	172.0 (148–198)	171.0 (147–193)	172.0 (147–198)
Weight, kg	72.70 (45.0–120.0)	76.00 (45.5–122.7)	73.75 (45.0–122.7)
Body mass index, kg/m^2	24.39 (18.0–38.7)	25.64 (17.5–42.0)	25.12 (17.5–42.0)
ASDAS-CRP, mean ± SD	3.8 ± 0.8	3.9 ± 1.1	3.9 ± 1.0
BASDAI (stratification factor), no. (%)			
4 ~ ≤8	92 (73.6)	95 (76.0)	187 (74.8)
>8–10	33 (26.4)	30 (24.0)	63 (25.2)
BASDAI score	6.8 (3.4–10.0)	6.6 (1.8–10.0)	6.7 (1.8–10.0)
BASFI score	6.3 (0.7–9.8)	6.3 (0.1–10.0)	6.3 (0.1–10.0)
BASMI score	4.0 (0.0–9.0)	4.0 (0.0–9.0)	4.0 (0.0–9.0)
Chest expansion, cm	3.0 (0.5–9.0)	2.5 (0.0–7.0)	3.0 (0.0–9.0)
SF-36 summary scores			
Physical component	34.1 (16.2–49.7)	33.1 (15.3–54.3)	33.4 (15.3–54.3)
Mental component	38.2 (15.1–63.7)	37.2 (12.5–63.6)	37.8 (12.5–63.7)
CRP, mg/dL	1.1 (0.0–13.0)	1.4 (0.0–17.4)	1.3 (0.0–17.4)
ESR, mm/h	33.0 (2.0–110.0)	34.0 (1.0–119.0)	34.0 (1.0–119.0)

Except where indicated otherwise, values are expressed as median (minimum–maximum). *ASDAS* Ankylosing Spondylitis Disease Activity Score, *BASDAI* Bath Ankylosing Spondylitis Disease Activity Index, *BASFI* Bath Ankylosing Spondylitis Functional Index, *BASMI* Bath Ankylosing Spondylitis Metrology Index, *CRP* C-reactive protein *ESR* erythrocyte sedimentation rate, *RP* reference product (i.e. reference infliximab), *SD* standard deviation, *SF-36* Short Form (36) Health Survey

versus 0.7 ± 1.0; week 30: 0.6 ± 1.4 versus 0.8 ± 1.2; week 54: 0.7 ± 1.4 versus 0.9 ± 1.1 for chest expansion).

Immunogenicity

The proportion of patients with ADAs was similar between the CT-P13 and RP groups at each time point (week 14: n = 11 (8.6 %) and n = 13 (10.7 %); week 30: n = 32 (25.0 %) and n = 25 (20.5 %); week 54: n = 25 (19.5 %) and n = 28 (23.0 %)). The vast majority of patients who were ADA-positive also had neutralizing activity in both the CT-13 and RP groups (week 14: n = 10 and n = 13; week 30: n = 31 and n = 24; week 54: n = 25 and n = 28).

Pharmacokinetics

A total of 223 (89.2 %) patients were included in the PK population (n = 113 and n = 110 in the CT-P13 and RP groups, respectively). C_{max} and C_{min} values were similar between the two treatment groups up to week 54 (Fig. 4).

The influence of ADAs on primary PK endpoints ($C_{max,ss}$ and AUC_τ) was also investigated. Figure 5 shows these endpoints by ADA titer level at week 30 in the CT-P13 and RP groups. There was a trend for both $C_{max,ss}$ and AUC_τ to be lower with higher ADA titer levels. This impact of ADAs on drug exposure was similar in the two treatment groups. In a related subgroup analysis, mean (coefficient of variation) C_{max} was comparable in the CT-P13 and RP groups at week 54 in both ADA-negative (142.98 (27.6) versus 135.27 (22.6) μg/mL, respectively) and ADA-positive (122.53 (31.1) versus 117.16 (25.6) μg/mL) patients.

Safety

Due to incorrect kits being dispensed, three patients randomly assigned to the RP treatment group received one dose of CT-P13 in this study. Therefore, the safety population comprised 128 and 122 patients in the CT-P13 and RP groups, respectively.

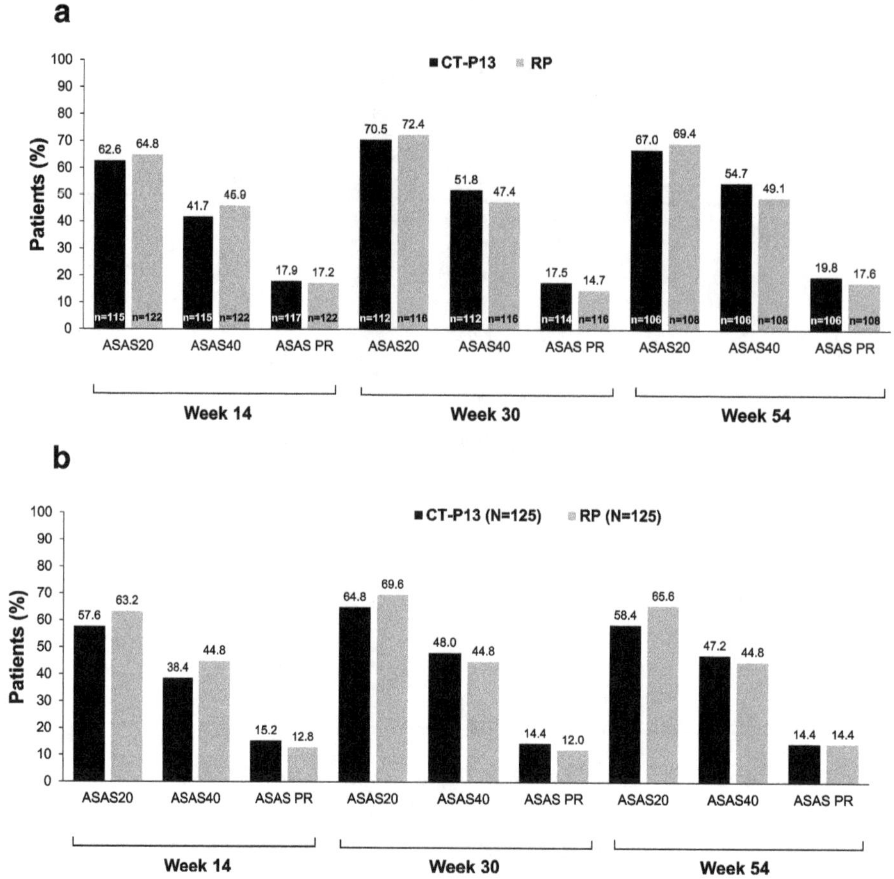

Fig. 2 Proportion of patients with an ASAS20 response, ASAS40 response and ASAS PR* up to week 54 by treatment in the **a** ITT population (MEX approach) and **b** ITT population (LOCF approach). "n = numbers" in the bar represent the denominator of patients assessed at each time point. *PR was defined as a value of <20 on a 0–100 scale in each of the following four domains: patient global assessment, pain, function, and inflammation. *ASAS* Assessment of Spondylo Arthritis international Society (ASAS20 and ASAS40, 20 % and 40 % response according to the ASAS International Working Group criteria for improvement), *ITT* intention-to-treat, *LOCF* last observation carried forward, *MEX* missing equals excluded, *PR* partial remission, *RP* reference product (i.e. reference infliximab)

The proportion of patients who experienced at least one TEAE was similar in the CT-P13 and RP groups (n = 95 (74.2 %) and 82 (67.2 %), respectively). Most TEAEs were mild or moderate in intensity. TEAEs considered by the investigator to be related to study treatment were reported in 64 (50.0 %) and 63 (51.6 %) patients, respectively. The most common of these events are shown in Table 2. Related TEAEs occurring in >4 % of patients were (for CT-P13) abnormal liver function test (n = 16 (12.5 %)), upper respiratory tract infection (n = 12 (9.4 %)), infusion-related reaction (n = 11 (8.6 %)) and latent TB (9 (7.0 %)), and (for RP) abnormal liver function test (n = 15 (12.3 %)), infusion-related reaction (n = 15 (12.3 %)), upper respiratory tract infection (n = 8 (6.6 %)) and latent TB (6 (4.9 %)). Infusion-related reactions affected more ADA-positive than ADA-negative patients in both treatment groups (CT-P13: 6/44 (13.6 %) versus 5/84 (6.0 %); RP: 11/39 (28.2 %) versus 4/83 (4.8 %)).

Two cases of active TB were reported in the CT-P13 group and one case was reported in the RP group. A single case of malignancy, which was considered to be unrelated to treatment, was reported in the CT-P13 group (basal cell carcinoma). The onset date of this event was unknown, but was believed to have started 2 years previously, based on the medical history of the patient (melanocyte nevus). Treatment for the event was excision of a skin nodule of the nose. The event was considered to have recovered/resolved according to the investigator.

The proportion of patients who experienced at least one serious AE (SAE) was similar between the CT-P13 and RP groups (n = 10 (7.8 %) and 8 (6.6 %), respectively), as was the proportion who had an SAE considered related to treatment (n = 4 (3.1 %) and 5 (4.1 %); see Additional file 1 for details of treatment-related SAEs). The number of patients with at least one TEAE leading to discontinuation was comparable between the CT-P13

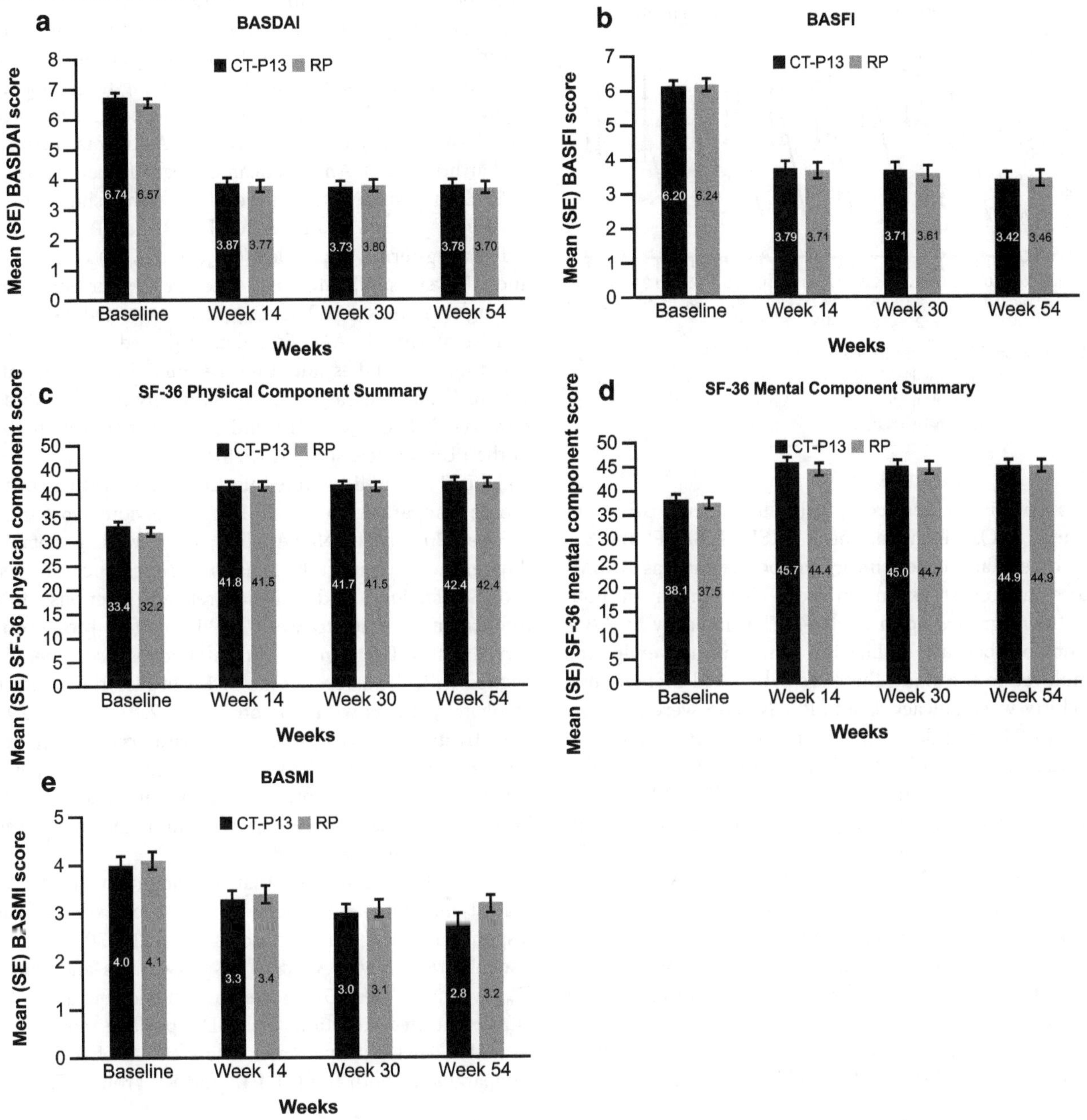

Fig. 3 Mean **a** BASDAI, **b** BASFI, **c** SF-36 Physical Component Summary, **d** SF-36 Mental Component Summary and **e** BASMI scores up to week 54 by treatment. *BASDAI* Bath Ankylosing Spondylitis Disease Activity Index, *BASFI* Bath Ankylosing Spondylitis Functional Index, *BASMI* Bath Ankylosing Spondylitis Metrology Index, *RP* reference product (i.e. reference infliximab), *SF-36* Short Form (36) Health Survey, *SE* standard error

and RP groups (n = 11 (8.6 %) and 9 (7.4 %), respectively). Of these, 9 (7.0 %) and 7 (5.7 %) were considered to be related to CT-P13 and RP, respectively. Overall, treatment-related events leading to discontinuation of more than one patient were TB in two patients from the CT-P13 group and one in the RP group, two abnormal liver function tests (one in each group), and infusion-related reactions in one patient from the CT-P13 group and five from the RP group. Two deaths occurred during the study, one in each treatment group. Both were due to car accidents and were considered not related to study treatment.

Discussion

PLANETAS was a multinational, randomized, double-blind biosimilar study that evaluated the equivalence of PK and comparability of efficacy and safety between CT-P13 and RP up to 54 weeks in patients with active AS.

Similar clinical efficacy was observed between CT-P13 and RP up to week 54. ASAS responses at weeks 30 and

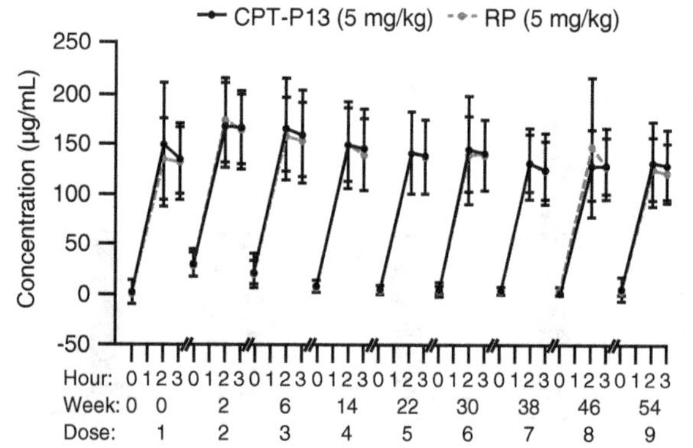

Fig. 4 Mean (SD) serum PK parameters of CT-P13 and RP (PK population). Note: values below the LLOQ have been set equal to the LLOQ. *LLOQ* lower limit of quantification, *PK* pharmacokinetics, *RP* reference product (i.e. reference infliximab), *SD* standard deviation

54, respectively, were comparable in the two treatment groups. PROs—including mean BASDAI, BASFI and SF-36 scores—and other efficacy endpoints such as BASMI score and chest expansion were also similar in both treatment groups up to week 54. The similarity in PROs is notable because, unlike the other efficacy endpoints employed in the study, these are patient-led evaluations.

Thirty-week efficacy data in PLANETAS were comparable to 24-week data from a pivotal placebo-controlled clinical study of RP in AS (ASSERT) [2, 13]. Analogously, the efficacy data seen here for CT-P13 at week 54 are in line with findings previously reported for RP in different clinical trials with a similar duration [15–17]. For example, in the current analysis, the ASAS20 responses and improvement of BASDAI and BASFI scores with CT-P13 at 54 weeks were 67 %, 3.1 and 2.9, respectively. Similar improvements in these measurements were also observed at weeks 48–58 in historical studies with RP (ASAS20 at week 58 = 75 %; BASDAI from 6.6 at week 0 to 2.4 at week 54; BASFI from 6.1 at baseline to 4.4 at week 48) [15–17]. While there are inherent limitations associated with comparing across trials due to differences in patient populations and methods, it is reassuring that the data for CT-P13 are generally in line with historical observations for RP. Long-term efficacy equivalence of CT-P13 and RP has also been established in a 54-week analysis of the PLANETRA study in rheumatoid arthritis (RA). An American College of Rheumatology (ACR)20 response was achieved in a highly similar proportion of patients treated with CT-P13 and RP [18].

The long-term PK profiles (C_{max} and C_{min}) of CT-P13 and RP were similar to each other in the current study through to week 54. The C_{max} data reported here are consistent with PLANETAS data reported at 30 weeks and those of studies adopting a similar RP dosing pattern in Crohn's disease [13, 19]. Similarity of PK was also observed between CT-P13 and RP in patients with RA in the PLANETRA study [12, 18].

CT-P13 was well tolerated up to week 54, with a safety profile comparable to that of RP. As previously reported at week 30 for PLANETAS [13], there was no notable difference between study arms in the incidence of AEs, SAEs, infections and infusion-related reactions; this trend continued up to week 54. The safety profile observed with CT-P13 in the current study is also generally aligned with the safety profile of RP in historical studies involving patients with AS and RA [1, 2, 15–17, 20–29]. One treatment-unrelated case of basal cell carcinoma was reported with CT-P13. It is believed that the malignancy started 2 years prior to study participation. Following appropriate treatment (excision), the event was considered to have resolved.

It is well documented that development of ADAs against infliximab is associated with decreased clinical response and drug serum concentration [13, 30–32]. We also observed lower ASAS20 response rates and lower C_{max} values at week 54, as well as a higher incidence of infusion-related reactions in ADA-positive compared with ADA-negative patients. These ADA effects were comparable in both the CT-P13 and RP groups. Further

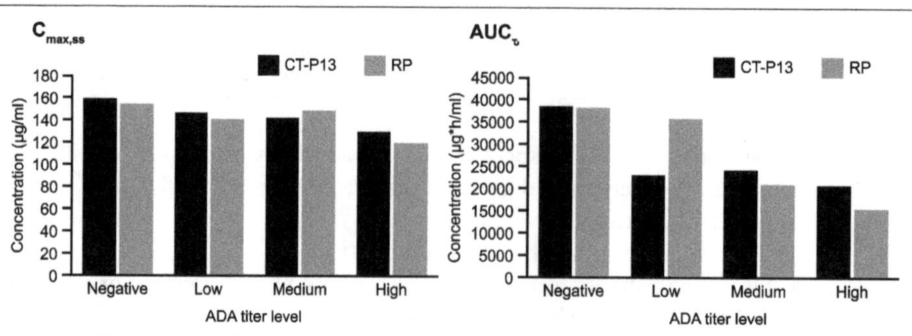

Fig. 5 Primary PK parameters ($C_{max,ss}$ and AUC_{τ}) by ADA titer level at week 30 (PK population). Note: titer levels were defined as low, medium and high titer based on tertile grouping of the data. *ADA* anti-drug antibodies, AUC_{τ} area under the concentration time curve over the dosing interval, at steady state between week 22 and week 30, $C_{max,ss}$ the observed maximum serum concentration at steady state between week 22 and week 30, *PK* pharmacokinetics, *RP* reference product (i.e. reference infliximab)

Table 2 Treatment-related adverse events reported in at least 1 % of all (total) patients, n (%)

	CT-P13 (n = 128)	RP (n = 122)	Total CT-P13 + RP (n = 250)
Abnormal liver function test	16 (12.5)	15 (12.3)	31 (12.4)
Infusion-related reaction	11 (8.6)	15 (12.3)	26 (10.4)
Upper respiratory tract infection	12 (9.4)	8 (6.6)	20 (8.0)
Latent tuberculosis	9 (7.0)	6 (4.9)	15 (6.0)
Urinary tract infection	5 (3.9)	4 (3.3)	9 (3.6)
Neutropenia	4 (3.1)	3 (2.5)	7 (2.8)
Elevated serum creatine phosphokinase	4 (3.1)	2 (1.6)	6 (2.4)
Rash	2 (1.6)	4 (3.3)	6 (2.4)
Headache	3 (2.3)	1 (0.8)	4 (1.6)
Herpes virus infection	1 (0.8)	3 (2.5)	4 (1.6)
Sinusitis	2 (1.6)	1 (0.8)	3 (1.2)
Tuberculosis	2 (1.6)	1 (0.8)	3 (1.2)

RP reference product (i.e. reference infliximab)

analysis of PK parameters with respect to ADA levels found a trend for both AUC_{τ}, and $C_{max,ss}$ to be lower with increasing ADA titer level, although a formal statistical inference was not made due to a limited statistical power.

Further extensions of the current study and the PLANETRA study were conducted to examine the efficacy and safety of switching treatment from RP to CT-P13 in patients with AS and RA, respectively. Additionally, a formal randomized double-blind 'switching' clinical trial is currently progressing in Norway. This trial ('NOR-SWITCH'; ClinicalTrials.gov identifier: NCT02148640) is comparing the safety and efficacy of switching from RP to CT-P13 versus continued treatment with RP in several indications, including RA. Data from the PLANETAS/PLANETRA extensions and NOR-SWITCH will provide further evidence on the ability to switch from RP to CT-P13.

The main limitation of this analysis is that PLANETAS was primarily designed to compare the PK profiles of CT-P13 and RP at 30 weeks. While prospectively planned, the longer-term efficacy, safety and PK data presented here are from a secondary analysis of the study.

Conclusions

This multinational, randomized, biosimilar study in patients with active AS demonstrated that CT-P13 and RP have highly comparable efficacy, safety, immunogenicity and PK profiles up to week 54. Together with the findings from the PLANETRA study in patients with RA, these data further demonstrate the similarity between CT-P13 and RP in diverse clinical settings.

Abbreviations

ADA: Anti-drug antibody; AE: Adverse event; AS: Ankylosing spondylitis; ASAS: Assessment of Spondylo Arthritis international Society; ASDAS: Ankylosing Spondylitis Disease Activity Score; AUC: Area under the curve; AUC_{τ}: Area under the concentration time curve over the dosing interval, at steady state between week 22 and week 30; BASDAI: Bath Ankylosing Spondylitis Disease Activity Index; BASFI: Bath Ankylosing Spondylitis Functional Index; BASMI: Bath Ankylosing Spondylitis Metrology Index; CI: Confidence interval; C_{max}: Maximum serum concentration; $C_{max,ss}$: Maximum serum concentration at steady state between week 22 and week 30; C_{min}: Minimum serum concentration; CRP: C-reactive protein; LOCF: Last observation carried forward; MEX: Missing equals excluded; OR: Odds ratio; PK: Pharmacokinetics; PRO: Patient-reported outcome; RA: Rheumatoid arthritis; RP: Reference product; SAE: Serious adverse event; SD: Standard deviation; SF-36: Short Form (36) Health Survey; TB: Tuberculosis; TEAE: Treatment-emergent adverse event; TNF: Tumor necrosis factor.

Competing interests

DHY and WP: Consultation for CELLTRION. FB reports consultancy fees from Gebro Pharma, and grants from Bioiberica, MSD, GSK, UCB, Roche, Pfizer, Celgene, Amgen, Grunenthal, Sanofi, Tedec-Meiji, and lecture fees from Bioiberica. SSH and SHL are full-time employees of CELLTRION. JBra has received honoraria for talks, advisory boards, paid consultancies or grants for studies from Abbvie (Abbott), Amgen, Boehringer Ingelheim, Bristol-Myers-Squibb, Celgene, CELLTRION, Centocor, Chugai, EBEWE Pharma, Janssen, Medac, MSD (Schering-Plough), Mundipharma, Novartis, Pfizer (Wyeth), Roche, Sanofi-Aventis and UCB. All other authors declare that they have no competing interests.

Authors' contributions

WP, DHY, JBra, SSH and SHL were involved in the conception and design of the study, and/or analysis and interpretation of data; drafting of the manuscript and revising it critically for important intellectual content; and final approval of the version to be published. JJ, JBrz, AG, VK, IGS, CA-M, WJOE, SWK, DA and FB were involved in the acquisition of data; drafting of the manuscript and revising it critically for important intellectual content; and final approval of the version to be published.

Acknowledgements

The authors wish to thank the patients and study personnel who made this trial possible, and the PLANETAS study investigators: Bulgaria; Rashkov R; Chile; Aguirre V, Gutierrez M, Miranda P; Korea (Republic of); Kim HY, Kim TH, Lee YA, Lim MJ, Park YB, Park YE, Song JS, Suh CH; Latvia; Mikazane H, Saulite-Kandevica D; Mexico; Araiza R, Cons Molina F, Morales-Torres J, Pacheco-Tena C, Gutierrez-Ureña S; Poland; Brzosko M, Hrycaj M, Jeka S, Korkosz M, Krogulec M, Piotrowski M, Ruzga Z, Wiland P; Portugal; Vaz Patto J; Spain; Díaz-González F; Ukraine; Amosova K, Dyadyk O, Kovalenko V, Lysenko G, Smiyan S, Ter-Vartanian S; USA; Ahn C.

The following ethical bodies approved the study in the centers involved: Bulgaria: Ethics Committee for Multi-centre Trials; Chile: Comité de Ética en Investigación Escuela de Medicina Pontificia Universidad Católica de Chile; Comite de Evaluacion de Etica Cientifico del Servicio de Salud Metropolitano Oriente; Comite de Etica de la Investigacion Servicio de Salud Valdivia; Colombia: Comité de Ética en Investigación Servimed; Comite de Etica de la Investigacion Riesgo de Fractura SA; Latvia: The Ethics Committee for Clinical Trials on Medicinal Products; Mexico: Comite de Investigacion y Etica del Hospital Central "Dr. Ignacio Morones Prieto"; Comité de Ética e Investigación Christus Muguerza del Parque SA de CV; Comite Bioetico para la Investigacion Clinica S.C. Institutional Review Board; Comité de Enseñanza, Investigación y Ética del Hospital Civil de Guadalajara Fray Antonio Alcalde; Comité de Etica e Investigación del Hospital Aranda de la Parra; Poland: Komisja Bioetyczna przy Okregowej Radzie Lekarskiej Wielkopolskiej Izby Lekarskiej w Poznaniu; Portugal: Comissão de Ética para a Investigação Clinica; Republic of Korea: Inha University Hosiptal IRB; Chungnam National University Hospital Institutional Review Board; Pusan National University Hospital Institutional Review Board; HanYang University Medical Center IRB; Kyung Hee University Medical Center IRB; Chung-Ang University Hospital IRB; IRB of Seoul St. Mary's Hospital, The Catholic University; Severance Hospital Institutional Review Board; Ajou University Hospital Institutional Review Board; Spain: CEIC de Galicia (SERGAS); CEIC Hospital Universitario de Canarias; Ukraine: Central Commission on Ethics Questions of the MoH of Ukraine. This work was funded by CELLTRION Inc. The funding body contributed to the design of the study and the collection, analysis, and interpretation of data; and reviewed drafts and the final version of the manuscript. The final decision to submit the manuscript was taken by the authors. Editorial support (writing assistance, assembling tables and figures, collating author comments, grammatical editing and referencing) was provided by Rick Flemming (Aspire Scientific Limited, Bollington, UK) and was funded by CELLTRION Healthcare Co., Ltd (Incheon, Republic of Korea).

Author details

[1]Inha University Hospital, Incheon, Republic of Korea. [2]Hanyang University Hospital, Seoul, Republic of Korea. [3]Linea Corporis, Warszawa, Poland. [4]Wojewodzki Szpital Zespolony w Elblagu, Elblag, Poland. [5]Institute of Urgent and Recovery Surgery, Donetsk, Ukraine. [6]University Hospital St. Marina, Varna, Bulgaria. [7]Prosalud y Cia Ltda, Santiago, Chile. [8]Hospital Central Dr. Ignacio Morones Prieto, San Luis Potosí, Mexico. [9]Servimed Empresa Unipersonal, Bucaramanga, Colombia. [10]Chungnam National University Hospital, Daejeon, Republic of Korea. [11]P. Stradina Clinical University Hospital, Riga, Latvia. [12]Hospital Universitario a Coruña, A Coruña, Spain. [13]CELLTRION, Incheon, Republic of Korea. [14]Rheumazentrum Ruhrgebiet, Herne, Germany.

References

1. Braun J, Brandt J, Listing J, Zink A, Alten R, Golder W, et al. Treatment of active ankylosing spondylitis with infliximab: a randomised controlled multicentre trial. Lancet. 2002;359:1187–93.
2. van der Heijde D, Dijkmans B, Geusens P, Sieper J, DeWoody K, Williamson P, et al. Efficacy and safety of infliximab in patients with ankylosing spondylitis: results of a randomized, placebo-controlled trial (ASSERT). Arthritis Rheum. 2005;52:582–91.
3. van der Heijde D, Sieper J, Maksymowych WP, Dougados M, Burgos-Vargas R, Landewe R, et al. 2010 Update of the international ASAS recommendations for the use of anti-TNF agents in patients with axial spondyloarthritis. Ann Rheum Dis. 2011;70:905–8.
4. Braun J, van den Berg R, Baraliakos X, Boehm H, Burgos-Vargas R, Collantes-Estevez E, et al. 2010 update of the ASAS/EULAR recommendations for the management of ankylosing spondylitis. Ann Rheum Dis. 2011;70:896–904.
5. Nast A, Mrowietz U, Kragballe K, de Jong EM, Puig L, Reich K, et al. Barriers to the prescription of systemic therapies for moderate-to-severe psoriasis—a multinational cross-sectional study. Arch Dermatol Res. 2013;305:899–907.
6. Putrik P, Ramiro S, Kvien TK, Sokka T, Pavlova M, Uhlig T, et al. Inequities in access to biologic and synthetic DMARDs across 46 European countries. Ann Rheum Dis. 2014;73:198–206.
7. World Health Organization. Expert Committee on Biological Standardization. Guidelines on evaluation of similar biotherapeutic products (SBPs). 2009. Available at: http://www.who.int/biologicals/areas/biological_therapeutics/BIOTHERAPEUTICS_FOR_WEB_22APRIL2010.pdf. Accessed 19 Feb 2015.
8. European Medicines Agency. Committee for Medicinal Products for Human Use (CHMP). Assessment report: Remsima (infliximab). 2013. Available at: http://www.ema.europa.eu/docs/en_GB/document_library/EPAR_-_Public_assessment_report/human/002576/WC500151486.pdf. Accessed 19 Feb 2015.
9. Jung SK, Lee KH, Jeon JW, Lee JW, Kwon BO, Kim YJ, et al. Physicochemical characterization of Remsima®. mAbs. 2014;6:1163–77.
10. European Medicines Agency. Committee for Medicinal Products for Human Use (CHMP). Guideline on Similar Biological Medicine Products (CHMP/437/04 Rev 1). 23 October 2014. Available at: http://www.ema.europa.eu/docs/en_GB/document_library/Scientific_guideline/2014/10/WC500176768.pdf. Accessed 2 July 2015.
11. U.S. Department of Health and Human Services; Food and Drug Administration; Center for Drug Evaluation and Research (CDER); Center for Biologics Evaluation and Research (CBER). Scientific Considerations in Demonstrating Biosimilarity to a Reference Product. Guidance for Industry. April 2015. Available at: http://www.fda.gov/downloads/Drugs/GuidanceComplianceRegulatoryInformation/Guidances/UCM291128.pdf. Accessed 2 July 2015.
12. Yoo DH, Hrycaj P, Miranda P, Ramiterre E, Piotrowski M, Shevchuk S, et al. A randomised, double-blind, parallel-group study to demonstrate equivalence in efficacy and safety of CT-P13 compared with innovator infliximab when coadministered with methotrexate in patients with active rheumatoid arthritis: the PLANETRA study. Ann Rheum Dis. 2013;72:1613–20.
13. Park W, Hrycaj P, Jeka S, Kovalenko V, Lysenko G, Miranda P, et al. A randomised, double-blind, multicentre, parallel-group, prospective study comparing the pharmacokinetics, safety, and efficacy of CT-P13 and innovator infliximab in patients with ankylosing spondylitis: the PLANETAS study. Ann Rheum Dis. 2013;72:1605–12.
14. van der Linden S, Valkenburg HA, Cats A. Evaluation of diagnostic criteria for ankylosing spondylitis. A proposal for modification of the New York criteria. Arthritis Rheum. 1984;27:361–8.
15. Braun J, Brandt J, Listing J, Zink A, Alten R, Burmester G, et al. Long-term efficacy and safety of infliximab in the treatment of ankylosing spondylitis: an open, observational, extension study of a three-month, randomized, placebo-controlled trial. Arthritis Rheum. 2003;48:2224–33.
16. Breban M, Ravaud P, Claudepierre P, Baron G, Henry YD, Hudry C, et al. Maintenance of infliximab treatment in ankylosing spondylitis: results of a one-year randomized controlled trial comparing systematic versus on-demand treatment. Arthritis Rheum. 2008;58:88–97.
17. Giardina AR, Ferrante A, Ciccia F, Impastato R, Miceli MC, Principato A, et al. A 2-year comparative open label randomized study of efficacy and safety of etanercept and infliximab in patients with ankylosing spondylitis. Rheumatol Int. 2010;30:1437–40.
18. Yoo DH, Racewicz A, Brzezicki J, Yatsyshyn R, Tobias-Arteaga E, Baranauskaite A, et al. A phase 3 randomised controlled trial to compare CT-P13 with infliximab in patients with active rheumatoid arthritis: 54 week results from the PLANETRA study. Ann Rheum Dis. 2013;72 Suppl 3:73 [OP0068].
19. US Food and Drug Administration. Infliximab Product Approval Information: Clinical Pharmacology Review 1999; Available at: http://www.fda.gov/downloads/Drugs/DevelopmentApprovalProcess/HowDrugsareDeveloped andApproved/ApprovalApplications/TherapeuticBiologicApplications/ucm107725.pdf. Accessed 20 Feb 2015
20. Maini RN, Breedveld FC, Kalden JR, Smolen JS, Davis D, Macfarlane JD, et al. Therapeutic efficacy of multiple intravenous infusions of anti-tumor necrosis factor alpha monoclonal antibody combined with low-dose weekly methotrexate in rheumatoid arthritis. Arthritis Rheum. 1998;41:1552–63.
21. Westhovens R, Yocum D, Han J, Berman A, Strusberg I, Geusens P, et al. The safety of infliximab, combined with background treatments, among patients with rheumatoid arthritis and various comorbidities: a large, randomized, placebo-controlled trial. Arthritis Rheum. 2006;54:1075–86.

22. Zhang F-C, Hou Y, Huang F, Wu D-H, Bao C-D, Ni L-Q, et al. Infliximab versus placebo in rheumatoid arthritis patients receiving concomitant methotrexate: a preliminary study from China. APLAR J Rheumatol. 2006;9:127–30.
23. Abe T, Takeuchi T, Miyasaka N, Hashimoto H, Kondo H, Ichikawa Y, et al. A multicenter, double-blind, randomized, placebo controlled trial of infliximab combined with low dose methotrexate in Japanese patients with rheumatoid arthritis. J Rheumatol. 2006;33:37–44.
24. Lipsky PE, van der Heijde DM, St Clair EW, Furst DE, Breedveld FC, Kalden JR, et al. Infliximab and methotrexate in the treatment of rheumatoid arthritis. Anti-Tumor Necrosis Factor Trial in Rheumatoid Arthritis with Concomitant Therapy Study Group. N Engl J Med. 2000;343:1594–602.
25. Schiff M, Keiserman M, Codding C, Songcharoen S, Berman A, Nayiager S, et al. Efficacy and safety of abatacept or infliximab vs placebo in ATTEST: a phase III, multi-centre, randomised, double-blind, placebo-controlled study in patients with rheumatoid arthritis and an inadequate response to methotrexate. Ann Rheum Dis. 2008;67:1096–103.
26. St Clair EW, van der Heijde DM, Smolen JS, Maini RN, Bathon JM, Emery P, et al. Combination of infliximab and methotrexate therapy for early rheumatoid arthritis: a randomized, controlled trial. Arthritis Rheum. 2004;50:3432–43.
27. Quinn MA, Conaghan PG, O'Connor PJ, Karim Z, Greenstein A, Brown A, et al. Very early treatment with infliximab in addition to methotrexate in early, poor-prognosis rheumatoid arthritis reduces magnetic resonance imaging evidence of synovitis and damage, with sustained benefit after infliximab withdrawal: results from a twelve-month randomized, double-blind, placebo-controlled trial. Arthritis Rheum. 2005;52:27–35.
28. Marzo-Ortega H, McGonagle D, Jarrett S, Haugeberg G, Hensor E, O'Connor P, et al. Infliximab in combination with methotrexate in active ankylosing spondylitis: a clinical and imaging study. Ann Rheum Dis. 2005;64:1568–75.
29. Van Den Bosch F, Kruithof E, Baeten D, Herssens A, de Keyser F, Mielants H, et al. Randomized double-blind comparison of chimeric monoclonal antibody to tumor necrosis factor alpha (infliximab) versus placebo in active spondylarthropathy. Arthritis Rheum. 2002;46:755–65.
30. Plasencia C, Pascual-Salcedo D, Nuno L, Bonilla G, Villalba A, Peiteado D, et al. Influence of immunogenicity on the efficacy of long-term treatment of spondyloarthritis with infliximab. Ann Rheum Dis. 2012;71:1955–60.
31. Wolbink GJ, Vis M, Lems W, Voskuyl AE, de Groot E, Nurmohamed MT, et al. Development of anti-infliximab antibodies and relationship to clinical response in patients with rheumatoid arthritis. Arthritis Rheum. 2006;54:711–5.
32. Baert F, Noman M, Vermeire S, Van Assche G, DH G, Carbonez A, et al. Influence of immunogenicity on the long-term efficacy of infliximab in Crohn's disease. N Engl J Med. 2003;348:601–8.

19

Evaluation of the impact of fibromyalgia in disease activity and treatment effect in spondyloarthritis

Natalia Bello[1,2], Adrien Etcheto[1,3], Caroline Béal[1], Maxime Dougados[1,3] and Anna Moltó[1,3*]

Abstract

Background: Fibromyalgia (FM) can coexist with Spondyloarthritis (SpA) leading to diagnostic and treatment dilemmas, especially in the presence of enthesitis. With this study we aimed to estimate the prevalence of FM in SpA and to compare the clinical/disease features and TNF inhibitors (TNFi) in patients with/without FM.

Method: FM was defined by a score = > 5/6 of the Fibromyalgia Rapid Screening Tool (FiRST). SpA patients (according to the rheumatologist) and consecutively consulting in the day care hospital but also in the outpatient clinic at the rheumatology department of a tertiary care university hospital were included. Demographics, disease characteristics, activity and severity and TNFi treatment were compared in patients with and without FM; retention rate of the first TNFi and associated factors were explored (Kaplan Meier and Cox regression).

Results: Of the 196 enrolled SpA patients, 42 (21.4 %) were positively screened for FM. No statistically significant differences in the prevalence of FM were found with regard to the fulfillment of the ASAS criteria for peripheral/axial SpA, nor with regard to the fulfillment of the imaging vs. clinical arm of the ASAS criteria. However, patients with coexisting FM presented significantly with more enthesitis, higher disease activity (BASDAI and VAS) and poorer function scores (BASFI). No differences were found with regard to the initiation of TNFi treatment (79.0 % vs. 70.0 %, respectively), but the retention rate of the first TNFi after 2 years was shorter in the group of patients with FM (28.1 % (95 % CI 12.5-44.0) vs. 41.7 % (95 % CI 32.2-51.3), $p = 0.01$).

Conclusion: This study confirms that coexistent FM in SpA might impact the patient-reported outcome indices for disease activity and function, and the retention rate of TNFi treatment.

Keywords: Spondyloarhtritis, Fibromyalgia, TNF alpha blockers treatment

Background

Spondyloarthritis (SpA) is a disease that includes a spectrum of chronic inflammatory entities involving the axial skeleton (sacroiliac joints and spine) and the peripheral joints, and sharing a number of clinical features such as arthritis, enthesitis, uveitis, dactylitis, psoriasis, and inflammatory bowel disease with a common genetic background, the human leukocyte antigen (HLA) B27 [1–4]. In 2009, the Assessment of the Spondyloarthritis International Society (ASAS) proposed a new set of classification criteria with the aim of recognizing patients with early axial SpA (axSpA) including for the first time the imaging of the sacroiliac joints (SIJ) by magnetic resonance imaging (MRI) and abnormal C-reactive protein (CRP) [5], and another set for SpA patients with predominantly peripheral manifestations (e.g., peripheral arthritis, enthesitis, and dactylitis) [6, 7]. The axSpA criteria allow the classification of patients with chronic back pain lasting for ≥3 months and occurring before 45 years of age, through two arms: the imaging arm in which patients present with sacroiliitis (either on radiographs or MRI) plus at least one additional SpA feature, and the clinical arm in which patients need to be HLA-B27 positive and present with two or more SpA characteristics.

However, the clinical arm has been criticized and is not well-recognized by our health authorities nor some

* Correspondence: anna.molto@aphp.fr
[1]Rheumatology Department, Cochin Hospital, AP-HP, París, France
[3]INSERM (U1153): Clinical Epidemiology and Biostatistics, PRES Sorbornne Paris-Cité, Paris, France

colleagues, despite the fact that it has been fully validated [8]. The main argument for such criticism is that this arm would allow the classification of SpA in patients without any objective sign of inflammation (abnormal CRP or presence of inflammatory lesions seen on MRI of the SIJ) or structural damage in the SIJ seen on pelvic radiographs [6, 9].

Indeed, although the ASAS criteria have been proven to be highly specific with acceptable sensitivity both for diagnosis and classifying SpA patients [10, 11], one could consider it inappropriate to apply them as a diagnostic tool in the absence of objective signs of structural damage or inflammation, due to the potential risk of misdiagnosing or over-diagnosing SpA in patients with other conditions (e.g., fibromyalgia (FM), especially in the presence of enthesitis [12].

FM is a complex chronic condition of unknown etiology being considered as a pain amplification syndrome associated with a central nervous system sensitization mechanism [13]. Its hallmark symptoms are chronic widespread musculoskeletal pain and generalized tender points, but other symptoms can be present, such as fatigue, sleep alterations and stiffness leading to significant physical disability and reduced quality of life [14, 15]. Its prevalence has been estimated at around 2–7 % of the general global population and is predominantly found in women [13]. FM can frequently be associated with other rheumatic diseases such as rheumatoid arthritis and Sjögren syndrome [16], and some studies have reported the prevalence of FM at 12.6–15.0 % in SpA, but studies are sparse [16–18]. This FM-SpA association may present diagnostic and treatment dilemmas because some SpA symptoms (e.g., pain at entheses, fatigue, stiffness, and tenderness) can be also found in FM [12, 19]. Few data are available to date, but it has already been reported that SpA patients with FM tend to present with higher self-reported disease activity indices (i.e., Bath Ankylosing Spondylitis Disease Activity Index (BASDAI)) making interpretation of disease activity and treatment response in SpA patients with concomitant FM very challenging [19–21].

In the absence of specific biomarkers for FM, diagnosis can currently be performed using the American College of Rheumatology (ACR) criteria (1990 ACR classification of FM and the ACR 2010 and modified 2010 diagnostic criteria (2011)) [14, 22, 23]. However, these criteria were developed for research and classification purposes, and are difficult to apply in daily practice because they are time consuming and require some training to be implemented [24]. Moreover, such criteria (i.e., ACR 1990) integrate tender points on physical examination that might reflect enthesitis in patients with SpA. Therefore, with the objective of identifying an easy and valid screening tool to facilitate the identification of FM patients in clinical practice and research, the self-reported Fibromyalgia Rapid Screening Tool (FiRST) [25] was developed, which has sensitivity of 90.5 % and specificity of 85.7 % [25] for the identification of FM patients.

All the above prompted us to conduct this study aiming to 1) estimate the prevalence of FM according to the FiRST in a population of patients with SpA and to compare the prevalence with regard to the arm fulfilled within the axial criteria (i.e., the imaging and clinical arms), and 2) compare the demographics/disease features, and TNF inhibitor (TNFi) treatment in terms of initiation and first TNFi retention rate, in patients with and without FM, respectively.

Methods

Study design

The completion of the FiRST, BASDAI and Bath Ankylosing Spondylitis Functional Index (BASFI) questionnaires were performed prospectively, and data on demographics and disease features were retrospectively retrieved from the medical files.

Study population

Patients aged ≥18 years were included, who were diagnosed with SpA (according to the rheumatologist) and were consecutively attending the day care hospital, but also the outpatient clinic at the rheumatology department of a tertiary care university hospital.

Data collection

FM was defined if the score was ≥5/6 in the FIRST questionnaire [25]. Medical files of each patient who completed the FiRST questionnaire were reviewed by two external investigators. The following information was collected: age, gender, smoking status (past, current, never), body weight and height, and the date of SpA diagnosis, all available items permitting the calculation of the fulfilment of the ASAS criteria; BASDAI [26], global visual analog scale (VAS) according to the patient, presence and number of current swollen joints diagnosed by a physician and CRP at the day of the visit were collected, and severity of the disease evaluated at the time of the visit using the BASFI [27]; SpA treatments since disease onset including information on non-steroidal anti-inflammatory drugs (NSAIDs), conventional disease-modifying antirheumatic drugs (cDMARD), and the type and number of TNFi, number of switches, start/end date and reason for discontinuation for each TNFi. Information on past or current use of psychotropic medications (i.e., myorelaxants, antidepressants, or anxiolytics), strong opioids [28, 29], and history of depression were collected. No imaging (i.e., ultrasound or MRI) was performed specifically for this study.

Ethics considerations

This study was not submitted to any ethical committee because it was performed using data collected in routine care. However, all patients gave their oral consent to use their data for this present study (as stated by French national official procedures for non-interventional studies).

Missing data handling

In the case of missing information patients were contacted by telephone to obtain such information. If CRP was not available on the day of the visit, the last available CRP measurement collected within the previous 6 months was used. Furthermore, if any of the answers to the FiRST questionnaire were missing, we only excluded the patients for whom the missing answers did not allow us to determine their group (with/without FM), e.g., a patient who positively answered three questions but did not answer the last three questions.

Statistical analysis

Continuous variables were reported by their mean and standard deviation (SD) and qualitative variables by frequency and percentage. Statistical significance was set at $p < 0.05$. The analysis was performed with the statistical software SAS 9.4.

Evaluation of the reliability of the FiRST questionnaire was performed. It was evaluated in a subset of 22 patients in two consecutive visits. These patients had stable disease (BASDAI between two visits: 0.22 (±1.32)) and no treatment changes. The average time between the two visits was 22 weeks (± 7.68). Reliability of the FM diagnosis according to the FiRST definition was assessed by prevalence-adjusted bias-adjusted kappa statistics (PABAK).

FM prevalence was estimated in the global SpA population, but also with regard to the ASAS classification criteria fulfilment (axial or peripheral) and to the fulfilment of the imaging vs. clinical arm of the ASAS criteria for axSpA. Demographics, disease characteristics, activity and severity were compared in the FM+/FM− groups by the *t* test and chi square (χ^2) test, as appropriate.

The percentage of patients who were ever exposed to a TNFi, the mean number of TNFi received, the mean duration of the first TNFi treatment and the reasons for discontinuation of each TNFi were assessed in the total population and compared in the FM+ /FM− groups. The retention rate of the first TNFi treatment in the FM+/FM− groups was estimated by survival analysis (Kaplan–Meier curves) and compared by the log-rank test. The predisposing factors for discontinuation of the first TNFi during the first 2 years were estimated by Cox regression models first by univariate and thereafter by multivariate analysis, including in the model only the variables that had a p value <0.10 in the univariate analysis, plus age and gender. Finally, the percentage of patients who received ≥3 TNFi within 12 months (*switchers*) in both groups was compared by the χ^2 test.

Results

Of the 213 patients who completed the FiRST questionnaire, 196 were retained for our analysis: patients without a confirmed diagnosis of SpA (n = 14) and patients who incompletely answered the questionnaire (n = 3) were excluded. The reliability of the FM diagnosis was good, with a PABAK = 0.64 (95 % CI 0.314; 0.958). In our SpA population, the prevalence of concomitant FM was 21.4 % (42/196).

Fibromyalgia prevalence according to the ASAS classification criteria

Figure 1 summarizes the prevalence of FM depending on the ASAS classification criteria. Of the 196 patients included in the analysis, 185 (94.4 %) met the ASAS criteria (182 (98.4 %) and 3 (1.6 %) axial and peripheral, respectively). For the ASAS criteria for axSpA, 150 patients (82.4 %) and 32 patients (17.6 %) fulfilled the imaging and clinical arms, respectively.

Prevalence of concomitant FM was greater in the group of patients not fulfilling the ASAS criteria, although this difference was not statistically significant (21.1 % vs. 30.0 %, not significant). More interestingly, no differences in the prevalence of FM were observed in the group of patients fulfilling the imaging and clinical arms of the ASAS criteria for axSpA (21.3 % vs. 19 %, not significant).

Demographics, disease characteristics, activity and severity were compared in the FM+ and FM− groups (see Table 1). These two groups were similar in terms of age, mean age at disease onset and smoking status. However, patients fulfilling the FM+ definition presented more frequently with enthesitis (59.5 % vs. 39.0 %, $p = 0.01$), a higher total BASDAI (4.7 (±2.3) vs. 2.6 (±1.9), $p < 0.01$), higher global VAS (5.9 (±2.4) vs. 3.0 (±2.5), $p < 0.01$) and higher BASFI (4.8 (±2.7) vs. 2.0 (±2.3), $p < 0.01$). No significant differences were found for treatment with non-steroidal anti-inflammatory drugs (NSAIDs) and conventional disease-modifying antirheumatic drugs (cDMARDs); as expected, the percentage of patients with either history of depression, or use of psychotropic medication or strong opioids was significantly higher in the FM+ group (67 % vs. 35 %, $p < 0.01$).

TNFi treatment

Table 2 summarizes TNFi treatment characteristics in our population. The percentage of patients ever exposed to TNFi did not differ between the FM+ vs. FM− groups (79 % vs. 70 %, respectively, not significant), whereas the percentage of switchers was significantly higher in the

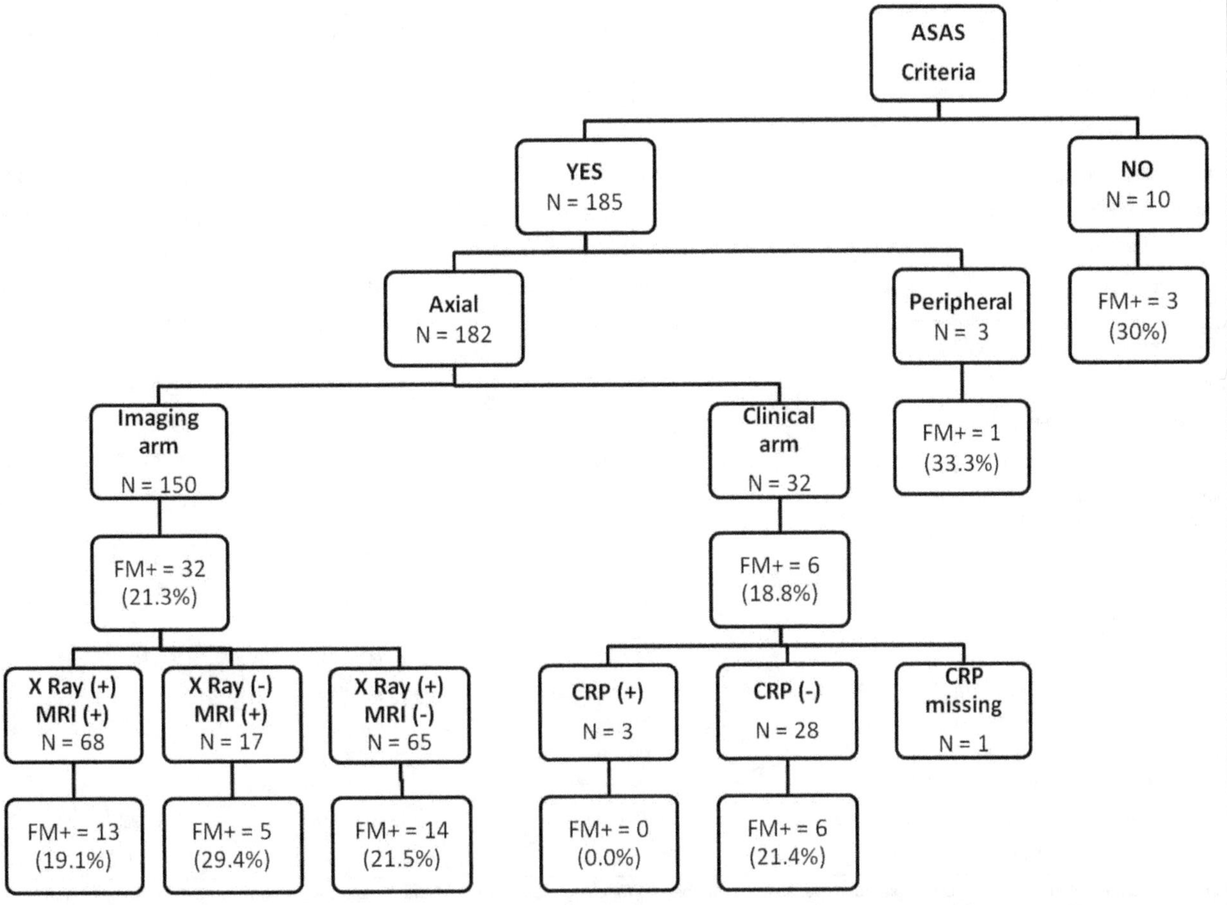

Fig. 1 Fibromyalgia (*FM*) in spondyloarthritis depending on the Assessment of the Spondyloarthritis International Society (*ASAS*) classification criteria and the arm fulfilled. *FM+* fibromyalgia defined by the Fibromyalgia Rapid Screening Tool (*FIRST*) questionnaire (i.e., FIRST ≥5/6), *XRay(+)* radiographic sacroiliitis, *MRI(+)* magnetic resonance imaging sacroiliitis, *CRP(+)* abnormal C-reactive protein (i.e., ≥6 mg/L)

FM+ group (15.2 % vs. 4.0 %, $p = 0.03$). Mean duration of the first TNFi was significantly shorter in the FM+ group (1.7 (± 2.4) vs. 3.5 (± 4.0) years, $p < 0.01$) (Table 2).

The retention rate of the first TNFi after 2 years was significantly shorter in the FM+ group: 28.1 % (95 % CI 12.5; 44.0) (n = 9) vs. 41.7 % (95 % CI 32.2; 51.3) (n = 43) of patients were still on TNFi treatment after 2 years in the FM+ and FM− groups, respectively ($p < 0.01$) (Fig. 2).

Univariate Cox analysis identified FM (hazard ratio (HR) 1.8, 95 % CI 1.1; 3.0), peripheral involvement (HR 1.6, 95 % CI 1.0; 2.6) and history of depression or psychotropic medications or strong opioids intake (HR 0.6, 95 % CI 0.4; 0.9) as associated factors for discontinuation of the first TNFi; however, on multivariate analysis only FM (HR 1.7, 95 % CI 1.0; 2.9) and peripheral involvement (HR 1.6, 95 % CI 1.0; 2.6) were independently associated with discontinuation of the first TNFi. Reasons for discontinuation of each TNFi were similar percentages in the two groups (p value not significant), inefficacy being the most frequent reason in the total population.

Discussion

To our best knowledge, this is the first study aiming to evaluate the prevalence of FM in a population of patients with SpA with regard to the fulfilment of the ASAS classification criteria, and our results show that no differences were found between the imaging and clinical arms of the ASAS criteria for axSpA. This finding is an argument in favor of the validity of such criteria, particularly for the clinical arm, which is still not fully accepted by some members of the scientific community. The phenotype of SpA patients with concomitant FM was more frequently female and presented more frequently with enthesitis, reporting greater disease activity and poorer function scores. These results are consistent with previous studies [16, 17, 20, 30, 31].

As SpA patients with coexisting FM frequently present with a higher disease activity score, the evaluation of disease activity and treatment effect might be challenging, and might lead to unnecessary initiation of a TNFi, dose escalations or switches. In our study, the percentage of patients initiating a TNFi did not differ in the FM+ and

Table 1 Demographic and disease characteristics of patients with and without fibromyalgia

	Total number of patients (n = 196)	Fibromyalgia+ (n = 42)	Fibromyalgia– (n = 154)	P
Age, years	43.0 (12.6)	41.4 (10.2)	43.4 (13.13)	0.21
Gender, female	59 (30.1 %)	17 (40.5 %)	42 (27.3 %)	0.10
Age at disease onset, years	29.9 (11.9)	28.7 (9.3)	30.2 (12.5)	0.40
Smoking status, ever smoked	106 (55.8 %)	23 (56.1 %)	83 (55.7 %)	0.96
HLA B27-positive	157 (82.2 %)	35 (83.3 %)	122 (81.9 %)	0.83
Radiographic sacroiliitis	134 (70.2 %)	27 (67.5 %)	107 (70.9 %)	0.68
Magnetic resonance imaging evidence of inflammatory lesions of the sacroiliac joints	88 (58.3 %)	20 (54.1 %)	68 (59.7 %)	0.55
Raised C-reactive protein*	39 (22.3 %)	8 (20.0 %)	31 (23.0 %)	0.69
Past history of, or current arthritis	72 (36.7 %)	12 (28.6 %)	60(39 %)	0.22
Past history of, or current enthesitis	85 (43.4 %)	25 (59.5 %)	60 (39 %)	0.01
Bath Ankylosing Spondylitis Disease Activity Index total (0–10)	3.0 (2.2)	4.7 (2.3)	2.6 (1.9)	<0.01
Global visual analog scale (0–10)	3.6 (2.8)	5.9 (2.4)	3.0 (2.5)	<0.01
Bath Ankylosing Spondylitis Functional Index (range 0–10)	2.6 (2.7)	4.8 (2.7)	2.0 (2.3)	<0.01
History of depression	42 (23.2 %)	16 (41.0 %)	26 (18.3 %)	<0.01
Past or current intake of psychotropic medications** or strong opioids	82 (41.8 %)	28 (66.7 %)	54 (35.1 %)	<0.01
Past or current intake of psychotropic medications or strong opioids or history of depression	82 (41.8 %)	28 (66.7 %)	54 (35.1 %)	<0.01
Non-steroidal anti-inflammatory drug intake, ever	193 (99.0 %)	42 (100.0 %)	151 (98.7 %)	1.00
Synthetic disease-modifying antirheumatic drug use, ever	104 (53.1 %)	23 (54.8 %)	81 (52.6 %)	0.80

All results are presented as mean ± SD for continuous variables or number (%) for categorical variables. Fibromyalgia + was defined as a Fibromyalgia Rapid Screening Tool (FiRST) score ≥5/6. * ≥ 6 mg/L; **myorelaxants, antidepressants or anxiolytics

FM– group, but patients with concomitant FM+ disease were more likely to switch to other TNFi treatments. Moreover, the retention rate of the first TNFi was shorter in the FM+ group and the presence of FM was independently associated with a first TNFi discontinuation. This confirms that the existence of concomitant FM in SpA might complicate the evaluation of treatment response [19, 20], and suggests that coexistence of FM should be carefully screened when initiating a TNFi and/or evaluating its treatment effect, especially in the presence of

Table 2 TNF inhibitor (TNFi) treatment in patients with and without fibromyalgia

	Total number of patients (n = 196)	Fibromyalgia+ (n = 42)	Fibromyalgia- (n = 154)	P
Patients who received at least one TNFi	141 (71.9 %)	33 (78.6 %)	108 (70.1 %)	0.28
Number of TNFi treatments	1.84 (1.0)	2.36 (1.1)	1.68 (0.9)	<0.01
Switchers*	9 (6.5 %)	5 (15.2 %)	4 (3.8 %)	0.03
First TNFi				
Mean duration of first TNFi treatment, years	3.0 (3.8)	1.7 (2.4)	3.5 (4.0)	<0.01
Reason for TNFi discontinuation:				
Inefficacy %	54 (69.2 %)	12 (54.6 %)	42 (75.0 %)	0.14
Toxicity %	4 (5.1 %)	2 (9.1 %)	2 (3.6 %)	0.76
Inefficacy + toxicity %	4 (5.1 %)	3 (13.6 %)	1 (1.8 %)	0.23
Others %	16 (20.5 %)	5 (22.7 %)	11 (19.6 %)	1.00

All results are presented as mean ± SD for continuous variables or number (%) for categorical variables. Fibromyalgia + was defined as a Fibromyalgia Rapid Screening Tool (FiRST) score ≥5/6. *Patients who received ≥3 TNFi within ≤12 months

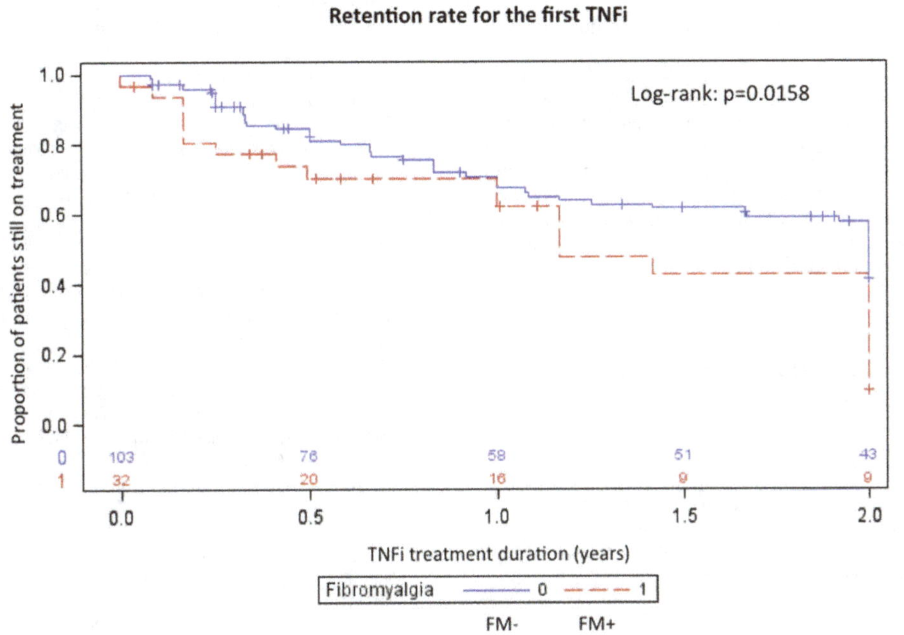

Fig. 2 Kaplan–Meier curve for retention rate of first TNF inhibitor (TNFi) during the first 2 years. *FM* fibromyalgia

peripheral and/or enthesitic symptoms and in the presence of very severe disease activity and patient-reported scores. In this sense the FiRST questionnaire represents an easy to use and valid tool that might be used in clinical practice before starting a TNFi, in particular in patients presenting with enthesitis.

Our study has some weaknesses but also some strengths. First the diagnosis of FM according to the rheumatologist was not collected. However, we verified the external validity of the FiRST in this SpA setting by confirming the greater use of psychotropic medication or strong opioids, or the history of depression in the group of patients positively screened as FM+ [32, 33]. Second, lower sensitivity of the FIRST when applied in an SpA population compared to the original study (66 % vs. 90 %) has been recently reported [34]; however, these data were not available at the time the study started. Furthermore we did not use the ACR criteria (1990 ACR classification of FM [14] - modified 2010 preliminary ACR criteria [22]) to validate our results on the prevalence of FM, but this was due to the complexity of applying such criteria in a daily practice setting [23]. Finally, one could consider that the sample size of our study was too small to draw definite conclusions, e.g., in the evaluation of the retention rate of the first TNFi, only nine patients were at risk after 18 months of follow up in the FM+ group.

Nevertheless, our study also has some strengths. First, our analyses were performed on a representative number of SpA patients in daily practice. Furthermore, to the best of our knowledge this is the first study aiming to evaluate the prevalence of FM according to the fulfilment of the ASAS classification criteria and its impact on TNFi treatment.

Conclusions

In summary, the similar percentages of FM in the different subgroups of the ASAS classification criteria might be a good argument in favor of the validity of these criteria, and in particular of the clinical arm. The coexistence of FM might impact the score of the instrument used to evaluate disease activity and severity, particularly in the patient-reported scores, and therefore might complicate the evaluation of treatment response. The implementation of the FiRST questionnaire might be helpful in clinical practice, especially in the presence of enthesitic symptoms. Other studies aiming to prospectively evaluate the impact of concomitant FM in SpA in the treatment effect of TNFi should allow us to confirm (or not) our findings.

Abbreviations

ACR: American College of Rheumatology; ASAS: Assessment of Spondyloarthritis International Society; axSpA: axial SpA; BASDAI: Bath Ankylosing Spondylitis Disease Activity Index; BASFI: Bath Ankylosing Spondylitis Functional Index; cDMARD: conventional disease-modifying antirheumatic drug; CRP: C-reactive protein; FiRST: Fibromyalgia Rapid Screening Tool; FM: fibromyalgia; MRI: magnetic resonance imaging; NSAID: non-steroidal anti-inflammatory drug; PABAK: prevalence-adjusted bias-adjusted kappa statistics; SIJ: sacroiliac joint; SpA: spondyloarthritis; TNFi: tumor necrosis factor inhibitor; VAS: visual analog scale.

Competing interests

There are no other benefits from commercial sources for the work reported in the manuscript, and no other financial/non-financial interests that any of the authors may have, which could create a potential conflict of interest or the appearance of a conflict of interest with regard to the work.

Authors' contributions

NB participated in the design of the study, data collection, design of the statistical analysis plan and drafted the manuscript. CB participated in data collection and critically reviewed the manuscript. AE participated in the design of the study and performed the statistical analysis and critically reviewed the manuscript. MD conceived the study, participated in the interpretation of data and critically reviewed the manuscript. AM conceived the study, participated in the interpretation of data, contributed to drafting the manuscript and critically reviewed it. All authors have given final approval of the version to be published and have agreed to be accountable for all aspects of the work in ensuring that questions related to the accuracy or integrity of any part of the work are appropriately investigated and resolved.

Acknowledgements

NB received a bursary for stays abroad from Sociedad Española de Reumatologia to conduct this study.

Author details

[1]Rheumatology Department, Cochin Hospital, AP-HP, París, France. [2]Rheumatology Department, Hospital General Universitario Gregorio Marañón, Madrid, Spain. [3]INSERM (U1153): Clinical Epidemiology and Biostatistics, PRES Sorbornne Paris-Cité, Paris, France.

References

1. Ehrenfeld M. Spondyloarthropathies. Best Pract Res Clin Rheumatol. 2012;26:135–45.
2. Garg N, van den Bosch F, Deodhar A. The concept of spondyloarthritis: Where are we now? Best Pract Res Clin Rheumatol. 2014;28:663–72.
3. Gladman DD. Clinical aspects of the spondyloarthropathies. Am J Med Sci. 1998;316:234–8.
4. Dougados M. Diagnostic features of ankylosing spondylitis. Br J Rheumatol. 1995;34:301–3.
5. Rudwaleit M, van der Heijde D, Landewé R, Listing J, Akkoc N, Brandt J, et al. The development of Assessment of SpondyloArthritis international Society classification criteria for axial spondyloarthritis (part II): validation and final selection. Ann Rheum Dis. 2009;68:777–83.
6. Dougados M, Baeten D. Spondyloarthritis. Lancet. 2011;377:2127–37.
7. Rudwaleit M, van der Heijde D, Landewé R, Akkoc N, Brandt J, Chou CT, et al. The Assessment of SpondyloArthritis International Society classification criteria for peripheral spondyloarthritis and for spondyloarthritis in general. Ann Rheum Dis. 2011;70:25–31.
8. Moltó A, Paternotte S, van der Heijde D, Claudepierre P, Rudwaleit M, Dougados M. Evaluation of the validity of the different arms of the ASAS set of criteria for axial spondyloarthritis and description of the different imaging abnormalities suggestive of spondyloarthritis: data from the DESIR cohort. Ann Rheum Dis. 2015;74(4):746–51.
9. Sieper J, Rudwaleit M, Baraliakos X, Brandt J, Braun J, Burgos-Vargas R, et al. The Assessment of SpondyloArthritis international Society (ASAS) handbook: a guide to assess spondyloarthritis. Ann Rheum Dis. 2009;68 Suppl 2:ii1–44.
10. Moltó A, Paternotte S, Comet D, Thibout E, Rudwaleit M, Claudepierre P, et al. Performances of the Assessment of SpondyloArthritis International Society axial spondyloarthritis criteria for diagnostic and classification purposes in patients visiting a rheumatologist because of chronic back pain: results from a multicenter, cross-sectional study. Arthritis Care Res. 2013;65:1472–81.
11. Tomero E, Mulero J, de Miguel E, Fernández-Espartero C, Gobbo M, Descalzo MA, et al. Performance of the Assessment of Spondyloarthritis International Society criteria for the classification of spondyloarthritis in early spondyloarthritis clinics participating in the ESPERANZA programme. Rheumatol (Oxford). 2014;53:353–60.
12. Roussou E, Ciurtin C. Clinical overlap between fibromyalgia tender points and enthesitis sites in patients with spondyloarthritis who present with inflammatory back pain. Clin Exp Rheumatol. 2012;30(6 Suppl 74):24–30.
13. Yunus MB. The prevalence of fibromyalgia in other chronic pain conditions. Pain Res Treat. 2012;2012:584573.
14. Wolfe F, Smythe HA, Yunus MB, Bennett RM, Bombardier C, Goldenberg DL, et al. The American College of Rheumatology 1990 Criteria for the Classification of Fibromyalgia. Report of the Multicenter Criteria Committee. Arthritis Rheum. 1990;33:160–72.
15. Atzeni F, Sallì S, Benucci M, Di Franco M, Alciati A, Sarzi-Puttini P. Fibromyalgia and arthritides. Reumatismo. 2012;64:286–92.
16. Haliloglu S, Carlioglu A, Akdeniz D, Karaaslan Y, Kosar A. Fibromyalgia in patients with other rheumatic diseases: prevalence and relationship with disease activity. Rheumatol Int. 2014;34:1275–80.
17. Salaffi F, De Angelis R, Carotti M, Gutierrez M, Sarzi-Puttini P, Atzeni F. Fibromyalgia in patients with axial spondyloarthritis: epidemiological profile and effect on measures of disease activity. Rheumatol Int. 2014;34:1103–10.
18. Azevedo VF, Paiva E dos S, Felippe LRH, Moreira RA. Occurrence of fibromyalgia in patients with ankylosing spondylitis. Rev Bras Reumatol. 2010;50:646–50.
19. Atzeni F, Boccassini L, Di Franco M, Alciati A, Marsico A, Cazzola M, et al. Chronic widespread pain in spondyloarthritis. Reumatismo. 2014;66:28–32.
20. Aloush V, Ablin JN, Reitblat T, Caspi D, Elkayam O. Fibromyalgia in women with ankylosing spondylitis. Rheumatol Int. 2007;27:865–8.
21. Marchesoni A, Atzeni F, Spadaro A, Lubrano E, Provenzano G, Cauli A, et al. Identification of the clinical features distinguishing psoriatic arthritis and fibromyalgia. J Rheumatol. 2012;39:849–55.
22. Wolfe F, Clauw DJ, Fitzcharles M-A, Goldenberg DL, Katz RS, Mease P, et al. The American College of Rheumatology preliminary diagnostic criteria for fibromyalgia and measurement of symptom severity. Arthritis Care Res. 2010;62:600–10.
23. Bennett RM, Friend R, Marcus D, Bernstein C, Han BK, Yachoui R, et al. Criteria for the diagnosis of fibromyalgia: validation of the modified 2010 preliminary American College of Rheumatology criteria and the development of alternative criteria. Arthritis Care Res. 2014;66:1364–73.
24. Wolfe F. Stop using the American College of Rheumatology criteria in the clinic. J Rheumatol. 2003;30:1671–2.
25. Perrot S, Bouhassira D, Fermanian J, Cercle d'Etude de la Douleur en Rhumatologie. Cercle d'Etude de la Douleur en Rhumatologie. Development and validation of the Fibromyalgia Rapid Screening Tool (FiRST). Pain. 2010;150:250–6.
26. Garrett S, Jenkinson T, Kennedy LG, Whitelock H, Gaisford P, Calin A. A new approach to defining disease status in ankylosing spondylitis: the Bath Ankylosing Spondylitis Disease Activity Index. J Rheumatol. 1994;21:2286–91.
27. Calin A, Garrett S, Whitelock H, Kennedy LG, O'Hea J, Mallorie P, et al. A new approach to defining functional ability in ankylosing spondylitis: the development of the Bath Ankylosing Spondylitis Functional Index. J Rheumatol. 1994;21:2281–5.
28. Jadad AR, Browman GP. The WHO analgesic ladder for cancer pain management. Stepping up the quality of its evaluation. JAMA. 1995;274: 1870–3.
29. World Health Organization. WHO's cancer pain ladder for adults. http://www.who.int/cancer/palliative/painladder/en/.
30. Heikkilä S, Ronni S, Kautiainen HJ, Kauppi MJ. Functional impairment in spondyloarthropathy and fibromyalgia. J Rheumatol. 2002;29:1415–9.
31. Tournadre A, Pereira B, Lhoste A, Dubost JJ, Ristori JM, Claudepierre P, et al. Differences between women and men with recent-onset axial spondyloarthritis: results from a prospective multicenter French cohort. Arthritis Care Res. 2013;65:1482–9.
32. Torta R, Pennazio F, Ieraci V. Anxiety and depression in rheumatologic diseases: the relevance of diagnosis and management. Reumatismo. 2014;66:92–7.
33. Wasserman RA, Brummett CM, Goesling J, Tsodikov A, Hassett AL. Characteristics of chronic pain patients who take opioids and persistently report high pain intensity. Reg Anesth Pain Med. 2014;39:13–7.
34. Fan A, Pereira B, Tournadre A, Tatar Z, Malochet-Guinamand S, Soubrier M, et al. Evaluation of the Fibromyalgia Rapid Screening Tool (FiRST) Questionnaire to Screen Fibromyalgia Associated with Inflammatory Rheumatic Disease [abstract]. Arthritis Rheumatol. 2015; 67 (suppl 10). http://acrabstracts.org/abstract/evaluation-of-the-fibromyalgia-rapid-screening-tool-first-questionnaire-toscreen-fibromyalgia-associated-with-inflammatory-rheumatic-disease/. Accessed date February 6, 2016.

20

The prevalence of vertebral fractures in spondyloarthritis: relation to disease characteristics, bone mineral density, syndesmophytes and history of back pain and trauma

Piet Geusens[1,2,3*], Liesbeth De Winter[1], Dana Quaden[1], Johan Vanhoof[3], Debby Vosse[3], Joop van den Bergh[2,4,5] and Veerle Somers[1]

Abstract

Introduction: An increased risk of vertebral fracture (VF) is one of the extra-articular manifestations of spondyloarthropathy (SpA). The prevalence of moderate to severe VFs visualized by radiography (Rx) in patients with SpA in daily practice is unknown until imaging of the full spine is available, as most VFs do not present with clinical signs and symptoms of an acute fracture.

Methods: We evaluated the prevalence of VFs (>25 % loss in height) on available Rx and dual-energy X-ray absorptiometry (DXA) images in 390 consecutive patients with SpA in daily practice. We assessed their association with disease characteristics, bone mineral density, the modified Stoke Ankylosing Spondylitis Spinal Score, and history of trauma.

Results: Forty-six patients (11.8 %) had Rx VF (56.4 % men, 93.5 % in the thoracic spine), and 44.5 % had multiple VFs. Compared with patients without VF, patients with VF were older (52.2 vs. 47.3 years, $p < 0.01$; range 25–84 years), had lower femoral neck T-scores (−1.1 vs. −0.7; $p < 0.05$), and had a marginally higher modified Stoke Ankylosing Spondylitis Spinal Score (11.7 vs. 7.0; $p = 0.06$). Among patients with VFs, 15.2 % had a history of trauma with acute back pain ($p < 0.001$ vs. no VF). The reliability of DXA for diagnosing radiographic VFs was high (κ 0.90).

Conclusions: Moderate to severe VFs are found in more than 10 % of patients with SpA before the age of 40 years in 5 % of women and 9 % in men. Most VFs are located in the thoracic region, are related to low femoral neck bone mineral density and to stiffening of the spine, and are only rarely related to trauma history. DXA is a useful alternative for diagnosing VFs.

Keywords: Spondyloarthropathy, Bone mineral density, Vertebral fracture, Vertebral fracture assessment

Introduction

An increased risk of vertebral fracture (VF) is one of the extra-articular manifestations of ankylosing spondylitis (AS) [1, 2] and other spondyloarthropathies (SpAs) [3, 4]. In population studies, it has been shown that the risk of radiographic and clinical VFs is increased in patients with AS [3, 5–9], even early in the disease [6, 10], and is also increased in those with inflammatory bowel disease (IBD) [3] and psoriatic arthritis (PsA) [4]. The prevalence of VFs has been studied in several surveys including 22–158 patients with AS in whom the prevalence of radiographic VFs ranged from 1.4 % to 58.0 %. Nevertheless, criteria for patient selection were variable in these studies (consecutive patients or patients selected on the basis of disease activity, occiput to wall distance (OWD), sex or age, and including clinical VFs or systematic evaluated morphometric VFs), as were the criteria for VF diagnosis (variable thresholds of vertebral height loss) [10–14].

* Correspondence: piet.geusens@scarlet.be
[1]Hasselt University, Biomedical Research Institute, and Transnationale Universiteit Limburg, Diepenbeek, Belgium, Martelarenlaan 42, 3500 Hasselt, Belgium
[2]Division of Rheumatology, Department of Internal Medicine, CAPHRI School for Public Health and Primary Care, Maastricht University Medical Center, Maastricht, P.O. Box 616, 6200 MD Maastricht, The Netherlands

Based on the increased rate of VF in AS, imaging of the spine is advocated in cases of significant change in the course of the disease [15, 16]. However, most VFs do not present with the clinical signs and symptoms of an acute fracture and are overlooked when back pain is interpreted as a disease flare of spondylitis. No data are available on the relationship between history of trauma and acute or chronic back pain in SpA.

Imaging of the spine is most often performed with conventional radiography (Rx), but Vertebral Fracture Assessment (VFA) using dual-energy X-ray absorptiometry (DXA) technology is of increasing interest because of its low radiation dose and high negative predictive value (NPV) [17], and it has also been studied in AS [13, 18, 19].

We evaluated the presence of VF using Rx and VFA in a non-academic rheumatology practice in a large cohort of patients with SpA in relation to disease characteristics, bone mineral density (BMD), syndesmophytes, and history of back pain and trauma.

Methods

Study population

A total of 390 consecutive ambulatory patients with SpA who were seen by six rheumatologists in an ambulatory non-academic rheumatology clinic were included between July 2013 and December 2013.

Diagnoses of AS, undifferentiated SpA, PsA, and IBD were made by the treating rheumatologists according to the criteria set forth in national and international guidelines [20]. This study was approved by the medical ethics committee of Ziekenhuisnetwerk Antwerpen (Belgium), and all patients provided informed consent before participation.

Bone mineral density

BMD was measured in the lumbar spine (anteroposterior projection), femoral neck, and total hip using DXA with standard procedures as recommended by the manufacturer (Lunar Prodigy Primo BX-1 L enCORE device, version 12.30; GE Healthcare Life Sciences, Chalfont St. Giles, UK). VFA imaging was performed using software provided by the manufacturer for this device.

Radiographic assessment and scoring

Lateral images of the thoracic and lumbar spine were semiquantitatively evaluated according to the Genant score for anterior, middle, and posterior height using available digital Rx and VFA images [21, 22]. VFA was performed using a semiquantitative (SQ) technique. Each Rx and VFA image was inspected visually by the treating rheumatologist to decide whether it contained a fracture in any of the visualized vertebrae and assigned a grade based on the Genant SQ scale, where grade 2 (moderate) is a reduction of 26–40 % and grade 3 (severe) a reduction of over 40 %. In case of doubt, vertebral heights were measured using the digital measuring device supplied by the provider of the digital Rx system. Only vertebral deformities >25 % were considered as a VF (grades 2 and 3), as this degree of deformity increases the specificity compared with a lesser degree of deformity [23].

On lateral spine radiographs, the cervical, lumbar and thoracic vertebrae were scored using the modified Stoke Ankylosing Spondylitis Spinal Score (mSASSS) as 0 (normal), 1 (erosion, sclerosis, or squaring), 2 (obvious syndesmophyte), and 3 (total bone bridge) [16]. The mSASSS according to Assessment of SpondyloArthritis international Society includes scoring of radiographs at the cervical and lumbar spine (range 0–72). In addition, the same scoring method was also used for the thoracic spine, and additional mSASSS was calculated for both the thoracic spine (range 0–72) and total spine (range 0–144).

Each of the six experienced rheumatologists performed scoring of mSASSS on radiographs and VFs on the radiographs and VFAs of their own patients. They were all experienced and trained in scoring VF, as well as in patients with SpA, at the yearly bone curriculum meetings of the Osteoporosis Working Group of the Royal Belgian Rheumatology Society. Therefore, no intra- or interreader reliability was tested.

Disease characteristics

Disease characteristics of patients included the Bath Ankylosing Spondylitis Disease Activity Index (BASDAI), Bath Ankylosing Spondylitis Functional Index (BASFI), Ankylosing Spondylitis Disease Activity Score (ASDAS), OWD, presence of human leukocyte antigen B27 (HLA-B27), and serum erythrocyte sedimentation rate (ESR) and C-reactive protein (CRP). All patients were asked about a history of falls and trauma and subsequent acute or chronic back pain.

Statistical analysis

We report descriptive statistics and comparisons between patients with and without a VF using analysis of variance (ANOVA) for continuous variables and cross-tabulation for dichotomous variables.

Univariable and multivariable logistic regression analyses were used to estimate the effects of factors that were significantly different between patients with and without a VF on the likelihood [expressed as odds ratio (OR) with 95 % confidence interval (CI)] that participants had a radiographic VF.

A reliability analysis using the κ statistic was performed to determine consistency between VFA and Rx in diagnosing VF. For the diagnostic value of VFA in identifying radiographic VF, we calculated sensitivity, specificity, positive predictive value (PPV), and NPV. Calculations were performed using IBM SPSS version 22 software (IBM, Armonk, NY, USA).

Results

Study population

The basic characteristics and BMD of the 390 patients with SpA are shown in Table 1. These included 175 (44.9 %) men and 215 (55.1 %) women, 286 (73.3 %) of whom had AS, 40 (10.3 %) of whom had PsA, 18 (4.6 %) of whom had IBD, and 46 (11.8 %) of whom had undifferentiated SpA. The patients' mean age was 47.9 years [standard deviation (SD) 11.9, range 21–84 years]. The mean time since first symptoms was 14.6 years (SD 10.7, range 1–60 years), and the mean time since diagnosis was 10.8 years (SD 9.9, range: 0–60 years). The mean difference between symptoms and diagnosis was 3.9 years (SD 5.8, range 0–33 years). HLA-B27 was present in 203 (62.8 %) of the 323 patients in whom this was evaluated. In addition, 168 (43.1 %) of the patients had undergone treatment with tumor necrosis factor blockers at the time of the survey.

Table 1 Basic characteristics of included patients with spondyloarthritis ($n = 390$)

Characteristics	Mean[a]	Range[b]
Age, yr	47.9 ± 11.9	21–84
Symptom duration, yr	14.6 ± 10.7	1–60
Disease duration, yr	10.8 ± 9.9	0–60
ESR, mm/h	9.0 ± 10.4	0–86
CRP, mg/L	3.8 ± 6.3	0–60
BASDAI	4.3 ± 2.3	0–10
BASFI	5.0 ± 8.0	0–83
ASDAS-ESR	2.2 ± 1.0	0–5
ASDAS-CRP	2.2 ± 1.1	0–5
mSASSS		
Cervical spine	3.7 ± 9.2	0–42
Thoracic spine	10.6 ± 20.4	0–72
Lumbar spine	3.9 ± 8.0	0–30
Cervical + lumbar spine	7.6 ± 15.9	0–72
Total spine	18.1 ± 34.4	0–144
T-score		
Lumbar spine	−0.2 ± 1.7	−4.3 to ±10.4
Femoral neck	−0.7 ± 1.1	−3.8 to ±4.7
Total hip	−0.4 ± 1.1	−3.2 to ±4.9

ESR erythrocyte sedimentation rate, *CRP* C-reactive protein, *BASDAI* Bath Ankylosing Spondylitis Disease Activity Index, *BASFI* Bath Ankylosing Spondylitis Functional Index, *ASDAS* Ankylosing Spondylitis Disease Activity Score, *mSASSS* modified Stoke Ankylosing Spondylitis Spinal Score

[a]Characteristics of patients with SpA are presented as mean absolute number ± standard deviation

[b]Range of absolute numbers for a given characteristic

The majority of patients had normal BMD (T-score −1.0 or higher) in the spine (79.7 %) and in the femoral neck (59.5 %), whereas 17.2 % and 36.4 % had a T-score between −1 and −2.5, respectively. Only a minority of patients had a T-score −2.5 or lower (3.1 % in the spine and 4.1 % in the femoral neck). BMD decreased with age in the femoral neck in women (−0.46; $p < 0.001$) and men (−0.31; $p < 0.001$), as well as in the spine in women (−0.26; $p < 0.001$), but it increased with age in the spine in men (0.27; $p < 0.001$) (Fig. 1).

The classical mSASSS (cervical + lumbar spine) was 7.6 (SD 15.9, range 0–72). The mSASSS for the thoracic spine was 10.6 (range 0–72), resulting in a total spine mSASSS score of 18.1 (SD 34.4, range 0–144). mSASSS >0 were found in the cervical spine in 30.1 % of patients, in the thoracic spine in 43.6 %, in the lumbar spine in 38.2 %, in the cervical and lumbar spine combined in 45.1 %, and in the total spine in 55.1 %.

By Rx, moderate to severe VFs were identified in 46 patients, of whom 25 (54.3 %) were men. Twenty patients (43.5 %) had more than one VF (18 had 2 VFs and 2 had 3 VFs), resulting in a total of 68 VFs. Of the 68 VFs, 62 (91.2 %) were located in the thoracic spine (Fig. 2). The prevalence was highest in IBD (22.2 %), followed by 12.2 % in AS and 10.0 % in PsA, and lowest in undifferentiated SpA (6.5 %).

Comparisons between patients with and without VF are shown in Table 2. Compared with patients without VF, patients with a VF were older (52.2 vs. 47.3 years, range 25–84 years; $p < 0.01$). They had a lower T-score in the femoral neck (−1.00 vs. −0.70; $p < 0.05$) and total hip (−0.74 vs. −0.27; $p < 0.05$), more peripheral joint disease (4.4 vs. 3.5; $p < 0.05$), a marginally higher classical (cervical + lumbar) mSASSS (11.7 vs. 7.0; $p = 0.06$), and a significantly higher thoracic mSASSS (16.2 vs. 9.8; $p < 0.05$).

Compared with patients with an mSASSS score of 0 at the level of BMD measurement (L2-L4), patients with mSASSS scores >0 had a significantly higher T-score in the spine (0.47 vs. 0.12; $p = 0.50$). In contrast, the T-score was significantly lower in the femoral neck (−1.01 vs. −0.60; $p < 0.001$) and in the total hip (−0.65 vs. −0.22; $p < 0.001$).

Univariable logistic regression analysis revealed the OR for VF (based on the significant differences in Table 2): age (OR 1.35 per 10-year increase, 95 % CI 1.08–1.62) (Fig. 3), duration of symptoms (OR 1.35 per 10-year increase, 95 % CI 1.08–1.61), thoracic mSASSS (OR 1.13 per 10-point increase, 95 % CI 1.00–1.25), and femoral neck T-score (OR 1.38 per 1 SD decrease, 95 % CI 1.01–1.88). In multivariable regression analysis including these factors, only age remained significant, with an OR of 1.35 (95 % CI 1.08–1.62) per 10-year increase in age.

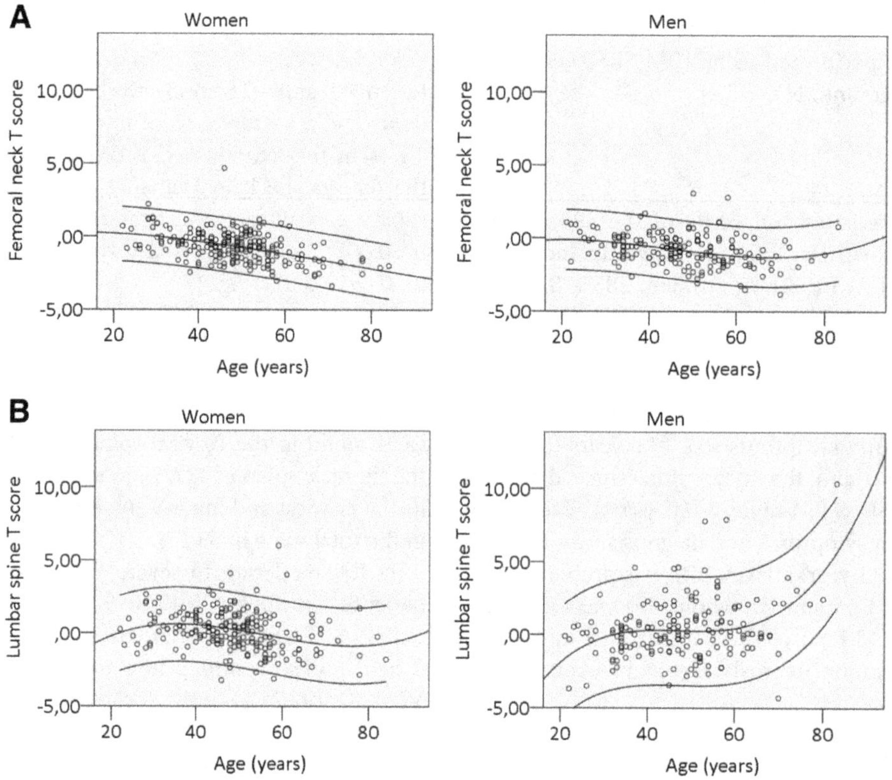

Fig. 1 Correlation between bone mineral density (of the femoral neck and lumbar spine) and age. Bone mineral density of patients with SpA is represented as T-score. T-scores are shown in the (**a**) femoral neck and (**b**) lumbar spine for both women (*left*) and men (*right*) according to their age (years). *Lines* represent the 95 % confidence intervals

A history of falls was reported by 15.1 % of patients, 17.4 % with and 14.8 % without a VF (not statistically significant). A history of trauma with subsequent acute back pain was reported by 15.2 % of patients, 15.2 % with and 2.6 % without a VF ($p = 0.001$). A history of trauma with subsequent chronic back pain was reported by 1.3 % of patients, 8.7 % with and 0.3 % without a VF ($p = 0.001$).

One patient had a history of spontaneous dorsal arch fracture at T10 without previous trauma, which was

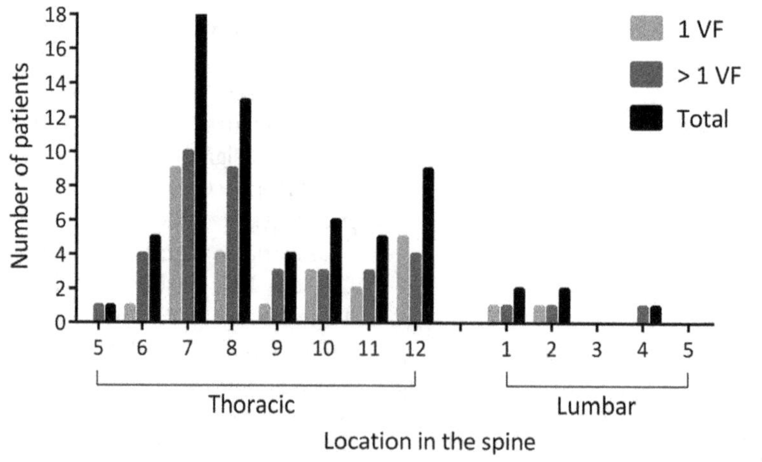

Fig. 2 Prevalence of vertebral fractures (VFs) in the thoracic and lumbar spine of patients with spondyloarthropathy (SpA). The occurrence of VFs is represented as the absolute number of patients with SpA with VFs in either the thoracic (T5-T12) or lumbar part of the spine (L1-L5) (*black*). The absolute number of patients with SpA with only one VF located in the thoracic or lumbar spine is shown with *light gray bars. Dark gray bars* represent patients with SpA with more than one VF located in the thoracic or lumbar spine

Table 2 Basic characteristics of patients with spondyloarthritis without ($n = 344$) and with ($n = 46$) one or more radiographic vertebral fractures >25 %

Characteristics	Patients without VF (n = 344)	Patients with VF (n = 46)	*p* value[a]
Age, yr[b]	47.3 ± 11.6	52.2 ± 13.1	<0.01
Symptom duration, yr[c]	14.1 ± 10.4	18.5 ± 12.4	<0.01
Disease duration, yr[d]	10.5 ± 9.6	12.5 ± 12.1	ns
ESR, mm/h	9.2 ± 10.7	8.0 ± 8.1	ns
CRP, mg/L	4.0 ± 6.5	2.9 ± 3.8	ns
BASDAI	4.3 ± 2.3	4.7 ± 2.2	ns
BASFI	5.0 ± 8.5	4.9 ± 2.9	ns
ASDAS-ESR	2.2 ± 1.0	2.4 ± 0.9	ns
ASDAS-CRP	2.2 ± 1.0	2.3 ± 1.0	ns
OWD	1.3 ± 4.2	2.5 ± 5.5	0.09
mSASSS			
Cervical spine	3.4 ± 8.5	5.8 ± 13.2	0.10
Thoracic spine	9.8 ± 19.6	16.2 ± 25.1	<0.05
Lumbar spine	3.6 ± 7.6	6.0 ± 10.3	<0.07
Cervical + lumbar spine	7.0 ± 15.0	11.7 ± 21.6	0.06
Total spine	16.8 ± 32.8	27.9 ± 43.5	<0.05
T-score			
Lumbar spine	0.25 ± 1.70	0.13 ± 1.50	ns
Femoral neck	−0.70 ± 1.06	−1.00 ± 0.97	<0.05
Total hip	−0.34 ± 1.09	−0.59 ± 1.04	ns

ESR erythrocyte sedimentation rate, *CRP* C-reactive protein, *BASDAI* Bath Ankylosing Spondylitis Disease Activity Index, *BASFI* Bath Ankylosing Spondylitis Functional Index, *ASDAS* Ankylosing Spondylitis Disease Activity Score, *mSASSS* modified Stoke Ankylosing Spondylitis Spinal Score, *TNF* tumor necrosis factor, *ns* not statistically significant, *VF* vertebral fracture, *OWD* Occiput to wall distance

Characteristics of patients with spondyloarthritis (SpA) are represented as mean absolute number ± standard deviation

[a]Means of characteristics were compared between patients with SpA without and with VF using analysis of variance. *p* value <0.05 was considered statistically significant.

[b]Mean age ± standard deviation in years

[c]Mean symptom duration ± standard deviation in years; time since first symptoms

[d]Mean disease duration ± standard deviation in years; time since diagnosis

diagnosed only after bone scintigraphy and magnetic resonance imaging and that healed spontaneously without complications other than temporarily increased back pain. Three patients (0.8 %) had a history of VF with neurologic complications: two after a cervical fracture and one after a lumbar fracture.

The reliability of Rx and VFA for diagnosing VF was found to be $\kappa = 0.898$ (standard error 0.036; $p < 0.001$) (Table 3). Rx VF could not be diagnosed on the basis of VFA in six patients, because the VFA images were of insufficient quality. In two patients, VFs were diagnosed with the use of VFA, and the VFs were also present on radiographs but with a deformity of <25 % on Rx.

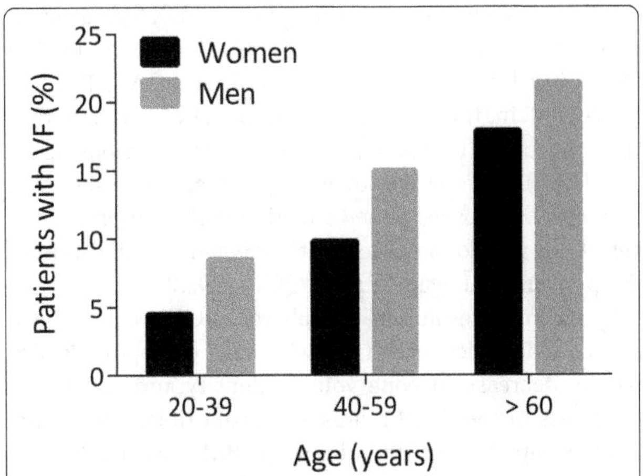

Fig. 3 Prevalence of vertebral fractures (VFs) according to age and sex of patients with spondyloarthropathy (SpA). The prevalence of VFs is shown as the percentage of men (*gray bars*) or women (*black bars*) of the total number of patients with SpA with VFs in three different age groups. Age groups were 20–39 years, 40–59 years, and 60 years and older

The analysis of the diagnostic value of VFA to detect VFs identified on Rx indicated sensitivity of 87 % (95 % CI 74–95 %), with specificity of 99 % (95 % CI 98–100 %), PPV of 95 % (95 % CI 84–99 %), and NPV of 98 % (95 % CI 96–99 %).

Discussion

In this large survey of VFs in 390 men and women with SpA, we found >10 % prevalence of moderate to severe VFs, already before the age of 30 years and within 5 years of symptoms.

The pathophysiology of VFs in SpA is complex [13, 24–26]. In AS, markers of bone resorption are increased in active disease and are related to low BMD and bone loss in the femoral neck and in the spine [27, 28]. Markers of bone formation are mostly normal in AS and not correlated with BMD [27]. Low BMD and bone loss

Table 3 Analysis of congruence between conventional radiography and Vertebral Fracture Assessment for diagnosing vertebral fractures

		Rx		
		VF	No VF	Total
VFA	VF	40	2	42
	No VF	6	342	348
	Total	46	344	390

VF vertebral fracture, *VFA* Vertebral Fracture Assessment

Patients with spondyloarthritis with or without VF who were diagnosed by radiography (Rx) or by VFA using dual X-ray energy absorptiometry are represented as absolute numbers. Agreement between VFA and Rx was excellent ($\kappa = 0.898$, standard error 0.036; $p < 0.001$). The diagnostic value of VFA in identifying Rx VF indicated sensitivity of 87 % [95 % confidence interval (CI) 74–95 %], specificity of 99 % (95 % CI 98–100 %), positive predictive value of 95 % (95 % CI 84–99 %), and negative predictive value of 98 % (95 % CI 96–99 %)

have been documented in the spine [by DXA and quantitative computed tomography (QCT)] and in the hip (by DXA) [29, 30]. Later in the course of AS, BMD is decreased in the hip (as shown by DXA) and within the vertebrae (by QCT), but not in the lumbar spine (by DXA). This is due to intervertebral syndesmophyte formation, periosteal bone formation with squaring of the vertebrae, ankylosis of the facet joints, and calcification of the perivertebral ligaments (by QCT) [29, 30].

Using high-resolution peripheral QCT, it has been shown that patients with AS who have osteoporosis also have a decrease in bone volume density and in cortical thickness in the distal radius and distal tibia, which correlated with trabecular volumetric BMD in the lumbar spine using QCT [31]. These studies suggest that patients with AS have a generalized loss of trabecular bone density. The clinical consequence is that this low BMD and bone loss are measurable by DXA in the spine and hip early in the disease, but only in the hip later in the disease course [24, 25].

Interestingly, in this study, the presence of VF was related to mSASSS and marginally to BMD measured by DXA in the femoral neck. This indicates that, in addition to a low BMD, an altered biomechanical performance of the vertebrae by the stiffening of the spine contributes to the occurrence of VF [13, 24, 25]. These results further support the European League Against Rheumatism (EULAR) recommendations on imaging in SpA, which state that in patients with axial SpA without syndesmophytes in the lumbar spine visualized by conventional Rx, osteoporosis should be assessed by hip DXA and anteroposterior spine DXA. In patients with syndesmophytes in the lumbar spine visualized by conventional Rx, osteoporosis should be assessed by hip DXA supplemented by either spine DXA in lateral projection or possibly QCT of the spine [32].

VFs do not occur uniformly along the spine, but, as shown in postmenopausal and senile osteoporosis, they occur more often in the midthoracic and thoracolumbar regions than elsewhere [33, 34], which is likely attributable to biomechanical factors. Apart from loading (body height, weight, muscle forces, movements such as bending), other factors play a role in VF, such as spinal curvature and the heterogeneity of BMD between vertebrae [35]. Furthermore, a wedged thoracic VF increases the biomechanical stresses in other vertebrae [36]. In view of the relationship between VF and mSASSS in this and other studies [14], stiffening of the spine in SpA also could contribute to VF risk. Segmental or generalized syndesmophyte formation (bamboo spine) transforms the flexible spine in a long stiff bone (with intravertebral osteoporosis as shown with computed tomography) with decreased biomechanical competence. Stiffening of the spine in AS can also explain why VFs in AS occur at unusual locations (cervical spine) with unusual characteristics (e.g., transdiscal and horizontal transvertebral fractures and fractures of the dorsal arch structures of the vertebrae, which was reported by one of our patients) and with severe neurologic deficits, which occurred in three patients (0.8 %) [24].

Patients with a VF more often had a history of acute and chronic back pain after trauma than did patients without a VF. However, this occurred only in a minority of patients with a VF (one of six patients), suggesting that most VFs in SpA are not the result of trauma. The clinical consequence is that a history of trauma helps to identify only a limited number of patients with a VF. According to the ASAS/EULAR recommendations, imaging of the spine is advocated in AS in cases of a significant change in the course of the disease [15, 16]. However, on the basis of the high prevalence of subclinical VFs, this recommendation could need adaption, as VFs can be diagnosed only when imaging of the spine is performed and can be present without a history of trauma or typical signs and symptoms of an acute fracture.

The agreement between digitized Rx and VFA in diagnosing VFs, as well as the high NPV [17–19], is of clinical interest. VFA missed six (12.5 %) of the radiographic VFs. This indicates that in the majority of patients with SpA, VFA will enable diagnosis of VFs using a much lower level of radiation than Rx. Earlier studies showed less congruent results, but this could have been due to measuring vertebral heights using a less reliable magnification loop on plain radiographic films instead of electronic aids on digitized radiographs in this study [18, 19].

In view of its high NPV, VFA allows selection of patients who will or who will not need Rx for diagnosing VFs [17–19, 23]. A prevalent VF is a strong predictor of future VFs and non-VFs. No fracture prevention studies are available in SpA. It is therefore indicated that patients with SpA and early bone loss, osteoporosis, and/or a prevalent VF should be considered candidates for antiresorptive drugs to prevent fractures.

The strength of this study is the large sample collection and the representativeness of the patient group in a peripheral non-academic rheumatology center, including a broad range of ages and representing both sexes. Interestingly, we found the overall prevalence of SpAs to be as common in women as in men. The dominant male prevalence in AS is well accepted. However, the gender distribution in our survey is in line with the finding that, in recent years, the gender ratio approached 1:1 in an AS patient survey in Germany [37] and in a population survey in the south of Sweden for SpAs [38]. This finding has been included in the ASAS mission statement on epidemiology of AS [39]. The reported data regarding prevalence of PsA according to gender is conflicting [38]. The incidence of Crohn's disease is similar between women and men, but the prevalence of IBD with SpA is unknown [40].

The finding that VFA using DXA has high sensitivity, specificity, PPV, and NPV compared with Rx is another strength with possible clinical consequences for screening. It indicates that VFA can be used as a prescreening tool for the presence of a VF in SpA, limiting the use of radiographs to patients with a VF on VFA, or when VFA is not of adequate quality to evaluate VFs.

A limitation of the study is the small number of patients with PsA and IBD. Furthermore, we chose only VFs with a deformity >25 % and not smaller deformities, as this would have increased sensitivity but decreased specificity for diagnosing a VF [23]. Therefore, the prevalence of VFs is even higher in this population when mild deformities are also included [14]. Last, the relationship between a history of trauma and the presence of VF should be interpreted with caution, as there is a possibility of recall bias of traumas.

Conclusions

Moderate to severe VFs are found in more than 10 % of patients with SpA, already before the age of 40 years in 5 % of women and 9 % of men and within 5 years of disease symptoms. Most VFs are located in the thoracic region, are subclinical, and are related to low femoral neck BMD and stiffening of the thoracic spine. VFA is helpful in selecting patients in whom Rx should be performed to diagnose a VF.

Abbreviations

ANOVA: Analysis of variance; AS: Ankylosing spondylitis; ASDAS: Ankylosing Spondylitis Disease Activity Score; BASDAI: Bath Ankylosing Spondylitis Disease Activity Index; BASFI: Bath Ankylosing Spondylitis Functional Index; BMD: Bone mineral density; CI: Confidence interval; CRP: C-reactive protein; DXA: Dual-energy X-ray absorptiometry; ESR: Erythrocyte sedimentation rate; EULAR: European League Against Rheumatism; HLA-B27: Human leukocyte antigen B27; IBD: Inflammatory bowel disease; mSASSS: Modified Stoke Ankylosing Spondylitis Spinal Score; NPV: Negative predictive value; OR: Odds ratio; OWD: Occiput to wall distance; PPV: Positive predictive value; PsA: Psoriatic arthritis; QCT: Quantitative computed tomography; Rx: Radiography; SD: Standard deviation; SpA: Spondyloarthropathy; SQ: Semiquantitative; TNF: Tumor necrosis factor; VF: Vertebral fracture; VFA: Vertebral Fracture Assessment.

Competing interests

The authors declare that they have no competing interests.

Authors' contributions

PG conceived of the study, participated in its conception and design, carried out the acquisition and analysis of data, and drafted and revised the manuscript. LW participated in interpreting the data and contributed to the writing and revision of the manuscript. DQ participated in the acquisition of data, helped to analyze and interpret the data, and contributed to drafting and revising the manuscript. JV participated in the conception and design of this study, helped to acquire and analyze the data, and participated in drafting and revising the manuscript. DV contributed to the conception and design of the study, participated in drafting the manuscript, and helped to revise the manuscript. JvdB contributed to the acquisition of the data, helped to draft the manuscript, and participated in revising the manuscript. VS made substantial contributions to the conception and design of the study, carried out the acquisition and analysis of data, and participated in drafting and revising the manuscript. All authors read and approved the final manuscript.

Acknowledgments

This study was supported by Hasselt University and Transnationale Universiteit Limburg, Maastricht University Medical Centre. It was also supported by an unrestricted grant from AbbVie for a non-interventional study survey.

Author details

[1]Hasselt University, Biomedical Research Institute, and Transnationale Universiteit Limburg, Diepenbeek, Belgium, Martelarenlaan 42, 3500 Hasselt, Belgium. [2]Division of Rheumatology, Department of Internal Medicine, CAPHRI School for Public Health and Primary Care, Maastricht University Medical Center, Maastricht, P.O. Box 616, 6200 MD Maastricht, The Netherlands. [3]ReumaClinic, Genk, Bretheistraat 149, 3600 Genk, Belgium. [4]Department of Internal Medicine, VieCuri Medical Centre, P.O. Box 1926, 5900 BX Venlo, The Netherlands. [5]Department of Internal Medicine, NUTRIM School for Nutrition, Toxicology and Metabolism, Maastricht University Medical Centre, P.O. Box 616, 6200 MD Maastricht, The Netherlands.

References

1. El Maghraoui A. Extra-articular manifestations of ankylosing spondylitis: prevalence, characteristics and therapeutic implications. Eur J Intern Med. 2011;22:554–60. doi:10.1016/j.ejim.2011.06.006.
2. Sieper J, Braun J, Rudwaleit M, Boonen A, Zink A. Ankylosing spondylitis: an overview. Ann Rheum Dis. 2002;61 Suppl 3:iii8–18.
3. Weiss RJ, Wick MC, Ackermann PW, Montgomery SM. Increased fracture risk in patients with rheumatic disorders and other inflammatory diseases—a case-control study with 53,108 patients with fracture. J Rheumatol. 2010;37:2247–50. doi:10.3899/jrheum.100363.
4. Pedreira PG, Pinheiro MM, Szejnfeld VL. Bone mineral density and body composition in postmenopausal women with psoriasis and psoriatic arthritis. Arthritis Res Ther. 2011;13:R16. doi:10.1186/ar3240.
5. Prieto-Alhambra D, Munoz-Ortego J, De Vries F, Vosse D, Arden NK, Bowness P, et al. Ankylosing spondylitis confers substantially increased risk of clinical spine fractures: a nationwide case-control study. Osteoporos Int. 2015;26:85–91. doi:10.1007/s00198-014-2939-3.
6. Cooper C, Carbone L, Michet CJ, Atkinson EJ, O'Fallon WM, Melton 3rd LJ. Fracture risk in patients with ankylosing spondylitis: a population based study. J Rheumatol. 1994;21:1877–82.
7. Vosse D, Landewé R, van der Heijde D, van der Linden S, van Staa TP, Geusens P. Ankylosing spondylitis and the risk of fracture: results from a large primary care-based nested case-control study. Ann Rheum Dis. 2009;68:1839–42. doi:10.1136/ard.2008.100503.
8. Muñoz-Ortego J, Vestergaard P, Rubio JB, Wordsworth P, Judge A, Javaid MK, et al. Ankylosing spondylitis is associated with an increased risk of vertebral and nonvertebral clinical fractures: a population-based cohort study. J Bone Miner Res. 2014;29:1770–6. doi:10.1002/jbmr.2217.
9. Robinson Y, Sanden B, Olerud C. Increased occurrence of spinal fractures related to ankylosing spondylitis: a prospective 22-year cohort study in 17,764 patients from a national registry in Sweden. Patient Saf Surg. 2013;7:2. doi:10.1186/1754-9493-7-2.
10. van der Weijden MA, Claushuis TA, Nazari T, Lems WF, Dijkmans BA, van der Horst-Bruinsma IE. High prevalence of low bone mineral density in patients within 10 years of onset of ankylosing spondylitis: a systematic review. Clin Rheumatol. 2012;31:1529–35. doi:10.1007/s10067-012-2018-0.
11. Geusens P, Vosse D, van der Linden S. Osteoporosis and vertebral fractures in ankylosing spondylitis. Curr Opin Rheumatol. 2007;19:335–9. doi:10.1097/BOR.0b013e328133f5b3.
12. Geusens P, Vosse D, van der Heijde D, Vanhoof J, van Tubergen A, Raus J, et al. High prevalence of thoracic vertebral deformities and discal wedging in ankylosing spondylitis patients with hyperkyphosis. J Rheumatol. 2001;28:1856–61.

13. Sambrook PN, Geusens P. The epidemiology of osteoporosis and fractures in ankylosing spondylitis. Ther Adv Musculoskelet Dis. 2012;4:287–92. doi:10.1177/1759720x12441276.
14. Ghozlani I, Ghazi M, Nouijai A, Mounach A, Rezqi A, Achemlal L, et al. Prevalence and risk factors of osteoporosis and vertebral fractures in patients with ankylosing spondylitis. Bone. 2009;44:772–6. doi:10.1016/j.bone.2008.12.028.
15. Sieper J, Rudwaleit M, Baraliakos X, Brandt J, Braun J, Burgos-Vargas R, et al. The Assessment of SpondyloArthritis international Society (ASAS) handbook: a guide to assess spondyloarthritis. Ann Rheum Dis. 2009;68 Suppl 2:ii1–44. doi:10.1136/ard.2008.104018.
16. Braun J, van den Berg R, Baraliakos X, Boehm H, Burgos-Vargas R, Collantes-Estevez E, et al. 2010 update of the ASAS/EULAR recommendations for the management of ankylosing spondylitis. Ann Rheum Dis. 2011;70:896–904. doi:10.1136/ard.2011.151027.
17. Chapurlat RD, Duboeuf F, Marion-Audibert HO, Kalpakcioglu B, Mitlak BH, Delmas PD. Effectiveness of instant vertebral assessment to detect prevalent vertebral fracture. Osteoporos Int. 2006;17:1189–95. doi:10.1007/s00198-006-0121-2.
18. Vosse D, Heijckmann C, Landewé R, van der Heijde D, van der Linden S, Geusens P. Comparing morphometric X-ray absorptiometry and radiography in defining vertebral wedge fractures in patients with ankylosing spondylitis. Rheumatology (Oxford). 2007;46:1667–71. doi:10.1093/rheumatology/kem135.
19. Scott-Russell A, Dennison E, Taylor P, Cooper C. Comment on: Comparing morphometric X-ray absorptiometry and radiography in defining vertebral wedge fractures in patients with ankylosing spondylitis. Rheumatology (Oxford). 2008;47:1107–9. doi:10.1093/rheumatology/ken133.
20. Bijlsma JWJ. EULAR textbook on rheumatic diseases. London: BMJ/EULAR; 2012.
21. Genant HK, Jergas M, Palermo L, Nevitt M, Valentin RS, Black D, et al. Comparison of semiquantitative visual and quantitative morphometric assessment of prevalent and incident vertebral fractures in osteoporosis. J Bone Miner Res. 1996;11:984–96. doi:10.1002/jbmr.5650110716.
22. Genant HK, Wu CY, van Kuijk C, Nevitt MC. Vertebral fracture assessment using a semiquantitative technique. J Bone Miner Res. 1993;8:1137–48. doi:10.1002/jbmr.5650080915.
23. Bonnyman AM, Webber CE, Stratford PW, MacIntyre NJ. Intrarater reliability of dual-energy X-ray absorptiometry-based measures of vertebral height in postmenopausal women. J Clin Densitom. 2012;15:405–12. doi:10.1016/j.jocd.2012.03.005.
24. Geusens P, Lems WF. Osteoimmunology and osteoporosis. Arthritis Res Ther. 2011;13:242. doi:10.1186/ar3375.
25. Roux C. Osteoporosis in inflammatory joint diseases. Osteoporos Int. 2011;22:421–33. doi:10.1007/s00198-010-1319-x.
26. Goldring SR. Osteoimmunology and bone homeostasis: relevance to spondyloarthritis. Curr Rheumatol Rep. 2013;15:342. doi:10.1007/s11926-013-0342-2.
27. Coiffier G, Bouvard B, Chopin F, Biver E, Funck-Brentano T, Garnero P, et al. Common bone turnover markers in rheumatoid arthritis and ankylosing spondylitis: a literature review. Joint Bone Spine. 2013;80:250–7. doi:10.1016/j.jbspin.2012.08.004.
28. Vosse D, Landewé R, Garnero P, van der Heijde D, van der Linden S, Geusens P. Association of markers of bone- and cartilage-degradation with radiological changes at baseline and after 2 years follow-up in patients with ankylosing spondylitis. Rheumatology (Oxford). 2008;47:1219–22. doi:10.1093/rheumatology/ken148.
29. Lee YS, Schlotzhauer T, Ott SM, van Vollenhoven RF, Hunter J, Shapiro J, et al. Skeletal status of men with early and late ankylosing spondylitis. Am J Med. 1997;103:233–41.
30. Lange U, Kluge A, Strunk J, Teichmann J, Bachmann G. Ankylosing spondylitis and bone mineral density—what is the ideal tool for measurement? Rheumatol Int. 2005;26:115–20. doi:10.1007/s00296-004-0515-4.
31. Klingberg E, Lorentzon M, Göthlin J, Mellström D, Geijer M, Ohlsson C, et al. Bone microarchitecture in ankylosing spondylitis and the association with bone mineral density, fractures, and syndesmophytes. Arthritis Res Ther. 2013;15:R179. doi:10.1186/ar4368.
32. Mandl P, Navarro-Compan V, Terslev L, Aegerter P, van der Heijde D. EULAR recommendations for the use of imaging in the diagnosis and management of spondyloarthritis in clinical practice. Ann Rheum Dis. 2015;74:1327–39. doi:10.1136/annrheumdis-2014-206971.
33. Delmas PD, van de Langerijt L, Watts NB, Eastell R, Genant H, Grauer A, et al. Underdiagnosis of vertebral fractures is a worldwide problem: the IMPACT study. J Bone Miner Res. 2005;20:557–63. doi:10.1359/jbmr.041214.
34. Melton 3rd LJ, Lane AW, Cooper C, Eastell R, O'Fallon WM, Riggs BL. Prevalence and incidence of vertebral deformities. Osteoporos Int. 1993;3:113–9.
35. Christiansen BA, Bouxsein ML. Biomechanics of vertebral fractures and the vertebral fracture cascade. Curr Osteoporos Rep. 2010;8:198–204. doi:10.1007/s11914-010-0031-2.
36. Okamoto Y, Murakami H, Demura S, Kato S, Yoshioka K, Hayashi H, et al. The effect of kyphotic deformity because of vertebral fracture: a finite element analysis of a 10° and 20° wedge-shaped vertebral fracture model. Spine J. 2015;15:713–20. doi:10.1016/j.spinee.2014.11.019.
37. Feldtkeller E, Bruckel J, Khan MA. Scientific contributions of ankylosing spondylitis patient advocacy groups. Curr Opin Rheumatol. 2000;12:239–47.
38. Haglund E, Bremander AB, Petersson IF, Strombeck B, Bergman S, Jacobsson LT, et al. Prevalence of spondyloarthritis and its subtypes in southern Sweden. Ann Rheum Dis. 2011;70:943–8. doi:10.1136/ard.2010.141598.
39. Assessment of SpondyloArthritis International Society. Mission statement. http://www.asas-group.org/mission-statement.php. Accessed 14 Oct 2015.
40. Lucendo AJ, Hervias D, Roncero O, Lorente R, Bouhmidi A, Angueira T, et al. Epidemiology and temporal trends (2000–2012) of inflammatory bowel disease in adult patients in a central region of Spain. Eur J Gastroenterol Hepatol. 2014;26:1399–407. doi:10.1097/meg.0000000000000226.

21

Is the current ASAS expert definition of a positive family history useful in identifying axial spondyloarthritis? Results from the SPACE and DESIR cohorts

Zineb Ez-Zaitouni[1*], Andrea Hilkens[1], Laure Gossec[2,3], Inger Jorid Berg[4], Robert Landewé[5], Roberta Ramonda[6], Maxime Dougados[7], Désirée van der Heijde[1] and Floris van Gaalen[1]

Abstract

Background: The Assessment of SpondyloArthritis international Society (ASAS) definition of a positive family history (PFH) of spondyloarthritis (SpA) includes the following diseases in first- or second-degree relatives: ankylosing spondylitis (AS), acute anterior uveitis (AAU), reactive arthritis (ReA), inflammatory bowel disease (IBD), and psoriasis. However, it is not known if a PFH for each of these diseases contributes to making a diagnosis of axSpA, sacroiliitis on imaging, or fulfilling the ASAS criteria in patients presenting with chronic back pain (CBP). Therefore, the aim of this study was to assess which SpA diseases in family members are associated with human leukocyte antigen B27 (HLA-B27) and axial spondyloarthritis (axSpA) in CBP patients.

Methods: CBP patients suspected of axSpA from the SPACE ($n = 438$) and the DESIR ($n = 647$) cohort were asked about the presence of SpA diseases in first- or second-degree relatives (AS, AAU, ReA, IBD, and psoriasis). The associations between a PFH and HLA-B27, sacroiliitis on imaging (magnetic resonance imaging (MRI) or radiographs), axSpA diagnosis, and ASAS classification in CBP patients were assessed.

Results: In the SPACE and the DESIR cohort, a PFH of AS (odds ratio (OR) 5.9 (95% confidence interval (CI) 3.5–9.9), and OR 3.3 (95% CI 2.1–5.2)) and a PFH of AAU (OR 9.8 (95% CI 3.3–28.9) and OR 21.6 (95% CI 2.9–160.1)) were significantly associated with presence of HLA-B27. Furthermore, in both cohorts a PFH of AS and a PFH of AAU were positively associated with fulfilment of the ASAS criteria, but not with sacroiliitis on imaging. In SPACE but not in DESIR a PFH of AAU was positively associated with axSpA diagnosis. In both cohorts a PFH of ReA, IBD, or psoriasis was not positively associated with HLA-B27 positivity, sacroiliitis on imaging, axSpA diagnosis, or meeting the ASAS criteria for axSpA.

Conclusions: In our cohorts, a PFH of AS or AAU is useful for case-finding of axSpA as this is correlated with HLA-B27 carriership. However, as a PFH of ReA, IBD, or psoriasis does not contribute to identifying axSpA in CBP patients, these data suggest that the widely used ASAS definition of a PFH of SpA should be updated.

Keywords: Family history, Ankylosing spondylitis, Acute anterior uveitis, Reactive arthritis, IBD, Psoriasis, Axial spondyloarthritis, Diagnostic work-up, Chronic back pain

* Correspondence: z.ez-zaitouni@lumc.nl
[1]Department of Rheumatology, Leiden University Medical Center, P.O. Box 9600, 2300 RC Leiden, The Netherlands
Full list of author information is available at the end of the article

Background

Axial spondyloarthritis (axSpA) is a chronic inflammatory disease mainly involving the spine and sacroiliac joints. Genetic risk factors play a role in axSpA with human leukocyte antigen B27 (HLA-B27) by far the strongest genetic risk factor for disease [1]. A positive family history (PFH) of SpA has been reported in up to 40% of ankylosing spondylitis (AS) patients and the risk to develop AS in HLA-B27-positive first-degree relatives of HLA-B27-positive AS patients has been estimated to be 16-times higher than that of HLA-B27-positive individuals in the general population [2–5]. As a result, familial aggregation of SpA is considered a risk indicator for the presence of axSpA in patients with chronic back pain (CBP) and is part of several SpA classification criteria sets [6–8].

In the Assessment of SpondyloArthritis international Society (ASAS) classification criteria for axSpA, a PFH of SpA is defined as the presence of any of the following diseases in first- or second-degree relatives: AS, acute anterior uveitis (AAU), reactive arthritis (ReA), inflammatory bowel disease (IBD), and psoriasis [8]. This PFH definition is also recommended in diagnosing axSpA, and is incorporated in several referral strategies for CBP patients used by nonrheumatologists [9, 10].

However, only three of these diseases have a documented HLA-B27 association (i.e., AS, AAU, and ReA) and two are not HLA-B27 associated (i.e., IBD and psoriasis) [11–13]. Thus, even though a PFH of SpA is a common finding in axSpA patients it is unknown whether a PFH of each of these diseases contributes equally well to making a diagnosis of axSpA in patients presenting with CBP.

In this study, we present data from two unique early axSpA cohorts: the multinational multicenter SPondyloArthritis Caught Early (SPACE) cohort and the French multicenter DEvenir des Spondylarthropathies Indifférenciées Récentes (DESIR) cohort. In these cohorts of CBP patients with a suspicion of axSpA we have investigated which of the SpA diseases present among family members were associated with HLA-B27, sacroiliitis on imaging, a clinical diagnosis of axSpA, and meeting the ASAS classification criteria for axSpA.

Methods

Patient cohorts

The SPACE cohort is a prospective study which includes patients with short-term CBP (≥3 months, ≤2 years, and an onset <45 years) at a minimum age of 16 years from five Rheumatology outpatient clinics in the Netherlands, Norway, and Italy. DESIR is a prospective longitudinal cohort running in 25 centers in France (clinicaltrials.gov, NCT01648907). Patients between the ages of 18 and 50 years with inflammatory back pain (IBP) according to the Calin [14] or Berlin [15] criteria, persisting ≥3 months but <3 years, were included. In addition, the treating rheumatologist had to have a substantial suspicion of axSpA (level of confidence ≥5 on a 0–10 rating scale, where 0 = not confident and 10 = very confident). A detailed description of both cohorts is provided elsewhere [16, 17].

Table 1 Baseline characteristics and clinical features of CBP patients in the SPACE ($n = 438$) and DESIR cohorts ($n = 647$)

Characteristic	SPACE $n = 438$	DESIR $n = 647$
Age, years	31.3 (8.3)	33.6 (8.6)
Symptom duration, months	13.4 (7.4)	18.1 (10.5)
Male	165 (38)	305 (47)
IBP	286 (66)	647 (100)*
Good response to NSAIDs[a]	181/420 (43)	515/643 (80)
Past history or current symptoms		
Peripheral arthritis	64 (15)	363 (56)
Dactylitis	24 (6)	83 (13)
Enthesitis	89 (20)	312 (48)
AAU	34 (8)	51 (8)
IBD	34 (8)	23 (4)
Psoriasis	51 (12)	97 (15)
Elevated CRP (mg/L)/ESR (mm)[b]	123 (28)	254 (39)
HLA-B27 positive	174/436 (40)	376/646 (58)
Sacroiliitis, radiography[c]	48/434 (11)	172 (27)
Sacroiliitis, MRI[c]	135/431 (31)	207/636 (33)
ASAS criteria for axSpA	203 (46)	410/634 (65)
Any positive family history[d]	185 (42)	249 (39)
PFH of AS	90 (21)	127 (20)
PFH of AAU	27 (6)	29 (5)
PFH of ReA	14 (3)	6 (1)
PFH of IBD	33 (8)	32 (5)
PFH of Psoriasis	83 (19)	129 (20)
Total number of SpA diseases in first- or second-degree relatives		
Number of patients with 1 disease	135 (73)	189 (76)
Number of patients with 2 diseases	39 (21)	47 (19)
Number of patients with ≥3 diseases	11 (6)	13 (5)

Unless specified otherwise, results are presented as mean ± SD or number (%)
*Inclusion criterion
[a]Back pain not present anymore or is much better 24–48 hours after a full dose of NSAID
[b]Values greater than the upper limit of normal
[c]Imaging based on local reading. of sacroiliac joints
[d]Presence in first- or second-degree relatives of any of the following: AS, AAU, ReA, IBD, or psoriasis
AAU acute anterior uveitis, *AS* ankylosing spondylitis, *ASAS axSpA* criteria, Assessment of Spondyloarthritis international Society criteria for axial Spondyloarthritis, *CBP* chronic back pain, *CRP* C-reactive protein, *ESR* erythrocyte sedimentation rate, *HLA-B27* human leucocyte antigen B27, *IBD* inflammatory bowel disease, *IBP* inflammatory back pain, *MRI* magnetic resonance imaging, *NSAID* non-steroidal anti-inflammatory drug, *PFH* positive family history, *ReA* reactive arthritis, *SpA* spondyloarthritis

Table 2 Association of family history manifestations with HLA-B27 in CBP patients in the SPACE (*n* = 438) and DESIR cohorts (*n* = 647)

	SPACE*				DESIR**			
	HLA-B27 + *n* = 174	HLA-B27− *n* = 262	OR (95% CI)	*P* value	HLA-B27 + *n* = 376	HLA-B27− *n* = 270	OR (95% CI)	*P* value
Any PFH	97	87	2.5 (1.7–3.8)	<0.001	158	91	1.4 (1.0–2.0)	0.032
AS	65	24	5.9 (3.5–9.9)	<0.001	100	27	3.3 (2.1–5.2)	<0.001
AAU	23	4	9.8 (3.3–28.9)	<0.001	28	1	21.6 (2.9–160.1)	0.003
ReA	5	9	0.8 (0.3–2.5)	0.745	1	5	0.1 (0.01–1.2)	0.075
IBD	12	21	0.9 (0.4–1.8)	0.666	17	15	0.8 (0.4–1.6)	0.551
Psoriasis	34	48	1.1 (0.6–1.8)	0.750	69	60	0.8 (0.5–1.2)	0.225

*Two patients with unknown HLA-B27 status
**One with patient unknown HLA-B27 status
AAU acute anterior uveitis, *AS* ankylosing spondylitis, *CBP* chronic back pain, *CI* confidence interval, *HLA-B27* human leukocyte antigen B27, *IBD* inflammatory bowel disease, *OR* odds ratio, *PFH* positive family history (manifestation in first- or second-degree relatives), *ReA* reactive arthritis

Both studies were approved by local medical ethics committees. All participants provided prior written informed consent.

Clinical data collection

All patients underwent a diagnostic work-up according to a fixed protocol which includes physical examination, laboratory assessments (HLA-B27, C-reactive protein (CRP), and erythrocyte sedimentation rate (ESR)), and magnetic resonance imaging (MRI) as well as radiographs of sacroiliac joints. The presence and history of clinical SpA features were assessed: IBP, good response to nonsteroidal anti-inflammatory drugs (NSAIDs), peripheral arthritis, dactylitis, enthesitis, AAU, IBD, and psoriasis. Patients were asked about the presence of any of the following SpA diseases in first- or second-degree relatives: AS, AAU, ReA, IBD, and psoriasis. For each SpA disease the possible answers were "yes", "no" or "unknown/uncertain". A PFH was defined as the presence of ≥1 SpA-related disease in first- (mother, father, sister, brother, daughter, son) or second-degree relatives (aunt, uncle, niece, nephew, grandmother, and grandfather) reported by the patient [8].

In the SPACE cohort, axSpA was diagnosed by the treating rheumatologist. In the DESIR cohort axSpA diagnosis was defined as the level of confidence regarding diagnosis of ≥8 on a 0–10 numerical rating scale (where 0 = not confident at all and 10 = very confident). The ASAS axSpA classification criteria were used to classify patients.

Data analysis

Baseline demographic and clinical characteristics are presented using descriptive statistics for both the SPACE and DESIR cohorts. The association between each PFH disease and HLA-B27 in patients was assessed using the Chi-squared test. Similar analyses were performed for the assessment of the association between each PFH disease and a clinical diagnosis of axSpA, sacroiliitis on imaging (defined as either sacroiliitis on MRI,

Table 3 Association of family history manifestations with the fulfilment of ASAS axSpA criteria in the SPACE cohort and DESIR cohorts

	Fulfilment of ASAS axSpA criteria			
	SPACE		DESIR	
	OR (95% CI)	P- value	OR (95% CI)	P- value
Any PFH	2.1 (1.4-3.1)	<0.001	1.3 (1.0-1.9)	0.091
AS	3.3 (2.0-5.3)	<0.001	2.1 (1.3-3.3)	<0.001
AAU	7.4 (2.5-21.7)	<0.001	5.0 (1.5-16.7)	0.009
ReA	0.6 (0.2-1.9)	0.421	0.3 (0.05-1.5)	0.132
IBD	1.1 (0.5-2.2)	0.798	0.8 (0.4-1.6)	0.521
Psoriasis	1.2 (0.8-2.0)	0.388	1.2 (0.8-1.8)	0.464

Any PFH, any family history manifestation in first- or second-degree relatives; *AS* ankylosing spondylitis, *AAU* acute anterior uveitis, *ReA* reactive arthritis, *IBD* inflammatory bowel disease, *OR* odds ratio, *95% CI* 95% confidence interval

Table 4 PFH of diseases in first- or second-degree relatives of CBP patients meeting the ASAS axSpA criteria, stratified according to HLA-B27 status

Positive family history	SPACE cohort *n* = 201*		DESIR cohort *n* = 409**	
	HLA-B27+	HLA-B27−	HLA-B27+	HLA-B27−
Any PFH	90 (45%)	14 (7%)	145 (35%)	24 (6%)
AS	59 (29%)	2 (1%)	92 (23%)	5 (1%)
AAU	22 (11%)	1 (1%)	26 (6%)	0 (0)
ReA	4 (1%)	1 (1%)	1 (0.2%)	1 (0.2%)
IBD	11 (6%)	5 (3%)	14 (3%)	5 (1%)
Psoriasis	32 (16%)	9 (5%)	65 (16%)	20 (5%)

*Two hundred and three patients fulfilled ASAS-criteria, two with unknown HLA-B27 status
**Four hundred and ten patients fulfilled ASAS-criteria, one with unknown HLA-B27 status
AAU acute anterior uveitis, *AS* ankylosing spondylitis, *ASAS axSpA* Assessment of Spondyloarthritis international Society criteria for axial spondyloarthritis, *HLA-B27* human leucocyte antigen B27, *IBD* inflammatory bowel disease, *PFH* postitive family history (manifestation in first- or second-degree relatives), *ReA* reactive arthritis

radiographs, or on both modalities by local reading), and the fulfilment of the ASAS axSpA classification criteria.

Statistical testing was performed using Stata SE v.14 (StataCorp LP, College Station, TX, USA).

Results

For the current analyses, 438 patients from the SPACE cohort and 647 patients from the DESIR cohort with complete data at baseline were used (Table 1). Several baseline characteristics differed between the two cohorts, mainly reflecting differences in inclusion criteria. In both cohorts, the distribution of all PFH diseases (AS, AAU, ReA, IBD, and psoriasis) in first- or second-degree relatives were similar.

In both the SPACE and DESIR cohort, any PFH, a PFH of AS, and a PFH of AAU were significantly associated with HLA-B27 in CBP patients (Table 2). In multivariable analyses, a PFH of AS or AAU were independently associated with HLA-B27 positivity (data not shown). However, in neither cohort was a PFH of ReA, IBD, or psoriasis associated with HLA-B27-positivity.

To investigate whether the presence of a PFH for any of the diseases in relatives is associated with sacroiliitis, a clinical diagnosis of axSpA, or a positive ASAS classification, similar analyses were performed. In both cohorts, neither 'any PFH' nor a separate PFH of a disease were associated with sacroiliitis (Additional file 1). In SPACE but not in DESIR a PFH of AAU was positively associated with axSpA diagnosis (Additional file 2). While a PFH of AS or AAU had a significant positive association with fulfilment of the ASAS criteria, such an association was not found for a PFH of ReA, IBD, or psoriasis in the SPACE and DESIR cohorts (Table 3).

In addition, the relative contribution of HLA-B27 was investigated among patients who were classified according to the ASAS criteria. A total of 203 (46%) patients from the SPACE cohort and 410 (63%) patients from the DESIR cohort fulfilled the ASAS criteria for axSpA, and 156 (77%) and 347 (85%) patients were HLA-B27 positive, respectively (Table 4). A PFH was reported more frequently in HLA-B27-positive patients than in HLA-B27-negative patients meeting the ASAS classification criteria (SPACE 45% vs 7% and DESIR 35% vs 6%).

Discussion

To our knowledge this is the first study to investigate the usefulness of the separate SpA diseases in a PFH as defined for the ASAS classification criteria. In two independent cohorts of predominantly Caucasoid Europeans, we found that in CBP patients suspected of axSpA a PFH of ReA, IBD, or psoriasis were neither associated with HLA-B27 positivity, nor with sacroiliitis, a diagnosis of axSpA, or fulfilment of the ASAS criteria. In contrast, a PFH of AS or AAU was strongly correlated with HLA-B27 carriership.

IBD and psoriasis are generally not HLA-B27-associated diseases, but ReA has been reported to be associated with HLA-B27 in a secondary care setting, although in population-based studies the prevalence of HLA-B27 in ReA was comparable to that of the general population [12, 18]. A possible explanation for the absence of the association between ReA and HLA-B27 in our study is that the (self)-reported prevalence of ReA in family members of patients in the SPACE and DESIR cohort was low, suggesting underreporting.

It is important to emphasize that the current study was performed in patients with predominantly axial symptoms. Although only a PFH of AS or AAU have been shown to be independently associated with HLA-B27, this does not mean that a PFH of the other SpA diseases is always irrelevant [19]. For example, the presence of psoriasis in relatives could be relevant in a patient with peripheral symptoms suspected of psoriatic arthritis [20].

A strength of this study is the use of two large early axSpA cohorts in which all patients were assessed following a similar protocol which allowed for replication of findings. Strikingly similar prevalences of PFH were found in both cohorts which adds to the credibility of the data. The major limitation of this study, however, is that the diagnosis in relatives (the PFH) is solely based on patients' information which may have led to either under- or overestimation of a PFH. However, this is similar to most clinical settings in which PFH is also mostly based on self-reporting. Moreover, subdividing a PFH into five different diseases meant that a PFH of, for instance, AAU or ReA was uncommon.

Conclusions

In conclusion, in our two cohorts a PFH of ReA, IBD, and psoriasis does not contribute to diagnosing axSpA in CBP patients suspected of axSpA. A PFH of AS or AAU may be useful in case-finding in low prevalence settings, such as general practice, as these are correlated with HLA-B27 carriership. When replicated, preferably in other regions of the world in patients with a different genetic background, it is justified to remove a PFH of ReA, IBD, and psoriasis from the current ASAS definition of a positive PFH relevant for axSpA.

Abbreviations

AAU: Acute anterior uveitis; AS: Ankylosing spondylitis; ASAS: Assessment of SpondyloArthritis international Society; axSpA: Axial spondyloarthritis; CBP: Chronic back pain; HLA-B27: Human leukocyte antigen B27; IBD: Inflammatory bowel disease; IBP: Inflammatory back pain; MRI: Magnetic resonance imaging; PFH: Positive family history; ReA: Reactive arthritis

Acknowledgements
The DESIR cohort was sponsored by the Département de la Recherche Clinique et du Développement de l'Assistance Publique–Hôpitaux de Paris. This study is conducted under the umbrella of the French Society of Rheumatology and INSERM (Institut National de la Santé et de la Recherche Médicale). The database management is performed within the Department of Epidemiology and Biostatistics (Professor Paul Landais, D.I.M., Nîmes, France). An unrestricted grant from Pfizer was allocated for the 10 years of the follow-up of the recruited patients. The authors thank the different regional participating centers: Pr. M. Dougados (Paris, Cochin B), Pr. A. Kahan (Paris, Cochin A), Pr. O. Meyer, Pr. P. Dieudé (Paris, Bichat), Pr. P. Bourgeois, Pr. L. Gossec (Paris, La Pitié Salpetrière), Pr. F. Berenbaum (Paris, Saint Antoine), Pr. P. Claudepierre (Créteil), Pr. M. Breban (Boulogne Billancourt), Dr. B. Saint-Marcoux (Aulnay-sous-Bois), Pr. P. Goupille (Tours), Pr. J-F. Maillefert (Dijon), Dr. X. Puéchal, Dr. E. Dernis (Le Mans), Pr. D. Wendling (Besançon), Pr. B. Combe (Montpellier), Pr. L. Euller-Ziegler (Nice), Pr. P. Orcel, Dr. P. Richette (Paris, Lariboisière), Pr. P. Lafforgue (Marseille), Dr. P. Boumier (Amiens), Pr. M. Soubrier (Clermont-Ferrand), Dr. N. Mehsen (Bordeaux), Pr. D. Loeuille (Nancy), Pr. R-M. Flipo (Lille), Pr. A. Saraux (Brest), Dr. S. Pavy (Le Kremlin Bicêtre), Pr. A. Cantagrel (Toulouse), Pr. O. Vittecoq (Rouen). The authors also thank URC-CIC Paris Centre for the coordination and monitoring of the study.

Funding
This work was supported by an unrestricted grant from MSD. MSD was not involved in the design of the study, acquisition, analysis, or interpretation of the data, or drafting the manuscript.

Authors' contributions
ZE-Z, DvdH, and FvG were responsible for study conception and design. ZE-Z, AH, LG, IJB, RL, RR, MD, and FvG were responsible for acquisition of the data. ZE-Z, AH, DvdH, and FvG participated in interpretation and analysis of the data. ZE-Z drafted and wrote the manuscript. ZE-Z, AH, LG, IJB, RL, RR, MD, DvdH, and FvG were involved in critically revising the manuscript for important intellectual content. All authors read and approved the final manuscript.

Authors' information
All authors read and approved this manuscript.

Competing interests
The authors declare that they have no competing interests.

Author details
[1]Department of Rheumatology, Leiden University Medical Center, P.O. Box 9600, 2300 RC Leiden, The Netherlands. [2]Sorbonne Universités, UPMC Univ Paris 06, GRC-08, Paris, France. [3]Rheumatology Department, Pitie-Salpétrière Hospital, AP-HP, Paris, France. [4]Department of Rheumatology, Diakonhjemmet Hospital, Oslo, Norway. [5]Department of Clinical Immunology and Rheumatology, Amsterdam Medical Center, Amsterdam, The Netherlands. [6]Rheumatology Unit, Department of Medicine DIMED, University of Padova, Padova, Italy. [7]Paris Descartes University, Hôpital Cochin, Assistance Publique-Hôpitaux de Paris, INSERM (U1153): Epidémiologie Clinique et Biostatistiques, PRES Sorbonne Paris-Cité, Paris, France.

References

1. Schlosstein L, Terasaki PI, Bluestone R, Pearson CM. High association of an HL-A antigen, W27, with ankylosing spondylitis. N Engl J Med. 1973;288(14):704–6.
2. Bedendo A, Glorioso S, Pasini CV, Fabiano F, Casara D, Cavallo A, Todesco S. A family study of ankylosing spondylitis. Rheumatol Int. 1984;5(1):29–32.
3. van der Linden SM, Valkenburg HA, de Jongh BM, Cats A. The risk of developing ankylosing spondylitis in HLA-B27 positive individuals. A comparison of relatives of spondylitis patients with the general population. Arthritis Rheum. 1984;27(3):241–9.
4. Said-Nahal R, Miceli-Richard C, Berthelot JM, Duche A, Dernis-Labous E, Le Blevec G, Saraux A, Perdriger A, Guis S, Claudepierre P, et al. The familial form of spondylarthropathy: a clinical study of 115 multiplex families. Groupe Francais d'Etude Genetique des Spondylarthropathies. Arthritis Rheum. 2000;43(6):1356–65.
5. Brown MA, Kennedy LG, MacGregor AJ, Darke C, Duncan E, Shatford JL, Taylor A, Calin A, Wordsworth P. Susceptibility to ankylosing spondylitis in twins: the role of genes, HLA, and the environment. Arthritis Rheum. 1997;40(10):1823–8.
6. Amor B, Dougados M, Mijiyawa M. Criteria of the classification of spondylarthropathies. Rev Rhum Mal Osteoartic. 1990;57(2):85–9.
7. Dougados M, van der Linden S, Juhlin R, Huitfeldt B, Amor B, Calin A, Cats A, Dijkmans B, Olivieri I, Pasero G, et al. The European Spondylarthropathy Study Group preliminary criteria for the classification of spondylarthropathy. Arthritis Rheum. 1991;34(10):1218–27.
8. Rudwaleit M, van der Heijde D, Landewe R, Listing J, Akkoc N, Brandt J, Braun J, Chou CT, Collantes-Estevez E, Dougados M, et al. The development of Assessment of SpondyloArthritis international Society classification criteria for axial spondyloarthritis (part II): validation and final selection. Ann Rheum Dis. 2009;68(6):777–83.
9. Poddubnyy D, van Tubergen A, Landewe R, Sieper J, van der Heijde D. Development of an ASAS-endorsed recommendation for the early referral of patients with a suspicion of axial spondyloarthritis. Ann Rheum Dis. 2015;74(8):1483–7.
10. van den Berg R, de Hooge M, Rudwaleit M, Sieper J, van Gaalen F, Reijnierse M, Landewe R, Huizinga T, van der Heijde D. ASAS modification of the Berlin algorithm for diagnosing axial spondyloarthritis: results from the SPondyloArthritis Caught Early (SPACE)-cohort and from the Assessment of SpondyloArthritis international Society (ASAS)-cohort. Ann Rheum Dis. 2013;72(10):1646–53.
11. Reveille JD. Genetics of spondyloarthritis—beyond the MHC. Nat Rev Rheumatol. 2012;8(5):296–304.
12. Aho K, Ahvonen P, Lassus A, Sievers K, Tilikainen A. HL-A antigen 27 and reactive arthritis. Lancet. 1973;2(7821):157.
13. Wakefield D, Chang JH, Amjadi S, Maconochie Z, Abu El-Asrar A, McCluskey P. What is new HLA-B27 acute anterior uveitis? Ocul Immunol Inflamm. 2011;19(2):139–44.
14. Calin A, Porta J, Fries JF, Schurman DJ. Clinical history as a screening test for ankylosing spondylitis. JAMA. 1977;237(24):2613–4.
15. Rudwaleit M, Metter A, Listing J, Sieper J, Braun J. Inflammatory back pain in ankylosing spondylitis: a reassessment of the clinical history for application as classification and diagnostic criteria. Arthritis Rheum. 2006;54(2):569–78.
16. van den Berg R, de Hooge M, van Gaalen F, Reijnierse M, Huizinga T, van der Heijde D. Percentage of patients with spondyloarthritis in patients referred because of chronic back pain and performance of classification criteria: experience from the Spondyloarthritis Caught Early (SPACE) cohort. Rheumatology (Oxford). 2013;52(8):1492–9.
17. Dougados M, d'Agostino MA, Benessiano J, Berenbaum F, Breban M, Claudepierre P, Combe B, Dargent-Molina P, Daures JP, Fautrel B, et al. The DESIR cohort: a 10-year follow-up of early inflammatory back pain in France: study design and baseline characteristics of the 708 recruited patients. Joint Bone Spine. 2011;78(6):598–603.
18. Leirisalo-Repo M, Hannu T, Mattila L. Microbial factors in spondyloarthropathies: insights from population studies. Curr Opin Rheumatol. 2003;15(4):408–12.
19. Rudwaleit M, van der Heijde D, Khan MA, Braun J, Sieper J. How to diagnose axial spondyloarthritis early. Ann Rheum Dis. 2004;63(5):535–43.
20. Reich K, Kruger K, Mossner R, Augustin M. Epidemiology and clinical pattern of psoriatic arthritis in Germany: a prospective interdisciplinary epidemiological study of 1511 patients with plaque-type psoriasis. Br J Dermatol. 2009;160(5):1040–7.

22

Work outcome in yet undiagnosed patients with non-radiographic axial spondyloarthritis and ankylosing spondylitis; results of a cross-sectional study among patients with chronic low back pain

Lonneke van Hoeven[1,2*], Annelies E. R. C. H. Boonen[3], Johanna M. W. Hazes[1] and Angelique E. A. M. Weel[1,2]

Abstract

Background: To understand the impact of yet undiagnosed non-radiographic axial spondyloarthritis (nr-axSpA) and ankylosing spondylitis (AS) on work outcomes in a cohort of patients with long-lasting chronic low back pain (CLBP).

Methods: Data were used from a primary care CLBP cohort that was established to understand the prevalence of nr-axSpA and AS. Clinical characteristics comprised measures of back pain (visual analogue scale), inflammation (C-reactive protein) and physical functioning (Roland Morris Disability Questionnaire (RMDQ)). Worker outcomes comprised a question on employment and the Work Productivity and Activity Impairment (WPAI) questionnaire, distinguishing absenteeism, presenteeism, and overall work impairment in those employed and activity impairment in all patients. For each disease subgroup, employment ratio compared to the general population was assessed by indirect standardization. Factors associated with work productivity were explored by zero inflated negative binomial (ZINB) regression models.

Results: Patients with CLBP ($n = 579$) were included (41% male, mean age 36 years), of whom 71 (12%) were identified as having nr-axSpA and 24 (4%) as having AS. The standardized employment ratios were 0.89 (95% CI 0.84–0.94), 0.97 (95% CI 0.85–1.09) and 0.81 (95% CI 0.56–1.06) for patients with CLBP, nr-axSpA and AS, respectively. Scores for the WPAI subdomains were not significantly different between patients with CLBP, nr-axSpA or AS. The ZINB models showed significant associations between visual analog scale (VAS) score for pain and RMDQ and work productivity.

Conclusion: The impact of yet undiagnosed nr-axSpA and AS on patients' work outcomes was substantial but was not significantly different from those of patients with long-standing CLBP. Variables significantly associated with reduced work productivity were VAS for pain and RMDQ score.

Keywords: Axial spondyloarthritis, Low back pain, Work participation, Patient reported outcome measures, Burden of disease

* Correspondence: l.vanhoeven@erasmusmc.nl
[1]Department of Rheumatology, Erasmus MC, Wytemaweg 80, 3015 CN Rotterdam, The Netherlands
[2]Department of Rheumatology, Maasstad Hospital, Maasstadweg 21, 3079 DZ Rotterdam, The Netherlands
Full list of author information is available at the end of the article

Background

Low back pain (LBP) is a major health and societal problem affecting more than 80% of adults at some point in their lives [1]. Between 10 and 28% of episodes of LBP persist for more than 12 weeks and become chronic complaints [2]. A study has shown that up to 24% of chronic LBP (CLBP) in young adults can be explained by axial spondyloarthritis (axSpA) [3]. AxSpA is an auto-inflammatory disease of the spine that is potentially treatable. Two subtypes of axSpA can be distinguished; in non-radiographic axSpA (nr-axSpA) either sacroiliitis is visible on magnetic resonance imaging (MRI) or human leukocyte antigen B27 (HLA-B27) is positive, and in addition one or two so-called SpA features are present [4]. In those with radiographic axSpA, structural changes are visible on the X-ray of the sacroiliac joints and this subtype corresponds to what is commonly known as ankylosing spondylitis (AS).

Although the new classification criteria for axSpA were developed to enhance early recognition and subsequently provide earlier and better treatment, the profile of those in whom the diagnosis of axSpA is wrongly missed is not completely elucidated. This is important, as it could provide insight into the reversible burden of the disease when diagnosis would have made earlier. Several studies report an overall comparable clinical burden in patients with AS and nr-axSpA [5, 6], however these patients were referred in prospective settings and not wrongly missed.

The clinical burden of a chronic inflammatory disease can be expressed in terms of disease activity and impaired function, but also in work participation [7]. The impact of undiagnosed axSpA on the patients' capacity to work is important from the perspective of the patient and their families [8], and from the societal perspective when calculating indirect costs to determine the economic burden of a disease and the possible return on investment by using case-finding strategies for axSpA patients. Moreover, such data can help us understand the level of support patients with axSpA might need to help them to remain active in the labor force and safeguard their career perspective.

Some data are already available on the impact of AS and axSpA on work participation. A review of work outcomes in AS indicates that patients with longstanding disease incur official work disability up to three times more frequently, and that there had already been substantial work loss at the time of diagnosis [9]. Also a recent study in patients with early axSpA reported that within only 5 years of diagnosis, 19% of patients with axSpA were not employed because of the axSpA [10]. Also, in those still working, 28% and 48% of the patients reported having sick leave and reduced productivity at work [10]. A recent medication trial in patients with nr-axSpA showed an improvement in worker productivity of 9.6 h/week in the patients with nr-axSpA who had a good response to their treatment (assuming a 40-hour working week) [11], suggesting that early recognition of axSpA might prevent adverse work outcomes. It is already known that CLBP has a significant impact not only on work productivity, but also on daily activities [12, 13].

The aim of this study was to investigate work outcomes in yet undiagnosed patients with nr-axSpA and AS among a cohort of patients with CLBP. The specific aims were to compare the employment of patients with AS, nr-axSpA and CLBP with the general population, to explore whether these diagnostic groups differed in sick leave and productivity at work and to explore which demographic and disease characteristics contributed to sick leave and productivity at work.

Methods

Study population

All patients from the second cross-sectional Case Finding Axial SpondyloArthritis (CaFaSpA 2) study were included [14]. The study was performed in 2011 and 2012 in the south-western part of the Netherlands. Ethics approval from the Medical Ethical Committee from the St. Elisabeth Hospital in Tilburg, the Netherlands was received. Written informed consent was obtained from all participants at the research center, before any assessment was performed.

Patients with CLBP ages 18-45 years were selected by ICPC code L03 (nonspecific low back pain) from general practice (GP) records and invited to participate if the CLBP had been present for at least 3 months. Participating patients were examined by a rheumatologist or an experienced research nurse, i.e. recording of medical history and physical examination, including identification of features of SpA. All assessments and definitions adhered to the descriptions in the Assessment of SpondyloArthritis International Society (ASAS) handbook [15]. Blood was drawn to determine HLA-B27 positivity, C-reactive protein (CRP) (normal range 1–10 mg/L) and erythrocyte sedimentation rate (ESR) (normal range 0–15 mm Hg/min). X-ray and MRI of the sacroiliac joints were obtained in all patients. A definitive diagnosis of sacroiliitis was made according to the ASAS MRI criteria [4] or the modified New York criteria for the X-ray [16], by one of three trained radiologists, who were blinded to the clinical outcomes, laboratory data and results of other imaging methods. The primary outcome of this study was to identify new patients with axSpA using the ASAS classification criteria [4]. None of the newly identified patients with axSpA had received any treatment with non-steroidal anti-inflammatory drugs (NSAIDs) or biologic agents.

Questionnaires

To assess disease severity patients completed the Bath AS Disease Activity Index (BASDAI) [17], Ankylosing Spondylitis Disease Activity Score (ASDAS-CRP) [17], a visual analog scale (VAS) for pain (range 0–10) and the Roland Morris Disability Questionnaire (RMDQ) [18]. The RMDQ was developed to measure limitations in physical functioning in patients with CLBP. It consists of questions about impairment and limitations in different activities due LBP. Patients indicate if a question is applicable to them (score = 1) or not (score = 0). The score can range from 0 to 24 and a higher score indicates a higher level of disability.

Socioeconomic status and worker productivity

All participants completed questions about their highest achieved educational level; low (elementary school), medium (high school) and high (university), current work status (employed, or not employed), and the number of working days and working hours per week in those employed. To assess whether a patient was work-disabled or not work-disabled, we asked the patient is there was an official disapproval of the insurance company doctors. Answers to an open question about occupation were classified into non-manual (administrative, scientific and managerial professions) and manual (industrial, commercial, servicing, transportation and agricultural) jobs, using the International Standard Classification of Occupation (ISCO)-08 major groups [19].

Finally, the Work Productivity and Activity Impairment (WPAI) questionnaire was completed, which evaluates four subdomains; absenteeism, presenteeism, work impairment and activity impairment, due to back problems in the past 7 days [20]. The subdomains are all expressed in percentages; absenteeism (percentage work time lost), presenteeism (percentage productivity loss at work), work impairment (absenteeism and presenteeism combined) and activity impairment (percentage activity loss). Higher percentages indicate worse outcomes.

Statistical analyses

The ASAS criteria were used to classify patients as having nr-axSpA, AS or as not fulfilling the criteria (CLBP). Sociodemographic and clinical characteristics were summarized as mean and standard deviation (SD) or as median and interquartile range (IQR) and compared between subgroups using the unpaired *t* test or Wilcoxon rank sum test for continuous variables and the chi-square or Fisher exact test for categorical data.

Indirect standardization (by gender and age categories of 5 years) was used to calculate employment ratios for the total population and each disease subgroup (AS, nr-axSpA and CLBP), in comparison to the general Dutch population. Employment data from the general Dutch population was provided by the Dutch Centraal Bureau voor Statistiek (CBS) [21]. Poisson 95% confidence intervals (CI) for standardized proportions were calculated.

Scores in the WPAI are presented first as the proportion of patients with any (>0%) absenteeism, presenteeism, work or activity impairment and next as the average percentage absenteeism, presenteeism and work and activity impairment. Absenteeism, presenteeism and activity impairment were calculated only in employed patients, activity impairment in all patients. Differences between subgroups in the proportions of patients who had any restriction were tested using the chi-square and Fisher exact test. Differences between subgroups in the level of restriction in each subdomain of the WPAI were tested using the Wilcoxon rank sum test.

To investigate which factors are associated with each of the four domains of worker productivity, zero inflated negative binomial (ZINB) models were used. Zero inflated models are needed to adjust for the excess zeros in productivity outcomes (percentage zeros: absenteeism 87%; presenteeism 50%; work impairment 39%; activity impairment 32% of all observations). ZINB models assume that the zeros can result from two different processes; [22] the "certain zeros" (or always zeros) which are accounted for in the zero inflated logistic part and the "possible zeros" that are accounted for in the count part. As in the count part the values are over dispersed (i.e. the variance was much larger than the mean), the negative binomial distribution was preferred, and to fit the four subdomains of the WPAI, zero-inflated models were used [23].

To create the multivariable ZINB models four different steps were taken. In step 1 gender and age were included in both the binomial and count part of the ZINB model. In the second step all the candidate covariates (disease: CLBP, nr-axSpA or AS; education level: low, intermediate, high; occupation: manual vs. non-manual; duration of LBP (years); VAS score for pain; CRP, RMDQ score, ASDAS-CRP score and BASDAI score) were tested in univariate analysis in both the binomial and count part of the ZINB. All variables that were significant at $p < 0.20$ were considered for multivariable analyses in step 3. However, ASDAS-CRP and BASDAI were not validated in patients with CLBP, and as moderate correlation was seen between the VAS score for pain and the BASDAI score it was decided to take the ASDAS-CRP and BASDAI scores out of the multivariable model. In step 4, the model was repeated with the covariates with p values <0.05 in the multivariable analysis.

A ZINB provides regression coefficients for both the logistic and the count part separately. A positive coefficient in the zero inflated (logistic) part of the ZINB means that an increase in that variable leads to a higher likelihood of resulting in a "certain zero"'. A negative coefficient in the count part of the ZINB means that an increase of that variable leads to a smaller chance of scoring a zero in the outcome (i.e. subdomain of the WPAI).

The analyses were performed using STATA version 13.0 software (Stata Corporation TX, USA).

Results

CaFaSpA cohort

The enrollment of patients in the CaFaSpA 2 study has previously been described [14]. Overall, 2597 patients (ages 18–45 years) with CLBP from 38 primary care practices were invited to participate: 1161 patients (45%) responded to the invitation, among whom 480 expressed no interest in participation and 102 did not fulfil the inclusion criteria. In total there were 579 patients with CLBP included in this study. The median duration of LBP was 7 years (IQR 3–15 years), 41% of the patients were male and the mean age was 36.0 years (SD 7.0) (Table 1). In total 95 patients (16.4%) were classified as having axSpA, and 24 of those (25%) fulfilled the classification criteria for AS and 71 (75%) for nr-axSpA. The majority (59 out of 71) of the patients in the nr-axSpA group was classified based on MRI abnormalities. The percentage of women in the AS group was higher (75%) compared to the nr-axSpA (58%) and CLBP group (58%), although this difference was not statistically significant ($p = 0.10$). Of the three disease subgroups, patients with AS (8%) were less highly educated compared to patients with CLBP (21%) or nr-axSpA (24%). The percentage of patients with a manual occupation in the nr-axSpA group was 46% compared to 29% in the AS group and 37% in the patients with CLBP.

Table 1 Demographics and clinical characteristics in study participants ($n = 579$)

	CLBP ($n = 484$)	Nr-axSpA ($n = 71$)	AS ($n = 24$)
Age, mean (SD) years[a]	35.6 (7.1)	36.8 (6.6)	38.6 (5.8)
Male sex, *n* (%)	202 (42)	30 (42)	6 (25)
LBP duration, mean (SD) years	9.2 (7.7)	9.6 (7.4)	9.3 (9.9)
Disease activity			
VAS pain, median (IQR)[b]	5 (3–7)	4 (2–5)	4.5 (2–7)
BASDAI, median (IQR)	4.2 (2.3–6)	3.9 (2.4–5.4)	5.3 (2.9–6.6)
ASDAS-CRP, median (IQR)[c]	2.3 (1.6–2.9)	2.3 (1.6–2.9)	2.8 (2.1–3.5)
RMDQ, median (IQR)[d]	7 (3–13)	6 (3–9)	12 (5–17)
Educational level[e]			
Low (elementary school) (%)	177 (38)	29 (41)	11 (46)
Medium (high school) (%)	194 (41)	24 (34)	11 (46)
High (university) (%)	101 (21)	17 (24)	2 (8)
Work status			
Employed, *n* (%)	342 (72.2)	55 (77.5)	15 (62.5)
Disability pension, *n* (%)	8 (1.7)	2 (2.8)	0 (0)
Number of hours working per week, mean (SD)[f]	33.1 (9.4)	34.6 (8.6)	27.9 (12.4)
Occupation in employed patients[f]			
Manual, *n* (%)	124 (37)	24 (46)	4 (29)
Non-manual, *n* (%)	208 (63)	28 (54)	10 (71)

CLBP chronic low back pain, *Nr-axSpA* non-radiographic axial spondyloarthritis, *AS* ankylosing spondylitis, *IQR* interquartile range, *LBP* low back pain, *VAS* visual analog scale, *BASDAI* Bath Ankylosing Spondylitis Disease Activity Index, *ASDAS-CRP* Ankylosing Spondylitis Disease Activity Score-C-reactive protein, *RMDQ* Rolland Morris Disability Questionnaire. [a]$p = 0.04$ for CLBP vs. AS; [b]$p = 0.04$ for CLBP vs. nr-axSpA; [c]$p = 0.01$ for CLBP vs. AS; [d]$p = 0.03$ for CLBP vs. AS; [e]total number of questionnaires about educational level: CLBP, $n = 472$ (12 missing), nr-axSpA, $n = 70$ (1 missing); [f]total number of questionnaires about occupation and working hours in employed patients: CLBP, $n = 332$ (10 missing), AS, $n = 14$ (1 missing), nr-axSpA, n = 52 (3 missing)

Work status

In total 342 out of 579 participants (72.4%) were employed. After adjusting for age, the likelihood of being employed was 0.92 (95% CI 0.86–0.99) and 0.88 (95%CI 0.81–0.94) for men and women, respectively, compared with the Dutch general population. Age-adjusted ratios for being employed, in patients with CLBP, nr-axSpA or AS were 0.89 (95% CI 0.84–0.94), 0.97 (95% CI 0.85–1.09) and 0.81 (95% CI 0.56–1.06), respectively. There were no patients with a disability pension in the newly identified AS group, while there were eight patients (1.7%) in the CLBP group and two patients (2.8%) in the newly identified nr-axSpA group.

WPAI questionnaire

Of the 342 employed patients with CLBP, 318 (93%) completed the WPAI questionnaire, compared to 14/15 patients with AS (93%) and 48/55 patients with nr-axSpA (87%). Of the employed patients with AS, 14% had been absent from work in the past 7 days, while this percentage was 10% and 12% in the employed patients with nr-axSpA and with CLBP, respectively (Table 2). Presenteeism was the most prevalent in patients with CLBP (59%), but the percentage presenteeism was the highest in the AS group at 59%. There were no significant differences in any of the four sub scores between patients with CLBP and patients with nr-axSpA, or between patients with CLBP and patients with AS.

ZINB models

Detailed results on the age-adjusted and gender-adjusted univariable regression can be found in Additional file 1, while the final multivariable model is presented in Table 3. In the final model the VAS score for pain and the RMDQ score were independently associated with the logistic part of each of the four domains of the WPAI. For the count part of the model, the VAS score for pain and the RMDQ score were independently associated with presenteeism, and work and activity impairment. This means that patients with pain and functional limitations are unlikely to have no restrictions in worker

Table 2 Worker productivity assessed by the WPAI for employed patients with CLBP, nr-axSpA or AS (18–45 years of age)

	CLBP (*n* = 318)	Nr-axSpA (*n* = 48)	AS (*n* = 14)
Absenteeism			
Absenteeism present, *n* (% (95% CI))	38 (12 (8–16))	5 (10 (4–23))	2 (14 (2–43))
Absenteeism, mean % (SD)	53 (31)	47 (43)	54 (59)
Presenteeism			
Presenteeism present, *n* (% (95% CI))	188 (59 (53–64))	23 (47 (34–61))	7 (53 (27–79))
Presenteeism, mean % (SD)	45 (28)	46 (32)	59 (34)
Work impairment			
Work impairment present, *n* (% (95% CI))	197 (62 (56–67))	25 (52 (37–67))	8 (57 (29–82))
Work impairment, mean % (SD)	49 (30)	48 (33)	62 (36)
Activity impairment[a]			
Activity impairment present, *n* (% (95% CI))	322 (68 (63–72))	45 (63 (51–75))	19 (79 (58–93))
Activity impairment, mean % (SD)	51 (27)	49 (28)	56 (34)

WPAI Worker Productivity and Activity Impairment Questionnaire, *CLBP* chronic low back pain, *nr-axSpA* non-radiographic axial spondyloarthritis, *AS* ankylosing spondylitis. There were no significant differences in any of the four sub scores between patients with CLBP and patients with nr-axSpA, or between patients with CLBP and patients with AS. [a]Calculated in all patients, not only in the employed patients (CLBP, *n* = 474; nr-axSpA, *n* = 71; AS, *n* = 24)

productivity (so unlikely to belong to the zero inflated part) and that increased pain and functional limitations are associated with more presenteeism, overall work impairment and activity impairment, but no absenteeism. In addition, lower educational level was associated with a likelihood of work impairment and level of overall work impairment, and with the level of presenteeism, and longer disease duration was associated with a decreased likelihood of work impairment.

As an example of the interpretation of the output of the ZINB model; for activity impairment the "inflated" (logit) model predicting the "certain zeros" indicates that if a patient was to increase their VAS pain score by one point, the odds that the patient will belong in the "certain zero" group (have no activity impairment) would be a factor of exp(-0.261) = 0.770. In other words, the higher a patient's VAS score the less likely the patient is to be a certain zero (have no activity impairment). On the other hand, the "count" part indicates that one point increase in the VAS pain score would increase activity impairment by a factor exp(0.079) = 1.082. Thus, the higher a patient's VAS score, the more activity impairment is present.

Discussion

To our knowledge this is the first study investigating the impact of yet undiagnosed nr-axSpA and AS on work outcomes within a group of patients with long-standing CLBP. The employment rate among our patients with CLBP was, as anticipated, lower than expected compared to the Dutch population of the same age and gender, and the lower employment rate was more pronounced in the patients with AS, although this was not significantly different. In addition the patients with AS reported the highest values of absenteeism, presenteeism and work and activity impairment, although the differences between patients with CLBP and nr-axSpA were not significant, perhaps due to the small

Table 3 Final results of the ZINB regression model testing associations between demographical and clinical parameters and the WPAI subdomains corrected for age and gender

	Absenteeism		Presenteeism		Work impairment		Activity impairment	
Parameter	Count	Logistic	Count	Logistic	Count	Logistic	Count	Logistic
Education level								
Intermediate			0.100 (0.195)		-0.051 (0.578)	0.844 (0.004)		
High			-0.228 (0.015)		-0.252 (0.017)	0.716 (0.029)		
Duration of LBP (years)						0.043 (0.012)		
VAS pain		-0.190 (0.008)	0.081 (0.000)	-0.165 (<0.001)	0.079 (<0.001)	-0.324 (<0.001)	0.079 (<0.001)	-0.261 (<0.001)
RMDQ		-0.188 (<0.001)	0.048 (<0.001)	-0.005 (0.744)	0.058 (<0.001)	-0.152 (<0.001)	0.044 (<0.001)	-0.106 (<0.001)

Only the significant regression coefficients are shown, with the *p* values in parentheses. The logistic part of the ZINB model is generated for the "certain zero" cases, predicting whether or not a patient would be in this group. At the same time the count part of the model is predicting the counts for those patients who are not certain zeros.

ZINB zero inflated negative binomial, *WPAI* Worker Productivity and Activity Impairment Questionnaire, *LBP* low back pain, *VAS* = visual analog scale, *RDMQ* Roland Morris Disability Questionnaire number of patients with AS in the study population. Pain and functional limitations were associated with higher likelihood of having any work impairment. Pain by itself was associated with level of presenteeism, overall work impairment and activity impairment.

A comprehensive comparison with the existing literature is difficult as this is the first study addressing patients with previously unrecognized axSpA. Further, there is only limited literature on work outcomes in patients with nr-axSpA [24], and last but not least, data on employment and sick leave are country-specific, as the socioeconomic environment plays an important role [25]. Notwithstanding, a comparison that can be made involves a recent study in Dutch patients with early axSpA (defined based on the ESSG criteria), which evaluated problems in work participation. This study showed a remarkable high percentage of employed patients with axSpA, namely 81% [10]. This employment rate is even higher than the employment rate of the Dutch general population in 2014, which was 74.8% in the age category of 15–45 years [21]. An explanation of this high employment rate can be the high percentage of male participants in this study, which was 69% or the relatively low median BASDAI score (3.0) that was reported by the participants.

Focusing on the variables that are associated with work productivity in patients with axSpA, they are reported equally within different studies and settings. Several studies reported that variables measuring pain, disease activity and physical functioning are associated with reduced work productivity [10, 26–29]. This association is not only found in axSpA but also in other rheumatic conditions such as rheumatoid arthritis [30].

The strength of this study is our study population, which provided an unique opportunity to investigate work outcomes in as yet undiagnosed patients with nr-axSpA and with AS and to compare the findings with those in patients with long-standing CLBP. Moreover, none of the patients with nr-axSpA or AS had been diagnosed or treated by a rheumatologist for their disease, so there was no treatment bias in assessing the impact of the disease on work outcomes. A further strength of this study is the use of the ZINB models to assess associations with work productivity; this is a very elegant statistical technique using a logistic and a count model at the same time, creating an optimal fit for our data with excessive zeros [23].

A limitation of our study is the cross-sectional design, which limits any conclusions about causality. The risk of sampling bias was minimized by using only simple inclusion criteria (age 18–45 years and CLBP lasting more than 3 months). We did not include coping in our analyses, therefore is it unclear to which extent coping plays a role in the self-reported questionnaires such as the VAS for pain and the RMDQ. Not all participants answered the questions on work outcomes; however, the response rate for those questionnaires was 92% and there were no difference in patients' characteristics between the responders and non-responders. Another potential limitation is that it is unclear why the patients with nr-axSpA or AS have not been recognized by their primary care physicians and referred to a rheumatologist; is this because their primary care physician had limited knowledge about axSpA and did not recognize those patients or because the patients had so far experienced few symptoms from their disease? The second reason seems unlikely, as the median BASDAI score was 3.9 and 5.2 in patients with nr-axSpA and AS, respectively. Also, selection bias towards more patients with more severe CLBP seems unlikely, as the median VAS score in our study is comparable to or even lower than VAS scores in other cohorts with low back pain [31]. Finally, the group of patients with AS only contained 24 patients, of whom only 15 were employed, making it hard to find significant differences between the AS, nr-axSpA and CLBP groups.

On this line it should be noted that there was a high percentage women in our AS sample (75%); no other AS cohorts are reported to have such a high percentage. A possible explanation can be that we used a different approach to including patients in our study; we only selected based on age and the presence of CLBP. In other cohorts patients have been selected by predefined features specific to axSpA, leading to the possibility that male participants are easier to include. On the other hand, this finding could be an indication that at this moment more female patients with AS are being missed by primary care physicians, indicating an opportunity to educate primary care physicians more thoroughly about axSpA.

It is important to conduct research on work productivity, absenteeism and presenteeism in as yet undiagnosed patients with axSpA, as they can be indicators of future work disability [32]. Our results show that there are significant associations between patient-reported outcome measurement (PROMs) such as pain and functional limitations and work productivity, but no associations between more objective variables such as age, gender, disease (CLBP, nr-axSpA or AS), manual occupation and work productivity; this leads to the cautious conclusion that the impact on work productivity is not disease-related but related to the degree of pain and physical limitations a patients experiences. This finding is encouraging as we know from previous studies that adequately treating patients with AS or nr-axSpA leads to an improvement in PROMs [33]. Moreover, after starting treatment, not only is an improvement in work participation reported, but also an improvement in unpaid work is reported in patients with AS and with nr-axSpA [11, 34]. A recent study in southern Sweden in patients with nr-axSpA showed a sustained improvement in work disability even two years after the start of treatment [35]. These findings emphasize that is important and useful to recognize patients suspected of having axSpA early and refer them to a rheumatologist.

Conclusions

Our findings demonstrate that the impact of as yet undiagnosed nr-axSpA and AS is substantial although the outcomes in work productivity were not significantly different from those in patients with long-standing CLBP. Variables associated with reduced work productivity were mainly PROMs such as VAS pain score and functional limitations measured by the RMDQ. Early recognition and subsequently adequate treatment of yet undiagnosed patients with nr-axSpA and with AS can potentially lead to maintaining optimal work productivity in patients with nr-axSpA and with AS and a reduction in indirect costs.

Abbreviations

AS: Ankylosing spondylitis; ASAS: Assessment of SpondyloArthritis International Society; ASDAS: Ankylosing Spondylitis Disease Activity Score; axSpA: Axial spondyloarthritis; BASDAI: Bath Ankylosing Spondylitis Disease Activity Index; CaFaSpA: Case Finding Axial Spondyloarthrits; CBS: Centraal Bureau Statistiek; CI: Confidence interval; CLBP: Chronic low back pain; CRP: C-reactive protein; ESR: Erythrocyte sedimentation rate; GP: General Practitioner; HLA-B27: Human leukocyte antigen B27; ICPC: International Classification of Primary Care; ISCO: International Standard Classification of Occupation; MRI: Magnetic resonance imaging; Nr-axSpA: Non-radiographic axial spondyloarthritis; RMDQ: Rolland Morris Disability Questionnaire; SD: Standard deviation; VAS: Visual analogue scale; WPAI: Work Productivity and Activity Impairment; ZINB: Zero inflated negative binomial

Acknowledgements

We gratefully thank all GPs and participants of this study. We thank our research nurse Esther Hofland, the participating radiologists, Helen Wieringa and Ferry Nobrega, the Diagnostic Centre Rotterdam, Schiedam and Voorschoten, Casper Webers for his statistical input and the staff of the research centre TDIOR BV.

Funding

This work was supported by an unrestricted grant from Abbvie (grant number: IMM-10-0147). The company had no influence on study design, collection of data, analysis or interpretation of data.

Authors' contributions

Conception or design of the work: LH, JH, AW. Data collection: LH, AW. Data analysis and interpretation: LH, AB, AW. Drafting the article: LH, AB, AW. Critical revision of the article: LH, AB, JH, AW. Final approval of the version to be published: LH, AB, JH, AW.

Competing interests

The authors declare that they have no competing interests.

Author details

[1]Department of Rheumatology, Erasmus MC, Wytemaweg 80, 3015 CN Rotterdam, The Netherlands. [2]Department of Rheumatology, Maasstad Hospital, Maasstadweg 21, 3079 DZ Rotterdam, The Netherlands. [3]Department of Rheumatology, Maastricht University Medical Centre, P. Debyelaan 25, 6229 HX Maastricht, The Netherlands.

References

1. Hoy D, Bain C, Williams G, March L, Brooks P, Blyth F, Woolf A, Vos T, Buchbinder R. A systematic review of the global prevalence of low back pain. Arthritis Rheum. 2012;64(6):2028–37.
2. Freburger JK, Holmes GM, Agans RP, Jackman AM, Darter JD, Wallace AS, Castel LD, Kalsbeek WD, Carey TS. The rising prevalence of chronic low back pain. Arch Intern Med. 2009;169(3):251–8.
3. van Hoeven L, Luime J, Han H, Vergouwe Y, Weel A. Identifying axial spondyloarthritis in Dutch primary care patients, ages 20-45 years, with chronic low back pain. Arthritis Care Res (Hoboken). 2014;66(3):446–53.
4. Rudwaleit M, van der Heijde D, Landewe R, Listing J, Akkoc N, Brandt J, Braun J, Chou CT, Collantes-Estevez E, Dougados M, et al. The development of Assessment of SpondyloArthritis International Society classification criteria for axial spondyloarthritis (part II): validation and final selection. Ann Rheum Dis. 2009;68(6):777–83.
5. Poddubnyy D, Brandt H, Vahldiek J, Spiller I, Song IH, Rudwaleit M, Sieper J. The frequency of non-radiographic axial spondyloarthritis in relation to symptom duration in patients referred because of chronic back pain: results from the Berlin early spondyloarthritis clinic. Ann Rheum Dis. 2012;71(12): 1998–2001.
6. Kiltz U, Baraliakos X, Karakostas P, Igelmann M, Kalthoff L, Klink C, Krause D, Schmitz-Bortz E, Florecke M, Bollow M, et al. Do patients with non-radiographic axial spondylarthritis differ from patients with ankylosing spondylitis? Arthritis Care Res (Hoboken). 2012;64(9):1415–22.
7. Kiltz U, van der Heijde D. Health-related quality of life in patients with rheumatoid arthritis and in patients with ankylosing spondylitis. Clin Exp Rheumatol. 2009;27(4 Suppl 55):S108–111.
8. Ramonda R, Marchesoni A, Carletto A, Bianchi G, Cutolo M, Ferraccioli G, Fusaro E, De Vita S, Galeazzi M, Gerli R, et al. Patient-reported impact of spondyloarthritis on work disability and working life: the ATLANTIS survey. Arthritis Res Ther. 2016;18:78.
9. Boonen A, van der Linden SM. The burden of ankylosing spondylitis. J Rheumatol Suppl. 2006;78:4–11.
10. van der Weijden MA, Boonen A, van der Horst-Bruinsma IE. Problems in work participation and resource use should not be underestimated in patients with early spondyloarthritis. J Rheumatol. 2014;41(12):2413–20.
11. van der Heijde D, Joshi A, Pangan AL, Chen N, Betts K, Mittal M, Bao Y. ASAS40 and ASDAS clinical responses in the ABILITY-1 clinical trial translate to meaningful improvements in physical function, health-related quality of life and work productivity in patients with non-radiographic axial spondyloarthritis. Rheumatology (Oxford). 2015;55(1):80–8.
12. Hoy D, March L, Brooks P, Blyth F, Woolf A, Bain C, Williams G, Smith E, Vos T, Barendregt J, et al. The global burden of low back pain: estimates from the Global Burden of Disease 2010 study. Ann Rheum Dis. 2014;73(6):968–74.
13. Froud R, Patterson S, Eldridge S, Seale C, Pincus T, Rajendran D, Fossum C, Underwood M. A systematic review and meta-synthesis of the impact of low back pain on people's lives. BMC Musculoskelet Disord. 2014;15:50.
14. van Hoeven L, Vergouwe Y, de Buck PD, Luime JJ, Hazes JM, Weel AE. External validation of a referral rule for axial spondyloarthritis in primary care patients with chronic low back pain. PLoS One. 2015;10(7):e0131963.
15. Sieper J, Rudwaleit M, Baraliakos X, Brandt J, Braun J, Burgos-Vargas R, Dougados M, Hermann KG, Landewe R, Maksymowych W, et al. The Assessment of SpondyloArthritis International Society (ASAS) handbook: a guide to assess spondyloarthritis. Ann Rheum Dis. 2009;68 Suppl 2:ii1–44.
16. Goie The HS, Steven MM, van der Linden SM, Cats A. Evaluation of diagnostic criteria for ankylosing spondylitis: a comparison of the Rome, New York and modified New York criteria in patients with a positive clinical history screening test for ankylosing spondylitis. Br J Rheumatol. 1985;24(3):242–9.

17. Zochling J. Measures of symptoms and disease status in ankylosing spondylitis: Ankylosing Spondylitis Disease Activity Score (ASDAS), Ankylosing Spondylitis Quality of Life Scale (ASQoL), Bath Ankylosing Spondylitis Disease Activity Index (BASDAI), Bath Ankylosing Spondylitis Functional Index (BASFI), Bath Ankylosing Spondylitis Global Score (BAS-G), Bath Ankylosing Spondylitis Metrology Index (BASMI), Dougados Functional Index (DFI), and Health Assessment Questionnaire for the Spondylarthropathies (HAQ-S). Arthritis Care Res (Hoboken). 2011;63 Suppl 11:S47–58.
18. Roland M, Morris R. A study of the natural history of back pain. Part I: development of a reliable and sensitive measure of disability in low-back pain. Spine (Phila Pa 1976). 1983;8(2):141–4.
19. ISCO-08: http://www.ilo.org/public/english/bureau/stat/isco/isco08/.
20. Reilly MC, Gooch KL, Wong RL, Kupper H, van der Heijde D. Validity, reliability and responsiveness of the Work Productivity and Activity Impairment Questionnaire in ankylosing spondylitis. Rheumatology (Oxford). 2010;49(4):812–9.
21. CBS: http://statline.cbs.nl/Statweb/. 2014.
22. Yau KKW, Wang K, Lee AH. Zero-inflated negative binomial mixed regression modeling of over-dispersed count data with extra zeros. Biom J. 2003;45(4):437–52.
23. Greene WH. Accounting for excess zeros and sample selection in Poisson and negative binomial regression models. 1994.
24. Boonen A, Sieper J, van der Heijde D, Dougados M, Bukowski JF, Valluri S, Vlahos B, Kotak S. The burden of non-radiographic axial spondyloarthritis. Semin Arthritis Rheum. 2015;44(5):556-62.
25. Wynne-Jones G, Cowen J, Jordan JL, Uthman O, Main CJ, Glozier N, van der Windt D. Absence from work and return to work in people with back pain: a systematic review and meta-analysis. Occup Environ Med. 2014;71(6):448–56.
26. Haglund E, Bremander A, Bergman S, Jacobsson LT, Petersson IF. Work productivity in a population-based cohort of patients with spondyloarthritis. Rheumatology (Oxford). 2013;52(9):1708–14.
27. Boonen A, Brinkhuizen T, Landewe R, van der Heijde D, Severens JL. Impact of ankylosing spondylitis on sick leave, presenteeism and unpaid productivity, and estimation of the societal cost. Ann Rheum Dis. 2010;69(6): 1123–8.
28. Boonen A, Chorus A, Miedema H, van der Heijde D, van der Tempel H, van der Linden S. Employment, work disability, and work days lost in patients with ankylosing spondylitis: a cross sectional study of Dutch patients. Ann Rheum Dis. 2001;60(4):353–8.
29. de Hooge M, Ramonda R, Lorenzin M, Frallonardo P, Punzi L, Ortolan A, Doria A. Work productivity is associated with disease activity and functional ability in Italian patients with early axial spondyloarthritis: an observational study from the SPACE cohort. Arthritis Res Ther. 2016;18(1):265.
30. Geuskens GA, Hazes JM, Barendregt PJ, Burdorf A. Predictors of sick leave and reduced productivity at work among persons with early inflammatory joint conditions. Scand J Work Environ Health. 2008;34(6):420–9.
31. Gordon A, Callaghan D, Spink D, Cloutier C, Dzongowski P, O'Mahony W, Sinclair D, Rashiq S, Buckley N, Cohen G, et al. Buprenorphine transdermal system in adults with chronic low back pain: a randomized, double-blind, placebo-controlled crossover study, followed by an open-label extension phase. Clin Ther. 2010;32(5):844–60.
32. Mau W, Listing J, Huscher D, Zeidler H, Zink A. Employment across chronic inflammatory rheumatic diseases and comparison with the general population. J Rheumatol. 2005;32(4):721–8.
33. Callhoff J, Sieper J, Weiss A, Zink A, Listing J. Efficacy of TNFalpha blockers in patients with ankylosing spondylitis and non-radiographic axial spondyloarthritis: a meta-analysis. Ann Rheum Dis. 2015;74(6):1241–8.
34. Barkham N, Coates LC, Keen H, Hensor E, Fraser A, Redmond A, Cawkwell L, Emery P. Double-blind placebo-controlled trial of etanercept in the prevention of work disability in ankylosing spondylitis. Ann Rheum Dis. 2010;69(11):1926–8.
35. Wallman JK, Joud A, Olofsson T, Jacobsson LT, Bliddal H, Kristensen LE. Work disability in non-radiographic axial spondyloarthritis patients before and after start of anti-TNF therapy: a population-based regional cohort study from southern Sweden. Rheumatology (Oxford). 2017.

23

The performance of different classification criteria sets for spondyloarthritis in the worldwide ASAS-COMOSPA study

Pauline Bakker[1*], Anna Moltó[2,3], Adrien Etcheto[3], Filip Van den Bosch[1,4], Robert Landewé[5,6], Floris van Gaalen[1], Maxime Dougados[2,3] and Désirée van der Heijde[1]

Abstract

Background: In this study, we sought to compare the performance of spondyloarthritis (SpA) classification criteria sets in an international SpA cohort with patients included from five continents around the world.

Methods: Data from the (ASAS) COMOrbidities in SPondyloArthritis (ASAS-COMOSPA) study were used. ASAS-COMOSPA is a multinational, cross-sectional study with consecutive patients diagnosed with SpA by rheumatologists worldwide. Patients were classified according to the European Spondyloarthropathy Study Group (ESSG), modified European Spondyloarthropathy Study Group (mESSG), Amor, modified Amor, Assessment of SpondyloArthritis international Society (ASAS) axial Spondyloarthritis (axSpA), ASAS peripheral spondyloarthritis (pSpA) and ClASsification criteria for Psoriatic Arthritis (CASPAR) criteria. Overlap between the classification criteria sets was assessed for patients with and without back pain. Furthermore, patients fulfilling different arms of the ASAS axSpA criteria (imaging arm, clinical arm, both arms) were compared on the presence of SpA features.

Results: A total of 3942 patients (5 continents, 26 countries) were included. The mean age was 43.6 years, 65.0% were male, 56.2% were human leucocyte antigen B27-positive and 64.4% had radiographic sacroiliitis (based on modified New York criteria). Of the patients, 85.5% were classified by the ASAS SpA criteria (87.7% ASAS axSpA, 12.3% ASAS pSpA). Fulfilment of the Amor, ESSG and CASPAR criteria was present in 83.3%, 88.4% and 21.6% of patients, respectively. Of the patients with back pain ($n = 3227$), most were classified by all three of Amor, ESSG and ASAS axSpA criteria (71.4%). Patients fulfilling the imaging arm and the clinical arm of the ASAS axSpA criteria had similar presentations of SpA features. In patients without back pain, overlap between classification criteria sets was seen, although to a lesser extent.

Conclusions: Most patients with a clinical diagnosis of axial SpA in the worldwide ASAS-COMOSPA study fulfil several classification criteria sets, and a substantial overlap between different criteria sets is seen, which suggests a high level of credibility of the criteria. Large inter-regional differences in the fulfilment of classification criteria were not found. Patients fulfilling the clinical arm were remarkably similar to patients fulfilling the imaging arm with respect to the presence of most SpA features.

Keywords: Spondyloarthritis, Classification criteria, Worldwide interregional differences

* Correspondence: p.a.c.bakker@lumc.nl
[1]Department of Rheumatology, Leiden University Medical Centre, P.O. Box 96002300 RC Leiden, The Netherlands
Full list of author information is available at the end of the article

Background

Spondyloarthritis (SpA) encompasses a group of interrelated rheumatic conditions: ankylosing spondylitis (AS), including earlier forms of the disease that do not yet exhibit definitive structural damage on radiographs; psoriatic arthritis (PsA); arthritis associated with inflammatory bowel disease (IBD); and reactive arthritis [1]. Because SpA may have a heterogeneous presentation, a correct diagnosis is challenging. Rheumatologists make a diagnosis on the basis of what they have been taught during rheumatology training. The 'art of diagnosing' starts with a list of potential differential diagnoses, from among which the trained clinician deducts the most appropriate disease based upon the recognition of the 'Gestalt' and exclusion of other diagnoses.

Classification serves a completely different purpose, and several classification criteria sets of SpA are available. These classification criteria should be applied only in patients who have been diagnosed with SpA by a rheumatologist, and they cannot be used as a check box to be ticked in order to make the diagnosis. But the components of classification criteria may remind the clinician of the clinical picture of the disease. Different criteria sets put an emphasis on different features, and we do not know to what extent different criteria sets have penetrated different parts of the world. Therefore, we do not know which sets have influenced clinicians in particular regions most or to what extent these various sets of criteria describe more or less similar patients. Consequently, we do not know if rheumatologists around the world diagnose patients with a similar clinical picture of the disease.

The European Spondyloarthropathy Study Group (ESSG) criteria and the Amor criteria were developed to classify patients with SpA as a whole [2, 3]. In clinical practice, rheumatologists tend to distinguish patients with SpA according to their primary clinical presentation as patients with predominantly axial or predominantly peripheral complaints (with some overlap between these subtypes). The Assessment of SpondyloArthritis international Society (ASAS) has developed new criteria to better accommodate this distinction [4, 5]. These criteria sets can classify patients with predominantly axial symptoms as having axial spondyloarthritis (axSpA) and patients with predominantly peripheral symptoms as having peripheral spondyloarthritis (pSpA). The ASAS axSpA criteria consist of two arms: the imaging arm classifies patients who have sacroiliitis visualised on conventional radiographs and/or bone marrow oedema on magnetic resonance imaging (MRI), and the clinical arm classifies patients with normal imaging results. In 2006, a specific classification criteria set for PsA was developed, known as the ClASsification criteria for Psoriatic ARthritis (CASPAR) [6].

Classification criteria are used to include patients in clinical trials, cohort studies and other types of research. These criteria are frequently validated in restricted patient populations. We took the opportunity to investigate if rheumatologists worldwide diagnosed similar types of patients as having SpA by testing if patients fulfil similar criteria sets in the Assessment of SpondyloArthritis international Society COMOrbidities in SPondyloArthritis (ASAS-COMOSPA) study. Our assumption was that the more criteria sets a patient fulfils, the higher the likelihood that a patient with a diagnosis of SpA truly has SpA. The ASAS-COMOSPA study provides a unique opportunity to investigate this research question because it is, to our knowledge, the first observational study with such a large, worldwide population of patients with SpA, with axial and/or peripheral symptoms included [7].

Methods

Study population

The ASAS-COMOSPA study is an observational, cross-sectional, multicentre study which has been introduced elsewhere [7]. Participating rheumatologists were asked to include consecutive patients with a diagnosis of SpA from routine care. These patients had to fulfil the ASAS axSpA or pSpA criteria, but fulfilment of the ASAS criteria was not checked before inclusion. All information required to judge the fulfilment of various criteria sets, including the ASAS criteria, was collected in a random order (not grouped by criteria set) in the case report form.

Patients from 26 participating countries in 6 regions across the world (Western Europe, Central Europe, North America, Latin America, North Africa and Asia) were included. Western Europe was represented by Belgium, France, Germany, Hungary, Italy, the Netherlands, Portugal, Spain and the United Kingdom. Poland, Russia, Turkey and Ukraine were grouped into Central Europe. North America encompasses Canada and the United States, and Argentina, Brazil, Colombia and Mexico were summarized as Latin America. North Africa comprised Egypt and Morocco. China, Japan, Korea, Singapore and Taiwan were grouped and referred to as Asia. Approval by the local medical ethics committees, as well as written informed consent from all patients, was obtained before inclusion.

Classification criteria

Patients were classified according to the following criteria sets: ESSG, Amor, ASAS SpA, ASAS axSpA, ASAS pSpA, imaging arm of ASAS axSpA, clinical arm of ASAS axSpA and CASPAR criteria [8]. The presence of either inflammatory back pain (IBP) or peripheral arthritis is a mandatory entry criterion of the ESSG criteria. According to the ESSG criteria, patients with at least one of the entry criteria in combination with one other minor criterion, such as enthesitis or psoriasis, are classified as having SpA [2]. Human leukocyte antigen B27 (HLA-B27) is *not* incorporated in this criteria set. The Amor criteria include a list of features with different weights, none of which is essential to classify a patient as having SpA, but a classification of SpA depends on the sum of weights [3]. Because patients in the COMOSPA study were not asked about the presence of balanitis, night pain and buttock pain, these items have not been taken into account, and therefore patients cannot collect points on these items in the Amor and ESSG criteria. The ESSG and Amor criteria were developed before MRI became widely available. In the present analysis, we also investigated the possibility of including inflammatory findings on MRI (ASAS definition [9]) as a feature in both the ESSG and Amor criteria, resulting in the modified Amor (mAmor) and modified European Spondyloarthropathy Study Group (mESSG) criteria.

The ASAS axSpA criteria consist of two arms, the imaging arm and the clinical arm, and can be applied only to patients with back pain of ≥3 months' duration and an age of onset <45 years [10]. In patients with sacroiliitis visualised on pelvic radiographs or MRI, at least one other SpA feature should be present in order to be classified as axSpA according to the imaging arm [4]. In HLA-B27-positive patients, at least two other additional SpA features should be present in order to be classified as axSpA according to the clinical arm [4]. In patients without current back pain but with current peripheral manifestations, the classification for peripheral SpA can be applied. If a patient satisfies the entry criterion (current arthritis, enthesitis or dactylitis), the patient should have at least one other SpA feature if this is a specific SpA feature or at least two SpA features for less specific features [5]. Altogether, when current back pain (as defined above) is the presenting symptom, the ASAS axial SpA criteria should be applied. If arthritis/enthesitis/dactylitis is the presenting symptom, the peripheral SpA criteria should be applied. Together, these two sets form the ASAS SpA criteria.

A separate classification criteria set has been developed for PsA: the CASPAR criteria [6]. To meet the CASPAR criteria, the stem of the criteria demands first the presence of inflammatory articular disease and a score of at least 3 points derived from the presence of features such as skin psoriasis, dactylitis, nail lesions or juxta-articular bone formation visualised on radiographs (each feature is assigned a certain number of points). All above-described criteria sets are depicted in Additional file 1.

Data analysis

Disease characteristics were described using descriptive statistics. The fulfilment of classification criteria was calculated for the cohort as a whole and thereafter per region. Subsequently, overlap between the different classification criteria was investigated and presented in Venn diagrams. This was done for patients with back pain and patients without back pain separately. Next, we looked in detail at the fulfilment of the ASAS axSpA criteria, comparing patients fulfilling only the clinical arm, patients fulfilling only the imaging arm and patients fulfilling both the clinical and imaging arms with regard to demographics and the presence of SpA features. Information on HLA-B27 must be available to be able to classify patients in the 'imaging arm-only' group, and information on imaging must be available to be able to classify patients in the 'clinical arm-only' group. IBM SPSS Statistics version 20.0 software (IBM, Armonk, NY, USA) was used for statistical analysis.

Results

In total, 3984 patients were included in the COMOSPA study, with a mean number of SpA features of 5.5 (SD 1.8). The most common missing items were MRI of the sacroiliac joints (missing in 1951 patients), the presence of juxta-articular bone formation (missing in 999 patients) and HLA-B27 status (missing in 882 patients). There were 251 patients (6.4%) for whom both sacroiliac joint MRI and radiographs were not performed and 180 patients (4.6%) for whom HLA-B27 in addition was missing.

On the other hand, information on extra-articular manifestations was missing in none of the cases. Arbitrarily, a maximum of 6 missing items (total number of items 18) per patient was accepted. Patients with 7 or more missing items ($n = 42$) were left out of the analysis, which brings the total number of patients for this analysis to 3942. To define SpA features as present or absent, in order to apply the classification criteria, missing items were regarded as absent.

Demographics and disease characteristics are depicted in Table 1. Patients had a mean age of 44 years, and 65% were male. In the total cohort (patients with available data), HLA-B27 positivity was seen in 56% (73.0%) of the patients, and 54% (57.7%) had an elevated C-reactive protein level. Regarding the presence of sacroiliitis visualised on imaging, 64% (70.0%) presented with sacroiliitis seen on radiographs and 34% (94.8%) with sacroiliitis seen on MRI.

Fulfilment of classification criteria

Most (92.6%) of the 3942 patients fulfilled the mESSG criteria. Fulfilment of Amor, mAmor, ESSG and ASAS criteria was all above 80% (Table 2). A minority (12.3%) of the patients fulfilled the ASAS pSpA criteria, whereas 21.6% of the patients fulfilled the CASPAR criteria. We emphasise that the criteria were

Table 1 Baseline characteristics

	Total patients (*n* = 3942)	Based on available data	Number of patients with missing items
Age at inclusion, years, mean ± SD	43.6 (13.9)		0
Male sex, *n* (%)	2563 (65.0%)		0
HLA-B27-positive, *n* (%)	2217 (56.2%)	72.0%	882
IBP, *n* (%)	3219 (81.7%)		52
Morning stiffness, *n* (%)	2497 (63.3%)		22
Enthesitis, *n* (%)	1354 (34.3%)		0
Dactylitis, *n* (%)	610 (15.5%)		3
Psoriasis, *n* (%)	843 (21.4%)		0
Uveitis, *n* (%)	771 (19.6%)		0
Peripheral arthritis, *n* (%)	2424 (61.5%)		0
IBD, *n* (%)	209 (5.3%)		0
Positive family history, *n* (%)	1475 (37.4%)		117
Good response to NSAIDs, *n* (%)	2433 (61.7%)	77.5%	803
Elevated CRP, *n* (%)	2109 (53.5%)	57.7%	287
Preceding infection, *n* (%)	271 (6.9%)		74
Sacroiliitis based on radiograph (mNY), *n* (%)	2539 (64.4%)	70.0%	341
Sacroiliitis based on MRI, *n* (%)	1326 (33.6%)	65.7%	1951
Rheumatoid factor-negative, *n* (%)	3177 (80.6%)	94.8%	613
Psoriatic nail dystrophy, *n* (%)	460 (11.7%)		28
Juxta-articular bone formation, *n* (%)	526 (13.3%)	17.7%	999

Abbreviations: IBP Inflammatory back pain according to Assessment of SpondyloArthritis international Society definition (reference), *IBD* Inflammatory bowel disease, *CRP* C-reactive protein, *ESR* Erythrocyte sedimentation rate, *HLA-B27* Human leucocyte antigen, *mNY* Modified New York criteria, *NSAID* Non-steroidal anti-inflammatory drug, *MRI* Magnetic resonance imaging

applied to all patients; only the patients with seven or more missing values were left out, and missing items were regarded as absent.

Most patients ($n = 1507$) were included in Western Europe (85 centres from 26 countries), followed by 1073 patients in Asia, 438 patients in Central Europe, 337 patients in Latin America, 337 patients in North Africa and 239 patients in North America. Regional differences in fulfilment of classification criteria are depicted in Table 3. When we looked in detail at the ASAS SpA criteria, we found that in Central Europe, 84% of the patients fulfilled the ASAS axial SpA criteria (ASAS peripheral criteria 5.3%), whereas in contrast, in North America, 51% of the patients fulfilled the axial SpA criteria (ASAS peripheral criteria 22.6%). In both Asia and Central Europe, a small minority of the patients fulfilled the ASAS pSpA criteria, and the axial complaints were by far the predominant symptoms. A relatively high percentage of patients fulfilled the CASPAR criteria in North America compared with the other regions. Less pronounced regional differences were seen regarding criteria sets that cover the whole spectrum of SpA, namely the Amor and ESSG criteria.

Overlap in classification criteria

Venn diagrams representing the overlap between the different criteria sets are shown in Figs. 1 and 2. Figure 1 reveals that the majority of the patients with back pain were classified by all three criteria sets: Amor, ESSG and ASAS axSpA criteria ($n = 2392$ [74.1%]). Most patients who fulfilled two criteria sets fulfilled both the ASAS axSpA criteria and the ESSG criteria ($n = 268$ [8.3%]). Few patients fulfilled only one criteria set. Most of the patients who were picked up by one criteria set only were classified by the ASAS axSpA criteria ($n = 179$ [5.5%] compared with 1.3% by the ESSG criteria only and 0.2% by the Amor criteria only). The major overlap of the criteria points to the typical clinical pattern of SpA the included patients have.

Regarding the patients without current back pain (peripheral complaints), again substantial overlap between the criteria was seen (ASAS pSpA, Amor, ESSG, CASPAR) (Fig. 2). Most of the patients fulfilled all four criteria sets ($n = 224$ [31.3%]). Subsequently, 125 patients (17.5%) fulfilled all criteria, except those for PsA-specific CASPAR criteria, which is not surprising, because the CASPAR criteria are focussed on the clinical disease PsA and not on other forms of pSpA. Only six patients (0.8%) fulfilled only

Table 2 Fulfilment of classification criteria

Classification criteria	Patients who fulfilled the classification criteria, *n* (%)
Amor	3282 (83.3%)
mAmor	3454 (87.6%)
ESSG	3485 (88.4%)
mESSG	3652 (92.6%)
ASAS SpA total	3370 (85.5%)
ASAS axial SpA, current back pain	2955 (87.7%)
Both arms (imaging & clinical)	1737 (58.8%)
mNY+	976 (56.2%)
MRI+	169 (9.7%)
Both	592 (34.1%)
Imaging arm only	984 (33.3%)
mNY+	539 (54.8%)
MRI+	245 (24.9%)
Both	200 (20.3%)
Clinical arm only	234 (7.9%)
ASAS peripheral SpA	415 (12.3%)
CASPAR	852 (21.6%)

Abbreviations: mAmor Modified Amor, *ESSG* European Spondylarthropathy Study Group, *mESSG* Modified European Spondyloarthropathy Study Group, *ASAS* Assessment of SpondyloArthritis international Society, *mNY* Modified New York, *MRI* Magnetic resonance imaging, *CASPAR* ClASsification criteria for Psoriatic ARthritis

the CASPAR criteria, and only four patients (0.6%) fulfilled only the ASAS pSpA criteria. Regarding overlap between the different criteria sets in the different regions, the same trends were seen, and no substantial inter-regional differences were found (data not shown).

Comparison between patients fulfilling the ASAS imaging arm split by presence of HLA-B27 and the clinical arm only

Disease characteristics of patients fulfilling the imaging arm or the clinical arm only are depicted in Table 4. In addition, characteristics of patients fulfilling the imaging arm are presented on the basis of the presence or absence of HLA-B27. Only patients who have data available on HLA-B27 and imaging are included in Table 4. There were more male patients in the HLA-B27-positive imaging arm (74.1%) than in the HLA-B27-negative imaging arm (50.4%) and the clinical arm (53.1%). Psoriasis was seen more frequently in the group of HLA-B27-negative patients fulfilling the imaging arm. On the contrary, enthesitis and dactylitis were relatively more common in the patients who fulfilled only the clinical arm. A positive family history was also more frequently seen in the clinical arm than in the imaging arm (independent of HLA-B27 status).

Discussion

Appropriate diagnostic criteria for axSpA and pSpA do not exist and, in the absence of an unequivocal gold standard, will never be developed, but various classification criteria are available. These classification criteria have in common that they have been developed using the external standard 'expert opinion'. But expert opinion is not an equivocal and homogeneous construct and may potentially integrate different pictures of the disease SpA.

The present study reveals that, in our cohort, most patients diagnosed as having SpA fulfilled multiple classification criteria sets, which adds to the credibility of the construct of SpA as a recognizable entity. Although the substantial overlap between the different criteria sets for patients with both axial and with peripheral symptoms could be expected, the fact that different criteria sets have been developed for different target populations (e.g., the ESSG, focussed on the whole concept of SpA; the ASAS axial SpA criteria for patients with SpA axial symptoms) could have precluded overlap in different regions of the world. In the present study, we have shown that the significant overlap was consistent all over the world, thus suggesting that rheumatologists worldwide use similar 'pictures' of what SpA is. In other words,

Table 3 Regional differences in fulfilment of classification criteria

	Number of patients included	Patients fulfilling Amor criteria, *n* (%)	Patients fulfilling mAmor criteria, *n* (%)	Patients fulfilling ESSG criteria, *n* (%)	Patients fulfilling mESSG criteria, *n* (%)	Total patients fulfilling ASAS SpA criteria, *n* (%)	Patients fulfilling ASAS axSpA criteria, *n* (%)	Patients fulfilling, ASAS pSpA criteria, *n* (%)	Patients fulfilling CASPAR criteria, *n* (%)
Western Europe	1507	1242 (82.4%)	1333 (88.5%)	1335 (88.6%)	1433 (95.1%)	1305 (86.6%)	1149 (76.2%)	156 (10.4%)	388 (25.7%)
Central Europe	438	342 (78.1%)	364 (83.1%)	402 (91.8%)	419 (95.7%)	391 (89.3%)	368 (84.0%)	23 (5.3%)	32 (7.3%)
North America	239	203 (84.9%)	205 (85.8%)	219 (91.6%)	219 (91.6%)	176 (73.6%)	122 (51.0%)	54 (22.6%)	120 (50.2%)
Latin America	348	290 (83.3%)	307 (88.2%)	314 (90.2%)	326 (93.7%)	280 (80.5%)	239 (68.7%)	41 (11.8%)	93 (26.7%)
North Africa	337	300 (89.0%)	310 (92.0%)	316 (93.8%)	324 (96.1%)	308 (91.4%)	260 (77.2%)	48 (14.2%)	94 (27.9%)
Asia	1073	905 (84.3%)	935 (87.1%)	899 (83.8%)	931 (86.8%)	910 (84.8%)	817 (76.1%)	93 (8.7%)	125 (11.6%)

Abbreviations: ASAS Assessment of SpondyloArthritis international Society, *axSpA* Axial spondyloarthritis, *CASPAR* ClASsification criteria for Psoriatic Arthritis, *ESSG* European Spondyloarthropathy Study Group, *mAmor* Modified Amor, *mESSG* Modified European Spondyloarthropathy Study Group, *pSpA* Peripheral spondyloarthritis, *SpA* Spondyloarthritis

Percentages relate to number of patients of that specific region

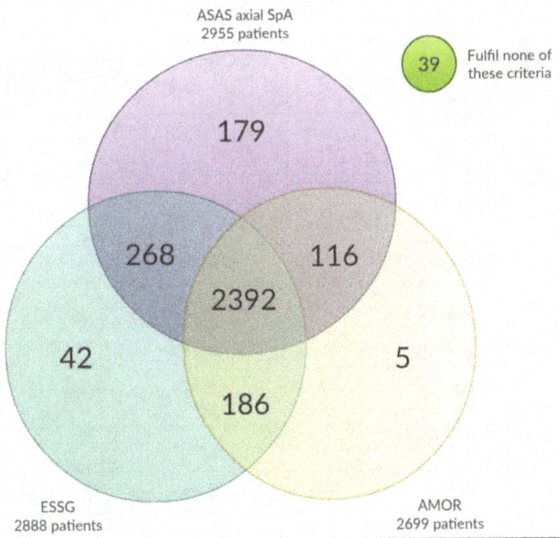

Fig. 1 Overlap between ESSG, AMOR, and axSpA criteria in patients with current back pain (*n* = 3227)

they operationalise the construct of SpA approximately similarly. In addition, the huge overlap (e.g., 74.1% of the patients fulfilled all three criteria sets, and only 7.6% fulfilled one set only) confirms that the criteria for SpA are highly credible.

As mentioned already, large interregional differences in the fulfilment of classification criteria were not found. This is remarkable in the light of all genetic and environmental differences, as well as differences in resources and health care systems around the world. In fact, it appears that the clinical picture—and consequently the diagnosis—of SpA is remarkably homogeneous around the world, despite all possible differences in, for example, genetic background, prevalence and medical training.

Of course, there were some notable differences. The most important one was that more patients with PsA and fewer patients with axial disease were included in North America than in other regions. We do not think this reflects a true difference in the prevalence of the different subtypes of the disease. This is supported by a recent systematic review that pooled population prevalence estimates for SpA, AS and PsA in geographic areas [11]. The prevalence of both the axial and peripheral subtypes was, on average, comparable in North America to other parts of the world. More likely, the difference could be due to local factors, such as a difference in areas of interest of the doctors including patients or referral centres for a certain disease. One reason may be the perception of PsA as belonging to SpA or not. It is well known that some rheumatologists view PsA as a separate entity and others view PsA as a subtype of SpA. Apparently, more doctors in North America than in other parts of the world consider patients with PsA as having SpA.

Regarding the inclusion criteria of the study, doctors were required to include patients with SpA only if they thought the patient would fulfil the ASAS SpA criteria (either peripheral or axial). However, fulfilment of the ASAS criteria was not formally checked before inclusion, as described in the Methods section above. When analysing the data, it became clear that only 85.5% of the patients actually did fulfil the ASAS SpA criteria, ranging from 73.6% in North America to 91.4% in North Africa. This implies that the large majority of patients with SpA are indeed covered by the criteria, pointing to high sensitivity but also indicating that doctors diagnose SpA in patients who do not fulfil the ASAS criteria. However, we would like to make a critical comment which relates to a limitation of the present study. The fact that rheumatologists were initially asked to include

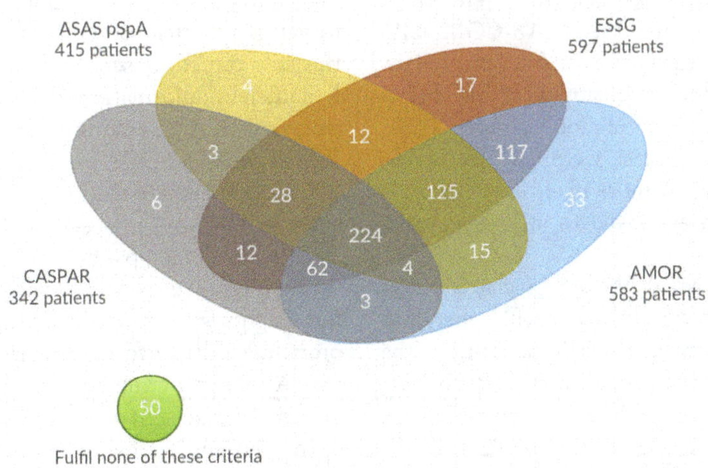

Fig. 2 Overlap between the ESSG, AMOR, CASPAR, and pSpA criteria in patients without current back pain (*n* = 715)

Table 4 Comparison between the imaging arm and clinical arm of the ASAS axSpA criteria, with the required presence of HLA-B27 and imaging

	Imaging arm (%), HLA-B27 always available		Clinical arm alone (%), imaging always available ($n = 98$)
	HLA-B27-positive ($n = 1746$)	HLA-B27-negative ($n = 546$)	
Age, years	40.3 (13.0)	42.7 (13.0)	42.8 (13.0)
Male sex	1294 (74.1%)	275 (50.4%)	52 (53.1)
IBP	1639 (93.3%)	529 (96.9%)	87 (88.8%)
Peripheral arthritis	904 (51.8%)	302 (55.3%)	57 (58.2%)
Psoriasis	147 (8.4%)	105 (19.2%)	14 (14.3%)
Uveitis	453 (25.9%)	49 (9.0%)	27 (27.6%)
Enthesitis	563 (32.2%)	164 (30.0%)	44 (44.9%)
Dactylitis	137 (7.8%)	55 (10.1%)	17 (17.3%)
IBD	73 (4.2%)	46 (8.4%)	6 (6.1%)
Positive family history	669 (38.3%)	166 (30.4%)	52 (53.1%)
Good response to NSAIDs	1180 (67.6%)	265 (48.5%)	64 (65.3%)
Elevated CRP	1094 (62.7%)	256 (46.9%)	41 (41.8%)

Abbreviations: HLA-B27 Human leucocyte antigen B27, *IBP* Inflammatory back pain, *IBD* Inflammatory bowel disease, *NSAID* Non-steroidal anti-inflammatory drug, *CRP* C-reactive protein

ASAS SpA patients (although fulfilment of the ASAS criteria was not met in all patients) could very well have led to an 'a priori' high percentage of ASAS classification criteria fulfilment. This could have led to an overestimation of performance of sensitivity of the criteria.

The ASAS classification criteria were developed in recent history. The criteria were validated in an international study of more than 600 patients with chronic back pain of unknown origin. In the ASAS study population, the ASAS criteria compared favourably with other previously established criteria sets with regard to sensitivity and specificity. In our study, if patients with axial symptoms were picked up by one criteria set only, of all sets tested, the ASAS axSpA criteria were most sensitive (although the others performed well, too). The latter could be due to the fact that the ASAS-COMOSPA study is not a cohort of early disease (as reflected by 65% modified New York criteria positivity). Prior studies have shown that performances of, for example, ESSG and Amor criteria in early disease were (slightly) worse than the ASAS criteria [12]. A more likely explanation is that the rheumatologists were asked to include patients fulfilling the ASAS criteria.

Although the imaging arm of the ASAS classification criteria is broadly recognized as highly specific, there has been debate on the validity of the clinical arm of the ASAS criteria, which has not been well received by different national and international health care systems. In the literature, it has been argued that patients fulfilling only the clinical arm of the ASAS axSpA criteria should not be considered as having 'true axSpA'. A reason why the clinical arm of the ASAS axSpA criteria has been developed is that MRI is not universally available. In our cohort, in which a large proportion of patients did not undergo MRI, our results demonstrate the value of the clinical arm of the ASAS criteria for scientific research. We found that patients fulfilling the clinical arm were remarkably similar to patients fulfilling the imaging arm with respect to the presence of many SpA features.

Strengths of the study are the multi-national cohort and the large number of patients included, which is unique, to our knowledge. Unfortunately, no control group was available, and therefore true specificity of the different classification criteria sets could not be calculated. Another limitation of the study is the relatively high number of missing values, especially when it comes to key items such as HLA-B27 and MRI. Unfortunately, this is a direct consequence of normal clinical practice: If sufficient information has been collected to make a diagnosis, further testing is often not performed (e.g., to save expenses).

We can conclude that, despite the heterogeneous character and varying prevalence of SpA as a disease across the world, similar patients are identified as having SpA by rheumatologists worldwide. Moreover, patients with the diagnosis of SpA usually fulfil multiple criteria sets, providing validity to the criteria, including the relatively new ASAS SpA criteria as well as to the concept of SpA. We emphasize that classification criteria for SpA were developed for use in epidemiological and clinical research and are not suitable for use as diagnostic tools in clinical practice.

Conclusions

Most patients diagnosed with SpA by rheumatologists in five continents across the world fulfilled multiple classification criteria sets. To our knowledge, this is the first study confirming the validity of the ASAS axSpA criteria in a large, worldwide population of patients. Patients fulfilling the clinical and/or imaging arms of the ASAS axSpA criteria have comparable SpA features.

For the first time, to our knowledge, the performance of the various SpA classification criteria sets is assessed in a worldwide setting with a very large number of patients included from five different continents. We also took the opportunity to phenotypically compare patients fulfilling the different arms of the ASAS axial SpA criteria in terms of demographics and presence of SpA features, among others.

Abbreviations

AS: Ankylosing spondylitis; ASAS: Assessment of SpondyloArthritis international Society; axSpA: Axial spondyloarthritis; CASPAR: ClASsification criteria for Psoriatic Arthritis; COMOSPA: COMOrbidities in SPondyloArthritis; ESSG: European Spondyloarthropathy Study Group; HLA-B27: Human leucocyte antigen B27; IBD: Inflammatory bowel disease; IBP: Inflammatory back pain; mAmor: Modified Amor; mESSG: Modified European Spondyloarthropathy Study Group; mNY: Modified New York criteria; MRI: Magnetic resonance imaging; NSAID: Non-steroidal anti-inflammatory drug; PsA: Psoriatic arthritis; pSpA: Peripheral spondyloarthritis; SpA: Spondyloarthritis

Acknowledgements

Not applicable.

Funding

The COMOSPA study was conducted under the umbrella of ASAS and was financially supported by unrestricted grants from AbbVie, Pfizer and UCB.

Authors' contributions

PB performed the statistical analyses and drafted the manuscript. DvdH supervised all procedures and gave methodological advice. All authors contributed to the acquisition and interpretation of the data, as well as the inclusion of patients. All authors read, revised, and approved the final manuscript.

Author's information

Not applicable.

Competing interests

The authors declare that they have no competing interests.

Author details

[1]Department of Rheumatology, Leiden University Medical Centre, P.O. Box 96002300 RC Leiden, The Netherlands. [2]Department of Rheumatology, Paris Descartes University, Hôpital Cochin, Paris, France. [3]Inserm (U1153), Clinical Epidemiology and Biostatistics, Paris, France. [4]Department of Rheumatology, Ghent University Hospital, Ghent, Belgium. [5]Department of Rheumatology, Amsterdam Medical Centre, Amsterdam, The Netherlands. [6]Atrium Medical Centre, Heerlen, The Netherlands.

References

1. Khan MA. Update on spondyloarthropathies. Ann Intern Med. 2002;136: 896–907.
2. Dougados M, van der Linden S, Juhlin R, Huitfeldt B, Amor B, Calin A, et al. The European Spondylarthropathy Study Group preliminary criteria for the classification of spondylarthropathy. Arthritis Rheum. 1991;34:1218–27.
3. Amor B, Dougados M, Mijiyawa M. Criteria of the classification of spondylarthropathies [in French]. Rev Rhum Mal Osteoartic. 1990;57:85–9.
4. Rudwaleit M, van der Heijde D, Landewé R, Listing J, Akkoc N, Brandt J, et al. The development of Assessment of SpondyloArthritis international Society classification criteria for axial spondyloarthritis (part II): validation and final selection. Ann Rheum Dis. 2009;68:777–83.
5. Rudwaleit M, van der Heijde D, Landewé R, Akkoc N, Brandt J, Chou CT, et al. The Assessment of SpondyloArthritis International Society classification criteria for peripheral spondyloarthritis and for spondyloarthritis in general. Ann Rheum Dis. 2011;70:25–31.
6. Taylor W, Gladman D, Helliwell P, Marchesoni A, Mease P, Mielants H, CASPAR Study Group. Classification criteria for psoriatic arthritis: development of new criteria from a large international study. Arthritis Rheum. 2006;54:2665–73.
7. Moltó A, Etcheto A, van der Heijde D, Landewé R, van den Bosch F, Bautista Molano W, et al. Prevalence of comorbidities and evaluation of their screening in spondyloarthritis: results of the international cross-sectional ASAS-COMOSPA study. Ann Rheum Dis. 2016;75:1016–23.
8. van der Linden S, Valkenburg HA, Cats A. Evaluation of diagnostic criteria for ankylosing spondylitis: a proposal for modification of the New York criteria. Arthritis Rheum. 1984;27:361–8.
9. Rudwaleit M, Jurik AG, Hermann KG, Landewé R, van der Heijde D, Baraliakos X, et al. Defining active sacroiliitis on magnetic resonance imaging (MRI) for classification of axial spondyloarthritis: a consensual approach by the ASAS/OMERACT MRI group. Ann Rheum Dis. 2009;68:1520–7.
10. Rudwaleit M, Khan MA, Sieper J. The challenge of diagnosis and classification in early ankylosing spondylitis: do we need new criteria? Arthritis Rheum. 2005;52:1000–8.
11. Stolwijk C, van Onna M, Boonen A, van Tubergen A. Global prevalence of spondyloarthritis: a systematic review and meta-regression analysis. Arthritis Care Res (Hoboken). 2016;68:1320–31.
12. van den Berg R, de Hooge M, van Gaalen F, Reijnierse M, Huizinga T, van der Heijde D. Percentage of patients with spondyloarthritis in patients referred because of chronic back pain and performance of classification criteria: experience from the Spondyloarthritis Caught Early (SPACE) cohort. Rheumatology (Oxford). 2013;52:1492–9. A published erratum appears in Rheumatology (Oxford). 2015;54:1336.

24

Mechanistic rationales for targeting interleukin-17A in spondyloarthritis

Siba P. Raychaudhuri[1,2*] and Smriti K. Raychaudhuri[1]

Abstract

The term spondyloarthritis (SpA) is used to describe a group of inflammatory autoimmune diseases, including ankylosing spondylitis and psoriatic arthritis, with common genetic risk factors and clinical features. SpA is clinically distinct from rheumatoid arthritis and typically affects the spine, sacroiliac joints, entheses, and, less commonly, peripheral joints. Although the pathogenesis of SpA is not fully understood, recent findings have identified the interleukin (IL)-17 pathway as a key mediator of disease pathogenesis. Clinical evidence for the efficacy of IL-17A inhibition by biologic agents was initially shown in patients with chronic plaque psoriasis, another autoimmune disease mediated by the IL-17 pathway. Subsequently, similar positive efficacy for inhibition of IL-17A was seen in patients with ankylosing spondylitis and psoriatic arthritis. Inhibition of IL-17A may also improve cardiovascular and metabolic comorbidities often found in patients with SpA because studies have linked these disorders to the IL-17 pathway. In this review, we will examine key preclinical studies that demonstrated the mechanistic role of IL-17A in the development SpA and discuss how these observations were translated into clinical practice.

Keywords: Spondyloarthritis, Review, Interleukin-17, IL-17A inhibition, Ankylosing spondylitis, Psoriatic arthritis, Preclinical studies, Clinical practice

Background

Spondyloarthritis (SpA) is a term used to describe a group of inflammatory autoimmune diseases that share common genetic risk factors and clinical features, including ankylosing spondylitis (AS), psoriatic arthritis (PsA), reactive arthritis, undifferentiated SpA, and enteropathic arthritis [1–6]. SpA typically affects the spine, sacroiliac joints, entheses, and peripheral joints. Hallmark features of SpA include enthesitis, focal inflammation, new bone formation and cartilage ossification that may lead to ankyloses [2, 4, 7–9]. Clinical phenotypes include inflammatory back pain, oligoarthritis, dactylitis, and extra-articular features such as uveitis, psoriasis, and inflammatory bowel disease (IBD) [5].

Worldwide estimates of the prevalence of SpA are variable. Available data suggest that SpA is relatively uncommon in Asian and Middle Eastern countries, affecting less than 0.9% of adult populations, while studies in European countries report SpA prevalence of between 0.3% and 1.9% [5]. According to data from the 2009–2010 US National Health and Nutrition Examination Survey (NHANES), it is estimated that SpA affects roughly 1% of the adult population in the US, which corresponds to between two million and three million people [6].

The exact pathogenesis of SpA is not well understood, but in recent years it has become clear that cytokines associated with innate and adaptive inflammatory immune responses play an important role in disease initiation and progression [2, 8, 9]. Cytokines produced by T-helper (Th)17 cells have been shown to contribute to pathogenic features of SpA, including joint erosion and inflammation, new bone formation, epidermal thickening, development of psoriatic skin lesions, pannus formation in joint capsules, synovial inflammation, and angiogenesis [7–12]. Specifically, preclinical studies using models of SpA have shown that expression of genes encoding proinflammatory cytokines including interleukin (IL)-17A, tumor necrosis factor (TNF)-α, and IL-23 is upregulated in affected joints [9, 13] and that IL-17 promotes

* Correspondence: sraychaudhuri@ucdavis.edu
[1]VA Medical Center Sacramento, Division of Rheumatology & Immunology, Sacramento, CA, USA
[2]Division of Rheumatology, Allergy & Clinical immunology, University of California School of Medicine, Davis, & VA Medical Center Sacramento, Sacramento, CA, USA

osteogenesis at inflamed sites (e.g., entheses) under conditions of mechanical stress, resulting in excess bone formation that is a key characteristic difference between SpA and rheumatoid arthritis (RA), which is characterized predominantly by bone erosion and resorption [14]. As such, the IL-17 pathway has been identified as a potential disease-modifying target for the treatment of SpA [9, 12, 15]. This article provides a review of the pathogenesis of SpA and the mechanistic rationales for targeting the IL-17A pathway based on its role in inflammation, cartilage damage, and bone changes.

Methods

Literature searches were conducted using PubMed to identify relevant articles and these results were supplemented by reference checking and with the authors' familiarity of the literature. Due to the large number of articles discussing IL-17A in SpA, a narrative review was deemed to be most appropriate for this manuscript.

IL-17A in the pathogenesis of SpA

IL-17 signaling has been identified as a key modulator of synovial inflammation and joint destruction in various arthropathies through its actions on synovial cells, osteoblasts, and chondrocytes (Fig. 1) [12]. Of the six members of the IL-17 cytokine family, IL-17A is the most well characterized, existing as a homodimer or as part of a heterodimer with IL-17F [8, 15]. Cellular production of IL-17 is complex and heterogeneous. Table 1 provides an overview of the diverse cellular sources of this cytokine. Notably, IL-17A and IL-17F are primarily produced by naive $CD4^+$ T cells that differentiate into Th17 cells in response to stimulation by IL-23 [8, 16]. In addition, IL-17A is produced by $CD8^+$ T cells, γδ T cells, natural killer cells, mast cells, neutrophils, and group 3 innate lymphoid cells [8]. Binding of IL-17A homodimers to the heterodimeric transmembrane IL-17 receptor (IL-17RA and IL-17RC) is a potent signal driving autoimmune inflammatory responses associated with arthritis-related tissue damage and joint destruction, as well as with mucocutaneous defense mechanisms against extracellular pathogens [8, 12, 14, 17, 18]. Furthermore, Th17 cells (IL-17A/IL-22) and its receptor system play important roles in osteoclast-mediated bone changes and cartilage destruction associated with inflammatory arthritis [2, 9, 14]. The IL-17 receptor is expressed by osteoclasts, osteoblasts, synoviocytes, and chondrocytes, and stimulation of IL-17A triggers Th17 cells, osteoblasts, and synovial fibroblasts to produce the receptor activator of nuclear factor-κB ligand (RANKL), which plays a vital role in production of osteoclasts and osteoclastic precursors [14].

Many basic research studies using in vitro and animal models have helped elucidate the roles of IL-17A and related cytokines in arthritis pathogenesis. Early mouse models of collagen-induced arthritis (CIA) identified IL-17 as a key contributor to RANKL-induced bone erosion and inflammatory joint destruction [19, 20]. Subsequently, tissue microscopy studies have shown that T cells with high levels of IL-23 receptors are present at the entheseal interface between tendon and bone of both axial and peripheral articular locations [9]. When IL-23

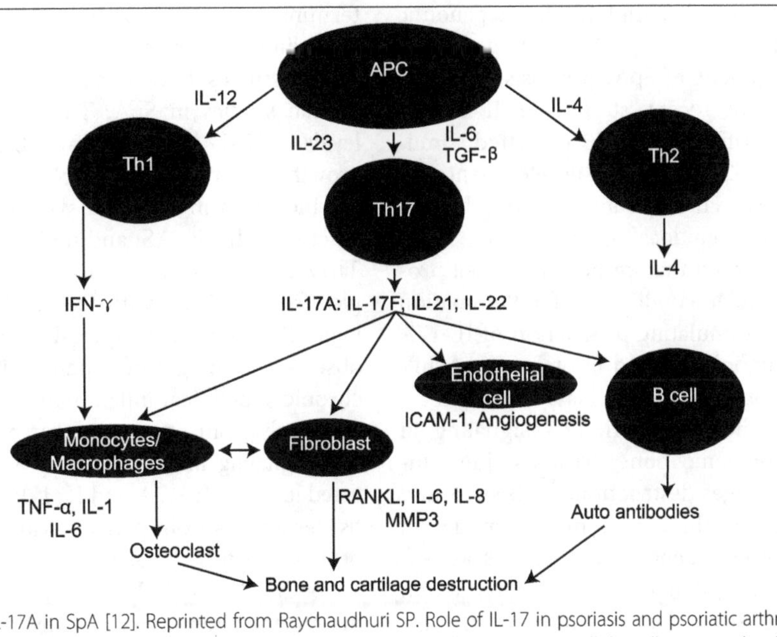

Fig. 1 Pathogenic role of IL-17A in SpA [12]. Reprinted from Raychaudhuri SP. Role of IL-17 in psoriasis and psoriatic arthritis. Clin Rev Allergy Immunol. 2013;44:183–93, with permission of Springer. *APC* antigen-presenting cell, *ICAM-1* intercellular adhesion molecule-1, *IL* interleukin, *IFN* interferon, *MMP3* matrix metalloproteinase 3, *TGF* transforming growth factor, *RANKL* receptor activator of nuclear factor-κB ligand, *Th* T-helper, *TNF* tumor necrosis factor

Table 1 Types of IL-17-producing cells [8, 12, 33, 36, 38, 76–80]

Cell type	Description
Adaptive Th17 cells	• A subset of activated CD4$^+$ T helper cells that produce high levels of IL-17A, IL-17F, and IL-22, and express IL-23R • CD4$^+$ TCRα/β$^+$ Th17 cells are a well characterized source of IL-17 that play a key role in immune inflammatory responses
Natural Th17 cells	• Subset of thymic Th17 cells that acquire effector function prior to peripheral antigen exposure • These cells have different TCR gene usage and signaling properties compared with conventional Th17 cells
γ/δ T cells	• Potent source of innate IL-17 produced independently of IL-6 • Properties are similar to Th17 cells (e.g., expression of CCR6, IL-23R, and RORγt); these cells also express TLR1, TLR2, and Dectin-1 • Levels of IL-17-producing γ/δ T cells increase during some types of bacterial infections • Different subsets of γ/δ T cells in the thymus produce either IL-17 or IFNγ • Major source of gut-protective IL-17, which acts independently from IL-23
iNKT cells	• Cells that express a restricted TCR that recognizes glycolipid antigens • May provide an alternative source of IL-17 when IL-6 is not present to stimulate Th17 cells • IL-17$^+$ cells express IL-23R and IL-1R1
Tc17 cells	• Subset of CD8$^+$ cells that produces IL-17 • May play a role in pathogenic skin and joint inflammation in psoriasis and PsA, respectively
ILC3s	• Subset of ILCs defined by their capacity to produce IL-17A and/or IL-22 • The role of ILCs in SpA and other forms of destructive arthritis is unclear because cell numbers are generally low
Neutrophils	• Source of IL-17 in effector phase of arthritis • Myeloperoxidase$^+$ and CD15$^+$ neutrophils have been identified as sources of IL-17 in facet joints of patients with SpA
Mast cells	• Primary source of IL-17$^+$ cells in synovial fluid of patients with SpA as a result of innate immune responses

CCR6 C-C chemokine receptor type 6, *IFN* interferon, *IL* interleukin, *ILC* innate lymphoid cell, *iNKT cells* invariant natural killer T cells, *PsA* psoriatic arthritis, *ROR* retinoic orphan receptor, *SpA* spondyloarthritis, *TCR* T-cell receptor, *Th* T-helper, *TLR* Toll-like receptor

levels were increased in cell cultures of these entheses, expression of IL-17A, IL-22, and bone morphogenic protein 7 increased, and IL-23 also induced severe enthesitis in animal models [9]. Initially, findings from genomic studies indicated that IL-23 receptor signaling plays a key role in the development of SpA, psoriasis, and IBD [21–24]. However, more recent studies in IL-17A$^{-/-}$ knockout mice have clarified that IL-23-mediated stimulation of IL-17A and IL-22 drives the development and severity of enthesitis [21]. Further substantiating the role of IL-17A in IL-23-induced local inflammation, Reinhardt and colleagues showed that entheseal γ/δ cell production is increased under conditions of inflammation and mechanical stress, stimulating production of IL-17A at anatomic sites commonly affected in SpA (e.g., Achilles tendon insertion, aortic root, and ciliary body) [25].

Further supporting the role of IL-17A signaling in the formation of pathogenic bone erosions, joint inflammation, and cartilage destruction, Lubberts and colleagues [26] observed that, in a mouse model of CIA, neutralization of endogenous IL-17A was associated with a decrease in systemic IL-6 and a reduction in cells that tested positive for RANKL and the inflammatory cytokine IL-1β. In addition, Adamopoulos and colleagues [27] observed that IL-17A gene transfer in a mouse model of CIA induced the expansion of osteoclast precursors and increased serum levels of biomarkers associated with bone resorption, including tartrate-resistant acid phosphatase 5b and carboxy-terminal collagen crosslinks.

Findings consistent with the results from basic research studies have been observed in several different human studies in SpA. These studies have shown that levels of IL-17A, IL-23, IL-6, IL-1β, IL-21, transforming growth factor (TGF)-β, TNF-α, and interferon (IFN)γ are increased in sera and synovial fluid of patients with reactive arthritis, AS, and undifferentiated SpA, and that Th17 cell levels are increased in peripheral blood samples from patients with PsA and AS [3, 28–31]. Pathologic Th17-cell overexpression of IL-17 has also been observed in the gut of patients with PsA, contributing to chronic subclinical inflammation [32].

A study from our group that highlights the role of IL-17A signaling in inflammatory arthritis showed that elevated levels of IL-17A and IL-17RA are present in synovial tissue samples from patients with PsA and, when cultures of these tissue samples were treated with an anti-IL-17RA antibody, IL-17A-induced expression of IL-8, IL-6, and matrix metalloproteinase (MMP)3 was decreased [33]. Another important study by Jansen and colleagues [34] showed that elevated levels of IL-17-producing CD4$^+$ T cells are present in patients with early, active axial SpA

Table 2 Differences between RA and SpA [8, 37]

RA	SpA
• Characterized primarily by symmetric polyarthritis and inflammation resulting in cartilage and bone destruction	• Oligo/polyarthritis is more often asymmetrical
• Axial involvement is rare	• Characterized primarily by axial disease of the sacroiliac joints and spine
• More common in women than men	• More common in men than women
• ACPA and RF antibodies are common	• ACPA and RF antibodies are absent
• Strong genetic association with HLA-DR	• Most common genetic involvement is HLA-B27
• Central clinical feature is synovitis	• Affects the axial skeleton and peripheral joints with synovial involvement, especially in entheses, bone, and bone marrow (osteitis)
• Driven by B- and/or T-cell autoreactivity	• Driven by innate immune cells (e.g., macrophages, PMN cells, mast cells)
• Macrophage effectors of synovial inflammation are driven predominantly by IFNγ	• Macrophage effectors of inflammation are driven predominantly by IL-17
• More pronounced hyperplasia of the synovial lining versus SpA	• Increased vascularity versus RA
• Extra-articular features include rheumatoid nodules, vasculitis, pneumonitis, scleritis	• Extra-articular features include IBD, psoriasis, uveitis, aortitis
• Little or no signs of tissue repair with joint damage	• Joint damage is characterized by new cartilage and bone formation (remodeling)

ACPA anti-citrullinated protein antibody, *HLA* human leukocyte antigen, *IBD* inflammatory bowel disease, *IFN* interferon, *IL* interleukin, *PMN* polymorphonuclear, *RA* rheumatoid arthritis, *RF* rheumatoid factor, *SpA* spondyloarthritis

with and without magnetic resonance imaging (MRI) abnormalities. Furthermore, Kenna and colleagues [35] observed that patients with active AS have increased levels of circulating γδ T cells that express IL-23R and produce IL-17, and a study by Noordenbos and colleagues [36] showed that synovial tissue from patients with SpA has increased levels of IL-17-expressing mast cells compared with tissue from patients with RA. Interestingly, this increase in IL-17 was not modulated by TNF-α blockade [36]. These studies highlight just a few key examples of the extensive research findings that have established IL-17A signaling as an important pathway in the development and progression of SpA.

Different roles of IL-17A in SpA and RA

While there are many similarities between the chronic spinal and joint inflammation observed in patients with RA and SpA, it is important to note that these diseases have several unique clinical, radiologic, serologic, and genetic features driven by different underlying pathogenic signaling pathways (Table 2) [8, 37]. Moreover, while many of the same cytokines are present in both RA and SpA, differential expression levels result in substantial differences in characteristic bone changes. In RA, TNF-α is the predominant proinflammatory cytokine, promoting RANKL-driven osteoclast erosion, as well as suppression of osteoblast formation [14]. In contrast, the IL-17A pathway plays a predominant role in the promotion of osteoclastogenesis in patients with SpA, and levels of circulating Th17 cells observed in the peripheral blood are much higher and more consistently observed than in patients with RA. Additionally, Th17 cells isolated from patients with SpA are more differentiated and polyfunctional than those from patients with RA [28]. These findings may be a result of different T-cell lineages in RA and SpA. For example, Menon and colleagues [38] observed that IL-17 in patients with PsA was predominantly produced by $CD8^+$-derived T cells (Tc17 cells), while IL-17A-producing T cells were only produced from the $CD4^+$ lineage in patients with RA. Furthermore, these authors observed that the frequency of synovial fluid $IL\text{-}17^+CD4^-$ T cells but not of $IL\text{-}17^+CD4^+$ T cells was associated with clinical measures of PsA disease activity [38].

Translation of IL-17 inhibition into clinical practice

There is currently an unmet need in the treatment of SpA [39]. Traditional disease-modifying antirheumatic drugs (e.g., methotrexate) are ineffective in spinal inflammatory arthritis and AS. While the TNF-α inhibitors etanercept, adalimumab, infliximab, certolizumab pegol, and golimumab have all demonstrated efficacy in AS and PsA, a substantial proportion of patients either do not respond at all or respond inadequately, while some patients are unable to tolerate these drugs [15, 39–41]. In recent years, other therapies used to treat RA have been investigated in AS, including the IL-1 receptor antagonist anakinra, the IL-6 inhibitor tocilizumab, the anti-CD20 antibody rituximab, and the costimulatory pathway inhibitor abatacept. However, none of these agents have demonstrated a meaningful clinical benefit in patients with AS [41].

It has been recognized that biologic agents with mechanisms of action other than TNF inhibition, which acts upstream of newer agents, would provide valuable alternatives for the treatment of SpA. However, until very recently there was a lack of alternatives to TNF-α inhibitors [39]. That changed with the approval of the IL-12/IL-23 antagonist ustekinumab, the phosphodiesterase 4 inhibitor apremilast, and the IL-17A inhibitor secukinumab for the treatment of PsA, and with the approval of secukinumab for the treatment of AS. Now, when patients fail to respond to one biologic due to lack of efficacy or poor tolerability, switching to another biologic with a different mechanism of action can be an effective treatment strategy [42, 43].

When choosing a biologic agent in SpA, it is reasonable to consider preclinical findings that support the mechanistic rationale for targeting IL-17A. IL-17A seems to be a more downstream effector of SpA pathogenesis than other cytokines (i.e., IL-23, TGF-β, IL-6, and IL-1β), which act upstream to trigger differentiation of Th17 cells in entheses and synovial tissue. Once activated, these Th17 cells stimulate production of downstream effector cytokines including IL-17 and IL-22, which contribute to inflammation, bone erosion, and bone fusion [2, 7, 9, 12, 27, 28, 33]. In addition to the good efficacy observed in SpA with this strategy, such downstream targeting may also be beneficial for patients with refractory SpA and those who are otherwise intolerant to other biologic therapies.

As clinical development programs for IL-17A inhibitors have progressed, findings from large-scale randomized controlled trials have supported the translation of IL-17A inhibition in SpA from bench to bedside. Positive findings have been observed in clinical studies of IL-17A inhibitors in psoriasis, PsA, and AS [44–49].

Psoriasis

The IL-17A inhibitor secukinumab is approved for the treatment of moderate-to-severe plaque psoriasis. In phase 3 clinical studies, secukinumab consistently provided substantial meaningful improvements in the signs and symptoms of moderate-to-severe chronic plaque psoriasis [44, 49]. In the pivotal ERASURE and FIXTURE studies, more than half of patients who received secukinumab 300 mg experienced a 90% improvement in Psoriasis Area and Severity Index (PASI90) scores at week 12, compared with 1% with placebo (ERASURE) and 21% with etanercept (FIXTURE) [44]. In the CLEAR phase 3 study, secukinumab 300 mg demonstrated superiority compared with ustekinumab for the primary endpoint of PASI90 at week 16 (79.0% vs 57.6% response rates, respectively; $p < 0.0001$) [49].

The IL-17A inhibitor ixekizumab was recently approved for the treatment of moderate-to-severe plaque psoriasis. In the UNCOVER-2 and UNCOVER-3 randomized controlled phase 3 studies, up to 71% of patients treated with ixekizumab achieved PASI90 at week 12, compared with 0.6% to 3.1% with placebo, and 18.7% to 25.7% with etanercept [45].

The anti-IL-17RA monoclonal antibody brodalumab was in late-stage development for the treatment of moderate-to-severe plaque psoriasis. Results of the phase 3 AMAGINE-1 study showed that, at week 12, PASI90 was achieved by 43% of patients treated with brodalumab 140 mg and by 70% of patients treated with brodalumab 210 mg, compared with 1% of patients in the placebo group [50]. In the AMAGINE-2 and AMAGINE-3 studies, brodalumab 210 mg demonstrated higher efficacy compared with ustekinumab based on week 12 PASI90 responses (70% vs 47% in AMAGINE-2, and 69% vs 48% in AMAGINE-3) [51]. However, the future of brodalumab development is uncertain based on observed events of suicidal ideation and behavior during clinical development [52].

Psoriatic arthritis

In early 2016, secukinumab received US Food and Drug Administration (FDA) approval for the treatment of active PsA. In the large-scale FUTURE 1 and FUTURE 2 phase 3 studies, patients received placebo or intravenous (IV) or subcutaneous (SC) induction dosing of secukinumab followed by SC maintenance dosing [46, 48]. At week 24 in FUTURE 1, at least 20% improvement in American College of Rheumatology response criteria (ACR20) responses were observed in 50% of patients receiving secukinumab 150 mg, 51% receiving secukinumab 75 mg, and 17% of patients receiving placebo ($p < 0.001$ for both comparisons with placebo) [48]. At week 24 in FUTURE 2, which had a mixed population of TNF-naive and TNF-experienced patients, ACR20 was achieved by 54% of patients receiving secukinumab 300 mg ($p < 0.0001$), 51% receiving secukinumab 150 mg ($p < 0.0001$), 29% receiving secukinumab 75 mg ($p = 0.0399$), and 15% of patients receiving placebo [46]. These improvements were sustained through 52 weeks of treatment [46, 48].

In the phase 3 SPIRIT-P1 trial of a TNF-naive population, significantly more patients achieved ACR20 with ixekizumab 80 mg once every 2 weeks (62%) and ixekizumab 80 mg once every 4 weeks (58%) than with placebo (30%; both $p \leq 0.001$) [53]. A clinical trial of ixekizumab in biologic-experienced patients with active PsA is ongoing (NCT02349295).

Ankylosing spondylitis

Secukinumab also recently received FDA approval for the treatment of active AS. In a randomized, double-blind, phase 2 study, 59% of patients treated with secukinumab achieved rapid, meaningful clinical improvement in AS symptoms compared with 24% of patients who received placebo [54]. These improvements were maintained for up to 2 years in patients who continued in an open-label extension of this study [55]. The benefits of secukinumab in patients with AS were confirmed in the phase 3 MEASURE 1 and MEASURE 2 studies [47]. In these randomized controlled trials, patients received placebo, or IV or SC loading doses of secukinumab followed by SC maintenance dosing. In MEASURE 1 and MEASURE 2, respectively, at least 20% improvement in Assessment of SpondyloArthritis International Society (ASAS20) response rates at week 16 were 61% in both studies in the secukinumab 150 mg group, 60% and 41% in the secukinumab 75 mg group, and 29% and 28% for patients who received placebo [47]. Improvement in signs and symptoms of AS occurred rapidly with secukinumab and were sustained over time. Secukinumab was also associated with improvements in physical functioning and health-related quality of life compared with placebo [47].

Studies of ixekizumab in biologic treatment-naive (COAST-V) and treatment-experienced (COAST-W) patients with AS are ongoing (NCT02696785 and NCT02696798).

Rheumatoid arthritis

As suggested by basic research studies characterizing the different roles of IL-17A in RA and SpA [38], results from clinical studies of IL-17A inhibitors in RA indicate that these agents may have limited therapeutic efficacy in this patient population [56, 57]. In separate phase 2 studies of secukinumab and ixekizumab in patients with RA, ACR20 response rates differed across the dose ranges studied, without a consistent dose–response relationship [56, 57]. In a 16-week phase 2 study of secukinumab, ACR20 response rates ranged from 36% to 54% in the active-treatment arms, compared with 34% with placebo [56]. In a second 52-week phase 2 study of secukinumab, ACR20 response rates were not significantly different between secukinumab and placebo (42.9% vs 40.9%), but significant improvements were observed in the secukinumab arm based on 28-joint Disease Activity Score (DAS28), global assessments of disease activity, pain assessments, and high-sensitivity C-reactive protein levels [58].

Among biologic treatment-naive patients in a phase 2 study of ixekizumab, ACR20 response rates ranged from 43% to 70%, compared with 35% for placebo. In this study, ACR20 response rates were significantly higher with ixekizumab 80 mg and 180 mg compared with placebo for patients with prior inadequate response to TNF-α inhibitors [57]. Patients in this study were eligible to enter a 48-week open-label extension. Patients in the extension who experienced clinical improvements during the initial 16-week study generally maintained these improvements through week 64 [59].

Based on findings from these phase 2 studies, it cannot be ruled out that a subset of patients with RA may experience clinical benefits from treatment with IL-17A inhibitors. However, a recent study investigating the relationship between genetic biomarkers and secukinumab treatment response in patients with RA found that the human leukocyte antigen (HLA)-DRB1*04 and HLA-DRB1* shared epitope allelic groups were not predictive of treatment response [60].

Safety profiles of secukinumab and ixekizumab

IL-17A inhibitors have been shown to have good overall safety profiles [61]. In psoriasis clinical trials, secukinumab's side-effect profile was similar to that of the TNF-α inhibitor etanercept and the IL-12/IL-23 antagonist ustekinumab, with no safety signals indicating an increased risk for serious adverse events of interest, including malignancy, infection, or induction of autoimmune diseases [44, 49]. In placebo-controlled studies of secukinumab in PsA and AS, the incidence and types of adverse events were similar between secukinumab and placebo, with a small increased risk for infections, including candidiasis [46–48]. Similarly, in the UNCOVER-2 and UNCOVER-3 psoriasis clinical studies, rates of serious adverse events were low and similar with ixekizumab and etanercept, and a small number of *Candida* infections were reported [45].

Management of comorbidities and extra-articular manifestations of SpA

It has been hypothesized, based on findings from recent research, that IL-17A inhibition may have beneficial effects on some of the common comorbidities observed in patients with SpA, as well as extra-articular symptoms of the disease, including uveitis and psoriasis [62]. Based on available data, Golden and colleagues [63] have speculated that the inflammation associated with increased levels of Th17 cells and their associated cytokines may initiate or worsen comorbidities, including atherosclerosis and metabolic syndrome; thus, it is logical to hypothesize that SpA treatments that modulate inflammatory responses in the Th17 pathway could have added benefits related to improvements in comorbidities.

In experiments performed by Barry and colleagues, prolonged elevations in IL-17RA, IL-17A, and IL-17F levels following myocardial ischemia/reperfusion injury in rats contributed to permanent cardiac damage [64]. In vivo experiments also showed that IL-17 neutralization reduced necrotic and apoptotic myocyte death, suggesting beneficial effects following human myocardial infarction [64].

Preclinical studies have linked increased IL-17 production with development of hypertension and endothelial dysfunction through promotion of oxidative stress in the kidneys and vasculature [65, 66]. These findings are supported by results from a clinical study that showed serum IL-17 levels were significantly higher in patients with prehypertension compared with normotensive controls [67]. Additionally, Hautefort and colleagues [68] observed that monocyte-derived dendritic cells in patients with idiopathic pulmonary arterial hypertension induced greater activation and proliferation of $CD4^+$-derived Th17 cells, resulting in higher levels of IL-17 compared with controls.

In a large-scale, case-controlled, genetic screening study in patients with coronary artery disease (CAD), Zhang and colleagues [69] found a significant association between specific *IL17A* single nucleotide polymorphisms (SNPs) and risk of CAD and acute myocardial infarction in a Chinese Han population. Similarly, Vargas-Alarcón and colleagues [70] found associations between two *IL17A* haplotypes and development of premature CAD in a Mexican population. In the group that developed premature CAD, polymorphisms were also associated with increased risks for central obesity, increased visceral abdominal fat, and metabolic syndrome. Interestingly, such increased risks for obesity may contribute to disease pathogenesis in SpA because activated white adipose tissue stimulates production of IL-17 and other proinflammatory cytokines [71].

In a randomized, placebo-controlled, phase 2a trial of patients with moderate-to-severe Crohn's disease, IL-17A inhibition with secukinumab did not meet its primary endpoint, and worsening of Crohn's disease was experienced by some patients [72]. However, in mechanistic studies, mixed findings have been reported for the role of IL-17 in the gut with both protective and proinflammatory effects observed [73] and additional research is required to fully understand the role of IL-17 in the gut. Although Crohn's disease has been reported in patients with AS treated with IL-17 inhibitors, a small number of individuals were affected (incidence rate of 0.7 cases per 100 patient-years in pooled secukinumab-group data from MEASURE 1 and MEASURE 2) [47]. Furthermore, in large, pooled studies of patients with psoriasis treated with IL-17 inhibitors, IBD was reported infrequently (incidence rate of 0.33 cases per 100 patient-years with secukinumab and incidence rate of 2.9 cases per 1000 patient-years with ixekizumab) [74, 75]. The risk of IBD with IL-17 inhibition is minimal.

Conclusions

In summary, there is ample evidence supporting the central role of IL-17A-secreting cells in inflammation, bone resorption/remodeling, and cartilage damage associated with SpA, and there are strong mechanistic rationales for targeting this pathway in SpA disease management. Findings from clinical studies support these rationales and indicate that biologic IL-17A inhibitors may provide effective and well-tolerated alternatives to other approved treatments for the management of SpA.

Abbreviations

ACR: American College of Rheumatology; AS: Ankylosing spondylitis; ASAS: Assessment of SpondyloArthritis International Society; CAD: Coronary artery disease; CIA: Collagen-induced arthritis; DAS28: 28-joint Disease Activity Score; FDA: Food and Drug Administration; HLA: Human leukocyte antigen; IBD: Inflammatory bowel disease; IFN: Interferon; IL: Interleukin; IL-17RA: Interleukin-17 receptor A; IL-17RC: Interleukin-17 receptor C; IV: Intravenous; MMP: Matrix metalloproteinase; NHANES: National Health and Nutrition Examination Survey; PASI: Psoriasis Area and Severity Index; PsA: Psoriatic arthritis; RA: Rheumatoid arthritis; RANKL: Receptor activator of nuclear factor-κB ligand; SC: Subcutaneous; SNP: Single nucleotide polymorphism; SpA: Spondyloarthritis; TGF: Transforming growth factor; Th: T-helper; TNF: Tumor necrosis factor

Acknowledgments

The authors were fully responsible for all content and editorial decisions and received no financial support or other form of compensation related to the development of this manuscript.

Funding

Technical assistance with editing and styling of the manuscript for submission was provided by Oxford PharmaGenesis Inc., and was funded by Novartis Pharmaceuticals Corporation.

Authors' contributions

SPR conceived of the concept for this review, and participated in its design and coordination, and drafted and reviewed the content of the manuscript. SKR conceived of the concept for this review, and participated in its design and coordination, and drafted and reviewed the content of the manuscript. Both authors read and approved the final manuscript.

Competing interests

The authors declare that they have no competing interests.

References

1. 2014 ACR/SAA/SPARTAN recommendations for the management of axial spondyloarthritis, including ankylosing spondylitis, and children with the enthesitis-related arthritis form of juvenile idiopathic arthritis. Project plan. http://www.rheumatology.org/Portals/0/Files/Axial%20SpA%20Project%20Plan.pdf. Accessed 30 Aug 2016.
2. Raychaudhuri SK, Saxena A, Raychaudhuri SP. Role of IL-17 in the pathogenesis of psoriatic arthritis and axial spondyloarthritis. Clin Rheumatol. 2015;34:1019–23.
3. Singh AK, Misra R, Aggarwal A. Th-17 associated cytokines in patients with reactive arthritis/undifferentiated spondyloarthropathy. Clin Rheumatol. 2011;30:771–6.
4. Wendling D. Treating to target in axial spondyloarthritis: defining the target and the arrow. Expert Rev Clin Immunol. 2015;11:691–3.
5. Stolwijk C, Boonen A, van Tubergen A, Reveille JD. Epidemiology of spondyloarthritis. Rheum Dis Clin North Am. 2012;38:441–76.

6. Reveille JD, Witter JP, Weisman MH. Prevalence of axial spondylarthritis in the United States: estimates from a cross-sectional survey. Arthritis Care Res (Hoboken). 2012;64:905–10.
7. Mitra A, Raychaudhuri SK, Raychaudhuri SP. Functional role of IL-22 in psoriatic arthritis. Arthritis Res Ther. 2012;14:R65.
8. Lubberts E. The IL-23-IL-17 axis in inflammatory arthritis. Nat Rev Rheumatol. 2015;11:415–29.
9. Sherlock JP, Joyce-Shaikh B, Turner SP, Chao CC, Sathe M, Grein J, et al. IL-23 induces spondyloarthropathy by acting on ROR-γt$^+$ CD3$^+$CD4$^-$CD8$^-$ entheseal resident T cells. Nat Med. 2012;18:1069–76.
10. Cai Y, Shen X, Ding C, Qi C, Li K, Li X, et al. Pivotal role of dermal IL-17-producing γδ T cells in skin inflammation. Immunity. 2011;35:596–610.
11. Numasaki M, Fukushi J, Ono M, Narula SK, Zavodny PJ, Kudo T, et al. Interleukin-17 promotes angiogenesis and tumor growth. Blood. 2003;101:2620–7.
12. Raychaudhuri SP. Role of IL-17 in psoriasis and psoriatic arthritis. Clin Rev Allergy Immunol. 2013;44:183–93.
13. Yamamoto M, Nakajima K, Takaishi M, Kitaba S, Magata Y, Kataoka S, et al. Psoriatic inflammation facilitates the onset of arthritis in a mouse model. J Invest Dermatol. 2015;135:445–53.
14. Rossini M, Viapiana O, Adami S, Idolazzi L, Fracassi E, Gatti D. Focal bone involvement in inflammatory arthritis: the role of IL17. Rheumatol Int. 2016;36:469–82.
15. Smith JA, Colbert RA. The interleukin-23/interleukin-17 axis in spondyloarthritis pathogenesis: Th17 and beyond. Arthritis Rheumatol. 2014;66:231–41.
16. Wendling D, Guillot X, Prati C. The IL-23/Th 17 pathway in spondyloarthritis: the royal road? Joint Bone Spine. 2015;82:1–4.
17. Conti HR, Gaffen SL. IL-17-mediated immunity to the opportunistic fungal pathogen candida albicans. J Immunol. 2015;195:780–8.
18. Gaffen SL. Structure and signalling in the IL-17 receptor family. Nat Rev Immunol. 2009;9:556–67.
19. Lubberts E, Joosten LA, Oppers B, van den Bersselaar L, Coenen-de Roo CJ, Kolls JK, et al. IL-1-independent role of IL-17 in synovial inflammation and joint destruction during collagen-induced arthritis. J Immunol. 2001;167:1004–13.
20. Lubberts E, van den Bersselaar L, Oppers-Walgreen B, Schwarzenberger P, Coenen-de Roo CJ, Kolls JK, et al. IL-17 promotes bone erosion in murine collagen-induced arthritis through loss of the receptor activator of NF-κB ligand/osteoprotegerin balance. J Immunol. 2003;170:2655–62.
21. Benham H, Rehaume LM, Hasnain SZ, Velasco J, Baillet AC, Ruutu M, et al. Interleukin-23 mediates the intestinal response to microbial β-1,3-glucan and the development of spondyloarthritis pathology in SKG mice. Arthritis Rheumatol. 2014;66:1755–67.
22. Duerr RH, Taylor KD, Brant SR, Rioux JD, Silverberg MS, Daly MJ, et al. A genome-wide association study identifies IL23R as an inflammatory bowel disease gene. Science. 2006;314:1461–3.
23. Cargill M, Schrodi SJ, Chang M, Garcia VE, Brandon R, Callis KP, et al. A large-scale genetic association study confirms IL12B and leads to the identification of IL23R as psoriasis-risk genes. Am J Hum Genet. 2007;80:273–90.
24. Wellcome Trust Case Control Consortium, Australo-Anglo-American Spondylitis Consortium (TASC), Burton PR, Clayton DG, Cardon LR, Craddock N, et al. Association scan of 14,500 nonsynonymous SNPs in four diseases identifies autoimmunity variants. Nat Genet. 2007;39:1329–37.
25. Reinhardt A, Yevsa T, Worbs T, Lienenklaus S, Sandrock I, Oberdörfer L, et al. Interleukin-23-dependent γ/δ T cells produce interleukin-17 and accumulate in the enthesis, aortic valve, and ciliary body in mice. Arthritis Rheumatol. 2016;68:2476–86.
26. Lubberts E, Koenders MI, Oppers-Walgreen B, van den Bersselaar L, Coenen-de Roo CJ, Joosten LA, et al. Treatment with a neutralizing anti-murine interleukin-17 antibody after the onset of collagen-induced arthritis reduces joint inflammation, cartilage destruction, and bone erosion. Arthritis Rheum. 2004;50:650–9.
27. Adamopoulos IE, Suzuki E, Chao CC, Gorman D, Adda S, Maverakis E, et al. IL-17A gene transfer induces bone loss and epidermal hyperplasia associated with psoriatic arthritis. Ann Rheum Dis. 2015;74:1284–92.
28. Jandus C, Bioley G, Rivals JP, Dudler J, Speiser D, Romero P. Increased numbers of circulating polyfunctional Th17 memory cells in patients with seronegative spondylarthritides. Arthritis Rheum. 2008;58:2307–17.
29. Singh R, Aggarwal A, Misra R. Th1/Th17 cytokine profiles in patients with reactive arthritis/undifferentiated spondyloarthropathy. J Rheumatol. 2007;34:2285–90.
30. Xueyi L, Lina C, Zhenbiao W, Qing H, Qiang L, Zhu P. Levels of circulating Th17 cells and regulatory T cells in ankylosing spondylitis patients with an inadequate response to anti-TNF-α therapy. J Clin Immunol. 2013;33:151–61.
31. Londono J, Romero-Sanchez MC, Torres VG, Bautista WA, Fernandez DJ, de Avila QA, et al. The association between serum levels of potential biomarkers with the presence of factors related to the clinical activity and poor prognosis in spondyloarthritis. Rev Bras Reumatol. 2012;52:529–44.
32. Ciccia F, Guggino G, Ferrante A, Raimondo S, Bignone R, Rodolico V, et al. Interleukin-9 overexpression and Th9 polarization characterize the inflamed gut, the synovial tissue, and the peripheral blood of patients with psoriatic arthritis. Arthritis Rheumatol. 2016;68:1922–31.
33. Raychaudhuri SP, Raychaudhuri SK, Genovese MC. IL-17 receptor and its functional significance in psoriatic arthritis. Mol Cell Biochem. 2012;359:419–29.
34. Jansen DT, Hameetman M, van Bergen J, Huizinga TW, van der Heijde D, Toes RE, et al. IL-17-producing CD4$^+$ T cells are increased in early, active axial spondyloarthritis including patients without imaging abnormalities. Rheumatology (Oxford). 2015;54:728–35.
35. Kenna TJ, Davidson SI, Duan R, Bradbury LA, McFarlane J, Smith M, et al. Enrichment of circulating interleukin-17-secreting interleukin-23 receptor-positive γ/δ T cells in patients with active ankylosing spondylitis. Arthritis Rheum. 2012;64:1420–9.
36. Noordenbos T, Yeremenko N, Gofita I, van de Sande M, Tak PP, Cañete JD, et al. Interleukin-17-positive mast cells contribute to synovial inflammation in spondylarthritis. Arthritis Rheum. 2012;64:99–109.
37. Lories RJ, Baeten DL. Differences in pathophysiology between rheumatoid arthritis and ankylosing spondylitis. Clin Exp Rheumatol. 2009;27:S10–4.
38. Menon B, Gullick NJ, Walter GJ, Rajasekhar M, Garrood T, Evans HG, et al. Interleukin-17 + CD8+ T cells are enriched in the joints of patients with psoriatic arthritis and correlate with disease activity and joint damage progression. Arthritis Rheumatol. 2014;66:1272–81.
39. Van den Bosch F, Deodhar A. Treatment of spondyloarthritis beyond TNF-alpha blockade. Best Pract Res Clin Rheumatol. 2014;28:819–27.
40. Colbert RA, Ward MM. 17 and 23: prime numbers for ankylosing spondylitis? Lancet. 2013;382:1682–3.
41. Toussirot E. Biologics in spondyloarthritis: TNFα inhibitors and other agents. Immunotherapy. 2015;7:669–81.
42. Lories RJ, de Vlam K. Tumour necrosis factor inhibitors in the treatment of psoriatic arthritis: a view on effectiveness, clinical practice and toxicity. Expert Opin Biol Ther. 2014;14:1825–36.
43. Rohekar S, Chan J, Tse SM, Haroon N, Chandran V, Bessette L, et al. 2014 Update of the Canadian Rheumatology Association/Spondyloarthritis Research Consortium of Canada treatment recommendations for the management of spondyloarthritis. Part II: specific management recommendations. J Rheumatol. 2015;42:665–81.
44. Langley RG, Elewski BE, Lebwohl M, Reich K, Griffiths CE, Papp K, et al. Secukinumab in plaque psoriasis—results of two phase 3 trials. N Engl J Med. 2014;371:326–38.
45. Griffiths CE, Reich K, Lebwohl M, van de Kerkhof P, Paul C, Menter A, et al. Comparison of ixekizumab with etanercept or placebo in moderate-to-severe psoriasis (UNCOVER-2 and UNCOVER-3): results from two phase 3 randomised trials. Lancet. 2015;386:541–51.
46. McInnes IB, Mease PJ, Kirkham B, Kavanaugh A, Ritchlin CT, Rahman P, et al. Secukinumab, a human anti-interleukin-17A monoclonal antibody, in patients with psoriatic arthritis (FUTURE 2): a randomised, double-blind, placebo-controlled, phase 3 trial. Lancet. 2015;386:1137–46.
47. Baeten D, Sieper J, Braun J, Baraliakos X, Dougados M, Emery P, et al. Secukinumab, an interleukin-17A inhibitor, in ankylosing spondylitis. N Engl J Med. 2015;373:2534–48.
48. Mease PJ, McInnes IB, Kirkham B, Kavanaugh A, Rahman P, van der Heijde D, et al. Secukinumab inhibition of interleukin-17A in patients with psoriatic arthritis. N Engl J Med. 2015;373:1329–39.
49. Thaci D, Blauvelt A, Reich K, Tsai TF, Vanaclocha F, Kingo K, et al. Secukinumab is superior to ustekinumab in clearing skin of subjects with moderate to severe plaque psoriasis: CLEAR, a randomized controlled trial. J Am Acad Dermatol. 2015;73:400–9.
50. Papp KA, Reich K, Paul C, Blauvelt A, Baran W, Bolduc C, et al. A prospective phase III, randomized, double-blind, placebo-controlled study of brodalumab in patients with moderate-to-severe plaque psoriasis. Br J Dermatol. 2016;175:273–86.
51. Lebwohl M, Strober B, Menter A, Gordon K, Weglowska J, Puig L, et al. Phase 3 studies comparing brodalumab with ustekinumab in psoriasis. N Engl J Med. 2015;373:1318–28.
52. Danesh MJ, Kimball AB. Brodalumab and suicidal ideation in the context of a recent economic crisis in the United States. J Am Acad Dermatol. 2016;74:190–2.

53. Mease PJ, van der Heijde D, Ritchlin CT, Okada M, Cuchacovich RS, Shuler CL, et al. Ixekizumab, an interleukin-17A specific monoclonal antibody, for the treatment of biologic-naive patients with active psoriatic arthritis: results from the 24-week randomised, double-blind, placebo-controlled and active (adalimumab)-controlled period of the phase III trial SPIRIT-P1. Ann Rheum Dis. 2016;76:79–87.
54. Baeten D, Baraliakos X, Braun J, Sieper J, Emery P, van der Heijde D, et al. Anti-interleukin-17A monoclonal antibody secukinumab in treatment of ankylosing spondylitis: a randomised, double-blind, placebo-controlled trial. Lancet. 2013;382:1705–13.
55. Baraliakos X, Borah B, Braun J, Baeten D, Laurent D, Sieper J, et al. Long-term effects of secukinumab on MRI findings in relation to clinical efficacy in subjects with active ankylosing spondylitis: an observational study. Ann Rheum Dis. 2016;75:408–12.
56. Genovese MC, Durez P, Richards HB, Supronik J, Dokoupilova E, Mazurov V, et al. Efficacy and safety of secukinumab in patients with rheumatoid arthritis: a phase II, dose-finding, double-blind, randomised, placebo controlled study. Ann Rheum Dis. 2013;72:863–9.
57. Genovese MC, Greenwald M, Cho CS, Berman A, Jin L, Cameron GS, et al. A phase II randomized study of subcutaneous ixekizumab, an anti-interleukin-17 monoclonal antibody, in rheumatoid arthritis patients who were naive to biologic agents or had an inadequate response to tumor necrosis factor inhibitors. Arthritis Rheumatol. 2014;66:1693–704.
58. Tlustochowicz W, Rahman P, Seriolo B, Krammer G, Porter B, Widmer A, et al. Efficacy and safety of subcutaneous and intravenous loading dose regimens of secukinumab in patients with active rheumatoid arthritis: results from a randomized phase II study. J Rheumatol. 2016;43:495–503.
59. Genovese MC, Braun DK, Erickson JS, Berclaz PY, Banerjee S, Heffernan MP, et al. Safety and efficacy of open-label subcutaneous ixekizumab treatment for 48 weeks in a phase II study in biologic-naive and TNF-IR patients with rheumatoid arthritis. J Rheumatol. 2016;43:289–97.
60. Burmester GR, Durez P, Shestakova G, Genovese MC, Schulze-Koops H, Li Y, et al. Association of HLA-DRB1 alleles with clinical responses to the anti-interleukin-17A monoclonal antibody secukinumab in active rheumatoid arthritis. Rheumatology (Oxford). 2016;55:49–55.
61. Xiong HZ, Gu JY, He ZG, Chen WJ, Zhang X, Wang JY, et al. Efficacy and safety of secukinumab in the treatment of moderate to severe plaque psoriasis: a meta-analysis of randomized controlled trials. Int J Clin Exp Med. 2015;8:3156–72.
62. Letko E, Yeh S, Foster CS, Pleyer U, Brigell M, Grosskreutz CL, et al. Efficacy and safety of intravenous secukinumab in noninfectious uveitis requiring steroid-sparing immunosuppressive therapy. Ophthalmology. 2015;122:939–48.
63. Golden JB, McCormick TS, Ward NL. IL-17 in psoriasis: implications for therapy and cardiovascular co-morbidities. Cytokine. 2013;62:195–201.
64. Barry SP, Ounzain S, McCormick J, Scarabelli TM, Chen-Scarabelli C, Saravolatz LI, et al. Enhanced IL-17 signalling following myocardial ischaemia/reperfusion injury. Int J Cardiol. 2013;163:326–34.
65. Trott DW, Harrison DG. The immune system in hypertension. Adv Physiol Educ. 2014;38:20–4.
66. Harrison DG. The immune system in hypertension. Trans Am Clin Climatol Assoc. 2014;125:130–8. discussion 138–40.
67. Yao W, Sun Y, Wang X, Niu K. Elevated serum level of interleukin 17 in a population with prehypertension. J Clin Hypertens (Greenwich). 2015;17:770–4.
68. Hautefort A, Girerd B, Montani D, Cohen-Kaminsky S, Price L, Lambrecht BN, et al. T-helper 17 cell polarization in pulmonary arterial hypertension. Chest. 2015;147:1610–20.
69. Zhang X, Pei F, Zhang M, Yan C, Huang M, Wang T, et al. Interleukin-17A gene variants and risk of coronary artery disease: a large angiography-based study. Clin Chim Acta. 2011;412:327–31.
70. Vargas-Alarcón G, Angeles-Martínez J, Villarreal-Molina T, Alvarez-León E, Posadas-Sánchez R, Cardoso-Saldaña G, et al. Interleukin-17A gene haplotypes are associated with risk of premature coronary artery disease in Mexican patients from the Genetics of Atherosclerotic Disease (GEA) study. PLoS One. 2015;10:e0114943.
71. Raychaudhuri SP. Comorbidities of psoriatic arthritis—metabolic syndrome and prevention: a report from the GRAPPA 2010 annual meeting. J Rheumatol. 2012;39:437–40.
72. Hueber W, Sands BE, Lewitzky S, Vandemeulebroecke M, Reinisch W, Higgins PD, et al. Secukinumab, a human anti-IL-17A monoclonal antibody, for moderate to severe Crohn's disease: unexpected results of a randomised, double-blind placebo-controlled trial. Gut. 2012;61:1693–700.
73. Xu XR, Liu CQ, Feng BS, Liu ZJ. Dysregulation of mucosal immune response in pathogenesis of inflammatory bowel disease. World J Gastroenterol. 2014;20:3255–64.
74. van de Kerkhof PC, Griffiths CE, Reich K, Leonardi CL, Blauvelt A, Tsai TF, et al. Secukinumab long-term safety experience: a pooled analysis of 10 phase II and III clinical studies in patients with moderate to severe plaque psoriasis. J Am Acad Dermatol. 2016;75:83–98. e4.
75. Reich K, Leonardi C, Langley RG, Warren RB, Bachelez H, Romiti R, et al. Inflammatory bowel disease among patients with psoriasis treated with ixekizumab: a presentation of adjudicated data from an integrated database of 7 randomized controlled and uncontrolled trials. J Am Acad Dermatol. 2016. doi: 10.1016/j.jaad.2016.10.027.
76. Kim JS, Jordan MS. Diversity of IL-17-producing T lymphocytes. Cell Mol Life Sci. 2013;70:2271–90.
77. Spits H, Artis D, Colonna M, Diefenbach A, Di Santo JP, Eberl G, et al. Innate lymphoid cells—a proposal for uniform nomenclature. Nat Rev Immunol. 2013;13:145–9.
78. Kugyelka R, Kohl Z, Olasz K, Mikecz K, Rauch TA, Glant TT, et al. Enigma of IL-17 and Th17 cells in rheumatoid arthritis and in autoimmune animal models of arthritis. Mediators Inflamm. 2016;2016:6145810.
79. Lee JS, Tato CM, Joyce-Shaikh B, Gulen MF, Cayatte C, Chen Y, et al. Interleukin-23-independent IL-17 production regulates intestinal epithelial permeability. Immunity. 2015;43:727–38.
80. Martin B, Hirota K, Cua DJ, Stockinger B, Veldhoen M. Interleukin-17-producing gammadelta T cells selectively expand in response to pathogen products and environmental signals. Immunity. 2009;31:321–30.

25

Does evaluation of the ligamentous compartment enhance diagnostic utility of sacroiliac joint MRI in axial spondyloarthritis?

Ulrich Weber[1,2,3*], Walter P. Maksymowych[4], Stanley M. Chan[5], Kaspar Rufibach[6], Susanne J. Pedersen[7], Zheng Zhao[8], Veronika Zubler[9], Mikkel Østergaard[7] and Robert GW Lambert[10]

Abstract

Introduction: Inflammation of the sacroiliac joints (SIJ) is a fundamental clinical feature of axial spondyloarthritis (SpA). The anatomy of the irregularly shaped SIJ is complex with an antero-inferior cartilaginous compartment containing central hyaline and peripheral fibrocartilage, and a dorso-superior ligamentous compartment. Several scoring modules to systematically assess SIJ magnetic resonance imaging (MRI) in SpA have been developed. Nearly all of them are based on the cartilaginous joint compartment alone. However, there are only limited data about the frequency of inflammatory lesions in the ligamentous compartment and their potential diagnostic utility in axial SpA. We therefore aimed to evaluate the ligamentous compartment on sacroiliac joint MRI for lesion distribution and potential incremental value towards diagnosis of SpA over and above the traditional assessment of the cartilaginous compartment alone.

Methods: Two independent cohorts of 69 and 88 consecutive back pain patients ≤50 years were referred for suspected SpA (cohort A) or acute anterior uveitis plus back pain (cohort B). Patients were classified according to rheumatologist expert opinion based on clinical, radiographic and laboratory examination as having nonradiographic axial SpA (nr-axSpA; n = 51), ankylosing spondylitis (n = 34), or nonspecific back pain (NSBP; n = 72). Five blinded readers assessed SIJ MRI globally for presence/absence of SpA. Bone marrow edema (BME) and fat metaplasia were recorded in the cartilaginous and ligamentous compartment. The incremental value of evaluating the ligamentous additionally to the cartilaginous compartment alone for diagnosis of SpA was graded qualitatively. We determined the lesion distribution between the two compartments, and the impact of the ligamentous compartment evaluation on diagnostic utility.

Results: MRI bone marrow lesions solely in the ligamentous compartment in the absence of lesions in the cartilaginous compartment were reported in just 0–2.0/0–4.0 % (BME/fat metaplasia) of all subjects. Additional assessment of the ligamentous compartment was regarded as essential for diagnosis in 0 and 0.6 %, and as contributory in 28.0 and 7.7 % of nr-axSpA patients in cohorts A and B, respectively. Concomitant BME in both compartments was evident in 11.6–42.0 % of nr-axSpA and 2.1–2.4 % of NSBP patients.

Conclusion: Assessing the ligamentous compartment on SIJ MRI provided no incremental value for diagnosis of axial SpA. However, concomitant BME in both compartments may help discriminate nr-axSpA from NSBP.

* Correspondence: ulrich.weber02@bluewin.ch
[1]King Christian 10th Hospital for Rheumatic Diseases, Gråsten, and Sygehus, Sønderjylland, Denmark
[2]Institute of Regional Health Research, University of Southern Denmark, Odense, Denmark
Full list of author information is available at the end of the article

Introduction

Inflammation of the sacroiliac joints (SIJ) is a fundamental clinical feature of axial spondyloarthritis (SpA), and sacroiliitis on magnetic resonance imaging (MRI) represents a major criterion in the Assessment of SpondyloArthritis International Society (ASAS) classification for axial SpA [1]. The anatomy of the irregularly curved SIJ is complex with an antero-inferior cartilaginous compartment, which contains central hyaline and peripheral fibrocartilage, and a dorso-superior ligamentous compartment [2, 3]. Small case series and anecdotal reports in patients with early spondyloarthritis suggest that inflammation starts in the subchondral bone marrow of the cartilaginous SIJ compartment [4–12].

Several scoring modules to systematically assess SIJ MRI in SpA have been developed. Nearly all of them are based on the cartilaginous joint compartment alone [13–19], and magnetic resonance images are acquired in a tilted semi-coronal plane running parallel to the posterior aspect of the sacrum. When scrolling from anterior to posterior through semi-coronal magnetic resonance images of the SIJ, the cartilaginous compartment is displayed on the first 5–6 MRI slices. The subsequent 1–2 slices have been termed "transitional" slices as they show both cartilaginous and ligamentous portions. The most posterior 3–4 slices depict the ligamentous compartment (Fig. 1). An assessment module of the SIJ developed by a Danish working group also scores inflammation in the bone marrow of the ligamentous SIJ compartment [20–22]. Magnetic resonance images for the Danish method are obtained not only in a semi-coronal but also in a semi-axial plane perpendicular to the long axis of the SIJ, which allows simultaneous assessment of the bone marrow in the ligamentous and cartilaginous compartments on the same image. However, there are only limited data about the frequency of inflammatory lesions in the ligamentous compartment and their incremental value towards diagnostic utility in axial SpA over and above the assessment of the cartilaginous compartment alone.

The goals of this study on SIJ MRI in two axial SpA inception cohorts were: (1) to systematically evaluate the frequency of bone marrow edema (BME) and fat metaplasia in the bone marrow of both the cartilaginous and ligamentous SIJ compartment by semi-coronal magnetic resonance images in SpA patients and controls; and (2) to assess the incremental value of the additional evaluation of the ligamentous compartment on diagnostic utility over and above the traditional assessment of the cartilaginous compartment alone in nonradiographic axial SpA (nr-axSpA) patients.

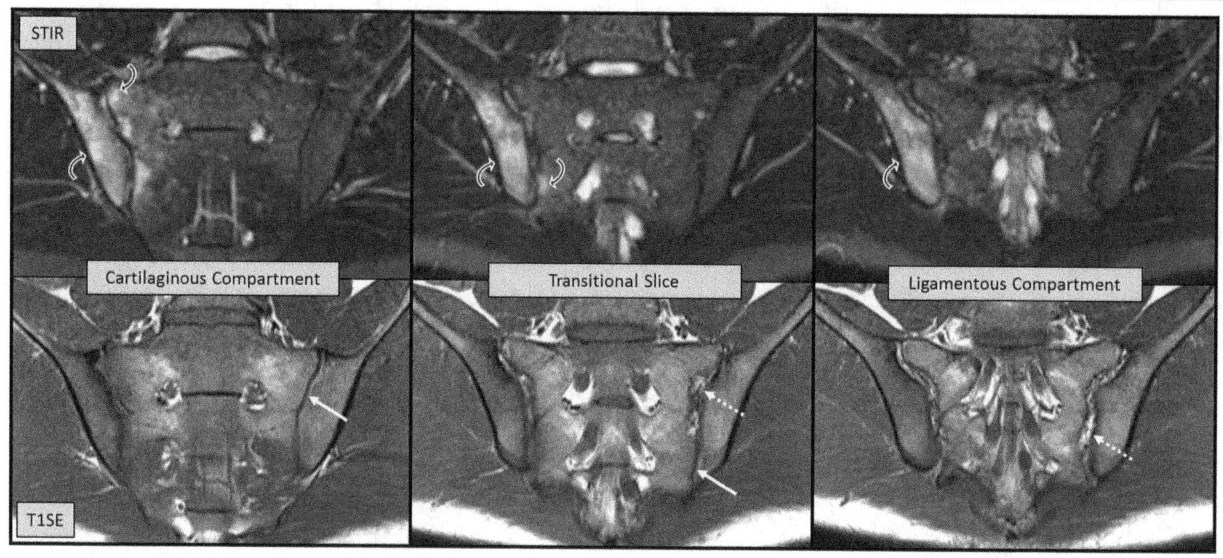

Fig. 1 MRI studies of a 22-year-old man, human leucocyte antigen B27-positive, with a 4-month history of inflammatory back pain. The radiographic modified New York criteria were not met, and C-reactive protein was 7 mg/l (reference limit ≤5 mg/l). The upper and lower rows show short tau inversion recovery (STIR) and corresponding T1 spin echo (T1SE) sequences, respectively. The left panel represents an MRI slice from the cartilaginous compartment (*solid white arrow* on T1SE), the right panel from the ligamentous compartment (*broken white arrow* on T1SE), and the central panel is a transitional slice containing parts of both the cartilaginous and ligamentous compartment (*solid and broken white arrows* on T1SE). The black and white pattern of the space between the ilium and the sacrum in the ligamentous compartment has its origin on the T1SE images in sacroiliac ligaments which have low MRI signal intensity surrounded by fat tissue which is bright on T1SE. On the STIR sequence, the ligamentous compartment is comprised of low signal ligaments and fat tissue as the fat signal is suppressed on STIR, and the bright signal relates to fluid in the lumen of blood vessels. In this patient with nonradiographic axial spondyloarthritis, bone marrow edema (*curved white and black arrows* on STIR) predominantly in the iliac part of the right sacroiliac joint extends from the cartilaginous into the ligamentous compartment

Methods

Subjects

The demographical and clinical characteristics of the study sample have been described elsewhere [23]. Two different approaches were used to recruit two inception cohorts of consecutive back pain patients aged ≤50 years newly referred to two university outpatient departments. Back pain patients referred by rheumatologists and primary care physicians for further evaluation of clinically suspected SpA were enrolled in cohort A (n = 69; University of Zurich). The same university clinic concomitantly recruited 20 age-matched healthy controls from hospital staff, defined by the Nordic questionnaire [24] and by absence of clinical features indicative for SpA. Patients of cohort B (n = 88; University of Alberta) presented with acute anterior uveitis (AAU) to a university ophthalmology department and were referred to rheumatology of the same university hospital for assessment of SpA if they indicated past or present back pain for ≥3 months on a structured questionnaire. Cohort A and B, being based on two different recruitment strategies, reflect more comprehensively the spectrum of SpA phenotypes seen in daily routine than would be by each cohort alone.

There is no standardized or generally accepted gold standard for imaging studies in axial SpA [25]. MRI cannot be used simultaneously for classification and for evaluating its diagnostic utility for reasons of conceptual circularity [26]. Rheumatologist expert opinion, which was consistently used as gold standard in three SpA classification criteria sets (Amor [27], European Spondylarthropathy Study Group (ESSG) [28], ASAS [1]), served as gold standard for diagnosis of axial SpA. In both inception cohorts, clinician expert opinion by one local rheumatologist (UW for cohort A and WPM for cohort B) based on clinical examination inclusive of standardized evaluation of inflammatory back pain according to Calin criteria [29] and of structured questionnaires on SpA-related features (modified Outcome in Ankylosing Spondylitis International Study (OASIS) protocol [30] for cohort A and Spondyloarthritis Research Consortium of Canada (SPARCC) protocol [31] for cohort B), pelvic radiographs and laboratory values (human leucocyte antigen B27 (HLA-B27), C-reactive protein (CRP)) served to classify the back pain patients as having nr-axSpA (n = 20 and 31 for cohorts A and B, respectively), ankylosing spondylitis (AS; n = 10 and 24 for cohorts A and B, respectively) and nonspecific back pain (NSBP; n = 39 and 33 for cohorts A and B, respectively). Two readers at each site independently categorized pelvic radiographs according to the modified New York criteria [32], and discrepancies were solved by consensus. Current or previous treatment with biologics was an exclusion criterion in both cohorts. The study protocols were approved by the local Ethics Review Boards (Ethics Committee of the University of Alberta, Edmonton, Canada; Kantonale Ethikkommission Zurich, Zurich, Switzerland) and written informed consent was obtained from the study participants.

Evaluation of magnetic resonance images

The technical parameters for short tau inversion recovery (STIR) and T1 spin echo (T1SE) sequences of semi-coronal MRI SIJ scans have been reported previously [17]. The MRI scans (1.5 T Avanto, Siemens Medical Solutions, Erlangen, Germany, for cohorts A and B) were read and scored independently by five blinded readers (one radiologist: VZ; four rheumatologists: SJP, UW, WPM and ZZ). The images of each cohort were evaluated separately in random order on electronic work stations, and MRI scores were entered into a customized online data entry module.

The evaluation of the cartilaginous compartment on SIJ MRI followed a standardized module [16, 17, 23] comprising two sections. The first section represented a global assessment indicating presence/absence of SpA according to both structural and active MRI features by viewing T1SE and STIR sequences simultaneously. The confidence in the global assessment was expressed by a numeric rating scale (NRS) score ranging from 0 (definitely nonSpA) to 10 (definitely SpA). The second section contained a detailed assessment recording BME and fat metaplasia according to standardized lesion definitions and a reference SIJ MRI set developed by consensus amongst study investigators [33]. BME and fat metaplasia in the bone marrow of the cartilaginous joint compartment were recorded as present/absent in each quadrant (upper and lower ilium, upper and lower sacrum) of each SIJ, based on evaluation of each MRI slice [17].

The assessment of the ligamentous compartment on SIJ MRI also comprised a global and a lesion-based section. Readers reported in the global section whether the additional evaluation of the ligamentous joint compartment provided an incremental value (expressed by the three categories "essential", "contributory" or "noncontributory") over and above the global assessment based on the cartilaginous joint compartment alone. Readers also recorded whether the additional evaluation of the ligamentous joint compartment changed diagnosis (from nonSpA to SpA or vice versa) or altered the confidence in a diagnosis of SpA based on MRI assessment of the cartilaginous compartment alone. The complex anatomy of the ligamentous joint compartment precluded an evaluation per joint quadrants. BME and fat metaplasia were recorded as present/absent if observed in bone marrow on any slice of the ligamentous compartment. Erosions were not scored in the ligamentous compartment because they cannot be discriminated reliably from physiological insertions of SIJ ligaments.

Statistical analysis

Data description

Differences in demographic and clinical characteristics between cohorts A and B were assessed by Fisher's exact test for nominal and Wilcoxon test for continuous variables. We calculated the mean percentage of patients and controls over five readers showing ≥1 BME or ≥1 fat metaplasia lesion (dichotomously indicating 'presence' or 'absence' of lesions) in the cartilaginous and ligamentous SIJ compartment, respectively.

Interobserver agreement on MRI lesions in both SIJ compartments

Interobserver reliability of MRI lesions was evaluated in both joint compartments because it might be expected that detection of lesions in the ligamentous compartment would be less reliable due to its more complex anatomy. Percent agreement (positive and negative concordance) among the 10 possible reader pairs for each group of study subjects, and weighted Cohen's kappa values for five readers jointly per cohort [34] were used to calculate the reproducibility of BME and fat metaplasia among the five readers for the cartilaginous and ligamentous SIJ compartments. Kappa values were not calculable for all categories of study subjects due to small sample sizes of n = 10–39 for nr-axSpA, AS, NSBP and healthy controls (HC) [35]. The inter-reader agreement was defined as slight, fair, moderate, substantial and almost perfect by values of the weighted Cohen's kappa $\kappa < 0.2$, $\kappa = 0.2\text{–} < 0.4$, $\kappa = 0.4\text{–} < 0.6$, $\kappa = 0.6\text{–} < 0.8$, and $\kappa = 0.8\text{–}1$, respectively [36]. For kappa values, we provide bootstrap confidence intervals based on 1000 bootstrap replications and computed at a confidence level of 95 %.

MRI lesions in the cartilaginous versus ligamentous joint compartment

We calculated the mean percentage of patients and controls over five readers who showed ≥1 MRI lesion both in the cartilaginous and ligamentous compartment, and in only one or in none of the two joint compartments, separately for BME and fat infiltration. The constellation of lesions observed solely in the ligamentous compartment without corresponding lesions in the cartilaginous compartment was further analyzed regarding agreement among the five readers.

Impact of the ligamentous joint compartment on classification

We calculated the mean percentage of patients and controls over five readers where the additional evaluation of the ligamentous compartment was regarded as essential, contributory or noncontributory for diagnosis of SpA versus nonSpA beyond the assessment of the cartilaginous compartment alone. We further analyzed whether the additional evaluation of the ligamentous compartment led to a switch in diagnosis (assessment of the cartilaginous compartment alone indicating nonSpA that changes to SpA by additional evaluation of the ligamentous compartment). We also assessed how often confidence in diagnosis of SpA increased from 5–7 to 8–10 following additional evaluation of the ligamentous compartment, and we expressed this as mean percentage of patients and controls over five readers.

We used R Core Team 2014, version 3.1.0, Vienna, Austria, for statistical analysis [37].

Results

Data description

Table 1 displays the characteristics of the two SpA inception cohorts representing a wide spectrum of SpA phenotypes. The two strategies to recruit patients with early SpA resulted in substantial demographical and clinical differences between the two cohorts, with cohort B having longer symptom duration and less disease activity. This disparity with regards to symptom duration, age of study participants and disease activity justified analysis of the two cohorts separately.

MRI bone marrow lesions were less frequent in the ligamentous than cartilaginous compartment, consistently across both cohorts, all study groups, and for both lesion types. Among nr-axSpA patients, BME in the ligamentous/cartilaginous compartment occurred in 42.0/83.0 % and 11.6/45.2 % for cohorts A and B, respectively, and fat metaplasia in 21.0/47.0 % and 25.2/43.9 %, respectively (Table 1). The same disparity was observed in AS patients, but with higher overall lesion frequencies. The disparity in MRI lesion frequency between the cartilaginous and the ligamentous compartment was particularly pronounced for BME in NSBP patients. In cohorts A and B, 27.7 and 27.9 % of NSBP patients had BME in the cartilaginous versus only 3.6 and 2.4 % in the ligamentous compartment, respectively.

In cohorts A and B, BME in the ligamentous compartment was recorded in 80.0 and 38.3 % of AS patients, respectively, compared to 42.0 and 11.6 % of nr-axSpA patients. Similarly, fat metaplasia in the ligamentous compartment was observed more often in AS (46.0 and 42.5 % for cohorts A and B, respectively) than in nr-ax-SpA (21.0 and 25.2 %, respectively) patients. However, a comparable difference in lesion frequency between AS and nr-axSpA groups was also recorded for the cartilaginous compartment. BME in the cartilaginous compartment was reported in 88.0 and 74.2 % of AS and 83.0 and 45.2 % of nr-axSpA patients in cohorts A and B, and fat metaplasia in 66.0 and 79.2 % of AS and 47.0 and 43.9 % of nr-axSpA patients.

Table 1 Demographical and clinical characteristics of two spondyloarthritis inception cohorts, and percentage of subjects with bone marrow edema or fat metaplasia in the cartilaginous and ligamentous compartments of the sacroiliac joints (mean percentage over five readers)

Cohort	A (n = 89)				B (n = 88)		
Recruitment mode	Suspected axial SpA by practising rheumatologists or PCP				AAU plus past or present back pain		
Group	nr-axSpA	AS	NSBP	HC	nr-axSpA	AS	NSBP
Number of subjects	20	10	39	20	31	24	33
Male:female (% male)	11:9 (55.0)	8:2 (80.0)	11:28 (28.2)	7:13 (35.0)	17:14 (54.8)	11:13 (45.8)	17:16 (51.5)
Age (years)	32.2 (12.3)	30.0 (9.5)*	32.7 (11.5)	30.6 (6.5)	36.2 (12.1)	41.5 (7.1)*	33.6 (15.7)
Symptom duration (years)	1.3 (1.8)*	3.9 (1.8)*	NA	NA	10.0 (14.0)*	12.5 (13.5)*	NA
HLA B27 positive (%)	12 (60.0)	9 (90.0)	ND	ND	24 (80.0)[b]	21 (87.5)	10 (55.6)[b]
BASDAI (NRS)	4.4 (3.1)[a]	5.4 (1.5)[a]	NA	NA	3.5 (4.4)	2.0 (3.4)[b]	NA
BASFI (NRS)	1.8 (3.9)*[a]	2.7 (1.5)[a]	NA	NA	0.8 (2.3)*	0.6 (2.8)[b]	NA
CRP (mg/l)	4.0 (4.5)[a]	5.0 (8.0)[a]	ND	ND	2.7 (5.2)	8.0 (8.7)[b]	0.9 (0.9)[b]
BME cart	83.0	88.0	27.7	34.0	45.2	74.2	27.9
BME lig	42.0	80.0	3.6	6.0	11.6	38.3	2.4
Fat cart	47.0	66.0	29.2	18.0	43.9	79.2	22.4
Fat lig	21.0	46.0	17.9	12.0	25.2	42.5	9.1

Values for patient characteristics are the median (interquartile range; expressed as difference between first and third quartile) unless otherwise stated

*$P \leq 0.05$ (Fisher's exact test) between cohorts A and B

[a]Cohort A: CRP values are based on 18, and BASDAI/BASFI values on 19 patients with nr-axSpA, respectively; BASDAI/BASFI and CRP values are based on 9 patients with AS

[b]Cohort B: HLA B27 values are based on 30 patients with nr-axSpA; BASDAI/BASFI and CRP values are based on 22 patients with AS; in NSBP patients, HLA B27 and CRP values are based on 18 subjects; the prevalence of HLA B27 in patients with AAU in general is 50–60 % [41]

AAU Acute anterior uveitis, *AS* Ankylosing spondylitis, *BASDAI* Bath Ankylosing Spondylitis Disease Activity Index, *BASFI* Bath Ankylosing Spondylitis Functional Index, *BME* Bone marrow edema, *Cart* Cartilaginous compartment of the sacroiliac joint, *CRP* C-reactive protein (reference range ≤5 mg/l), *Fat* Fat metaplasia, *HC* Healthy control, *HLA B27* Human leucocyte antigen B27, *Lig* Ligamentous compartment of the sacroiliac joint, *NA* Not applicable, *ND* Not done, *nr-axSpA* Nonradiographic axial spondyloarthritis, *NRS* Numeric rating scale, *NSBP* Nonspecific back pain, *PCP* Primary care physician

Interobserver agreement on MRI lesions in both joint compartments

Agreement by percent concordance among 10 possible reader pairs for BME and fat metaplasia showed no systematic discrepancies between the two joint compartments across both cohorts (Table 2). In cohort A, Cohen's kappa over five readers jointly for BME was substantial and comparable for the cartilaginous (kappa = 0.66) and ligamentous (kappa = 0.68) compartment. In cohort B, kappa for BME was substantial in the cartilaginous compartment (0.64), but fair for the ligamentous compartment (0.37). In cohorts A and B, Cohen's kappa for fat metaplasia was moderate in the cartilaginous compartment (0.40/0.51 in cohorts A and B, respectively) and fair for the ligamentous compartment (0.36/0.39 in cohorts A and B, respectively).

MRI lesions in the cartilaginous versus ligamentous joint compartment

MRI lesions occurring concomitantly in the cartilaginous and ligamentous SIJ compartment were recorded more frequently in AS than in nr-axSpA patients, both for BME and fat metaplasia and across both cohorts A and B (BME: 80.0 and 37.5 % in AS, and 42.0 and 11.6 % in nr-axSpA; fat metaplasia: 42.0 and 41.7 % in AS, and 21.0 and 25.2 % in nr-axSpA, respectively) (Table 3). By contrast, concomitant BME in both joint compartments was consistently very rare in controls of both cohorts A and B (NSBP patients 2.1 and 2.4 %; healthy controls in cohort A 4.0 %). Thus, the constellation of concomitant BME lesions in both the cartilaginous and ligamentous compartment showed more frequently in nr-axSpA (42.0 and 11.6 %) than in NSBP patients (2.1 and 2.4 %) in cohorts A and B. BME or fat metaplasia lesions solely in the ligamentous compartment were virtually absent for all groups of study subjects across both cohorts (0–2.0 % for BME and 0–4.0 % for fat metaplasia, respectively), and they were never recorded at the same site by more than one out of five readers.

Impact of the ligamentous joint compartment on diagnosis

The additional evaluation of the ligamentous compartment for diagnosis of SpA versus nonSpA over and above the assessment of the cartilaginous compartment alone was regarded as essential by one single reader in one nr-axSpA patient of cohort B enhancing the confidence in a diagnosis of SpA from 7 to 10 on a NRS ranging from 0–10 (Table 4). Otherwise none of the ligamentous joint assessments in any of the two cohorts

Table 2 Agreement as percent concordance among 10 possible reader pairs for each group of study subjects (kappa values for five readers jointly per cohort)

Cohort	A (n=89)				B (n=88)		
Group	nr-axSpA	AS	NSBP	HC	nr-axSpA	AS	NSBP
Number of subjects	20	10	39	20	31	24	33
Percent concordance among 10 reader pairs[a]							
Total (positive/negative)							
BME cart	88.0 (77.0/11.0)	88.0 (82.0/6.0)	78.5 (16.9/61.5)	85.0 (26.5/58.5)	78.1 (34.2/43.9)	78.3 (63.3/15.0)	86.7 (20.6/66.1)
BME lig	78.0 (31.0/47.0)	92.0 (76.0/16.0)	93.8 (0.5/93.3)	89.0 (0.5/88.5)	87.7 (5.5/82.3)	61.7 (19.2/42.5)	97.0 (0.9/96.1)
Fat cart	69.0 (31.5/37.5)	64.0 (48.0/16.0)	74.9 (16.7/58.2)	74.0 (5.0/69.0)	76.8 (32.3/44.5)	70.8 (64.6/6.3)	76.4 (10.6/65.8)
Fat lig	77.0 (9.5/67.5)	64.0 (28.0/36.0)	82.1 (9.0/73.1)	86.0 (5.0/81.0)	77.4 (13.9/63.5)	60.8 (22.9/37.9)	89.1 (3.6/85.5)
Kappa value for five readers jointly (95 % CI)[b]							
BME cart	0.66 (0.56–0.75)				0.64 (0.53–0.72)		
BME lig	0.68 (0.55–-0.79)				0.37 (0.26–0.45)		
Fat cart	0.40 (0.32–0.49)				0.51 (0.42–0.60)		
Fat lig	0.36 (0.25–0.45)				0.39 (0.25–0.51)		

[a]Percent concordance among 10 possible reader pairs (100 % = 10 concordant reader pairs); Total = positive and negative concordance for presence/absence of BME or fat metaplasia in the cartilaginous and ligamentous compartment of the sacroiliac joints
[b]Weighted Cohen's kappa values for all five readers jointly
AS Ankylosing spondylitis, *BME* Bone marrow edema, *Cart* Cartilaginous compartment of the sacroiliac joint, *CI* 95 % confidence interval, *Fat* Fat metaplasia, *HC* Healthy control, *Lig* Ligamentous compartment of the sacroiliac joint, *nr-axSpA* Nonradiographic axial spondyloarthritis, *NSBP* Nonspecific back pain, *R* Reader, *RP* Reader pair

were reported to be essential by the five readers. In only 28.0 and 7.7 % of nr-axSpA patients in cohorts A and B, respectively, was the evaluation of the ligamentous compartment considered contributory to diagnosis. The additional assessment of the ligamentous compartment was regarded as noncontributory for diagnosis in 72.0 and 91.6 % of nr-axSpA patients in cohorts A and B.

Table 3 Bone marrow edema and fat metaplasia in the cartilaginous versus ligamentous sacroiliac joint compartment (mean percentage of subjects over five readers)

Cohort	A (n=89)				B (n=88)		
Group	nr-axSpA	AS	NSBP	HC	nr-axSpA	AS	NSBP
Number of subjects	20	10	39	20	31	24	33
BME cart+/lig+	42.0	80.0	2.1	4.0	11.6	37.5	2.4
BME cart+/lig−	41.0	8.0	25.6	30.0	33.5	36.7	25.5
BME cart−/lig+	0	0	1.5[a]	2.0[a]	0	0.8[a]	0
BME cart−/lig−	17.0	12.0	70.8	64.0	54.8	25.0	72.1
Fat cart+/lig+	21.0	42.0	17.4	12.0	25.2	41.7	8.5
Fat cart+/lig−	26.0	24.0	11.8	6.0	18.7	37.5	13.9
Fat cart−/lig+	0	4.0[b]	0.5[b]	0	0	0.8[b]	0.6[b]
Fat cart−/lig−	53.0	30.0	70.3	82.0	56.1	20.0	77.0

[a]BME cart−/lig+: three NSBP patients and two HC by one single reader in cohort A; one AS patient by one reader in cohort B
[b]Fat cart−/lig+: two AS and one NSBP patient by three different readers in cohort A; one AS and one NSBP patient by two different readers in cohort B
AS Ankylosing spondylitis, *BME* Bone marrow edema, *Cart* Cartilaginous compartment of the sacroiliac joint, *Fat* Fat metaplasia, *HC* Healthy control, *Lig* Ligamentous compartment of the sacroiliac joint, *nr-axSpA* Nonradiographic axial spondyloarthritis, *NSBP* Nonspecific back pain

None of the ligamentous joint assessments led to a change in diagnosis.

Discussion

In two SpA inception cohorts reflecting routine practice with broad variation of symptom duration and disease activity, assessment of the ligamentous compartment on SIJ MRI provided no incremental value for diagnosis of axial SpA compared to the traditional evaluation of the cartilaginous SIJ compartment alone. Redundancy of MRI lesions in the ligamentous and cartilaginous compartment is the most likely explanation: nearly all SpA and control subjects having BME and/or fat metaplasia in the bone marrow of the ligamentous SIJ compartment showed the same lesion also in the cartilaginous compartment. However, concomitant BME in the cartilaginous and ligamentous compartments was observed more frequently in nr-axSpA than in NSBP patients (sensitivity/specificity 0.42/0.98 and 0.12/0.98 for cohorts A and B, respectively), which may assist towards discrimination of the two conditions (Figs. 1 and 2).

Lesions in the ligamentous SIJ compartment were more frequently reported in AS than in nr-axSpA patients. This observation is in agreement with the findings of an earlier retrospective study, which reported BME in enthesial SIJ structures more commonly in AS (40–86 %) than in patients with early undifferentiated SpA (26–43 %) [10]. A study recruiting 37 patients who fulfilled the ESSG criteria showed a statistically significant association of ligamentous SIJ inflammation with AS according to the

Table 4 Impact of assessment of the ligamentous sacroiliac joint compartments on diagnosis of SpA versus nonSpA (mean percentage of subjects over five readers)

Cohort	A (n=89)				B (n=88)		
Group	nr-axSpA	AS	NSBP	HC	nr-axSpA	AS	NSBP
Number of subjects	20	10	39	20	31	24	33
Lig essential for diagnosis of SpA vs Non-SpA	0	0	0	0	0.6[c]	0	0
Lig contributory for diagnosis of SpA vs Non-SpA	28.0	64.0	2.1	1.0	7.7	26.7	0
Lig non-contributory for diagnosis of SpA vs Non-SpA	72.0	36.0	97.9	99.0	91.6	73.3	100
Lig inducing change in diagnosis[a]	0	0	0	0	0	0	0
Lig inducing increase in confidence in diagnosis[b]	0	0	0	0	0.6[c]	0	0

[a]Change in diagnosis: assessment of the cartilaginous compartment alone indicating nonSpA (confidence 0–5) changed to SpA (confidence 5–10) by additional evaluation of the ligamentous compartment
[b]Increase in confidence of diagnosis: confidence in diagnosis of SpA increased from 5–7 to 8–10 following additional evaluation of the ligamentous compartment
[c]One nr-axSpA patient by one reader in cohort B
AS Ankylosing spondylitis, *HC* Healthy control, *Lig* Ligamentous compartment of the sacroiliac joint, *nr-axSpA* Nonradiographic axial spondyloarthritis, *NSBP* Nonspecific back pain, *SpA* Spondyloarthritis

modified New York criteria [21]. These earlier data suggested that inflammation in the ligamentous SIJ compartment may be indicative of longstanding rather than early disease. However, our findings question this hypothesis as we observed a comparable difference in lesion frequency between nr-axSpA and AS groups also in the cartilaginous compartment suggesting an overall accumulation of inflammatory lesions in both compartments over time. Only a follow-up study assessing both SIJ compartments longitudinally has the potential to clarify this issue.

Agreement for BME was substantial both in the cartilaginous and ligamentous compartment (kappa for five readers jointly 0.66 and 0.68, respectively) in cohort A. In cohort B, agreement was substantial in the cartilaginous compartment (kappa 0.64) and fair in the ligamentous compartment (kappa 0.37), the latter finding possibly attributable to a much lower frequency of ligamentous BME lesions compared to cohort A. A Dutch study on SIJ MRI in 68 patients with inflammatory back pain, but lacking a control group, showed comparable agreement on BME in the cartilaginous compartment (kappa for two readers for right/left SIJ 0.73/0.65), but a lower agreement in the ligamentous compartment (kappa for right/left SIJ 0.49/0.38) [38]. In our study, agreement for fat metaplasia in both joint compartments was lower than for BME.

An additional assessment of the ligamentous SIJ compartment provided no incremental value for diagnosis of axial SpA nor for confidence with this diagnosis over

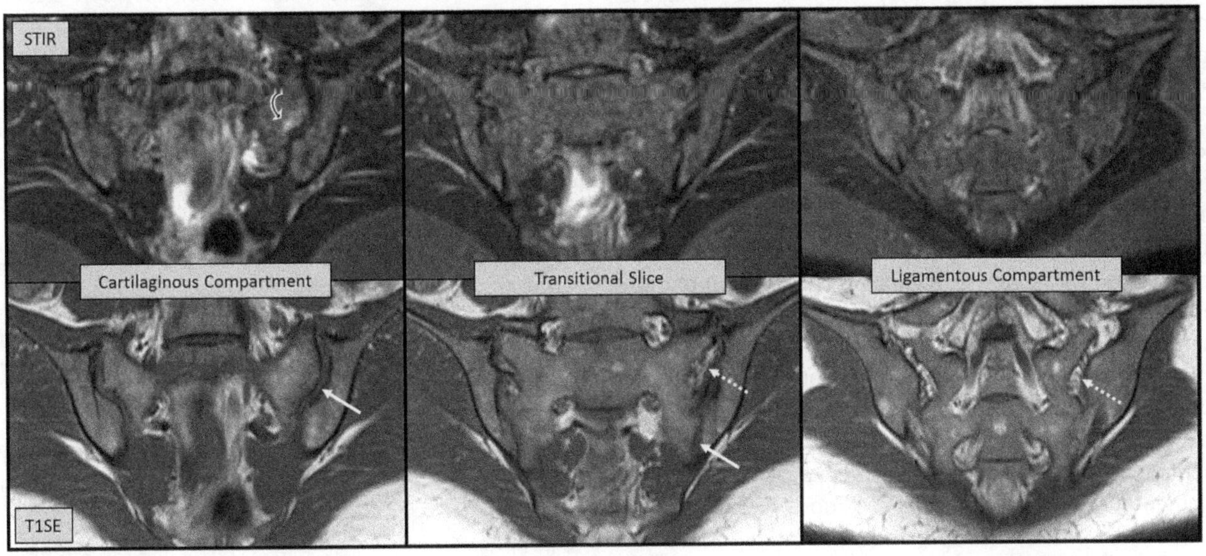

Fig. 2 Thirty-one-year-old woman with remitting mechanical back pain over several years. The sacral part of the left sacroiliac joint in the cartilaginous compartment demonstrates increased signal intensity compatible with bone marrow edema (*curved white and black arrows* on STIR), which is not visible on the transitional slice nor in the ligamentous compartment. See legend to Fig. 1 for details on the structure of the figure. *STIR* short tau inversion recovery, *T1SE* T1 spin echo

and above the traditional approach, in which only the cartilaginous compartment of the SIJ is evaluated. This finding is most likely due to a nearly complete redundancy between ligamentous and cartilaginous SIJ MRI lesions. There was virtually no isolated inflammation in the ligamentous SIJ compartment alone without associated lesions in the cartilaginous compartment. This observation is in line with the results of a previous report in which only 1 of 37 patients fulfilling the ESSG criteria showed isolated inflammation of just the ligamentous SIJ compartment [21]. However, in our study, concomitant BME lesions both in the cartilaginous and ligamentous compartment showed more frequently in nr-axSpA (12–42 %) than in NSBP patients (2 %). If confirmed by other studies, this MRI feature may facilitate the clinically often challenging discrimination between the two conditions.

A study limitation shared with most other evaluation modules of SIJ MRI is the lack of additional semi-axial slices, as proposed by the Danish working group [3, 20–22, 39]. Semi-axial slices running perpendicularly to the long axis of the SIJ, in contrast to the traditional semi-coronal imaging of the SIJ, may permit a more precise anatomical localization of MRI lesions by simultaneous visualization of both compartments and their anatomical border on the same image [3, 20]. Both sequences viewed together facilitate the identification of normal MRI features and variants that may mimic SpA-associated inflammatory SIJ lesions on the semi-coronal plane alone [3], such as normal vascular structures mimicking BME or the normal variant of a bipartite ilium suggesting erosion by semi-coronal slices only [2]. An additional semi-axial plane may also help to recognize partial volume artifacts between the cartilaginous and the ligamentous compartment, which may be misinterpreted as erosion on semi-coronal images alone [40].

However, data are lacking whether additional semi-axial slices facilitate evaluation of the ligamentous compartment leading to enhanced diagnostic utility of SIJ MRI in nr-axSpA. Two of our findings, that question a potentially relevant role of additional semi-axial slices, are the low frequency of ligamentous SIJ inflammation in early disease, and the very high association of inflammatory features in both compartments. Another challenge is the technically difficult assessment of the ligamentous compartment. Its irregular contour prevents a quadrant-based evaluation similar to the cartilaginous compartment, and defining a reproducible demarcation where the ligamentous compartment ends posteriorly is challenging.

Conclusion

Assessment of MRI bone marrow lesions in the ligamentous SIJ compartment provided no incremental value towards diagnosis of nr-axSpA. Moreover, it did not enhance confidence in the diagnosis over and above the traditional evaluation of the cartilaginous compartment alone, when using semi-coronal images. The most likely explanation was a high level of redundancy with MRI BME and fat metaplasia lesions occurring concomitantly in the ligamentous and cartilaginous compartments. However, BME observed simultaneously in both SIJ compartments might facilitate the clinically relevant discrimination between nr-axSpA and NSBP patients because the latter showed concomitant inflammation in both compartments only very rarely.

Abbreviations

AAU: Acute anterior uveitis; AS: Ankylosing spondylitis; ASAS: Assessment of SpondyloArthritis International Society; BME: Bone marrow edema; CRP: C-reactive protein; ESSG: European Spondylarthropathy Study Group; HC: Healthy controls; HLA B27: Human leucocyte antigen B27; MRI: Magnetic resonance imaging; nr-axSpA: Non-radiographic axial spondyloarthritis; NRS: Numeric rating scale; NSBP: Nonspecific back pain; OASIS: Outcome in Ankylosing Spondylitis International Study; SIJ: Sacroiliac joints; SpA: Spondyloarthritis; SPARCC: Spondyloarthritis Research Consortium of Canada; STIR: Short tau inversion recovery; T1SE: T1 spin echo.

Competing interests

The authors declare that they have no competing interests.

Authors' contributions

UW drafted the study design, acquired clinical data, was an MRI reader, performed the statistical analysis, and drafted the manuscript. WPM drafted the study design, acquired clinical data, was an MRI reader, and helped draft the manuscript. SMC participated in drafting the study design, acquired clinical data, and helped draft the manuscript. KR participated in drafting the study design, performed the statistical analysis, and helped draft the manuscript. SJP participated in drafting the study design, was an MRI reader, and helped draft the manuscript. ZZ participated in drafting the study design, was an MRI reader, and helped draft the manuscript. VZ participated in drafting the study design, was an MRI reader, and helped draft the manuscript. MØ participated in drafting the study design and the manuscript. RGWL drafted the study design and helped draft the manuscript. All authors take responsibility for interpretation of data. All authors read and approved the final manuscript.

Authors' information

KR is founder and owner of Rufibach rePROstat and is an employee of F. Hoffmann-La Roche, Basel, Switzerland.

Acknowledgements

The authors thank the patients and the healthy volunteers for their participation; Tracey Clare, Clinical Research Manager, Department of Radiology, University of Alberta; Paul Filipow, Data Manager, Edmonton, Canada, and Joel Paschke, Information Manager Canadian Research Education (CaRE) Arthritis, Edmonton, Canada for coordinating the Web-based MRI scoring module.

Funding statement

The Canadian Arthritis Society: National Research Initiative Award. Alberta Innovates Health Solutions. Walter L. and Johanna Wolf Foundation, Zurich, Switzerland.

Author details

[1]King Christian 10th Hospital for Rheumatic Diseases, Gråsten, and Sygehus, Sønderjylland, Denmark. [2]Institute of Regional Health Research, University of Southern Denmark, Odense, Denmark. [3]Department of Rheumatology, Balgrist University Hospital, Zurich, Switzerland. [4]Department of Medicine, University of Alberta, Edmonton, AB, Canada. [5]Department of Ophthalmology, University of Alberta, Edmonton, Alberta, Canada. [6]Rufibach rePROstat, Biostatistical Consulting and Training, Engelgasse 123, 4052 Basel, Switzerland. [7]Copenhagen Center for Arthritis Research Center for Rheumatology and Spine Diseases, Rigshospitalet, Glostrup, and, Department

of Clinical Medicine, University of Copenhagen, Copenhagen, Denmark.
[8]Department of Rheumatology, PLA General Hospital, Beijing, China.
[9]Department of Radiology, Balgrist University Hospital, Zurich, Switzerland.
[10]Department of Radiology and Diagnostic Imaging, University of Alberta, Edmonton, Alberta, Canada.

References

1. Rudwaleit M, van der Heijde D, Landewé R, Listing J, Akkoc N, Brandt J, et al. The development of Assessment of SpondyloArthritis international Society classification criteria for axial spondyloarthritis (part II): validation and final selection. Ann Rheum Dis. 2009;68:777–83.
2. Puhakka KB, Melsen F, Jurik AG, Boel LW, Vesterby A, Egund N. MR imaging of the normal sacroiliac joint with correlation to histology. Skeletal Radiol. 2004;33:15–28.
3. Egund N, Jurik AG. Anatomy and histology of the sacroiliac joints. Semin Musculoskelet Radiol. 2014;18:332–40.
4. Ahlström H, Feltelius N, Nyman R, Hällgren R. Magnetic resonance imaging of sacroiliac joint inflammation. Arthritis Rheum. 1990;33:1763–9.
5. Murphey MD, Wetzel LH, Bramble JM, Levine E, Simpson KM, Lindsley HB. Sacroiliitis: MR imaging findings. Radiology. 1991;180:239–44.
6. Hanly JG, Mitchell MJ, Barnes DC, MacMillan L. Early recognition of sacroiliitis by magnetic resonance imaging and single photon emission computed tomography. J Rheumatol. 1994;21:2088–95.
7. Bollow M, Braun J, Hamm B, Eggens U, Schilling A, König H, et al. Early sacroiliitis in patients with spondyloarthropathy: evaluation with dynamic gadolinium-enhanced MR imaging. Radiology. 1995;194:529–36.
8. Remy M, Bouillet P, Bertin P, Leblanche AF, Bonnet C, Pascaud JL, et al. Évaluation de l'imagerie par résonance magnétique (IRM) pour la détection de sacro-iliite au cours des stades précoces des spondylarthropathies séronégatives. Rev Rhum Ed Fr. 1996;63:677–83.
9. François RJ, Gardner DL, Degrave EJ, Bywaters EGL. Histopathologic evidence that sacroiliitis in ankylosing spondylitis is not merely enthesitis. Arthritis Rheum. 2000;43:2011–24.
10. Muche B, Bollow M, François RJ, Sieper J, Hamm B, Braun J. Anatomic structures involved in early- and late-stage sacroiliitis in spondyloarthritis: a detailed analysis by contrast-enhanced magnetic resonance imaging. Arthritis Rheum. 2003;48:1374–84.
11. Bollow M, Hermann KGA, Biedermann T, Sieper J, Schöntube M, Braun J. Very early spondyloarthritis: where the inflammation in the sacroiliac joints starts. Ann Rheum Dis. 2005;64:1644–6.
12. Weber U, Pfirrmann CWA, Kissling RO, MacKenzie CR, Khan MA. Early spondyloarthritis in an HLA-B27-positive monozygotic twin pair: a highly concordant onset, sites of involvement, and disease course. J Rheumatol. 2008;35:1464–6.
13. Hermann KGA, Braun J, Fischer T, Reisshauer A, Bollow M. Magnetic resonance tomography of sacroiliitis: anatomy, histological pathology, MR-morphology, and grading [in German]. Radiologe. 2004;44:217–28.
14. Maksymowych WP, Inman RD, Salonen D, Dhillon SS, Williams M, Stone M, et al. Spondyloarthritis Research Consortium of Canada magnetic resonance imaging index for assessment of sacroiliac joint inflammation in ankylosing spondylitis. Arthritis Rheum (Arthritis Care Res). 2005;53:703–9.
15. Marzo-Ortega H, McGonagle D, O'Connor P, Hensor EM, Bennett AN, Green MJ, et al. Baseline and 1-year magnetic resonance imaging of the sacroiliac joint and lumbar spine in very early inflammatory back pain. Relationship between symptoms, HLA-B27 and disease extent and persistence. Ann Rheum Dis. 2009;68:1721–7.
16. Maksymowych WP, Dhillon SS, Chiowchanwisawakit P, Pedersen SJ, Martinez B, Østergaard M, et al. Development and validation of web-based training modules for systematic evaluation of active inflammatory lesions in the spine and sacroiliac joints in spondyloarthritis. J Rheumatol. 2009;36 Suppl 84:48–57.
17. Weber U, Lambert RGW, Østergaard M, Hodler J, Pedersen SJ, Maksymowych WP. The diagnostic utility of magnetic resonance imaging in spondylarthritis. An international multicenter evaluation of one hundred eighty-seven subjects. Arthritis Rheum. 2010;62:3048–58.
18. Althoff CE, Sieper J, Song IH, Haibel H, Weiss A, Diekhoff T, et al. Active inflammation and structural change in early active axial spondyloarthritis as detected by whole-body MRI. Ann Rheum Dis. 2013;72:967–73.
19. Maksymowych WP, Wichuk S, Chiowchanwisawakit P, Lambert RG, Pedersen SJ. Development and preliminary validation of the Spondyloarthritis Research Consortium of Canada magnetic resonance imaging sacroiliac joint structural score. J Rheumatol. 2015;42:79–86.
20. Puhakka KB, Jurik AG, Egund N, Schiøttz-Christensen B, Stengaard-Pedersen K, van Overeem HG, et al. Imaging of sacroiliitis in early seronegative spondylarthropathy. Assessment of abnormalities by MR in comparison with radiography and CT. Acta Radiol. 2003;44:218–29.
21. Madsen KB, Jurik AG. Magnetic resonance imaging grading system for active and chronic spondyloarthritis changes in the sacroiliac joint. Arthritis Care Res (Hoboken). 2010;62:11–8.
22. Arnbak B, Jensen TS, Manniche C, Zejden A, Egund N, Jurik AG. Spondyloarthritis-related and degenerative MRI changes in the axial skeleton—an inter- and intra-observer agreement study. BMC Musculoskelet Disord. 2013;14:274.
23. Weber U, Østergaard M, Lambert RGW, Pedersen SJ, Chan SM, Zubler V, et al. Candidate lesion-based criteria for defining a positive sacroiliac joint MRI in two cohorts of patients with axial spondyloarthritis. Ann Rheum Dis. 2014; doi:10.1136/annrheumdis-2014-205408.
24. Kuorinka I, Jonsson B, Kilbom A, Vinterberg H, Biering-Sorensen F, Andersson G, et al. Standardised Nordic questionnaires for the analysis of musculoskeletal symptoms. Appl Ergon. 1987;18:233–7.
25. Weber U, Maksymowych WP. Advances and challenges in spondyloarthritis imaging for diagnosis and assessment of disease. Curr Rheumatol Rep. 2013;15:345.
26. Landewé RBM. Magnetic resonance imaging in the diagnosis of ankylosing spondylitis: be aware of gold standards and circularity. J Rheumatol. 2010;37:477–8.
27. Amor B, Dougados M, Mijiyawa M. Criteria for the classification of spondyloarthropathies [in French]. Rev Rhum Mal Osteoartic. 1990;57:85–9.
28. Dougados M, van der Linden S, Juhlin R, Huitfeldt B, Amor B, Calin A, et al. The European Spondylarthropathy Study Group preliminary criteria for the classification of spondylarthropathy. Arthritis Rheum. 1991;34:1218–27.
29. Calin A, Porta J, Fries JF, Schurman DJ. Clinical history as a screening test for ankylosing spondylitis. JAMA. 1977;237:2613–4.
30. Ciurea A, Scherer A, Exer P, Bernhard J, Dudler J, Beyeler B, et al. Tumor necrosis factor α inhibition in radiographic and nonradiographic axial spondyloarthritis: results from a large observational cohort. Arthritis Rheum. 2013;65:3096–106.
31. Gladman DD, Rahman P, Cook RJ, Shen H, Zummer M, Thomson G, et al. The spondyloarthritis research consortium of Canada registry for spondyloarthritis. J Rheumatol. 2011;38:1343–8.
32. Van der Linden S, Valkenburg HA, Cats A. Evaluation of diagnostic criteria for ankylosing spondylitis. A proposal for modification of the New York criteria. Arthritis Rheum. 1984;27:361–8.
33. CaRE Arthritis (Canadian Research and Education) website. URL https://www.carearthritis.com/Research_Collaborations.php.
34. Conger A. Integration and generalisation of kappas for multiple raters. Psychol Bull. 1980;88:322–8.
35. Flight L, Julious SA. The disagreeable behaviour of the kappa statistic. Pharmaceut Statist. 2015;14:74–8.
36. Landis J, Koch G. The measurement of observer agreement for categorical data. Biometrics. 1977;33:159–74.
37. R Core Team. R: A language and environment for statistical computing. Vienna, Austria: R foundation for statistical computing; 2014. http://www.R-project.org/.
38. Heuft-Dorenbosch L, Weijers R, Landewé R, van der Linden S, van der Heijde D. Magnetic resonance imaging changes of sacroiliac joints in patients with recent-onset inflammatory back pain: inter-reader reliability and prevalence of abnormalities. Arthritis Res Ther. 2006;8:R11.
39. Madsen KB, Schiøttz-Christensen B, Jurik AG. Prognostic significance of magnetic resonance imaging changes of the sacroiliac joints in spondyloarthritis—a follow-up study. J Rheumatol. 2010;37:1718–27.
40. Wittram C, Whitehouse GH. Normal variation in the magnetic resonance imaging appearances of the sacroiliac joints: pitfalls in the diagnosis of sacroiliitis. Clin Radiol. 1995;50:371–6.
41. Martin TM, Rosenbaum JT. An update on the genetics of HLA B27-associated acute anterior uveitis. Ocul Immunol Inflam. 2011;19:108–14.

Permissions

All chapters in this book were first published in AR&T, by BioMed Central; hereby published with permission under the Creative Commons Attribution License or equivalent. Every chapter published in this book has been scrutinized by our experts. Their significance has been extensively debated. The topics covered herein carry significant findings which will fuel the growth of the discipline. They may even be implemented as practical applications or may be referred to as a beginning point for another development.

The contributors of this book come from diverse backgrounds, making this book a truly international effort. This book will bring forth new frontiers with its revolutionizing research information and detailed analysis of the nascent developments around the world.

We would like to thank all the contributing authors for lending their expertise to make the book truly unique. They have played a crucial role in the development of this book. Without their invaluable contributions this book wouldn't have been possible. They have made vital efforts to compile up to date information on the varied aspects of this subject to make this book a valuable addition to the collection of many professionals and students.

This book was conceptualized with the vision of imparting up-to-date information and advanced data in this field. To ensure the same, a matchless editorial board was set up. Every individual on the board went through rigorous rounds of assessment to prove their worth. After which they invested a large part of their time researching and compiling the most relevant data for our readers.

The editorial board has been involved in producing this book since its inception. They have spent rigorous hours researching and exploring the diverse topics which have resulted in the successful publishing of this book. They have passed on their knowledge of decades through this book. To expedite this challenging task, the publisher supported the team at every step. A small team of assistant editors was also appointed to further simplify the editing procedure and attain best results for the readers.

Apart from the editorial board, the designing team has also invested a significant amount of their time in understanding the subject and creating the most relevant covers. They scrutinized every image to scout for the most suitable representation of the subject and create an appropriate cover for the book.

The publishing team has been an ardent support to the editorial, designing and production team. Their endless efforts to recruit the best for this project, has resulted in the accomplishment of this book. They are a veteran in the field of academics and their pool of knowledge is as vast as their experience in printing. Their expertise and guidance has proved useful at every step. Their uncompromising quality standards have made this book an exceptional effort. Their encouragement from time to time has been an inspiration for everyone.

The publisher and the editorial board hope that this book will prove to be a valuable piece of knowledge for researchers, students, practitioners and scholars across the globe.

List of Contributors

Karel Pavelka
Institute of Rheumatology and Department of Rheumatology, 1st Faculty of Medicine, Charles University, Prague, Czech Republic

Alan Kivitz
Altoona Center for Clinical Research, Duncansville, PA, USA

Eva Dokoupilova
Medical Plus, s.r.o., Uherske Hradiste, Czech Republic

Ricardo Blanco
Division of Rheumatology, Hospital Universitario Marqués de Valdecilla, Santander, Spain

Marco Maradiaga
Centro de Investigación de Tratamientos Innovadores de Sinaloa, Culiacán, México

Hasan Tahir
Barts Health NHS Trust, London, UK

Luminita Pricop, Aimee Readie and Brian Porter
Novartis Pharmaceuticals Corporation, East Hanover, NJ, USA

Yang Liu
Xi'an No.5 Hospital, Xi'an, People's Republic of China

Jiawen Xu
Department of Clinical Medicine, Health Science Center, Xi'an Jiaotong University, Xi'an, People's Republic of China

Mats Andersson
Novartis Pharma AG, Basel, Switzerland

Smriti K. Raychaudhuri
VA Medical Center Sacramento, Division of Rheumatology & Immunology, Sacramento, CA, USA

Siba P. Raychaudhuri
VA Medical Center Sacramento, Division of Rheumatology & Immunology, Sacramento, CA, USA
Division of Rheumatology, Allergy & Clinical immunology, University of California School of Medicine, Davis, & VA Medical Center Sacramento, Sacramento, CA, USA

Pauline Bakker, Floris van Gaalen and Désirée van der Heijde
Department of Rheumatology, Leiden University Medical Centre, RC Leiden, The Netherlands

Filip Van den Bosch
Department of Rheumatology, Leiden University Medical Centre, RC Leiden, The Netherlands
Department of Rheumatology, Ghent University Hospital, Ghent, Belgium

Anna Moltó and Maxime Dougados
Department of Rheumatology, Paris Descartes University, Hôpital Cochin, Paris, France
Inserm (U1153), Clinical Epidemiology and Biostatistics, Paris, France

Adrien Etcheto
Inserm (U1153), Clinical Epidemiology and Biostatistics, Paris, France

Robert Landewé
Department of Rheumatology, Amsterdam Medical Centre, Amsterdam, The Netherlands
Atrium Medical Centre, Heerlen, The Netherlands

Johanna M. W. Hazes
Department of Rheumatology, Erasmus MC, Wytemaweg 80, 3015 CN Rotterdam, The Netherlands

Lonneke van Hoeven and Angelique E. A. M. Weel
Department of Rheumatology, Erasmus MC, Wytemaweg 80, 3015 CN Rotterdam, The Netherlands
Department of Rheumatology, Maasstad Hospital, Maasstadweg 21, 3079 DZ Rotterdam, The Netherlands

Annelies E. R. C. H. Boonen
Department of Rheumatology, Maastricht University Medical Centre, P. Debyelaan 25, 6229 HX Maastricht, The Netherlands

Zineb Ez-Zaitouni, Andrea Hilkens, Désirée van der Heijde and Floris van Gaalen
Department of Rheumatology, Leiden University Medical Center, 2300 RC Leiden, The Netherlands

Laure Gossec
Sorbonne Universités, UPMC Univ Paris 06, GRC-08, Paris, France
Rheumatology Department, Pitie-Salpétrière Hospital, AP-HP, Paris, France

Inger Jorid Berg
Department of Rheumatology, Diakonhjemmet Hospital, Oslo, Norway

Robert Landewé
Department of Clinical Immunology and Rheumatology, Amsterdam Medical Center, Amsterdam, The Netherlands

Roberta Ramonda
Rheumatology Unit, Department of Medicine DIMED, University of Padova, Padova, Italy

Maxime Dougados
Paris Descartes University, Hôpital Cochin, Assistance Publique-Hôpitaux de Paris, INSERM (U1153): Epidémiologie Clinique et Biostatistiques, PRES Sorbonne Paris-Cité, Paris, France

Agnes Hartl, Joachim Sieper and Uta Syrbe
Department of Gastroenterology, Infectiology and Rheumatology, Charité Universitätsmedizin Berlin, Hindenburgdamm 30, 12203 Berlin, Germany

Denis Poddubnyy
Department of Gastroenterology, Infectiology and Rheumatology, Charité Universitätsmedizin Berlin, Hindenburgdamm 30, 12203 Berlin, Germany
German Rheumatism Research Centre, Charitéplatz 1, 10117 Berlin, Germany

Joachim Listing
German Rheumatism Research Centre, Charitéplatz 1, 10117 Berlin, Germany

Kay-Geert Hermann
Department of Radiology, Charité Universitätsmedizin Berlin, Charitéplatz 1, 10117 Berlin, Germany

Martin Rudwaleit
Klinikum Bielefeld Rosenhöhe, An der Rosenhöhe 27, 33647 Bielefeld, Germany

Jiangcan Hao, Wenyu Wang, Yan Wen, Awen He, Qianrui Fan, Xiong Guo and Feng Zhang
Key Laboratory of Trace Elements and Endemc Diseases of National Health and Family Planning Commission, School of Public Health, Health Science Center, Xi'an Jiaotong University, Xi'an, People's Republic of China

Nilasha Ghosh and Eric M. Ruderman
Northwestern University Feinberg School of Medicine, 675 North St. Clair, Suite 14-100, Chicago, IL 60611, USA

Caroline Béal
Rheumatology Department, Cochin Hospital, AP-HP, París, France

Natalia Bello
Rheumatology Department, Cochin Hospital, AP-HP, París, France
Rheumatology Department, Hospital General Universitario Gregorio Marañón, Madrid, Spain

Adrien Etcheto, Maxime Dougados and Anna Moltó
Rheumatology Department, Cochin Hospital, AP-HP, París, France
INSERM (U1153): Clinical Epidemiology and Biostatistics, PRES Sorbornne Paris-Cité, Paris, France

Liesbeth De Winter, Dana Quaden and Veerle Somers
Hasselt University, Biomedical Research Institute, and Transnationale Universiteit Limburg, Diepenbeek, Belgium, Martelarenlaan 42, 3500 Hasselt, Belgium

Piet Geusens
Hasselt University, Biomedical Research Institute, and Transnationale Universiteit Limburg, Diepenbeek, Belgium, Martelarenlaan 42, 3500 Hasselt, Belgium
Division of Rheumatology, Department of Internal Medicine, CAPHRI School for Public Health and Primary Care, Maastricht University Medical Center, Maastricht, 6200 MD Maastricht, The Netherlands
ReumaClinic, Genk, Bretheistraat 149, 3600 Genk, Belgium

Jürgen Braun
Rheumazentrum Ruhrgebiet, Herne, Germany

Matthew L. Stoll, S. Lou Bridges Jr, Maria I. Danila, Ranjit Kumar, Randy Q. Cron, Casey D. Morrow and Elliot J. Lefkowitz
University of Alabama at Birmingham, Birmingham, AL, USA

Pamela F. Weiss
Children's Hospital of Philadelphia, Philadelphia, PA, USA

Jennifer E. Weiss
Hackensack University Medical Center, Hackensack, NJ, USA

Peter A. Nigrovic
Boston Children's Hospital and Brigham and Women's Hospital, Boston, MA, USA

Barbara S. Edelheit
Connecticut Children's Medical Center, Hartford, CT, USA

Charles H. Spencer
Nationwide Children's Hospital, Columbus, OH, USA

Marilynn G. Punaro
Texas Scottish Rite Hospital, Dallas, TX, USA

Kenneth Schikler
University of Louisville, Louisville, KY, USA

Andreas Reiff
Children's Hospital of Los Angeles, Los Angeles, CA, USA

Pamela F. Weiss
Department of Pediatrics, Division of Rheumatology, Children's Hospital of Philadelphia, Philadelphia, PA, USA
Center for Pediatric Clinical Effectiveness (CPCE), Children's Hospital of Philadelphia, Philadelphia, PA, USA
Center for Clinical Epidemiology and Biostatistics, Perelman School of Medicine at the University of Pennsylvania, Philadelphia, PA, USA
The Children's Hospital of Philadelphia, Roberts Center for Pediatric Research, 2716 South Street, Room 11121, Philadelphia, PA 19146, USA

Nancy A. Chauvin and David M. Biko
Department of Radiology, Children's Hospital of Philadelphia, Philadelphia, PA, USA

Timothy G. Brandon
Department of Pediatrics, Division of Rheumatology, Children's Hospital of Philadelphia, Philadelphia, PA, USA
Center for Pediatric Clinical Effectiveness (CPCE), Children's Hospital of Philadelphia, Philadelphia, PA, USA

Rui Xiao
Center for Clinical Epidemiology and Biostatistics, Perelman School of Medicine at the University of Pennsylvania, Philadelphia, PA, USA

Walter P. Maksymowych
Department of Medicine, University of Alberta, Edmonton, AB, Canada
Canadian Research and Education (CaRE) Arthritis Organization, Edmonton, AB, Canada

Jacob L. Jaremko
Department of Radiology and Diagnostic Imaging, University of Alberta, Edmonton, AB, Canada

Robert G. Lambert
Department of Radiology and Diagnostic Imaging, University of Alberta, Edmonton, AB, Canada
Canadian Research and Education (CaRE) Arthritis Organization, Edmonton, AB, Canada

DJoel Paschke
Canadian Research and Education (CaRE) Arthritis Organization, Edmonton, AB, Canada

Désirée van der Heijde
Leiden University Medical Center, Leiden 2300 RC, The Netherlands

Joachim Sieper
Charité Universitätsmedizin Berlin, Berlin, Germany

Walter P. Maksymowych and Robert G. Lambert
University of Alberta, Edmonton, AB, Canada

Su Chen, Jaclyn K. Anderson and Aileen L. Pangan
AbbVie Inc., North Chicago, IL, USA

Maja Hojnik
AbbVie Inc., Ljubljana, Slovenia

Sungsin Jo, Young Lim Lee, Suman Kang, Bitnara Lee and Tae-Hwan Kim
Department of Rheumatology, Hanyang University Hospital for Rheumatic Diseases, 222-1, Wangsimni-ro, Seongdong-gu, Seoul 04763, Republic of Korea

Sang-Cheol Bae
Department of Rheumatology, Hanyang University Hospital for Rheumatic Diseases, 222-1, Wangsimni-ro, Seongdong-gu, Seoul 04763, Republic of Korea
Clinical Research Center for Rheumatoid Arthritis (CRCRA), Seoul, Republic of Korea

Sung Eun Wang
Hanyang Biomedical Research Institute, Hanyang University, Seoul, Republic of Korea

Jinil Han
Gencurix, Inc, Hanhwan Bizmetro 1, Guro 3-dong, Guro-gu, Seoul, Republic of Korea

Il-Hoon Sung
Department of Orthopedic Surgery, Hanyang University Hospital, Seoul, Republic of Korea

Ye-Soo Park
Department of Orthopedic Surgery, Hanyang University Hospital, Guri, Republic of Korea

Miranda van Lunteren, Sofia Ramiro, Désirée van der Heijde and Floris A. van Gaalen
Department of Rheumatology, Leiden University Medical Center, Leiden, the Netherlands

Augusta Ortolan
Department of Rheumatology, Leiden University Medical Center, Leiden, the Netherlands
Rheumatology Unit, Department of Medicine (DIMED), University of Padua, Padua, Italy

Roberta Ramonda
Rheumatology Unit, Department of Medicine (DIMED), University of Padua, Padua, Italy

Robert B. M. Landewé
Department of Rheumatology, Amsterdam Rheumatology and Immunology Center, Amsterdam, the Netherlands
Department of Rheumatology, Zuyderland Medical Center, Heerlen, the Netherlands

Hanne Dagfinrud
Department of Rheumatology, Diakonhjemmet Hospital, Oslo, Norway

Lennart T. H. Jacobsson
Department of Rheumatology, University of Gothenburg, Gothenburg, Sweden

Marta Arévalo, Jordi Gratacós Masmitjà, Mireia Moreno, Joan Calvet, Cristobal Orellana and Marta Larrosa
Rheumatology Department, Consorci Corporació Sanitària Parc Taulí, Institut d'Investigació i Innovació Parc Taulí I3PT, Universitat Autònoma de Barcelona, Parc Taulí s/n, 08208 Sabadell, Barcelona, Spain

Desirée Ruiz, Carmen Castro and Pilar Carreto
Rheumatology Department, Hospital General Universitario Reina Sofía/IMIBIC/Universidad de Córdoba, Córdoba, Spain

Lucy Law and Jeanette Beckman Rehnman
Department of Public Health and Clinical Medicine, Rheumatology, Umeå University, 901 87 Umeå, Sweden

Helena Forsblad-d'Elia
Department of Public Health and Clinical Medicine, Rheumatology, Umeå University, 901 87 Umeå, Sweden
Department of Rheumatology and Inflammation Research, Sahlgrenska Academy at University of Gothenburg, 405 30 Gothenburg, Sweden

Anna Deminger, Eva Klingberg and Lennart T. H. Jacobsson
Department of Rheumatology and Inflammation Research, Sahlgrenska Academy at University of Gothenburg, 405 30 Gothenburg, Sweden

Janneke J. de Winter, Leonieke J. van Mens and Robert Landewé
Department of Clinical Immunology and Rheumatology, Amsterdam Rheumatology and immunology Center, Academic Medical Center/ University of Amsterdam, Meibergdreef 9, 1105, AZ, Amsterdam, The Netherlands

Dominique L. Baeten
Department of Clinical Immunology and Rheumatology, Amsterdam Rheumatology and immunology Center, Academic Medical Center/ University of Amsterdam, Meibergdreef 9, 1105, AZ, Amsterdam, The Netherlands
Department of Experimental Immunology, Academic Medical Center/University of Amsterdam, Amsterdam, The Netherlands

Désirée van der Heijde
Department of Rheumatology, Leiden University Medical Center, Leiden, The Netherlands

Natasja Stæhr Gudmann, Morten Asser Karsdal, Anne-Christine Bay-Jensen, Yi He and Anne Sofie Siebuhr
Nordic Bioscience Biomarkers and Research, Herlev Hovedgade 207, Herlev 2730, Denmark

Heidi Lausten Munk and Peter Junker
Department of Rheumatology, Odense University Hospital, Odense, Denmark

Anne Friesgaard Christensen
Department of Rheumatology, Vejle Hospital, Vejle, Denmark

Anne Gitte Loft
Department of Rheumatology, Vejle Hospital, Vejle, Denmark
Department of Rheumatology, Aarhus University Hospital, Aarhus, Denmark

Leif Ejstrup
Department of Rheumatology, Esbjerg Hospital, Esbjerg, Denmark

Grith Lykke Sørensen
Institute of Molecular Medicine, University of Southern Denmark, Odense, Denmark

Ulf Lindström, Mats Dehlin and Lennart Jacobsson
Department of Rheumatology and Inflammation Research, Institute of Medicine, Sahlgrenska Academy, University of Gothenburg, Guldhedsgatan 10A, 405 30 Gothenburg, Sweden

Sofia Exarchou
Section of Rheumatology, Department of Clinical Sciences, Lund University, 221 85 Lund, Sweden

Elisabeth Lie
Diakonhjemmet Hospital, Vinderen, 0319 Oslo, Norway.

Helena Forsblad-d'Elia
Institution of Public Health and Clinical Medicine/ Rheumatology, Umeå University, 901 87 Umeå, Sweden

Johan Askling
Rheumatology Unit & Clinical Epidemiology Unit, Department of Medicine Solna, Karolinska Institutet, Solna 171 76, Stockholm, Sweden

Karel Pavelka, Ladislav Senolt, Marketa Husakova and Hana Hulejova
Department of Rheumatology, First Faculty of Medicine, Charles University and Rheumatology Institute, Prague, Czech Republic

Andrea Levitova and Maja Spiritovic
Department of Rheumatology, First Faculty of Medicine, Charles University and Rheumatology Institute, Prague, Czech Republic
Charles University, Faculty of Physical Education and Sport, Prague, Czech Republic

Robert D. Inman
Department of Immunology, University of Toronto, Toronto, ON, Canada
Department of Medicine, University of Toronto, Toronto, ON, Canada

Xenofon Baraliakos and Jürgen Braun
Department of Rheumatology, Rheumazentrum Ruhrgebiet Herne, Ruhr-University Bochum, Herne, Germany

Kay-Geert A. Hermann
Department of Radiology, Charité Medical School, Berlin, Germany

Atul Deodhar
Division of Arthritis & Rheumatic Diseases, Oregon Health & Science University, Portland, OR, USA

Désirée van der Heijde
Department of Rheumatology, Leiden University Medical Center, Leiden, The Netherlands

Stephen Xu
Department of Biostatistics, Janssen Research & Development, LLC, Spring House, PA, USA

Benjamin Hsu
Department of Immunology, Janssen Research & Development, LLC, Spring House, PA, USA.

Meliha C. Kapetanovic and Pierre Geborek
Section of Rheumatology, Department of Clinical Sciences Lund, Lund University, Lund, Sweden

Ingemar F. Petersson
Section of Rheumatology, Department of Clinical Sciences Lund, Lund University, Lund, Sweden
Section of Orthopedics, Department of Clinical Sciences Lund, Lund University, Lund, Sweden

Lars Erik Kristensen
Section of Rheumatology, Department of Clinical Sciences Lund, Lund University, Lund, Sweden
The Parker Institute, Department of Rheumatology, Copenhagen University Hospital, Frederiksberg and Bispebjerg, Denmark

Johan K. Wallman
Section of Rheumatology, Department of Clinical Sciences Lund, Lund University, Lund, Sweden
Reumatologiska kliniken, Skånes Universitetssjukhus Lund, Kioskgatan 3, 22185 Lund, Sweden

Won Park
Inha University Hospital, Incheon, Republic of Korea

Dae Hyun Yoo
Hanyang University Hospital, Seoul, Republic of Korea

Janusz Jaworski
Linea Corporis, Warszawa, Poland

Jan Brzezicki
Wojewodzki Szpital Zespolony w Elblagu, Elblag, Poland

Andriy Gnylorybov
Institute of Urgent and Recovery Surgery, Donetsk, Ukraine

Vladimir Kadinov
University Hospital St. Marina, Varna, Bulgaria

Irmgadt Goecke Sariego
Prosalud y Cia Ltda, Santiago, Chile

Carlos Abud-Mendoza
Hospital Central Dr. Ignacio Morones Prieto, San Luis Potosí, Mexico

William Jose Otero Escalante
Servimed Empresa Unipersonal, Bucaramanga, Colombia

Seong Wook Kang
Chungnam National University Hospital, Daejeon, Republic of Korea

Daina Andersone
P. Stradina Clinical University Hospital, Riga, Latvia

Francisco Blanco
Hospital Universitario a Coruña, A Coruña, Spain

Seung Suh Hong and Sun Hee Lee
CELLTRION, Incheon, Republic of Korea

Joop van den Bergh
Division of Rheumatology, Department of Internal Medicine, CAPHRI School for Public Health and Primary Care, Maastricht University Medical Center, Maastricht, 6200 MD Maastricht, The Netherlands
Department of Internal Medicine, VieCuri Medical Centre, 5900 BX Venlo, The Netherlands

Department of Internal Medicine, NUTRIM School for Nutrition, Toxicology and Metabolism, Maastricht University Medical Centre, 6200 MD Maastricht, The Netherlands

Johan Vanhoof and Debby Vosse
ReumaClinic, Genk, Bretheistraat 149, 3600 Genk, Belgium

Ulrich Weber
King Christian 10th Hospital for Rheumatic Diseases, Gråsten, and Sygehus, Sønderjylland, Denmark
Institute of Regional Health Research, University of Southern Denmark, Odense, Denmark
Department of Rheumatology, Balgrist University Hospital, Zurich, Switzerland

Walter P. Maksymowych
Department of Medicine, University of Alberta, Edmonton, AB, Canada

Stanley M. Chan
Department of Ophthalmology, University of Alberta, Edmonton, Alberta, Canada

Kaspar Rufibach
Rufibach rePROstat, Biostatistical Consulting and Training, Engelgasse 123, 4052 Basel, Switzerland

Susanne J. Pedersen and Mikkel Østergaard
Copenhagen Center for Arthritis Research Center for Rheumatology and Spine Diseases, Rigshospitalet, Glostrup, and, Departmentof Clinical Medicine, University of Copenhagen, Copenhagen, Denmark

Zheng Zhao
Department of Rheumatology, PLA General Hospital, Beijing, China

Veronika Zubler
Department of Radiology, Balgrist University Hospital, Zurich, Switzerland

Robert GW Lambert
Department of Radiology and Diagnostic Imaging, University of Alberta, Edmonton, Alberta, Canada

www.ingramcontent.com/pod-product-compliance
Lightning Source LLC
LaVergne TN
LVHW080735210926
848485LV00003B/559